UNDERSTANDING GLOBAL HEALTH

Edited by

William H. Markle, MD, FAAFP, DTM&H
Clinical Associate Professor Family Medicine
University of Pittsburgh School of Medicine
Program Director Family Medicine Residency
University of Pittsburgh Medical Center
McKeesport, Pennsylvania

Melanie A. Fisher, MD, MSc
Professor of Medicine, Section of Infectious Diseases
Director of the International Health Program
Robert C. Byrd Health Sciences Center
West Virginia University
Morgantown, West Virginia

Raymond A. Smego, Jr., MD, MPH, FACP, FRCP, DTM&H
Associate Dean for International Medical Education
Professor of Medicine, Infectious Diseases & International Health
Robert C. Byrd Health Sciences Center of West Virginia University
Associate Dean for Clinical Affairs
Oman Medical College
Sohar, Sultanate of Oman

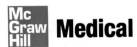 **Medical**

New York   Chicago   San Francisco   Lisbon   London   Madrid   Mexico City
New Delhi   San Juan   Seoul   Singapore   Sydney   Toronto

The McGraw-Hill Companies

Understanding Global Health

Copyright © 2007 by The McGraw-Hill Companies, Inc. All rights reserved. Printed in the United States of America. Except as permitted under the United States Copyright Act of 1976, no part of this publication my be reproduced or distributed in any form or by any means, or stored in a data base or retrieval system, without prior written permission of the publisher.

1 2 3 4 5 6 7 8 9 0   DOC/DOC   0 9 8 7

ISBN-13: 978-0-07-148784-9
ISBN-10 :   0-07-148784-0

Notice

Medicine is an ever-changing science. As new research and clinical experience broaden our knowledge, changes in treatment and drug therapy are required. The authors and the publisher of this work have checked with sources believed to be reliable in their efforts to provide information that is complete and generally in accord with the standards accepted at the time of publication. However, in view of the possibility of human error or changes in medical sciences, neither the authors nor the publisher nor any other party who has been involved in the preparation or publication of this work warrants that the information contained herein is in every respect accurate or complete, and they disclaim all responsibility for any errors or omissions or for the results obtained from use of the information contained in this work. Readers are encouraged to confirm the information contained herein with other sources. For example and in particular, readers are advised to check product information sheet included in the package of each drug they plan to administer to be certain that the information contained in this work is accurate and that changes have not been made in the recommended dose or in the contraindications for administration. This recommendation is of particular importance in connection with new or infrequently used drugs.

This book was set in Adobe Garamond by International Typesetting and Composition.
The editors were Karen Davis, James Shanahan, and Laura Libretti.
The production supervisor was Phil Galea.
Project management was provided by International Typesetting and Composition.
The index was prepared by Kevin Broccoli.
The cover designer was Aimee Davis.
Photo credit: Christoph Wilhelm/GettyImages.
RR Donnelley was printer and binder.

This book is printed on acid-free paper.

Library of Congress Cataloging-in-Publication Data

Understanding global health / edited by William H. Markle, Melanie A. Fisher, Raymond A. Smego, Jr.
    p. ; cm.
Includes bibliographical references.
ISBN-13: 978-0-07-148784-9 (pbk. : alk. paper)
ISBN-10: 0-07-148784-0 (pbk. : alk. paper)
1. World health.
[DNLM: 1. World Health. 2. Public Health. WA 530.1 U545 2007] I. Markle, William H. II. Fisher, Melanie A.
III. Smego, Raymond A.
RA441.U415 2007
362.1—dc22

2007022940

Contents

[†]Deceased.

Authors

Lisa V. Adams, MD (*Chapter 8*)
Assistant Professor, Section of Infectious Disease and
    International Health, Department of Medicine,
    and Coordinator, Global Health Initiative,
    Dartmouth Medical School
Hanover, New Hampshire
Lisa.V.Adams@Dartmouth.edu

Onil Bhattacharyya, MD, PhD (*Chapter 15*)
Research Fellow
Department of Family and Community Medicine
Faculty of Medicine, University of Toronto
Li Ka Shing Knowledge Institute
St. Michael's Hospital, University of Toronto
Toronto, Ontario
Onil.bhattacharyya@utoronto.ca

John H. Bryant, MD (*Chapter 16*)
Johns Hopkins School of Public Health
Baltimore, MD
Tropical Institute for Community Health and
    Development
Kisumu, Kenya
jbryant@wcbr.us

Thuy D. Bui, MD (*Chapter 2*)
Assistant Professor of Medicine
University of Pittsburgh School of Medicine
Division of General Internal Medicine
Medical Director, Program for Healthcare to
    Underserved Populations
Pittsburgh, Pennsylvania
buit@upmc.edu

Kevin Chan, MD, MPH, FAAP, FRCPC
    (*Chapter 14*)
Assistant Professor, Department of Pediatrics
Faculty of Medicine, Hospital for Sick Children, and
University of Toronto
Fellow, Munk Centre for International Studies
University of Toronto
Toronto, Ontario
kevinjchan@aol.com

Monika Doshi, MPH (*Chapter 4*)
Research Associate
University of Manitoba
Bangalore, Karnataka
mdoshi@jhsph.edu

Sheri Fink, MD, PhD (*Chapter 9*)
Visiting Scientist, Francois-Xavier Bagnoud Center
    for Health and Human Rights
Senior Fellow, Harvard Humanitarian Initiative
Harvard School of Public Health
Boston, Massachusetts
sherifink@aol.com

Jeffrey K. Griffiths, MD, MPH&TM (*Chapter 5*)
Director, Global Health
Associate Professor of Public Health, Medicine,
    Nutrition, and Civil and Environmental
    Engineering
Department of Public Health and Family Medicine
Tufts University School of Medicine
Boston, Massachusetts
Jeffrey.Griffiths@tufts.edu

Wayne A. Hale, MD, MS, FABFP, CAQ Geriatrics
    (*Chapter 11*)
Associate Professor, Department of Family Medicine
University of North Carolina at Chapel Hill
Moses Cone Health System Family Medicine
    Residency Program
Area Health Education Centers
Greensboro, North Carolina
wayne.hale@mosescone.com

Cynthia Haq, MD (*Chapter 7*)
Professor of Family Medicine and Population Health
    Sciences
Director, Center for Global Health
University of Wisconsin, School of Medicine and
    Public Health
Madison, Wisconsin
clhaq@wisc.edu

Jané D. Joubert, MA (*Chapter 11*)
Specialist Scientist
Burden of Disease Research Unit
South African Medical Research Council
Cape Town, South Africa
jane.joubert@mrc.ac.za

Sebastiana Kalula, MBChB, MRCP, MMed, MPhil
(*Chapter 11*)
Clinical Head of Division of Geriatric Medicine
Department of Medicine
Institute of Aging in Africa
University of Cape Town, South Africa
Sebastiana.Kalula@uct.ac.za

Rashida A. Khakoo, MD, MACP (*Chapter 12*)
Professor of Medicine, West Virginia School of
Medicine
Chief, Section of Infectious Diseases Department
of Medicine
Robert C. Byrd Health Sciences Center
West Virginia University
Morgantown, West Virginia
rkhakoo@hsc.wvu.edu

Amir A. Khaliq, MBBS, MSHS, MPH, PhD
(*Chapter 1*)
Associate Professor of Public Health
Health Administration & Policy
College of Public Health
University of Oklahoma Health Sciences Center
Oklahoma City, Oklahoma
amir-khaliq@ouhsc.edu

Ron Laporte, PhD (*Chapter 13*)
Professor of Epidemiology
Director, Disease Monitoring and
Telecommunications
WHO Collaborating Centre
Pittsburgh, Pennsylvania
Ronlaporte@aol.com

Judy Lewis, MPhil (*Chapter 4*)
Professor, Department of Community Medicine
University of Connecticut School of Medicine
Farmington, Connecticut
LewisJ@nso.uchc.edu

Faina Linkov, PhD (*Chapter 13*)
Research Assistant Professor of Medicine
Division of Hematology and Oncology
University of Pittsburgh Cancer Institute
Pittsburgh, Pennsylvania
fyL1@pitt.edu

William H. Markle, MD, FAAFP, DTM&H
(*Chapter 2*)
Clinical Associate Professor Family Medicine
University of Pittsburgh School of Medicine
Program Director Family Medicine Residency
University of Pittsburgh Medical Center
McKeesport, Pennsylvania
marklew@upmc.edu

Christopher Martin, MD, MSc (*Chapter 3*)
Associate Professor of Community Medicine and
Medicine
Department of Community Medicine
West Virginia University School of Medicine
Morgantown, West Virginia
cmartin@hsc.wvu.edu

Jeffry P. McKinzie, MD, FACEP (*Chapter 10*)
Assistant Professor of Emergency Medicine &
Pediatrics
Director, Division of International & Travel
Medicine
Vanderbilt University
Nashville, Tennessee
jeff.mckinzie@vanderbilt.edu

Alain J. Montegut, MD (*Chapter 7*)
Associate Professor
Director, Global Health Primary Care Initiative
Department of Family Medicine Boston University
Boston, Massachusetts
Alain.Montegut@bmc.org

Thomas E. Novotny, MD, MPH (*Chapter 17*)
Professor in Residence, Department of Epidemiol-
ogy and Biostatistics
Director, International Programs, Office of Medical
Education
Education Coordinator, UCSF Global Health
Sciences
University of California, San Francisco, California
novotnyt@globalhealth.ucsf.edu

Leon Piterman, MBBS, MMed, MEDSt, MRCP(UK), FRACGP (*Chapter 7*)
Professor of General Practice
Head, School of Primary Health Care
Monash University, East Bentley
Victoria, Australia
leon.piterman@med.monash.edu.au

Clydette Powell, MD, MPH (*Chapter 6*)
Associate Professor (Adjunct)
Department of Pediatrics
George Washington University School of Medicine
Washington, DC
CPowell@USAID.gov

Debra Rothenberg, MD, PhD (*Chapter 7*)
Assistant Program Director, Family Medicine
    Residency Program
Department of Family Medicine
Maine Medical Center
Portland, Maine
rothed@mmc.org

Arif R. Sarwari, MD, MSc (*Chapter 12*)
Associate Professor
Associate Program Director, Internal Medicine
    Residency Program
West Virginia University School of Medicine
Section of Infectious Diseases, Department of Medicine
Robert C. Byrd Health Sciences Center
Morgantown, West Virginia
asarwari@hsc.wvu.edu

Raymond A. Smego, Jr., MD, MPH, FACP, FRCP, DTM&H (*Chapter 1*)
Associate Dean for International Medical Education
Professor of Medicine, Infectious Diseases &
    International Health
Robert C. Byrd Health Sciences Center of
    West Virginia University
Associate Dean for Clinical Affairs
Oman Medical College
Sohar, Sultanate of Oman
rsmego@hsc.wvu.edu

Gary Snyder, MS (*Chapter 13*)
Associate Vice President, Communications and
    Marketing
Adjunct Professor, Arnold School of Public Health
University of South Carolina
Columbia, South Carolina
Adjunct Faculty Member, Tropical Disease Institute
Ohio University
gsnyder@gwm.sc.edu

Mark Stinson, MD[†] (*Chapter 9*)
Contra Costa Regional Medical Center
Martinez, California

Anvar Velji, MD, FRCP(c), FACP (*Chapter 16*)
Cofounder Global Health Education Consortium
    Chief Infectious Disease
Kaiser Permanente, South Sacramento
Clinical Professor of Medicine
University of California
Davis, California
anvarali.velji@kp.org

Edward Winant, PE, PhD (*Chapter 5*)
Environmental Engineer
Canaan Valley Institute
Davis, West Virginia
ed.winant@canaanvi.org

Godfrey B. Woelk, BSc (Soc), MCOMMH, PhD (*Chapter 8*)
Professor of Epidemiology
Department of Community Medicine,
    College of Health Sciences
University of Zimbabwe
Harare, Zimbabwe
gwoelk@gmail.com

David Zakus, BSc, MES, MSc, PhD (*Chapter 15*)
Director, Centre for International Health
Associate Professor, Departments of Public Health
    Sciences & Health Policy, Management and
    Evaluation
Faculty of Medicine, University of Toronto
Toronto, Ontario
davidzakus@cs.com

[†]Deceased.

Foreword

For most of the past century, the spread of mysterious, frightening diseases has been occurring mainly in the poorer parts of the planet. It is not until now that AIDS, after having been primarily identified as a "Third World," specifically African, condition, has briefly made its way to the highest level of political agendas. Meanwhile, malaria, tuberculosis, and malnutrition remain among the leading causes of death in the poorest countries.

The northern high-income G8 members and the Organization for Economic Co-operation and Development (OECD) countries have lived for decades as though they were immune to at least three of the hardship afflictions— famines, epidemics, and wars in their territory.

Severe acute respiratory syndrome (SARS), avian influenza, and bioterrorism have suddenly placed those countries on a similar level to rural China in the eyes of much of the world. These epidemic threats have evidenced the interdependent nature of society—from family and cultural events to transportation systems bringing us to work and bringing tourists to our countries—and to the smooth workings of a complex economy that is highly dependent on the good will and good commerce of other jurisdictions. The role of the public health system is critical within this rhythmic interchange between societies, providing enough trained people, resources, and built-in reserves to surveil, recognize, interpret, and respond to the blips on the epidemiological radar screen that signal a potential epidemic.

But SARS, avian influenza, and bioterrorism clearly do not constitute just a medical problem. What SARS and avian influenza also highlight is the extent to which public health—and, most importantly, perceptions and actions half a world away— influence the health of the political governments and the economy.

I was invited to attend the L20 Conference "HIV/AIDS, and Other Infectious Diseases" held on November 12–13, 2004, at the University for Peace Campus in San Jose, Costa Rica.[1] Besides having the honor to meet colleagues from all around the world,

I was impressed by the concern shown by the higher-income countries in building a "bio-shield" as an active defense of their territory against the new epidemic threats. The debate was crucial for my understanding of the current political concerns related to these global health issues. Many of us clearly recognized the agenda of self-interest advocated by the G8 countries. This conclusion was addressed in the final report of the L20 Conference:

"There was the concern that not all infections but selected infectious diseases were being discussed, with implicit criteria for selecting. Does the term "global infectious diseases" refer only to those acute and epidemic diseases that pose a potential threat to the developed world—HIV/AIDS, SARS, Ebola, possibly tuberculosis and influenza? What about other acute epidemic infections, largely confined to the developing world such as cholera and typhoid, or non-acute or non-epidemic infections again confined to the developing world such as yellow fever, malaria and schistosomiasis? If so, countries beyond the G8 will be quick to recognize the self-interested nature of such an agenda. Governments of poorer countries may agree, on the surface, to support the building of a "bio-shield" in order to obtain much needed funding, but their commitment to actually implementing yet another donor-led scheme designed to benefit rich countries is soon likely to flounder. The initiative needs to be framed in a way that there is true "buy in."[2]

It is necessary to reflect on some of the less obvious pathways and effects of globalization, and this book is an important contribution to such reflections. In Chapter 2, Bui and Markle clearly address this need given the current globalization juncture and conjunction of many changes in health policy: *"We are at the critical junction in global health where efforts to reform health systems and to control risk factors will require the commitment and coordination of policy makers, researchers, health ministries, the World Health Organization, the World Bank, private donors, and*

---

[1]For more information about L20 and the Infectious Diseases conference, documents refer to www.l20.org/libraryitem.php? libraryId=7 and www.l20.org/publications/7_hM_ID_participants.pdf.

[2]HIV/AIDS and Other Infectious Diseases. Final Report. University of Peace, San Jose, Costa Rica, November 2004. www.l20.org/libraryitem.php?libraryID=7.

nongovernmental organizations to improve the health of those who survive beyond childhood around the world." The authors pursue the logic of globalization with a knowledgeable academic spirit.

The solid argument for presenting this book to health professions students is that we truly live in an interdependent world and need to evaluate policies and decisions in one place in order to understand effects in another. In the future health professionals must be aware of this interdependency in order to improve their competencies and to build a "new professional and social commitment that is ethics oriented and that promotes a better world."

To the best of our knowledge, this book represents the first attempt to bring together a set of data from the global health situation describing the north and south in the major domains known to influence or to be essential components of health, health care, and health systems: education, nutrition, economics, medical assistance readiness and mitigation for war and catastrophes, women and children's health, ethics, professional education, and the environmental aspects. It evaluates each of these areas from the clinical and public health perspectives, while presenting data from each region and numerous countries as valuable case studies. In addition to providing a rigorous and well-referenced set of data for researchers and activists, it is also an innovative presentation of what is effectively a global health textbook for health professions students.

Sadly, the reader can draw a general conclusion that the current dominant vision is that world disparities within societies are not conducive to early improvement in the dismal health situation of most of the world's population. This is evident in a simple count of "promises kept versus promises broken," such as in the Health for All for Year 2000 Alma Ata declaration launched in 1978 in Kazakhstan, Soviet Union, and, more recently, G8 countries' explicit commitments made in official communiqués. The main challenge remains: how to place human health and well-being at the center of development.

For much of the world's population, the ability to lead a healthy life is limited by the direct and indirect effects of poverty. Almost half of the world's population lives on an income of US$2 per day or less (World Bank, 2001). Vulnerabilities too often magnify one another. Lack of access to health care is just one of these vulnerabilities. Among the many consequences is the fact that communicable diseases continue to comprise a significant portion of the burden of diseases in the developing world, as it has been clearly described in most chapters of this book.

We need to emphasize that many people outside the industrialized world now face a double burden of disease, as they are exposed not only to communicable diseases associated with poverty and an inadequate health care infrastructure, but also to noncommunicable diseases, such as diabetes, and to industrial pollution associated with rapid transitions to patterns of production and consumption that are more typical of the industrialized world.

This book provides an invaluable foundation for addressing this challenge. We hope that health professionals students, researchers, as well as other colleagues, will continue the work begun here, notably through analyzing the dynamics and processes through which the documents under examination have been produced, and discussing these dynamics as an ongoing curriculum requirement.

Each chapter displays information for fruitful debate. The components presented by the authors have inspired me to reflect very carefully on the global health situation. There are two elements that I wish to point out: (1) the need for optimizing the use of the scarce resources of middle- and low-income countries for the purpose of modifying their epidemiological profile and improving the quality of life, which also implies (2) the proper use of the available scientific information, which in turn implies increasing the capacity of sensible scientific production in both the biomedical and social contexts of the countries with the lowest incomes, and also the global need for establishing a "bias-free framework." It is worth mentioning what some authors have called these elements' "social epidemiology" in Latin America; and "eco-social epidemiology" in the United States and Europe. We agree with Krieger that "embodiment" is a key word of the new epidemiology glossary. The evidence shows the importance of epidemiologists' recognizing embodied expressions of social experiences. It is highlighted by Sapolsky's accounts of researchers overlooking how the sizes of both the adrenal and thymus glands are affected by chronic poverty and stress, thereby creating what Brunner has termed "biology of inequality."

A recent global health research forum publication states that to cut a swathe through the layers of tools that researchers and policy makers have had to apply in the past to avoid sexism, racism, ableism, classism, casteism, ageism, and endless other "isms" in their work, the forum offers their *BIAS FREE* framework as an integrative approach to explore and remove the compounding layers of bias that derive from any social hierarchy. *BIAS FREE* stands for Building an Integrative Analytical System for Recognizing and Eliminating in-Equities and is the statement of a goal, not of an achievement.[3]

The case of tuberculosis is a good example of the need for optimizing the use of the scarce resources of middle- and low-income countries and the proper use of the available scientific information in the global realm. Farmer in his book *Infectious Diseases and Inequalities* argues that tuberculosis is misclassified as reemerging. "Emerging from where?" he asks, and argues: "Tuberculosis is said to be another emerging disease, in which case, emerging is synonymous with reemerging. Its recrudescence is often attributed to the advent of HIV—the Institute of Medicine lists an increase in immunosuppressed populations as the sole factor facilitating the resurgence of tuberculosis—and the emergence of drug resistance."[4]

A global analysis does not suggest major decreases in the importance of tuberculosis as a cause of death. Tuberculosis has retreated in certain populations, maintained a steady state in others, and still surged forth in others, remaining as one of the world's leading infectious causes of adult deaths.

The L20 conference on infectious diseases final report states:

"Tuberculosis was ignored for two decades, despite continuing to kill millions in the developing world, until the early 1990s when tuberculosis rates began to rise again in deprived communities in high-income countries, and drug- resistant forms of tuberculosis began to pose a risk."[5]

Many attempts have been made to assure an effective medical intervention. Adams and Woelk, in Chapter 8, describe the situation about DOT (Directly Observed Treatment), "once a cornerstone to tuberculosis treatment". Nowadays, it has been the subject of "much heated debate" in the international tuberculosis control community. Considered a heavy burden on health care systems and impractical in rural or remote areas, DOT is being challenged.

Moreover, Volmink and Garner[6] in a Cochrane Collaboration Systematic Review have analyzed the results. Results from the review of ten randomized controlled trials (RCT) (ten RCT and 3985 participants) in low-, average- and high-income countries do not guarantee in any way that the DOT, as compared to the self-administered treatment, has a quantitatively significant effect on the cure or the completion of the treatment in persons receiving treatment for tuberculosis.

Granted, the discovery of effective anti-tuberculosis therapies has saved the lives of hundreds of thousands of tuberculosis patients, many in industrialized countries. But tuberculosis—once the leading cause of death among young adults in the industrialized world—was already in decline there well before the 1943 discovery of streptomycin. In other words, that action in the health care sector is only one of the influences on a population's health.

High-income countries have been able to collect a great deal of information on issues such as misuse of scientific information in clinical work and in the design of health policies. This mishandling has resulted in unnecessary deaths, as well as delayed the adoption of actions that may have prevented death or disability.

Even when using the lower estimates, deaths due to medical errors exceed the number attributable to the eighth leading cause of death in the United States. "More people die in a given year as a result of medical errors than from motor vehicle accidents (43,458), breast cancer (42,297), or AIDS (16,516)."[7]

Such information biases emerge for different reasons, one of them being the inadequate reading of the interdependent character of global health problems, and the other relating to the access and use of the best scientific information for clinical practice. The original question is: As new tests and therapies and interventions are developed, how do physicians and policy makers decide which to adopt? Without a clear, consistent framework, these decisions are typically driven by the practice patterns of local "opinion leaders," advertising, pharmaceutical representatives, specialists (who may see a different spectrum of patients), and other potentially biased sources. The result is a huge variation in practice patterns among regions, countries, and even cities within the same country.

[3]Burke MA, Eichler M. *The BIAS FREE Framework: A practrical tool for identifying and eliminating social biases in health research.* Geneva: Global Forum for Health Research, 2006.

[4]Farmer P. *Infections and Inequalities* Berkeley, CA: University of California Press, 1998.

[5]HIV/AIDS and Other Infectious Diseases. Final Report. University of Peace, San Jose, Costa Rica, November 2004. www.l20.org/libraryitem.php?libraryID=7.

[6]Volmink J, Garner P. Directly Observed Treatment for Tuberculosis. (*Revision Cochrane traducida*) In: *La Biblioteca Cochrane Plus*, 2007 Número 1. Oxford: Update Software Ltd from Cochrane Library Wiley & Son, 2007.

[7]Kohn LT, Corrigan JM, Donaldson MS, eds. To Err Is Human: Building a Safer Health System. Washington DC: Committee on Quality of Health Care in America, Institute of Medicine, Nat Acad Press, 2000.

In 1973, a small study demonstrated that steroids given to women expected to deliver prematurely reduced the likelihood of death in their infants. Six further studies in the next ten years showed mixed results, primarily because they were all quite small. Had a meta-analysis been done in 1983, it would have shown that the overall results of all the trials combined supported a beneficial effect of the steroids. However, it took another decade and seven more studies before these results were accepted and began to change practice. Had a systematic review of the literature been performed in 1983, it might have changed practice much sooner and saved thousands of lives of premature infants.

Therefore, it is clear that governments worldwide need evidence-based information around which interventions could best achieve the social goal of public health. Canada's recently published response to the WHO Commission on Social Determinants of Health states that ". . . Canadians, in general, enjoy very good health, but some Canadians are not as healthy as others. Major health disparities persist between various groups in Canadian society. Key health inequalities are associated with factors such as socioeconomic status, Aboriginal heritage, gender and geographic location. For example, when compared to Canadians more generally, First Nations and Inuit peoples have a life expectancy of 5–10 years less. Many of the consequences of these health inequalities are avoidable, including preventable early death, disease, and disability, and are costly for the health system and society in general. . . ." they state that the key insight underpinning the work of the Commission is that action in the health care sector is only one of the influences on a population's health. The Commission has the broader aim of improving the circumstances in which people live and work. The Commission will work to catalyze change among others by organizing knowledge and compiling evidence of successful interventions and policies; furthermore, within the Five Action plan components, *The Knowledge Networks*,[8] Nine Knowledge Networks (KNs) will synthesize knowledge on effective interventions, with a focus on low-income countries, and will issue recommendations to inform policy, action, and leadership.

The reading of scientific information and the transformation of the clinical practice and health policy designs, as we have already seen, have taken some time in countries where most of the knowledge is generated, but in developing countries, incorporating the new knowledge to the practice is even slower. For instance, there are still some practices being used that scientific knowledge has proven to be harmful, such as the use of prophylactic lidocaine for handling myocardial infarction, which was reported to cause a significant number of deaths in the United States, and that a meta-analysis showed, during the 1900s,[9] was associated with mortality rates in patients who had experienced a myocardial infarction.

This is due, among other things, not only to the limited access to up-to-date scientific publications, to language barriers, and currently, to the limited access to Internet and electronic media,[10] but also to the long proven and known—both in high- and low-resource countries—limitation of professionals for incorporating the new scientific information to daily practice. One effort to meet this challenge is the Epidemiology Supercourse, available free around the world, detailed by Linkov and LaPorte in Chapter 13. Another variable that also plays a significant role is the adoption of clinical practices more as a result of the influence of the pharmaceutical industry than from a proven clinical efficacy. For example, in the public health sector of a Central American country, the choice medication for an antiplatelet drug is clopidogrel instead of aspirin, which, with very few exceptions, has proven to have beneficial effects similar or superior to clopidrogrel[11] and with a lesser cost for the system.

In the reality of the globalized world we share and live in, the availability of complex tools for teamwork is a formidable advantage. As an ending to this Foreword, I would like to quote an inspiring thought contained in the pages of this very same book. Fink and Stinson talk in Chapter 9 about the essential need of evidence-based medicine and public health skills, even in extremely difficult scenarios, such as war, catastrophes and relief interventions: "Whether or not the aims of the work are narrowly or broadly defined, practitioners need excellent technical skills in evidence-based medicine and public health to avoid doing more harm than good."

---

[8]www.who.int/social_determinants/strategy/en/.

[9]Antman E, Lau J, Kupelnick B, et al. A comparison of results of meta-analyses of randomized control and recommendations of clinical experts. Treatments for myocardial infarction. *JAMA* 1992;2:240.

[10]Tristan, M. La barreras para el acceso a la informacion cientifica en centroamerica. Memoria Conferencia Anual de la Red Cochrane Iberoamerican. 2003; Buenos Aires, Argentina.

[11]Clinical Evidence On Line. www.clinicalevidence.com.

We shall continue to call for a comprehensive and strong response to this most urgent issue facing global health. This book presents a comprehensive analysis of global health and further reinforces our conviction that we cannot wait any longer to widen societal debate on the topic and propose global policies for action.

Mario Tristan, MSc, PhD, DTM&H
Director-General
IHCAI Foundation
International Health Central American Institute
Foundation
Cochrane Centre of Central America Branch of
the Iberoamerican Cochrane Centre
San Jose, Costa Rica

Foreword

Tolstoy, in *Anna Kerenina*, expressed the view that a person's moral universe should be demarked by the distance that can be walked, or at most, ridden. Tolstoy's view of a geographic perimeter to morality was best explained by Stephen Toulmin:[1]

> As he [Tolstoy] saw matters, genuinely moral relations can exist only between people who live, work, and associate together ... by taking a train, a moral agent leaves the sphere of truly moral actions for a world of strangers, toward whom he or she has few real obligations and with whom dealings can be only casual or commercial.... What Tolstoy rightly emphasized is the sharp difference that exists between moral relations with our families, intimates, and immediate neighbors or associates, and our moral relations with complete strangers.

Other ethicists, like Hans Jonas in the *Imperative of Responsibility*, have considered an orthogonal dimension of morality, that being its temporal perimeter.[2] Jonas insisted that human survival depends on our efforts to care for the future of our planet. He formulated a new and distinctive long term view of morality,

> Act so that the effects of your action are compatible with the permanence of genuine human life.

Global Health can certainly be viewed through a lens of morality. Some like Tolstoy might take a restrictive view, and others like Jonas an expansive view. This framework leads to intriguing questions about the spatial and temporal boundaries of our horizons of responsibility to other human beings, and the ethical corollaries of such boundary definitions and their implications for global health. However, a variety of other alternative motivations are commonly and legitimately offered for involvement in global health, including enlightened self interest, religious commitment, political advantage, and even adventurism. Such alternative justifications need not provoke weighty ethical questions. One need only remember that the pioneering global health worker David Livingston offered Christianity, commerce, and civilization, as his own motivations, to appreciate the evolving nature of diverse philosophical justifications for global health.[3]

This marvelous introductory textbook, *Understanding Global Health*, edited by William H. Markle, Melanie A. Fisher, and Raymond A. Smego, successfully presents a comprehensive introduction to Global Health for the naïve but interested reader (and who isn't naïve about at least some aspects of global health?). No explicit philosophical justifications are offered about why global health should be pursued (morality, self-interest, etc), because such a staked-out position is irrelevant to this text. The authors simply set out to impart an understanding of global health, and do so admirably in this book through a combination of thoughtful overall organization, well written individual chapters, ample illustrations, and useful tips and resources. Although this is a multi-authored volume, the chapters fit together remarkably well, with no needless overlap and no obvious internal dissonance. While the book is written by three medical doctors, and is generally slanted toward medical students and trainees, this is by no means a medical text. Almost half the chapters are devoted to epidemiology, environment, economics, ethics, and other public health-oriented topics. My own favorite chapter is that on "Global Health Communications, Social Marketing, and Emerging Communication Technologies" (Chapter 13). Another exemplary chapter is "Education and Careers in Global Health" (Chapter 17), an important topic I have never seen covered in another text, but professionally done here.

A host of synonyms have been used over the past few decades to label this growing field, including "international health", or "geographic medicine", or "tropical medicine." Such older terms persist in the names of many contemporary academic departments and institutes. However, the term "global health" used in the title of this text best captures the real spirit. Perhaps John Donne said it best (in 1624, ironically, just as the modern nation-state emerged in Europe):

> No man is an island, entire of itself...any man's death diminishes me, because I am involved in mankind; and therefore never send to know for whom the bell tolls; it tolls for thee.[4]

The distinction, of course, is that the key actors in global health are individual human beings working cooperatively with other human beings; neither nations nor geographic areas nor medical specialties are the primary actors.

Global health can be a valuable organizing principle. Some dramatic health threats, such as the emergence of epidemics like AIDS, SARS, and influenza, are easy for the public and for policy makers to understand and support as global health issues, both from the vantage of the rich and the poor countries. For other emerging health issues, however, global cooperation may be just as crucial, but the path forward less clear. One such emerging health issue is the astonishing increase in overall global life expectancy (from 47 years in 1950 to 65 years in 2005, and to a projected 75 years in 2050), with attendant world-wide changes in employment, dependency relationships, and health care needs.[5] Another area of certain change but uncertain impact is global weather and climate: social displacements from rising ocean levels and damage from extreme weather events will surely occur, but the net adverse effects of global warming on contagious diseases (will influenza, a winter disease, decline?) are far from clear.[6]

Some future global health changes are predictable and imminent, while others may be indistinct and uncertain. Regardless, I am confident that *Understanding Global Health* will provide the next generation of health professionals with a readable, authoritative, and practical volume to approach these current and future problems in global health. And I am optimistic that most readers will not only become informed and educated by this well-crafted volume, but they will also be inspired by it.

REFERENCES

1. Toulmin S. *The tyranny of principles.* Hastings Center Rep., Volume 11, No. 6, pages 31–39 (1981).
2. Hans Jonas. *The Imperative of Responsibility: In Search of Ethics for the Technological Age.* Chicago: University of Chicago Press, 1984.
3. David Livingstone. Speech at Cambridge University, 1857. www.cooper.edu/humanities/classes/coreclasses/hss3/d_livingstone.html
4. John Donne. The Complete Poetry and Selected Prose of John Donne. Edited by Charles M. Coffin. Random House, United States, 1994.
5. United Nations, Department of Economic and Social Affair. *World Population Prospects: The 2004 Revision.* United Nations, New York, 2005.
6. National Research Council. *Under the Weather: Climate, Ecosystems, and Infectious Diseases.* Report Chair Donald S. Burke. National Academy Press, Washington D.C., 2001.

Donald S. Burke, MD
Dean, Graduate School of Public Health
and Associate Vice Chancellor for Global Health
University of Pittsburgh
Pittsburgh, Pennsylvania

Preface

For some, the term *global health* conjures up images of strange, exotic places and customs. For others, it brings to mind images of suffering, lack of health care and lack of resources. Still others recall interactions with international colleagues who have contributed to research and knowledge. There are various definitions of global health. The older term, international health, brought to mind health limited by borders, with the self-interest of individual countries in the forefront. Diseases were not studied until they were felt to actually be important for the country in question. The old tropical disease institutions were often started with the idea of protecting the militaries that were going from the developed countries to the developing world.

Of course, today borders mean little. Diseases that one hears about in some far-off, remote corner of the world can soon be on a plane to your hometown. Thus, the view of health and health care today must be all encompassing, transcend borders, and truly fit to elevate the health of all people everywhere. Our own view is that global health represents the interests, activities, and data that are derived from and affect the health of the world as a whole and all mankind. As you read this book, our hope is that you will begin to see global health in new ways, and your role as a health team member and a world citizen in a new light.

We believe that this new book will be useful to students and learners of all ages whether they are beginning their study of global health or already working in this field. We want it to be useful to anyone wishing to expand their knowledge and gain new ideas, and to apply those ideas to the care of both patients and populations. We have included learning objectives and study questions in all chapters to best contribute to the learning and instruction experience in global medicine and health.

We have managed to bring together a truly remarkable group of authors and contributors for this text. Each one has extensive experience working globally, and each has a wealth of expertise in his or her own topic. The text explores the current burden of disease in the world, how health is determined, and the problems faced by the people and their health care workers around the world. The basics of epidemiology are included, as well as sections on ethics for those interested in international research. Basic issues in global health such as maternal and child health, primary health care, cross-cultural health care, and environmental health are covered thoroughly. Some very important current issues, such as emerging infectious diseases, drug resistance, HIV, tuberculosis, injuries, and nutritional problems, are explored in depth. More advanced topics are also included, such as the chapters on global health manpower needs, financing global health, and the communications revolution. There is special attention to the global demographic transition and the problems of aging, and the difficulties of people caught up in wars and disasters. These are new and important topics for our changing world. Finally, there is a chapter on training and opportunities for work in the global health sector.

We are indebted to the chapter authors for taking time from their very busy schedules and contributing their knowledge and scholarship to this book. Most of the authors are members of the Global Health Education Consortium (GHEC), an outstanding organization of medical educators dedicated to furthering knowledge in the field of global health. We also want to acknowledge Jim Shanahan from McGraw-Hill, who has tirelessly supported and pushed forward this work.

A sad note is that one of the authors, Dr. Mark Stinson, passed away unexpectedly in California before publication. Mark was a tireless worker for the underserved and had extensive experience in many of the world's hot spots. He put a lot of work into Chapter 9 and was very excited to see this book in production. He is greatly missed by all who knew him.

Invariably, in a book of this nature there will be some errors or inaccuracies. Although we have tried to proofread and double-check each chapter, we wish to take responsibility for anything that is incorrect. Some items may even be outdated by the time the book is actually published, and for this we really have no control. Certain areas within the field of global health can change rapidly.

We trust this book will contribute to a better understanding and awareness of and a greater empathy for the needs and health problems of people around our world. We hope that the reader will discover a greater desire to help contribute to solutions and progress toward better and more equitable world health. In our role as medical educators, we see great interest among students and residents in what is happening around the world. They wish to be involved and to make a difference. Most of us writing in this book began our work in global health with a certain degree of idealism. Fortunately, we still have that idealism even as it has matured and been tempered by reality. The idea of "health for all" still rings as something that is possible and that must be accomplished.

We hope this book can serve to help a new generation move closer to making this vision come true.

William H. Markle
Melanie A. Fisher
Raymond A. Smego, Jr.

Global Health: Past, Present, and Future

1

Amir Abdul Khaliq and Raymond A. Smego, Jr.

LEARNING OBJECTIVES

- *Understand the history of global health and the public health interventions that have led to the current state of world health*
- *Enumerate the major health problems and threats facing the world today*
- *Propose solutions for the various problems faced by health workers around the world*

public health *n. The science and practice of protecting and improving the health of a community, as by preventative medicine, health education, control of communicable diseases, application of sanitary measures, and monitoring of environmental hazards.*

—The American Heritage Dictionary

The collective personal health of a population is the public health. At the turn of the 20th century, the life expectancy for a citizen living in the United States was 45.2 years, and the five leading causes of death were influenza and pneumonia, tuberculosis, diarrhea and enteritis, heart disease, and stroke (Figure 1-1). Median survival for persons residing in less developed regions was even less, and worldwide the most important public health problems were largely infectious in nature. However, 100 years later the public health for the entire planet had dramatically improved. In 2004, the average Japanese was living 82 years, the average American 78 years, and the average Costa Rican 77 years (Figure 1-2). Even impoverished parts of the world in Africa, Asia, and Latin America saw tremendous public health gains in the 20th century. Unfortunately, the gains in some

developing countries marred by poverty and political strife have been less than dramatic. In 2004, the average life expectancy of a person in Kenya was 51 years, in Bangladesh 62 years, and in Guatemala 68 years. Sadly, the ongoing human immunodeficiency virus/acquired immunodeficiency syndrome (HIV/AIDS) pandemic, with its epicenter in Africa during the 1980s and 1990s, has contributed to huge setbacks in longevity in much of the African continent and elsewhere in the 25 years since its recognition. For example, the life expectancy for a Ugandan man was approximately 47.4 years in 1980–1985, 39.7 years in 1985–1990, and 38.9 years in 1995–2000. In 2004, the life expectancy of a Ugandan man had improved but was still only 48 years.

The leading causes of mortality in the United States today are heart disease, cancer, stroke, chronic lung disease, and unintentional injury. Pneumonia, influenza, and HIV/AIDS account for only 4.5% of the annual deaths. Globally, both communicable (e.g., pneumonia, diarrheal disease, HIV/AIDS, tuberculosis, and malaria) and noncommunicable diseases constitute the list of major public health priorities as developing countries in Asia, Africa, and Latin America continue their developmental, demographic, and epidemiologic transitions (Table 1-1). In Bayesian fashion, global populations are trading one set of diseases for another. In many countries, improved socioeconomic and public health conditions that led to a reduction in infectious disease–related morbidity and mortality have resulted in the introduction of lifestyle diseases such as obesity, coronary artery disease, hypertension, and other diseases related to excessive eating, smoking, alcohol consumption, and illicit drug use.

Scientific, social, cultural, economic, and political factors all contribute to the overall wellness of a community, be it local or international. All around the world, the impact of disease-oriented medical care on the overall health status of a country is relatively small compared with the collective contributions made by improved living conditions, including nutrition, sanitation, housing, education, and income.

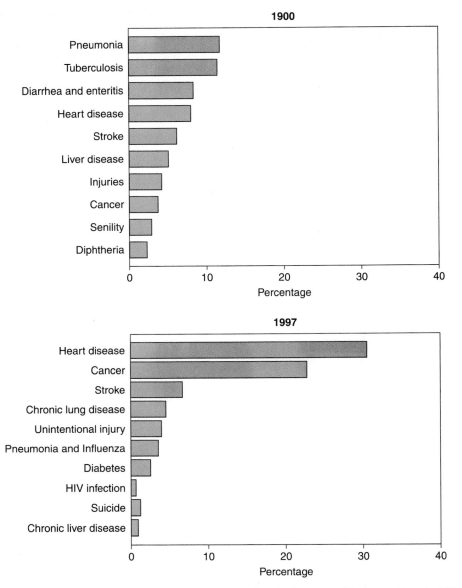

Figure 1-1. The ten leading causes of death as a percentage of all deaths: United States, 1900 and 1997. From the Centers for Disease Control and Prevention. Achievements in Public Health, 1900–1999: Control of Infectious diseases. *MMWR* 48;621–29:1999. (Reproduced with permission.)

PUBLIC HEALTH MILESTONES

From scientific discoveries to public policies, there have been numerous innovations and advances in public health throughout human history that have improved the quality and longevity of life around the globe. Public health is credited with adding almost 30 years to the life expectancy of people in the United States in the last century, and more than 22 years elsewhere in the world.

In 1999, the Centers for Disease Control and Prevention (CDC) formulated its list of ten great public health achievements in the 20th century as a testament to the remarkable evolution of the health of the world.[1] An expanded list of public health milestones is shown in Table 1-2. Dating back to ancient civilizations, there is evidence of societies working to improve the health of the general public. The Babylonian sewage systems were among the first designed to protect the water supply from

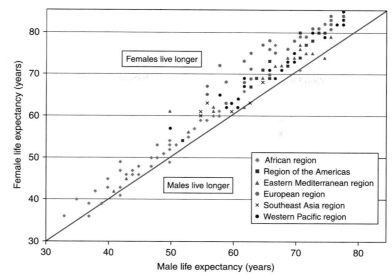

Figure 1-2. Life expectancy at birth for males and females, countries by WHO region, 2003. From the World Health Organization. http://www.who.int/healthinfo/statistics/maps_graphshealthstatus/en/index2.html. (Reproduced with permission.)

Table 1-1. Major global public health problems and threats, 2006.

Infectious diseases
   Tuberculosis (including multidrug-resistant TB)
   Malaria
   Acute lower respiratory infections in childhood
   Childhood diarrheas
   New and emerging infectious diseases

'Transition' diseases
   Cardiovascular disease
   Obesity
   Other lifestyle diseases related to smoking, alcohol,
      illicit drug use, etc.
   Mental and psychosocial illnesses

World hunger
Displaced and refugee populations
Maternal mortality
Motor vehicle injury and mortality
Occupational workplace safety
Landmines

Environmental and social determinants of public health
   Population growth
   Global climate change and natural disasters
   Pollution (air, water, other)
   Governmental corruption
   Political instability
   Regional conflict
   Nuclear threats
   Biological/chemical terrorism
   Economic divergence (inequity)

Table 1-2. Selected public health milestones during the 20th century.

Immunizations
Control of infectious diseases
Pasteurization
Fluoridation of drinking water
Maternal-child interventions
Family planning
Wastewater systems
Prevention and treatment of heart disease and stroke
Motor vehicle safety
Workplace safety
Safer and healthier foods
Tobacco control
Reducing firearm-related injuries
Preventing birth defects

contamination and disease. The innovation of pasteurization, discovered by Louis Pasteur in the 1860s, has helped to ensure the safety of food supplies throughout the world and keep them free of disease-causing organisms. In 1980, smallpox was officially eradicated from the planet, and although polio and measles have not been eradicated yet, the world is making progress towards elimination and for protecting children and communities from these once debilitating diseases.

In all parts of the globe there is an evolving health transition from first-generation diseases (e.g., common childhood infections, malnutrition, and reproductive risks) to second-generation diseases (e.g., cardiovascular and cerebrovascular diseases, cancers, and degenerative diseases) and to third-generation diseases (e.g., violence, drug abuse, and mental and psychosocial illness).[2]

Control of Infectious Diseases

The 19th century shift in population from countryside to cities that accompanied industrialization and immigration led to overcrowding in poor housing served by inadequate or nonexistent public water supplies and waste-disposal systems. These conditions resulted in repeated outbreaks of cholera, dysentery, tuberculosis, typhoid fever, influenza, yellow fever, and malaria. This global urbanization accelerated dramatically during the last four decades of the 20th century. In 1960, an estimated 70% of the world's population lived in rural areas; today, almost the same percentage live in cities and large metropolitan areas and are at risk for large-scale disease outbreaks. In 1994, the city of Shanghai, China, experienced an outbreak of viral hepatitis A involving more than 400,000 cases. Throughout the Indian subcontinent, virtually every major city has experienced outbreaks of viral hepatitis E linked to contaminated municipal water systems, involving up to 200,000 persons per outbreak.

Public health control of infectious diseases after 1900 was based on the 19th century discovery of microorganisms as the cause of many serious diseases such as cholera and tuberculosis.[3,4] Disease control resulted from improvements in sanitation and hygiene, the discovery of antibiotics, and the implementation of universal childhood vaccination programs. Scientific and technologic advances played a major role in each of these areas and are the foundation for today's disease surveillance and control systems. In Western countries, the incidence of many infectious diseases began to markedly decline by 1900 because of public health improvements, implementation of which continued into the 20th century.

In many urban and rural areas of Asia, Africa, and Latin America, basic public health services such as provision of clean drinking water, sewage and solid waste disposal, food safety, and public education about hygienic practices (e.g., food handling and handwashing) are still lacking or inadequate. These deficiencies contribute to a continued global burden of major waterborne and foodborne diseases such as acute diarrheal illness (responsible for approximately 1.9 million deaths every year), viral hepatitis, enteric fever, and brucellosis. One-third of the world's population suffers from diseases caused by unsafe food, and many of these people experience long-term complications or death. Furthermore, animal and pest control programs are inadequate worldwide and contribute to the persistence of diseases such as malaria, rabies, viral encephalitis, trypanosomiasis, plague, and anthrax.

In Western countries, deaths from infectious diseases declined markedly during the 20th century. In particular, there has been a sharp drop in infant and child mortality and a 29.2-year increase in life expectancy. For example, in the United States in 1900, 30.4% of all deaths occurred among children younger than 5 years; in 1997, that percentage was only 1.4%. In 1900, the three leading causes of death were pneumonia, tuberculosis, and diarrhea and enteritis, which (together with diphtheria) caused one-third of all deaths. Of these deaths, 40% were among children younger than 5 years. In 1997, heart disease and cancers accounted for 54.7% of all deaths, with less than 5% attributable to pneumonia, influenza, and HIV infection.

Despite this remarkable progress, infectious diseases remain among the greatest threats to persons living in poorer developing regions of the world. 60 percent of children who die under the age of five die because of pneumonia, diarrhea, or measles. Even as the number of tuberculosis cases is at an all-time low in the United States, the global prevalence of tuberculosis is at an all-time high, with about 8 million new cases and 3 million deaths annually. HIV/AIDS has become the most devastating epidemic in human history, supplanting the 1918 influenza pandemic that resulted in 20 million deaths. Since 1981, an estimated 30 million lives have been lost to HIV/AIDS, and almost 40 million more persons are believed to be infected worldwide, especially in sub-Saharan Africa, India, and Southeast Asia. This pandemic is still in progress. In addition, more than 20 new diseases were discovered in the last 25 years (Table 1-3), demonstrating the volatility of infectious diseases and the unpredictability of disease emergence. Many of the emerging infectious diseases, such as avian flu, severe acute respiratory syndrome (SARS), and hemolytic uremic syndrome, are zoonotic.

Immunizations

Vaccines are probably the greatest achievements of biomedical science and public health in history. At the beginning of the 20th century, infectious diseases exacted an enormous toll on the global population. Currently, vaccine-preventable diseases remain prevalent causes of child and adult mortality in Asia, Africa, and parts of Latin America.

In 1900, few effective measures existed to treat and prevent infectious diseases. Although the first vaccine against smallpox was developed in 1796, more than 100 years later its use was not widespread enough to fully control the disease. Four other vaccines—against rabies, typhoid, cholera, and plague—were developed late in the 19th century but were not used widely by 1900. Since 1900, vaccines have been developed or licensed against 22 other diseases (Table 1-4). In 1974, when the Expanded Programme on Immunization (EPI) was launched by the

Table 1-3. Newly recognized pathogens or diseases since 1981.

Avian influenza
Acanthamebiasis
Australian bat Lyssavirus
Babesiosis
Bartonella henselae
Coronaviruses/Severe acute respiratory syndrome (SARS)
Ehrlichiosis
Hantavirus pulmonary syndrome
Helicobacter pylori
Hendra or equine morbilli virus
Hepatitis C virus
Hepatitis E virus
HIV/AIDS
Human herpesvirus 8
Human herpesvirus 6
Human T-cell lymphotropic virus I
Human T-cell lymphotropic virus II
Borrelia burgdorferi
Microsporidia
  Encephalitozoon cuniculi
  Encephalitozoon hellem
  Enterocytozoon bieneusi
Nipah virus disease
Parvovirus B19
Variant Creutzfeldt-Jakob disease

Table 1-4. Vaccine-preventable diseases, by year of vaccine development or US licensure, 1798–2005.

Disease	Year
Smallpox[a]	1798[b]
Rabies	1885[b]
Typhoid	1896[b]
Cholera	1896[b]
Plague	1897[b]
Diphtheria[a]	1923[b]
Pertussis[a]	1926[b]
Tetanus[a]	1927[b]
Tuberculosis	1927[b]
Influenza	1945[c]
Yellow fever	1953[c]
Poliomyelitis[a]	1955[c]
Measles[a]	1963[c]
Mumps[a]	1967[c]
Rubella[a]	1969[c]
Anthrax	1970[c]
Meningitis	1975[c]
Pneumococcal	1977[c]
Adenovirus	1980[c]
Hepatitis B[a]	1981[c]
Haemophilus influenzae type b[a]	1985
Japanese B encephalitis	1992[c]
Hepatitis A	1995[c]
Varicella[a]	1995[c]
Lyme disease	1998[c]
Rotavirus[a]	1998[c],2006[d]
Human Papilloma virus	2005[c]

[a]Vaccine recommended for universal use in US children. For smallpox, routine vaccination ended in 1971.
[b]Vaccine developed (i.e., first published results of vaccine usage).
[c]Vaccine licensed for use in the United States. Withdrawn from the market in 2001.
[d]Live oral pentavalent vaccine.
From Centers for Disease Control and Prevention. Achievements in public health, 1900–1999: impact of vaccines universally recommended for children—United States, 1990–1998. *MMWR* 1999;48; 243–248. (Reproduced with permission.)

World Health Organization (WHO), less than 5% of the world's children were immunized against the six initial target diseases—diphtheria, tetanus, pertussis (whooping cough), polio, measles, and tuberculosis—during their first year of life. Until then, immunization programs had been largely restricted to industrialized countries, and even there were only partially implemented. By 1990, and again in the most recent statistics (after a slight interim drop in coverage rates), almost 80% of the 130 million children born each year were immunized before their first birthday. As coverage for each of the childhood vaccines has increased—now involving over 500 million immunization contacts with children every year—there has been a corresponding drop in the incidence of disease. The EPI (which today includes yellow fever and hepatitis B vaccines) now prevents the deaths of at least 3 million children a year. In addition, at least 750,000 fewer children are blinded, physically disabled, or mentally retarded as a result of vaccine-preventable diseases.

During the 20th century, substantial achievements were made in the control of many vaccine-preventable diseases.[5] The dramatic 95% or greater decline in morbidity from nine vaccine-preventable diseases (smallpox and the EPI diseases mentioned previously for which vaccines had been recommended for universal use in children as of 1990) and their complications attest to the remarkable efficacy of immunizations. Poliomyelitis caused by wild-type viruses

has been nearly eliminated, and cases of measles and *Haemophilus influenzae* type b (Hib) invasive disease among children younger than 5 years have been reduced to record low numbers. As is true for other public health interventions, national and international efforts to promote vaccine use depend on public health infrastructure, economics, and political stability and political will. With the proper mind-set and establishment of priorities, even large or poor countries can achieve remarkable rates of vaccination coverage for their populations.

The success of vaccination programs in the United States and Europe inspired the 20th century concept of disease eradication—the idea that a selected disease could be eliminated from all human populations through global cooperation. In 1980, after a decade-long campaign involving 33 nations, smallpox was eradicated worldwide, approximately a decade after it had been eliminated from the United States and the rest of the Western Hemisphere. Polio and dracunculiasis have the possibility of being eradicated in the near future.

Despite the dramatic declines in vaccine-preventable diseases, such diseases persist, particularly in developing countries, and several challenges face vaccine delivery worldwide. National treasuries and vaccine delivery systems must be capable of successfully implementing an increasingly complex vaccination schedule. An American child requires 15 to 19 doses of vaccine by age 18 months to be protected against 11 childhood diseases.[6] In addition, future immunization challenges are presented by the recent licensure of new vaccines such as the seven-valent conjugated pneumococcal vaccine, tetravalent meningococcal vaccines, and the human papilloma virus vaccine. Anticipated new vaccines include those for influenza, parainfluenza, and chronic diseases (e.g., gastric ulcers, and cancer caused by *Helicobacter pylori*, and rheumatic heart disease that occurs as a sequel to group A streptococcal infection). In the 1990s, given constrained national health care resources, many developing countries were forced to analyze their infectious diseases epidemiologies and choose between adding Hib or hepatitis B vaccine to their national EPI programs.

Clinical trials are under way for a vaccine to prevent and/or treat HIV infection. The global immunization challenge of this century will be finding a way to finance provision of an effective HIV vaccine for the world's masses who need it most. Creative and innovative strategies to fund the worldwide distribution of an effective HIV vaccine, when it becomes available, are being aggressively discussed with potential funders such as the World Bank, the World Monetary Fund, and the Gates foundation. The number of persons who will be candidates for an HIV vaccine will depend on whether the immunobiologic is strictly preventive or is therapeutic.

International partnerships involving affluent industrialized nations, the WHO, and Rotary International are seeking to eradicate polio in the near future. Efforts to accelerate control of measles, which causes approximately 1 million deaths each year, and to expand rubella vaccination programs are also under way around the world. The use of existing vaccines in routine childhood vaccination programs worldwide must be expanded, and successful introduction of new vaccines must occur as they are developed. Such efforts regarding infectious disease control and prevention can benefit both rich and poor countries by decreasing disease importations from developing countries. In the West, millions of cases of potentially preventable influenza, pneumococcal disease, and hepatitis B occur each year in adolescent and adult populations. Many new vaccines will be targeted at these age groups.

Antimicrobial Drug Resistance

Antibacterial antibiotics have been in civilian use for more than 60 years and have saved the lives of millions of persons with streptococcal and staphylococcal infections, gonorrhea, syphilis, and other infections. Drugs have also been developed to treat viral diseases (e.g., herpes and HIV infection), fungal diseases (e.g., candidiasis and aspergillosis), and parasitic diseases (e.g., malaria). Penicillin, discovered fortuitously by Sir Alexander Fleming in 1928, was not developed for medical use until the 1940s, but it soon changed the face of medicine. The drug quickly became a widely available medical product that provided effective treatment of previously incurable bacterial illnesses, with a broader spectrum and fewer side effects than sulfa drugs.

The increased development and use of antimicrobial agents has hastened the development of drug resistance. The emergence of drug resistance in many microorganisms is reversing some of the therapeutic miracles of the last 50 years and underscores the importance of disease prevention. Antimicrobial multidrug resistance is a serious and growing problem worldwide for community-based infections caused by *Plasmodium* species, *Mycobacterium tuberculosis*, *Streptococcus pneumoniae*, *Salmonella* and *Campylobacter* species, *Neisseria gonorrhoeae*, *Helicobacter pylori*, and HIV, as well as for nosocomial infections due to staphylococci, enterococci, Enterobacteriaceae, *Clostridium difficile*, and systemic fungi. (See Chapter 12 for more information.)

Future Challenges to the Control of Infectious Diseases

Successes in reducing morbidity and mortality from infectious diseases during the first three quarters of the 20th century led to complacency about the need for continued research into the treatment and control of infectious microbes. However, the global appearance of AIDS, the emergence of multidrug-resistant tuberculosis (MDR-TB), and an overall increase in infectious disease mortality during the 1980s and early 1990s have provided additional evidence that as long as microbes can evolve, new diseases will appear.

Molecular genetics has provided valuable insights into the remarkable ability of microorganisms to evolve, adapt, and develop drug resistance in an unpredictable and dynamic fashion. Resistance genes are transmitted from one bacterium to another on plasmids, and viruses evolve through replication errors and reassortment of

ZIMBABWE: A CASE STUDY OF AN HIV-RAVAGED COUNTRY

As mentioned previously, public health is generally the result of a summation of the scientific, social, cultural, economic, and political variables within a population. The HIV/AIDS pandemic has had an unprecedented impact on the fabric of individual nations and on the evolution of the planet as a whole because it has targeted the most economically and socially productive members of society as well as claimed the futures of maternally infected infants. This case study of one country in sub-Saharan Africa, Zimbabwe, illustrates the interplay of national and international factors that can lead to public health devastation.

Zimbabwe (formerly Rhodesia) achieved its independence from Britain in 1980; since that time, the Zimbabwe African National Union-Patriotic Front has been in power under the presidency of Robert Mugabe. Officially, Zimbabwe has a population of 13 million people, although actual population figures are thought to be much lower. 56 percent of the population live on less than US $1 a day, and 80% live on less than US $2 a day.

Zimbabwe is experiencing one of the world's worst HIV epidemics, and the level of HIV infection is one of the highest in the world, with about 25% of 15 to 49-year-olds infected. About 1.82 million of the nation's 14 million people are living with HIV or AIDS. The overall HIV prevalence, once as high as 34% in 2000, has recently declined to 21.6%. Over 3,200 people die each week from AIDS, and AIDS-related illnesses account for about three-fourths of hospital admissions. As a result, life expectancy in Zimbabwe has fallen to 33 years, from a historical high of 61 years in 1990. An estimated 1.3 million orphans and 1.8 million Zimbabweans are living with HIV and AIDS. Approximately one-third of all the country's teachers and over half of Zimbabwe's soldiers are HIV seropositive.

Since the late 1990s, the decline of Zimbabwe's once flourishing economy, in spite of well-developed infrastructure and financial systems, has gravely affected a large segment of the population. Unemployment is reportedly more than 70%, and the number of people living in poverty, also currently estimated at more than 70%, is increasing. Hyperinflation has reduced purchasing power. Real gross domestic product (GDP) has declined by 30% in the last 5 years, and annual inflation rates reached a record 1,000% in May 2006. Such continued high inflation hampers development, hitting the poor hardest. Agricultural production has plummeted in the last 6 years; for example, between 2000 and 2004, the national cattle herd shrank by 90%, and the production of flue-cured tobacco declined from 237 million kilograms to 70 million kilograms. The frequency of acute malnutrition declined in 2004, partly as a result of large-scale food aid, although the situation in some areas continues to worsen. On the Human Development Index, Zimbabwe ranks 147th of 177 countries.

Agriculture is the most important sector of the Zimbabwean economy but has been severely disrupted by land resettlement. This has led to a collapse in investor confidence and the flight of capital. Lack of foreign exchange has led to critical shortages in fuel and other imported commodities, including power. The cost of schooling has risen dramatically, posing serious challenges for low-income families. The decline in inward investment and development assistance is further compromising the prospects for economic recovery.

Food shortages affect up to half the population of Zimbabwe. A national vulnerability assessment in November 2005 estimated that 2.8 million Zimbabweans would face food shortages in the "hungry season" (January through March) leading up to the next harvest. Following much better rains, the harvest in 2006 was expected to be better than that in 2005. Due to hyperinflation, even when food is available it is unaffordable to many. However, the impact of chronic illness, localized flooding, and the high price of seeds and fertilizer will mean that many people will require assistance later in the year.

The International Monetary Fund (IMF) suspended payments to Zimbabwe in 2000, following the government's decision to abandon IMF public spending guidelines (including payments to war veterans, the cost of which amounted to 3% of GDP). The country went into arrears at the World Bank in 2000 and at the IMF the following year, effectively cutting off cooperation with either institution. The country is crippled by governmental corruption up to the presidential level; according to Transparency International's 2003 Corruption Perception Index, Zimbabwe ranked 106 of 133 on the global list of most corrupt nations.

Despite these obstacles, Zimbabwe is on track to achieve the Millennium Development Goal (MDG) target on HIV and AIDS, namely, to "have halted by 2015, and begun to reverse, the spread of HIV/AIDS." Declining HIV prevalence is likely to be a result of high mortality rates and changes in sexual behavior. Most of Zimbabwe's other MDGs are unlikely to be achieved by 2015 unless the political and social situation improves dramatically. Child and maternal mortality indicators show a steadily worsening situation, exacerbated by HIV/AIDS.

Current foreign aid priorities include tackling HIV/AIDS (including increasing access to antiretroviral therapy), food insecurity (including increasing individuals' access to seeds and fertilizers, nutrition gardens, and safe water), and support to orphans and vulnerable children (including school feeding and home-based care programs).

---

gene segments and by crossing species barriers. Recent examples of microbial evolution include the development of a virulent strain of avian influenza in Hong Kong (1997–1998) and the multidrug-resistant W strain of *M. tuberculosis* in the United States in 1991. The emergence of Vancomycin-Intermediate *Staphylococcus aureus* (VISA) and vancomycin-resistant *S. aureus* (VRSA) has become a major cause of global concern among clinicians and microbiologists.

For continued success in controlling infectious diseases, the global public health system must prepare to address diverse challenges, including the emergence of new infectious diseases, the reemergence of old diseases (sometimes in drug-resistant forms), large foodborne outbreaks, and acts of bioterrorism. Continued protection of health requires improved capacity for disease surveillance and outbreak response at the local, state, national, and global levels; the development and dissemination of new laboratory and epidemiologic methods; continued antimicrobial and vaccine development; and ongoing research into environmental factors that facilitate disease emergence.[7] The global public health response to the SARS outbreak in 2004 demonstrated unprecedented cooperation in surveillance and the dissemination of information. Ongoing research into the possible role of infectious agents (e.g., *Chlamydia trachomatis*, viruses) in causing or intensifying certain chronic diseases such as type 1 diabetes mellitus, some cancers, and atherosclerotic heart disease is also imperative.

MAJOR PUBLIC HEALTH CHALLENGES FOR THE FUTURE

World Hunger and Poverty

In 2000, WHO's Millennium Development Goals to be achieved by 2015 were endorsed by 189 countries; these goals include reducing by half the 1.2 billion people in the world who live on less than US $1 per day and the 852 million people who suffer from hunger on a daily basis.[8] It is estimated that every day more than 16,000 children die from hunger-related causes (one child every 5 seconds). Hunger is the most extreme manifestation of poverty, where individuals or families cannot afford to meet their most basic need for food. Hunger manifests itself in many ways other than starvation and famine. Undernourishment negatively affects people's health, productivity, sense of hope, and overall well-being. Lack of food can stunt growth, heighten susceptibility to illness, slow thinking, sap energy, hinder fetal development, and contribute to mental retardation. Economically, the constant securing of food consumes valuable time and energy, allowing less time for work and earning income. Socially, the lack of food erodes relationships and feeds shame so that those most in need of support are often least able to call upon it.

Poor nutrition and caloric deficiencies cause nearly one in three people to die prematurely or have disabilities, according to the WHO.[9] Pregnant women, nursing mothers, and children are among the groups most at risk for undernourishment. Every year, nearly 11 million children die before they reach their 5th birthday. Almost all of these deaths occur in developing countries, three-fourths of them in sub-Saharan Africa and South Asia, the two regions that also suffer from the highest rates of hunger and malnutrition. Most of these deaths are attributed not to outright starvation but to diseases that opportunistically afflict vulnerable children with host defenses weakened by hunger. Each year, more than 20 million low-birth-weight babies are born in developing countries. These babies risk dying in infancy, and those who survive often suffer lifelong physical and cognitive disabilities.

The four most common childhood illnesses are diarrhea, acute respiratory illness, malaria, and measles. Each of these illnesses is both preventable and treatable. Yet, poverty interferes with parents' access to immunizations and medicines. Chronic undernourishment superimposed on insufficient treatment greatly increases a child's risk of death. In the developing world, 27% of children younger than 5 years are moderately to severely underweight, 10% are severely underweight, 10% are moderately to severely wasted or seriously below weight-for-height, and an overwhelming 31% are moderately to severely stunted or seriously below normal height-for-age.[10]

HIV/AIDS

The HIV/AIDS epidemic has become a major obstacle in the fight against hunger and poverty in developing countries. Because the majority of HIV-infected persons with AIDS are young adults who normally harvest crops, food production has dropped dramatically in countries with high HIV/AIDS prevalence rates. In half of the countries in sub-Saharan Africa, per capita economic growth is estimated to be falling by between 0.5% and 1.2% each year as a direct result of AIDS. Infected adults also leave behind children and elderly relatives who have little means to provide for themselves. In 2003, 12 million children were newly orphaned in southern Africa, a number expected to rise to 18 million in 2010.[11] Since the epidemic began, 30 million people have died from AIDS, and more than 15 million children have lost at least one parent to the disease. The UNICEF term *child-headed households*, meaning minors orphaned by HIV/AIDS who are raising their siblings, illustrates the gravity of the situation.[11,12] Approximately 60% of the 40 million HIV-infected people in the world today live in sub-Saharan Africa (Figure 1-3).

Each year, another 5 million people become infected with HIV and more than 3 million people die of AIDS. Despite these figures, only a small minority of persons in need are receiving antiretroviral therapy (Figure 1-4), although the situation has improved since the advent of generic antiretroviral drug production and national scale-up drug distribution programs. WHO's Millennium Development Goal was to provide 3 million people in developing countries with antiretroviral treatment by the end of 2005.

Infant and Maternal Mortality

Child mortality is closely linked to poverty. Improvements in public health services are critical to childhood

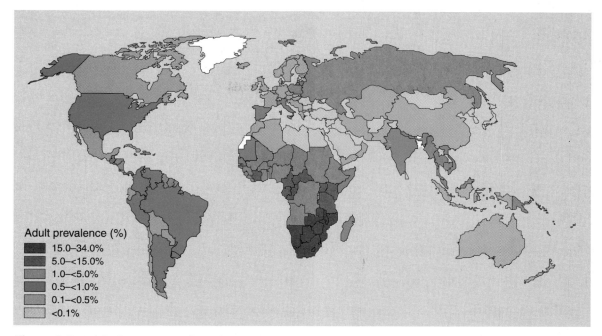

Figure 1-3. Adults (15–49 years of age) living with HIV (%), end 2005. From the World Health Organization. 2006 report on the global AIDS epidemic. (Reproduced with permission.)

survival, including safe water, better sanitation, and (especially for girls and mothers) education. In the United States from 1915 through 1997, the infant mortality rate declined more than 90%, to 7.2 per 1,000 live births; from 1900 through 1997, the maternal mortality rate declined almost 99%, to less than 0.1 reported death per 1,000 live births (7.7 deaths per 100,000 live births in 1997)—and the United States ranks only 25th among developed countries in infant mortality and 21st in maternal mortality (Figure 1-5). In stark contrast, in the Central African Republic in 2000, for every 1,000 live births 120 infants died and 179 children under age 4 died, and 1,100 of every 100,000 women died of pregnancy-related complications. Each year worldwide, almost 10.5 million children die before their 5th birthday.[13]

Geographical region	Number of people receiving ARV therapy (lowestimate – high estimate)	Estimated need	Coverage
Sub-Saharan Africa	810,000 (730,000–890 000)	4,700,000	17%
Latin America and the Caribbean	315,000 (295,000–335 000)	465,000	68%
East, South and South-East Asia	180,000 (150,000–210 000)	1,100,000	16%
Europe and Central Asia	21,000 (20,000–22 000)	160,000	13%
North Africa and the Middle East	4,000 (3,000–5 000)	75,000	5%
Total	1 330,000 (1,200,000–1 460 000)	6.5 million	20%

Figure 1-4. Antiretroviral coverage in low- and middle-income countries, by region, as of December 2004. From the World Health Organization. Progress on global access to antiretroviral therapy. March 21, 2007. http://www.who.int/hiv/facts/cov1205/en/index.html. (Reproduced with permission.)

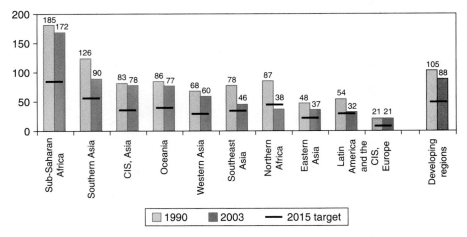

Figure 1-5. Under-five mortality rate per 1,000 live births, 1990 and 2003.

Worldwide, in 1960 one child in five died before age 5. By 1990, the rate had fallen to one in ten. Such progress gave hope that child mortality could be cut by two-thirds by 2015. But advances slowed in the 1990s, and only northern Africa, Latin America, the Caribbean, and Southeast Asia maintained their rapid pace. In these regions, economic growth, better nutrition, and better access to health care have helped spur improvements in child survival (Table 1-5). Regional averages, however, mask differences from country to country and disparities among socioeconomic groups. Important progress has also been observed in the Middle East, central and eastern Europe, the former Soviet Union, and South Asia (around a 30% reduction between 1990 and 2004). Unfortunately, substantial progress has not been observed in Africa, with only a 10% decline since 1990 and much less than that observed between 1970 and 1990. Almost 100 countries, including over 40 in sub-Saharan Africa, are not on track to reach WHO's 2015 Millennium Development Goal of two-thirds reduction in the under-five mortality rate observed in 1990.

One hundred years ago, most obstetrical deliveries and surgical interventions around the world were performed without following the principles of asepsis. As a result, large numbers of maternal deaths were caused by sepsis following delivery or illegally induced abortion, with the remaining deaths primarily attributed to hemorrhage and toxemia. Today, the complications of pregnancy and childbirth are still a leading cause of death and disability among women of reproductive age in the poorest regions of the world.[14,15] It is estimated that around 529,000 women die each year from maternal causes (especially intractable hemorrhage,. sepsis, complications of unsafe abortion, prolonged or obstructed labor, and eclampsia), and many more suffer injuries, infection, and disabilities during pregnancy or childbirth.

Poor obstetrical education and delivery practices are mainly responsible for the high numbers of maternal deaths, most of which are preventable. In many poor countries, obstetrical services are primarily provided by poorly trained or untrained medical practitioners (for example, in the Central African Republic only 44% of babies are delivered by skilled attendants). Most births occur at home with the assistance of midwives or traditional birth attendants. In much

Table 1-5. Environmental and medical interventions contributing to the decline in infant mortality in the 20th century.

Improvements in standards of living
Reduction in vaccine-preventable diseases
Control of milkborne diseases
Improvements in nutrition
Declining fertility rates
Longer birth spacing
Advances in clinical medicine
    Discovery of antibiotics and fluid and electrolyte therapies
    Technologic advances in neonatal medicine
Improvements in access to health care
Increases in surveillance and monitoring of disease
Placing of infants on their back
Regionalization of perinatal services
Improvements in education levels

of the world, consistent access to antenatal and postnatal care, which benefits both mother and fetus, is inadequate or lacking.

The foundations for maternal risk are often laid in girlhood. Women whose growth has been stunted by chronic malnutrition are vulnerable to obstructed labor. Anemia predisposes to hemorrhage and sepsis during delivery and has been implicated in at least 20% of post-partum maternal deaths in Africa and Asia. The risk of childbirth is even greater for women who have under-gone female genital mutilation; an estimated 2 million girls are mutilated every year.

Motor Vehicle Safety

Each year, road traffic accidents claim 1.2 million lives worldwide and injure or disable as many as 50 million more.[16] Road traffic accidents are the second leading cause of death worldwide among persons aged 5 to 29 years. Previous studies have shown that casualty and fatality rates in developing countries are higher than in the West. Furthermore, in the Middle East gulf countries, injury and death rates are much higher than in develop-ing countries with comparable vehicle ownership levels. For example, in the United Kingdom and United States in 2004 there were 0.72 and 1.51 road traffic fatalities per hundred million vehicle kilometers, respectively, whereas the United Arab Emirates recorded a dispropor-tionate 3.33 deaths per hundred million kilometers.[17] In 2004, road traffic mortality in Oman was 28 per 100,000 population, far in excess of the global average of 19 per 100,000 persons, and more than one-third of those who died were younger than 25 years.

Over the past two decades, research has provided a clear understanding of the circumstances surrounding motor vehicle injuries in children and the demographic risk and protective factors that influence the likelihood that a child will be injured. Riding unrestrained is the single most important risk factor for death and injury among children in motor vehicle accidents. In the United States in 2000, 47% of motor vehicle fatalities among oc-cupants younger than 5 years involved children who were not restrained. In most developing countries, infant and child safety seat usage is even lower.

Occupational Workplace Safety

Workplace safety is a serious concern in many parts of the world, where workers face significant health and safety risks during the course of trying to earn a living. Major unintentional occupation-related illnesses, in-juries, and deaths occur as a result of motor vehicle–related accidents, mining-related exposures and accidents, machine-related accidents, construction exposures and accidents, agriculture/forestry/fishing-related accidents, transportation/communications/public utilities–related

incidents, electrocutions, falls, and homicides. Workplace fatalities, injuries, and illnesses remain at unacceptably high levels and involve an enormous unnecessary health burden, suffering, and economic loss amounting to 4% to 5% of global GDP.[18]

In the United States, data from the National Safety Council from 1933 through 1997 indicate that deaths from unintentional work-related injuries declined 90%, from 37 per 100,000 workers to 4 per 100,000.[19,20] The corresponding annual number of deaths decreased from 14,500 to 5,100. During the same period, the workforce more than tripled, from 39 million to approximately 130 million. Workers in developing countries, however, have not achieved the same levels of workplace protec-tion as in the West. Globally, workers continue to die from preventable injuries sustained on the job. According to the latest International Labor Organization estimates for the year 2000, there are 2.0 million work-related deaths worldwide each year. WHO estimates that only 10% to 15% of workers have access to a basic standard of occupational health services. Mining remains the most hazardous industry worldwide.

Coronary Heart Disease and Stroke

An estimated 16.7 million deaths—or 29.2% of total global deaths—result from the various forms of cardiovas-cular disease (CVD): ischemic or coronary heart disease, cerebrovascular disease or stroke, hypertension, heart fail-ure, and rheumatic heart disease. Of these, 7.2 million deaths are due to ischemic heart disease, 5.5 million to stroke, and an additional 3.9 million to hypertensive and other heart conditions.[21] At least 20 million people survive heart attacks and strokes every year, with a sig-nificant proportion of them requiring costly clinical care, which puts a huge burden on long-term care re-sources. CVD affects people in their midlife years, un-dermining the socioeconomic development not only of affected individuals but also of families and nations. Lower socioeconomic groups generally have a greater prevalence of risk factors, diseases, and mortality in de-veloped countries. A similar pattern is emerging as the CVD epidemic matures in developing countries as well.

Cardiovascular diseases are no longer only diseases of the developed world. In 2005, some 80% of all CVD deaths worldwide took place in developing low- and middle-income countries, and these countries accounted for 86% of the global CVD disease burden. More than 60% of all coronary heart disease occurs in developing countries, partly as a result of increasing longevity, urban-ization, and lifestyle changes. It is estimated that by 2010, CVD will be the leading cause of death in devel-oping countries. Furthermore, CVD is responsible for 10% of disability-adjusted life years (DALYs) lost in low- and middle-income countries and 18% in high-income countries. DALYs represent healthy years lost and indicate the total burden of a disease as opposed to simply the resulting death. The global burden of coronary heart disease is projected to rise from 46 million DALYs in 1990 to 82 million in 2020. The rise in CVD reflects a significant combination of unhealthy dietary habits, reduced physical activity levels, and increased tobacco consumption worldwide as a result of industrialization, urbanization, economic development, and food market globalization.

More than half of the deaths and disability from heart disease and strokes each year can be reduced by a combination of simple, cost-effective, national efforts and individual actions to reduce major risk factors such as high blood pressure, diabetes mellitus, high cholesterol, obesity, and smoking. Obesity is one of the newest global epidemics, especially in developed and transitional countries. Because of obesity's association with cardiovascular disease and diabetes, obesity control and weight loss must be considered an important global strategy to improve the health and well-being of people all over the world.

In the West, major milestones in the management of angina pectoris and heart attack, including expensive or invasive interventions such as diagnostic coronary angiography, thrombolytic therapy, statins, IIb/IIIa platelet receptor blocker drugs, percutaneous transluminal coronary angioplasty, coronary artery stenting, coronary artery bypass grafting, and ventricular assist devices, have resulted in impressive declines in mortality from these conditions in the past two decades. The technologic future holds even more promise for cardiovascular disease treatment. However, these diagnostic and therapeutic services are largely inaccessible to the majority of populations living in Asia, Africa, and Latin America. No matter what advances are made in high-technology medicine, major global reductions in death and disability from cardiovascular disease will only come from preventive measures involving modification of risk factors, not from cure. The most cost-effective methods of reducing risk are population-wide interventions combining effective economic, educational, and broad health promotion policies and programs emphasizing the dietary intake of fats, cessation of smoking, and salt restriction.

The WHO, in collaboration with the CDC, is presently working to provide actionable information to develop and implement appropriate national and international policies related to the global epidemic of heart attack and stroke. As part of such efforts, the WHO has produced *The Atlas of Heart Disease and Stroke*, which addresses the problem of heart disease and stroke in a clear and accessible format for a wide audience. This highly valuable reference material has been designed for use by policy makers, national and international organizations, health professionals, and the general public. This picturesque atlas is in six parts: cardiovascular disease, risk factors, the burden, action, the future and the past, and world tables.[22]

Displaced and Refugee Populations

Under the United Nations (UN) Convention on the Status of Refugees, a refugee is defined as a person who, "owing to a well-founded fear of being persecuted for reasons of race, religion, nationality, membership in a particular social group, or political opinion, is outside the country of his nationality, and is unable to, or, owing to such fear, is unwilling to avail himself of the protection of that country." Internally displaced persons (IDPs) are people who have similarly been forced from their homes but have not crossed an internationally recognized state border. At the beginning of 2005, 13.4 million refugees were recognized by the UN. Although the overall number of refugees worldwide has decreased in recent years, increases have occurred in Africa, Asia, and the Pacific. Together, women and children make up approximately 80% of the refugee population.[23] The UN High Commissioner for Refugees (UNHCR) reports that, on average, refugees will spend 17 years outside of their home country.

In 2004, approximately 25,000,000 IDPs were displaced by conflict in 48 countries: 36% were located in camps or centers, 15% were living in urban areas, and 49% were either dispersed in rural areas or living in an unknown type of settlement.[24] More than half of the world's displaced people live in Africa, and nearly half live in countries experiencing ongoing conflict. Children and adolescents under the age of 18 account for nearly half this number, with 13% being under the age of 5.

Refugees and internally displaced individuals face daunting economic, social, and health risks that accompany displacement (Table 1-6). Relief programs target

Table 1-6. Factors that place refugees and internally displaced persons at risk for serious public health and humanitarian consequences.

Displacement and separation from families
Social instability
Increased mobility
Sexual and gender-based violence
Exploitation and abuse (including HIV/AIDS)
Poverty and food insecurity
Lack of access to health services, education, and
    basic assistance
Lack of linguistically and culturally appropriate health
    information
Forced labor or slavery
Forcible recruitment into armed groups
Trafficking
Abduction
Detention and denial of access to asylum or family-
    reunification procedures

---

the specific needs of women, children and adolescents, older refugees, and particular ethnic or social groups. Unaccompanied children and those with only one parent are at greatest risk, since they lack the protection, physical care, and emotional support provided by the family.[25,26] Safety and well-being is especially difficult in the presence of armed elements among displaced or refugee populations. Furthermore, many IDPs and self-settled refugees are in countries where the government is either indifferent or actively hostile to their assistance and protection needs. In at least 13 countries in recent years, including Myanmar, Sudan, Uganda, and Zimbabwe, state forces or government-backed militia have attacked displaced and other civilian populations.

Landmines

More than 80 countries, located in every region in the world, are affected by landmines or unexploded ordnance or both. Some of the most mine-contaminated countries include Afghanistan, Angola, Burundi, Bosnia and Herzegovina, Cambodia, Chechnya, Colombia, Iraq, Lebanon, Nepal, and Sri Lanka.[27,28] Other countries with landmines, such as Myanmar, India, and Pakistan, provide little public information about the extent of their problem.

Over the past decades, landmine deaths and injuries have totaled in the hundreds of thousands. The precise number of still-buried, undetonated explosive devices is unknown. An estimated 15,000 and 20,000 new landmine-related casualties occur each year, translating into 1,500 new casualties each month, more than 40 new casualties a day, or at least 2 new casualties per hour. Most casualties are civilians, and most live in countries that are now at peace. In Cambodia, for example, over 45,000 landmine injuries were recorded between 1979 and 2005, and some 20,000 people were killed by landmines during this same period. More than 75% of the total casualties were civilians.

Landmines indiscriminately kill or maim civilians, soldiers, peacekeepers, and aid workers alike. Antipersonnel landmines are still being laid today, and together with mines from previous conflicts, claim victims each day in every corner of the globe. The situation has improved in recent years, but a global mine crisis remains and a mine-free world is a long way off.

Environmental and Social Determinants of Public Health

POPULATION GROWTH

Population structures and dynamics have profound potential implications for world health in the 21st century. In the last century the world experienced an unprecedented increase in population, from 1.7 billion in 1900 to almost 6.5 billion in 2000. By the end of the present century, growth projections suggest that world population will be between 8 to 20 billion persons. Urbanization will be accelerated, and international migration may be the most important demographic feature of the 21st century.

In the ensuing decades, aging of the population in America, Japan, China, India, and elsewhere will have dramatic social and economic ramifications on health and health care. Demographic changes worldwide will affect every aspect of the quality of life, including the environment, food, economy, schools, jobs, and health. In all countries there will be a further health transition from first-generation diseases to second- and third-generation diseases. The ability of the world to feed itself will depend not only on food production but also on "population choices in the quality, style, distribution, and pattern of human consumption".[2]

GLOBAL CLIMATE CHANGE AND NATURAL DISASTERS

Global Warming The earth's surface has undergone unprecedented warming over the last century, particularly over the last two decades. Every year since 1992 has been on the current list of the 20 warmest years on record. In its 2001 report, the Intergovernmental Panel on Climate Change (IPCC) stated that "there is new and stronger evidence that most of the warming observed over the last 50 years is attributable to human activities"[29] and that global warming has altered natural patterns of climate.

Carbon dioxide from the burning of fossil fuels and clearing of land has been accumulating in the atmosphere, where it acts like a blanket keeping the earth warm and heating up the surface, oceans, and atmosphere (the greenhouse effect). Current levels of carbon dioxide are higher than at any time during the last 650,000 years. The world's oceans have absorbed about 20 times as much heat as the atmosphere over the past half-century, leading to higher temperatures not only in surface waters but also in water 1,500 feet below the surface. Some observed climatic, physical, and ecological changes include an increase in global average surface temperature of about 0.8°C (1.4°F) in the 20th century, a rise in global average sea level and an increase in ocean water temperatures, and increased rainfall and other precipitation levels in certain regions of the world.[30,31] Scientists predict that continued global warming on the order of 1.4°C to 5.8°C (2.5°–10.4°F) over the next 100 years (as projected in the IPCC's Third Assessment Report) is likely to result in the following:

- A rise in sea level between 3.5 and 34.6 inches (9–88 cm), leading to more coastal erosion, flooding during storms, and permanent inundation
- Severe stress on many forests, wetlands, alpine regions, and other natural ecosystems

- Greater threats to human health as mosquitoes and other disease-carrying insects and rodents spread diseases over larger geographic regions
- Disruption of agriculture in some parts of the world due to increased temperature, water stress, and sea-level rise in low-lying areas such as Bangladesh or the Mississippi River delta.

Natural Disasters Natural disasters have been important sources of human morbidity and mortality throughout history, in every region of the world. Floods, earthquakes, hurricanes, tornadoes, fires, and other disasters wreak havoc on global populations each year. The tsunami that struck 11 countries in South Asia in December 2004 resulted in devastation of staggering proportions: more than 150,000 people dead (especially in Indonesia and Sri Lanka), tens of thousands of people missing, thousands of miles of destroyed coastline, and loss of livelihood for millions of distraught survivors. Although this catastrophe was unusually vast, it was a classic natural disaster in several ways, uncomplicated by war or terrorism. The short-term public health needs of the surviving population were familiar (albeit massive): water, sanitation, food, shelter, and appropriate medical care administered to persons remaining in place and the thousands who were living in self-settled displaced communities.[32]

In addition to the instantaneous devastation, in many natural disasters the number of casualties may increase by as much as twofold as a result of the spread of communicable diseases in the crowded communities that are often created in the aftermath. The public health model for natural disasters highlights a cycle of preparedness, mitigation, response, and recovery. Short-term interventions after large-scale natural disasters include supplying the recommended 20 liters of water per person per day and ensuring that there are adequate, culturally appropriate sanitation facilities to prevent outbreaks of cholera, dysentery, and hepatitis A; targeted measles vaccination in unvaccinated populations, with vitamin A supplementation when indicated; control of vector-borne illnesses such as malaria and dengue through early treatment and mosquito-control measures; early diagnosis and treatment of acute respiratory and gastrointestinal infections, particularly among infants and young children; delivery of adequate amounts of culturally appropriate emergency food rations; counseling for survivors experiencing grief, loss, and guilt; and epidemic surveillance to detect the early appearance of communicable diseases. The longer-term recovery and rehabilitation needs in disaster-affected areas are less understood than the short-term needs, but are typically strategic rather than logistic in nature and involve a transition from emergency relief activities to sustainable reconstruction and development activities.

ENVIRONMENTAL POLLUTION

Indoor Air Pollution More than 3 billion people worldwide continue to depend on solid fuels, including biomass fuels (wood, dung, straw, and agricultural residues) and coal, for their energy needs. Cooking and heating with solid fuels on open fires or traditional stoves results in high levels of indoor air pollution. Indoor smoke contains a range of health-damaging pollutants, such as small particles, carbon monoxide, nitrous oxides, sulfur oxides (especially from coal), formaldehyde, and carcinogens (such as benzo[a]pyrene and benzene). Particulate pollution levels may be 20 times higher than accepted guideline values. There is consistent evidence that exposure to indoor air pollution can lead to acute lower respiratory infections (ALRIs) in children younger than 5, particularly pneumonia (ALRIs represent the single most important cause of death in children younger than 5 years and account for at least 2 million deaths annually in this age group), and to chronic obstructive pulmonary disease and lung cancer (where coal is used) in adults.

According to *The World Health Report 2005*, indoor air pollution is responsible for 1.6 million deaths, mostly of women and children, in developing countries, and is estimated to cause 3.1% of the overall burden of disease in developing countries and 2.7% globally (Figure 1-6).[33] In most societies, it is women who

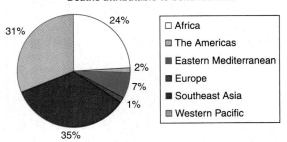

Deaths attributable to solid fuel use

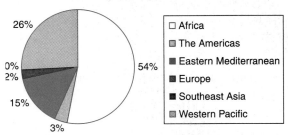

DALYs attributable to solid fuel use

Figure 1-6. Deaths and disability adjusted life years (DALYs) attributable to solid fuel use. From (Reproduced with permission.)

cook and spend time near the fire, and in developing countries they are typically exposed to these very high levels of indoor air pollution for between 3 and 7 hours per day over many years. Young children are often carried on their mother's back during cooking. Consequently, they spend many hours breathing smoke from early infancy. Emerging evidence suggests that indoor air pollution in developing countries may also increase the risk of other important child and adult health problems, including asthma, otitis media and other acute upper respiratory infections, low birth weight and perinatal mortality, tuberculosis, nasopharyngeal and laryngeal cancer, cataracts (blindness), and cardiovascular disease.

Clearly, some of the world's regions rely heavily on solid fuel use at the household level, whereas others have made an almost complete transition to cleaner fuels, such as gas and electricity. For example, more than 75% of the population in India, China, and nearby countries and 50% to 75% of people in parts of South America and Africa continue to cook with solid fuels. These differences in household solid fuel use patterns are reflected in an unequal share of the disease burden due to indoor air pollution, with Africa, Southeast Asia, and the Western Pacific region shouldering the biggest death toll. More than half of the total DALYS lost due to exposure to indoor air pollution occur in Africa, highlighting the urgent need to intervene. WHO has developed a comprehensive Program on Indoor Air Pollution to support developing countries.

Water Pollution An important fraction of the burden of water-related diseases (in particular, water-related vector-borne diseases) is attributable to the way in which water resources are developed and managed. In many parts of the world, the adverse health impacts of dam construction, irrigation development, and flood control include an increased incidence of malaria, Japanese encephalitis, schistosomiasis, lymphatic filariasis, and other diseases. Other health issues indirectly associated with water resource development include nutritional status, exposure to agricultural pesticides and their residues, and accidents/injuries. The WHO's Water, Sanitation and Health Program focuses on drinking water quality, bathing waters, water resources quality, and wastewater use.

Water-related infectious diseases are a major cause of morbidity and mortality worldwide, and newly recognized pathogens and new strains of established pathogens are being discovered that present important additional challenges to both the water and public health sectors. Between 1972 and 1999, 35 new agents of disease were discovered, and many more have reemerged. Among these are several pathogens that may be transmitted through water.

POLITICAL INSTABILITY, REGIONAL CONFLICT, AND GOVERNMENTAL CORRUPTION

Some have suggested that improvement in the health status of populations, particularly those in developing countries, can occur only through sociopolitical change, a global outlook, and local empowerment. International aid agencies and voluntary groups are important partners in this effort. However, lack of national and international political will and geopolitical stability are major barriers in this regard. At all levels, there has been a global failure to address the root causes of poverty, disease, and homelessness. Even though there is widespread recognition of the inextricable link between health and development, global and national efforts to address the challenges of access to and distribution of resources have fallen woefully short.

Effective public health infrastructure depends critically on strong economies. Unfortunately, developing countries around the globe have track records of widespread corruption that siphons billions of dollars from their economies each year, thereby diverting valuable financial assets that could be used for preventive and curative health care services. Various forms of corruption are generally related to nondemocratic political systems and political instability.[34] Protracted civil and regional conflicts lead to the socioeconomic instability of a nation, which invariably affects the health and welfare of its citizens.

BIOLOGIC AND CHEMICAL TERRORISM

For decades, but especially since the attacks of September 11, 2001, the world has been preparing itself for bioterrorism, that is, the deliberate release of viruses, bacteria, or other biologic agents designed to cause illness or death in people, animals, or plants. Biologic agents can be spread through air, water, or food; some potential bioterrorism agents, such as smallpox virus and hemorrhagic fever viruses, can be spread from person to person. These agents are classified into three categories according to their transmissibility and the severity of illness or death they cause (Table 1-7).[35] Category A agents are microorganisms or toxins that pose the highest risk to public health and global security, and category C agents are those that are considered emerging threats.

Category A

- Many are easily spread or transmitted from person to person
- Result in high death rates and have the potential for major public health impact
- Might cause public panic and social disruption
- Require special action for public health preparedness

Table 1-7. Microbial agents with bioterrorism potential.

Category A	Category B (*cont.*)

Bacillus anthracis (anthrax)
Clostridium botulinum (botulism)
Yersinia pestis (plague)
Variola major (smallpox) and other pox viruses
Francisella tularensis (tularemia)
Viral hemorrhagic fever viruses
  Arenaviruses
    LCM, Junin, Machupo, Guanarito, and Lassa fever
      viruses
  Bunyaviruses
  Hantaviruses
    Rift Valley fever virus
  Flaviviruses
    Dengue virus
  Filoviruses
    Ebola virus
    Marburg virus
	Bacteria
	  Diarrheagenic *Escherichia coli,* pathogenic *Vibrio* spp.,
	    Shigella spp., *Salmonella* spp., *Listeria monocyto-*
	    genes, Campylobacter jejuni, Yersinia enterocolitica
	Viruses
	  Caliciviruses, hepatitis A virus
	Protozoa
	  Cryptosporidium parvum, Cyclospora cayetanensis,
	    Giardia lamblia, Entamoeba histolytica, Toxoplasma
	    gondii, microsporidia
	Viral encephalitis viruses
	  West Nile, LaCrosse, California encephalitis, Venezuelan
	    equine encephalitis, Eastern equine encephalitis,
	    Western equine encephalitis, Japanese B encephalitis,
	    and Kyasanur forest viruses

Category B	**Category C**
Burkholderia pseudomallei (melioidosis) *Coxiella burnetii* (Q fever) *Brucella* species (brucellosis) *Burkholderia mallei* (glanders) Ricin toxin (of *Ricinus communis*) Epsilon toxin (of *Clostridium perfringens*) Staphylococcal enterotoxin B *Rickettsia prowazekii* (typhus fever) Food- and waterborne pathogens	Nipah virus and additional hantaviruses Tickborne hemorrhagic fever viruses Crimean-Congo hemorrhagic fever virus Tickborne encephalitis viruses Yellow fever Multidrug-resistant *Mycobacterium tuberculosis* Influenza Other rickettsiae Rabies virus Severe acute respiratory syndrome–associated coronavirus (SARS-CoV)

From National Institute of Allergy and Infectious Diseases (NIAID) Biodefense Research. NIAID category A, B, and C pathogens. http://www3.niaid.nih.gov/biodefense/bandc_priority.htm.

Category B

- Are moderately easy to spread
- Result in moderate illness rates and low death rates
- Require specific enhancements of existing laboratory capacity and enhanced disease monitoring

Category C

- Are easily available
- Are easily produced and spread
- Have the potential for high morbidity and mortality rates and major health impact

Chemical terrorism refers to the intentional release of a hazardous chemical into the environment for the purpose of public harm. Types and categories of potential chemical warfare agents include biotoxins, blister agents/vesicants, blood agents, caustics (acids), choking/lung/pulmonary agents, incapacitating agents, long-acting anticoagulants, metallic poisons, nerve agents, organic solvents, toxic alcohols, and vomiting agents. Protection of the global public heath from biologic and chemical terrorism involves well-orchestrated disaster preparedness including improved education, disease recognition, surveillance, and emergency notification by first responders, clinicians, laboratories, and public health workers.

NUCLEAR THREATS

The possibility of regional or global nuclear conflict looms as an ominous public health threat in the 21st century. Major industrialized countries such as the United States, Russia, England, France, and Germany have had nuclear capabilities for decades, but it is likely that newer nuclear-capable nations such as India, Pakistan, and Israel and nuclear-striving North Korea and Iran pose much greater nuclear risks to world populations.

ECONOMIC DISPARITIES

The world is witnessing huge economic transformations in all countries. Private markets and free trade, although highly efficient, are never equitable, and the 21st century will continue to see both a convergence in the rates of improvement of life expectancies and a divergence in the capacity for income generation between countries, as the rich become richer and the poor get poorer. Finally, global health will be influenced by national debates regarding the inclusion of education and health care in the concept of basic human rights, similar to social, political, and religious rights.

STUDY QUESTIONS

1. Trace the rise and fall of the importance of infectious diseases to global health and enumerate the new infectious threats in the world.

2. How have sanitation, environmental health, and attention to basic necessities such as food and water improved global health, and how are they threatened today?

3. Take one global health challenge from this chapter and expand on its causes, trends, and the corrective action needed, taking into account resources in the developing world.

REFERENCES

1. Centers for Disease Control and Prevention. Ten great public health achievements—United States, 1900–1999. *MMWR* 1999;48:241–243.

2. Chen LC. World population and health. In: Institute of Medicine, ed. *2020 Vision: Health in the 21st Century*. New York: National Academies Press, 1996:16–23.

3. Hinman A. 1889 to 1989: a century of health and disease. *Public Health Rep* 1990;105:374–380.

4. Centers for Disease Control and Prevention. Achievements in public health, 1900–1999: control of infectious diseases. *MMWR* 1999;48:621–629. http://www.cdc.gov/mmwrhtml/mm4829a1.htm.

5. Centers for Disease Control and Prevention. Achievements in public health, 1900–1999: impact of vaccines universally recommended for children—United States, 1990–1998. *MMWR* 1999;48;243–248.

6. Centers for Disease Control and Prevention. Recommended childhood and adolescent immunization schedule—United States, 2006. *MMWR* 2006;54(52):Q1–Q4. http://www.cdc.gov/mmwr/preview/mmwrhtml/mm5451-Immunizationa1.htm.

7. National Center for Infectious Diseases. *Emerging Infectious Diseases: A Strategy for the 21st Century.* Atlanta, GA: US Department of Health and Human Services, 1998.

8. Food and Agriculture Organization of the United Nations. *State of Food Insecurity in the World 2005.* ftp://ftp.fao.org/docrep/fao/008/a0200e/a0200e00.pdf.

9. UNICEF. *State of the World's Children 2005: Childhood Under Threat.* New York: UNICEF, 2004. http://www.uniceforg/sowc05/english/fullreport.html.

10. UNICEF. HIV/AIDS and children. http://www.unicef.org/aids/index_action.html.

11. Lamptey PR, Johnson JL, Khan M. *The Global Challenge of HIV and AIDS.* Washington, DC: Population Reference Bureau, 2006. Population Bulletin 61, no. 1. http://www.prb.org/pdf06/61.1GlobalChallenge_HIVAIDS.pdf.

12. World Health Organization. *Central African Republic.* http://www.who.int/disasters/repo/15100.pdf.

13. UNICEF. Child mortality. May 2006. http://www.childinfo.org/areas/childmortality/.

14. AbouZahr C, Wardlaw T. Maternal mortality at the end of the decade: what signs of progress? *Bull World Health Organ* 2001;79(6):561–573.

15. World Health Organization. *Maternal Mortality in 2000: Estimates Developed by WHO, UNICEF and UNFPA.* Geneva: World Health Organization, 2004.

16. World Health Organization, Regional Office for the Eastern Mediterranean. WHO launches the *World Report on Road Traffic Injury Prevention.* Press Release no. 10. July 12, 2005.

17. Bener A, Crundall D. Road traffic accidents in the United Arab Emirates compared to Western countries. *Adv Transport Studies* 2005;A6:5–12.

18. World Health Organization. Occupational health. http://www.who.int/occupational_health/en/.

19. Centers for Disease Control and Prevention. Achievements in public health, 1900–1999: improvements in workplace safety—United States, 1900–1999. *MMWR* 1999;48:461–469.

20. National Safety Council. *Accident Facts.* Itasca, IL: National Safety Council, 1998.

21. Mackay J, Mensah GA. Global burden of coronary heart disease. In: *The Atlas of Heart Disease and Stroke.* Geneva: World Health Organization and Centers for Disease Control and Prevention, 2004. http://www.who.int/entity/cardiovascular_diseases/en/cvd_atlas_13_coronaryHD.pdf.

22. Mackay J, Mensah GA. *The Atlas of Heart Disease and Stroke.* Geneva: World Health Organization and Centers for Disease Control and Prevention, 2004. http://www.who.int/cardiovascular_diseases/resources/atlas/en/.

23. United Nations High Commissioner for Refugees. *UNHCR Global Appeal 2006.* Geneva: UNHCR. http://www.unhcr.org/cgi-bin/texis/vtx/template?page=publ&src=static/ga2006/ga2006toc.htm.

24. Internal Displacement Monitoring Centre http://www.internal-displacement.org/8025708F004CE90B/(httpPages)/22FB1D4E2B196DAA802570BB005E787C?OpenDocument&count=1000

25. United Nations High Commissioner for Refugees. *Refugee Children.* Report of the Global Consultations on International Protection, 4th meeting, EC/GC/02/9, 25 April 2002, p. 1.

26. Joint United Nations Programme on HIV/AIDS (UNAIDS) and the United Nations High Commissioner for Refugees. *Strategies to Support the HIV-Related Needs of Refugees and Host Populations.* Geneva: UNAIDS, 2005.

27. International Campaign to Ban Landmines. http://www.icbl.org/country.

28. International Campaign to Ban Landmines. *Landmine Monitor Report 2005: Toward a Mine-Free World.* Ottawa, Ontario: Mines Action Canada, 2005. http://www.icbl.org/lm/2005/report.html.

29. Intergovernmental Panel on Climate Change. *Climate Change 2001: IPCC Third Assessment Report.* New York: Cambridge University Press, 2002.

30. U.S. National Aeronautics and Space Administration Goddard Institute for Space Studies. Global temperature trends: 2005 summation. January 2006. http://data.giss.nasa.gov/gistemp/2005.

31. U.S. National Oceanic and Atmospheric Administration National Climate Data Center. *Climate of 2005: Annual Report.* http://www.ncdc.noaa.gov/oa/climate/research/2005/ann/global.html.

32. VanRooyen M, Leaning J. After the tsunami—facing the public health challenges. *N Engl J Med* 2005;352:435–438.

33. World Health Organization. Indoor air pollution and health. Fact Sheet no. 292. June 2005. http://www.who.int/mediacentre/factsheets/fs292/en/.

34. Transparency International. http://www.transparency.org/. Accessed faqs on corruption www.transparency.org/news_room/ faq/corruption_faq

35. National Institute of Allergy and Infectious Diseases (NIAID) Biodefense Research. NIAID category A, B, and C pathogens.http://www3.niaid.nihgov/biodefense/bandc_priority.htm.

The Global Burden of Disease

2

Thuy D. Bui and William H. Markle

LEARNING OBJECTIVES

- *Understand why it is important to measure health and disease*
- *Understand the attributes of mortality, morbidity, and disability as they apply to burden of disease*
- *Become familiar with various composite measures of burden of disease, their relative strengths and weaknesses, and how they are used in public health literature, World Health Organization (WHO) reports, and the lay press*
- *Understand how data on global health measures affect policy change and development and their limitations*
- *Apply the global burden of disease study to understanding poverty and global health inequalities*

RATIONALE FOR COMPOSITE INDICATORS

Measuring the impact of diseases on populations is a prerequisite for determining effective ways to reduce the burden of illness. Traditional methods of quantifying disease in populations, such as incidence, prevalence, mortality, birth rate, and infant mortality rate, do not capture nonfatal health outcomes. In the past three decades, significant international effort has been put into the development of composite indicators that include both mortality and morbidity measures in order to make judgments about the health of populations and to identify which interventions would have the greatest effect.

The growth of aging populations and the increase of associated chronic diseases, particularly in the more developed regions, have partially provided an impetus to examine nonfatal health outcomes and the associated quality of life. Disability and suffering are difficult to quantify because they involve complex, subjective notions of pain, discomfort, and emotional distress that are interpreted within a social and cultural context. Prior work on health-related quality of life measures, measures of utility or preference-weighted time, and the 1980 World Health Organization's International Classification of Impairment, Disability and Handicaps provided some of the framework for the development of morbidity measures that would be incorporated into summary measures of population health. This framework recognized four dimensions:

1. Diseases
2. Impairments of functional abilities (loss or abnormality of psychological, physiological, or anatomical structure or function)
3. Disabilities (restriction or lack of ability to perform an activity of daily living)
4. Handicaps or limitation in social participation (social disadvantage resulting from an impairment or disability)

The benefits of having a common currency to measure the magnitude of health problems include the following abilities:

- Comparing the health of populations
- Monitoring trends over time
- Conducting cost-effectiveness analyses
- Measuring the population-wide benefits of health interventions

Implicit in the applications of these measures are the ability to assess global health inequalities; to inform debates on priorities for health service delivery and for planning, research, and development in the health sector; and to improve public health curricula and training.[1]

Capturing timely accurate data is a particular concern, especially in resource-poor settings. Mortality information is probably the most widely available kind of health information, obtained through death certificates and registries, but even this type of data is found to be incomplete and unreliable. An adult who presents with fever, diarrhea, and hypotension to a district hospital and dies before any definitive diagnostic testing, may have died from malaria, dysentery, sepsis, and/or AIDS. Data about morbidity presented in the literature are often based on self-perceived or observed assessments, household surveys, and interview information. As this chapter examines the methods used to assess the global burden of disease, keep in mind that all measures of population health involve choices and value judgments in both their construction and their application.[2]

HEALTH EXPECTANCIES AND HEALTH GAPS

There are two types of composite measures—health gaps and health expectancies. Figure 2-1 illustrates a typical survivorship curve for a hypothetical population.[1] The area under the middle curve (black dashed line) is divided into two components: H, which represents health expectancy (time lived in full health), and D, which represents time lived at each age in some defined level of disability. Life expectancy at birth [the middle curve (black dashed line)] is simply H + D. The top curve (blue unbroken line) signifies an ideal goal of full health until death for the population. The area G between the middle curve (life expectancy) and the top curve is equivalent to premature mortality. A health gap is then area G and some function of area D. How you define area D (disability weights) is a major issue wrestled with by the various composite measures. This chapter touches on disability-free life expectancy (DFLE) and health-adjusted life expectancy (HALE) as examples of health expectancy measures and focuses on

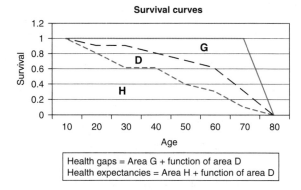

Figure 2-1. Health expectancy, health gap, and survivorship curves for a hypothetical population. From Murray CJL, Salomon J, Mathers CD, Lopez AD, eds. *Summary Measures of Population Health.* Geneva: World Health Organization, 1999. (Adapted with permission.)

disability-adjusted life years (DALYs) and healthy life years (HeaLYs) as examples of health gap measures.

SIX COMPOSITE INDICATORS FOR BURDEN OF DISEASE ASSESSMENT

Health Expectancies

POTENTIAL YEARS OF LIFE LOST

Potential years of life lost (PYLL) is a simple summary measure of premature mortality defined as the total number of years lost through the failure of individuals to live their expected number of years. The advantage of PYLL over crude mortality rates is that the crude mortality rate is weighted by the large number of deaths occurring in older people. PYLL allows decision makers and others to selectively evaluate leading causes of mortality in younger age groups. For example, if we define premature death as death before age 65, a person dying at age 52 from heart disease would represent 13 PYLL. The major limitation of the PYLL approach is that it does not count death at or above the potential (age 65 or 75 years) and hence cannot measure the benefits of health interventions in this age group. Moreover, morbidity and disability are not considered in this indicator. The US Centers for Disease Control and Prevention (CDC) has published tables of years of potential life lost (YPLL, which is the same as PYLL) before age 75 years by race and ethnicity, by leading causes, by risk factors such as tobacco or alcohol abuse, and by specific disease.

Example: Alcohol-Attributable Deaths In 2001, the CDC estimated 2.3 million YPLLs in the United States related to excessive alcohol consumption, making alcohol the third leading preventable cause of deaths in the country.[3] Alcoholic liver disease is the leading *chronic* cause of alcohol-attributable deaths (AAD), and motor vehicle crashes are the leading *acute* cause of AAD. Seventy-four percent of the total YPLLs were among males, and 12% among persons younger than 21 years. As a risk factor, alcohol resulted in relatively more years of life lost compared with tobacco because alcohol-attributable deaths, particularly those caused by injuries, primarily affect youth and young adults. Globally, alcohol consumption has increased in recent decades, with most of that increase in developing countries.

DAYS OF HEALTHY LIFE LOST

The concept of days of healthy life lost (DHLL) was developed by the Ghana Health Assessment Project Team in 1981. This measure partitions the total days of healthy life lost of a person into those lost due to premature death and those lost due to permanent and temporary disability before death. Obviously, the data requirements of the DHLL (estimation of incidence, case fatality, case disability, average age of onset and duration, and the local expectation of life for various disease categories) are high and are not readily available from routinely collected health data. Assessing disability severity requires community and expert-based consensus in a participatory process. Different assumptions will result in differential effects on the data results. This is still considered a landmark study in the creation of composite measures of disease burden.

QUALITY-ADJUSTED LIFE YEAR

Quality-adjusted life year (QALY) is a measure of the value of health outcomes that incorporates both lives saved and patients' valuations of quality of life in alternative health states into a single index number. The QALY calculation is derived from the change in utility value (individual preference for different nonfatal health outcomes) induced by the treatment multiplied by the duration of the treatment effect to provide the number of QALYs gained. QALYs can then be incorporated with medical costs to arrive at a final common denominator of cost/QALY, or the cost-utility analysis. This parameter can be used to compare the cost-effectiveness of any treatment. A year of perfect health is considered equal to 1.0 QALY. The value of a year of ill health is discounted. For example, a year bedridden might have a value equal to 0.5 QALY. Extending someone's life for a year at one-half full health is equal to 0.5 QALY, which is also equal to extending two people's lives by a year at one-fourth full health! An improvement in health from 0.4 to 0.6 QALY is numerically equivalent to an improvement from 0.7 to 0.9.

To compute the average QALYs attained by an individual with a certain disease or illness, cross-sectional surveys using health-related quality of life instruments can be used along with stationary population actuarial techniques. For example, a woman who is healthy in her first 60 years of life with a health-related quality of life (HRQL) valued at 0.95 experiences severe pneumonia with complications that decreases her HRQL to 0.7 until her death at age 62. Although she lives to age 62, she only attains 58 QALYs in her life path: $(0.95 \times 60) + (0.7 \times 2)$.

There are many formulations for calculating QALYs. QALYs are linked to a particular health status measuring instrument and depend on the reliability and validity of that instrument. The vast research on QALY confirms inconsistencies in values derived for similar or equivalent health states or illnesses due to variations in individual perception, group experience, scaling properties, and the differential sensitivity and reliability of the measures. QALY does not really indicate the comparative burden of various conditions and diseases.

Health-related quality of life (HRQL) utility measures apply the time trade-off method to assess preferences to create QALYs. This requires the respondents to value health states by making explicit what they would be willing to sacrifice in terms of time or risk of death in order to return to better or perfect health. The Health Utility Index (HUI), the EuroQoL EQ-5D, the World Health Organization Quality of Life (WHOQoL), and the SF-36 include key domains such as physical, psychological and social role function, health perceptions, and symptoms (Table 2-1). Respondents are asked to indicate their level of health on a scale for each question. Weights are then used to score the responses to the various domains.

Example: The Cost-Effectiveness of Combination Antiretroviral Therapy for HIV Disease in the United States According to Freedberg and associates, life expectancy adjusted for the quality of life increased from 1.53 for untreated patients to 2.91 years for those receiving the three-drug cocktail for AIDS in the United States. The drugs increased average total per-person lifetime medical costs from $45,000 to $77,000 (including health care costs due to longer life), which worked out to a cost of $23,000 per quality-adjusted year of life gained as compared with no therapy—slightly less (or more cost-effective) than thrombolytic therapy in suspected myocardial infarction.[4] We will look at the cost-effectiveness of HIV/AIDS interventions in Africa later.

Example: The Cost-Effectiveness of Treating Hepatitis C Infection Six and 12 months of interferon-alpha treatment gained 0.25 QALYs at an incremental cost of $1,000 and 0.37 QALYs at an incremental cost of $1,900, respectively.[5] Thus, although 6 months of interferon-alpha therapy was less efficacious than 12 months of therapy, it was more cost-effective ($4,000 per QALY gained compared with $5,000 per QALY gained). Nonetheless, in patients younger than 60, both 6 and

Table 2-1. Key domains of utility measures.

HUI	SF-36	EuroQol EQ-5D	WHOQoL
Vision	Physical function (PF)	Mobility	Physical health
Hearing	Role—physical (RP)	Self-care	Psychological
Speech	Bodily pain (BP)	Usual activities	Level of independence
Ambulation	General health (GH)	Pain/discomfort	Social relations
Dexterity	Vitality (VT)	Anxiety/depression	Environment
Emotion	Social function (SF)		Spirituality/religion/personal beliefs
Cognition	Role—emotional (RE)		
Pain	Mental health (MH)		

HUI, Health Utility Index; WHOQoL, World Health Organization Quality of Life project.

12 months of therapy compared favorably with other established medical interventions, such as screening mammography and cholesterol reduction programs. Important variables affecting the cost-effectiveness of interferon-alpha treatment included the cost and efficacy of interferon-alpha, the cost of treatment for decompensated cirrhosis, and the quality of life in patients with chronic hepatitis C—areas where additional data are needed.

HEALTH EXPECTANCIES

The health expectancy measure combines information on length of life and quality of life. It estimates the number of years the average person of a given age can expect to live in a certain state of health. Health expectancies can be categorized into two main classes:

- Those that use dichotomous health state weights, such as disability-free life expectancy (DFLE), which uses a weight of 1 for states of health with no disability and a weight of 0 for states of health with any level of disability above the threshold
- Those that use health state valuations for an exhaustive set of health states—polychotomous or continuous weights, such as disability-adjusted life expectancy

(DALE), known better as health-adjusted life expectancy (HALE)

Various methods exist for calculating health expectancies. The Sullivan method is the only one for which data are widely available. It requires only a population life table (Table 2-2), which can be constructed for a population using the observed mortality rates at each age for a given time period and prevalence data for each type of disability at each age and the weight assigned to each type of disability. Such prevalence rates can be obtained readily from cross-sectional health or disability surveys carried out for a population at a point in time. The appendix to this chapter provides a more detailed explanation of the Sullivan method to calculate DFLE. The Sullivan method is criticized for not producing a pure period indicator. The prevalence rates are partly dependent on earlier health conditions of each age cohort; therefore, it is not capable of detecting sudden changes in population health.

Health expectancies can also be calculated using multistate life tables so that they can be based only on currently measured mortality, incidence, and remission and not on prevalence. The International Network on Health

Table 2-2. Abridged life table for the total population: United States, 2002.

Age	Probability of dying between ages x and $(x+n)$ $_nq_x$	Number surviving to age x l_x	Number dying between ages x and $(x+n)$ $_nd_x$	Person-years lived between ages x and $(x+n)$ $_nL_x$	Total number of person-years lived above age x T_x	Expectation of life at age x e_x
0–1	0.006971	100,000	697	99,389	7,725,787	77.3
1–5	0.001238	99,303	123	396,921	7,626,399	76.8
5–10	0.000759	99,180	75	495,706	7,229,477	72.9
10–15	0.000980	99,105	97	495,311	6,733,771	67.9
15–20	0.003386	99,008	335	494,345	6,238,460	63.0
20–25	0.004747	98,672	468	492,189	5,744,116	58.2
25–30	0.004722	98,204	464	489,871	5,251,927	53.5
30–35	0.005572	97,740	545	487,395	4,762,056	48.7
35–40	0.007996	97,196	777	484,164	4,274,661	44.0
40–45	0.012066	96,419	1,163	479,362	3,790,497	39.3
45–50	0.017765	95,255	1,692	472,292	3,311,135	34.8
50–55	0.025380	93,563	2,375	462,186	2,838,843	30.3
55–60	0.038135	91,188	3,478	447,838	2,376,658	26.1
60–65	0.058187	87,711	5,104	426,603	1,928,820	22.0
65–70	0.088029	82,607	7,272	395,866	1,502,217	18.2
70–75	0.133076	75,335	10,025	352,791	1,106,350	14.7
75–80	0.201067	65,310	13,132	294,954	753,560	11.5

$_nq_x$ is the probability, at age x, of dying in the interval x to $(x+n)$, computed from $2mn/(2+mn)$; m is the age-specific death rate/1,000, and n = interval width.
l_x is the number alive at the beginning of the interval (applied to a hypothetical group of 100,000 newborns).
$_nd_x$ is the number dying between age x and $(x+n) = {}_nq_x \times l_x$.
$_nL_x$ is the total person-years lived in each age interval $(T_x - T_{x+n})$, which is roughly $n(l - d/2)$ for all age groups except the first and the last.
T_x is the total years remaining at each age, obtained by cumulating the L column backward, from bottom to top.
e_x is the average expectation of life = T/l.
From Arias E. *United States Life Tables, 2002.* Hyattsville, MD: National Center for Health Statistics, 2004. National Vital Statistics Reports 53, no. 6.

Expectancies (REVES/Reseau Esperance de Vie en Sante) has developed and promoted the concept and methods of health expectancies, which have been adopted by the European Union (EU) member states to monitor trends in health across the EU.

The World Health Report first provided HALE indicators for WHO member states in 2000. Global life expectancy at birth in 2000 was 65 years, which represented an increase of almost 6 years over the past two decades. Global HALE at birth in 2000 was 56 years. Figure 2-2 features estimates of the healthy life expectancy at birth of selected countries for 2002. The WHO undertook a multicountry survey study (MCSS) in 2000–2001 using a new health status instrument based on the International Classification of Functioning, Disability and Health, which seeks information from a representative sample of respondents on their current states of health according to seven core domains. To overcome the problem of comparability of self-reported health data, the WHO survey instrument used performance tests and vignettes to calibrate self-reported health in each of the core domains. The measurement of time spent in poor health is derived from estimates of severity-adjusted prevalences for health conditions by age and sex from the Global Burden of Disease 2000 study and the surveys from the MCSS with adjustments for dependent comorbidity.

Of note, there is considerable lack of consistency in the use of terminology in disability surveys and lack of standardization in health state descriptions. North American countries have used the term *functional limitation* for disability, and *disability* for handicap or participation restriction. An international agreement for a standardized disability survey instrument would provide a consistent definition and measure of health status. The World Health Survey, undertaken by the WHO since 2003, utilizes a health status instrument that incorporates severity levels and is cross-culturally valid. Its results will contribute to future analysis of healthy life expectancy.[6]

Although there are still relatively few countries for which the measure can be compared, HALE is considered a reasonable candidate for a single summary measure of population health because its severity-weighted disability measure is less subject to the problems of self-report or threshold definition and because it is comprehensible and intuitive. However, it is difficult to relate health expectancies back to disease and risk factor causes because all disease and injury contributes to the risk of death or disability at each age, and the health expectancy is a weighted sum of these risks across all ages in a population life table. Moreover, the gains in health expectancies for specific disease elimination or prevention are not additive. Elimination of two or more diseases simultaneously results in a larger gain in health expectancies than the sum of the gains from elimination of each disease on its own. Health expectancies are quite inelastic to disease elimination in low-mortality countries. The complete elimination of cancer in Australia would result in an additional 2.1 healthy years of life for Australian females, which is less than a 3% increase on the current value of 75 years for HALE at birth.[7]

There is a linear correlation across countries between life expectancy at birth (LE) and HALE, suggesting the effect of compression of morbidity when moving from low to high life expectancy as all the years gained are healthy years. Comparable longitudinal cross-population data for specific populations will confirm whether compression of morbidity is occurring in low-mortality populations. Some researchers have questioned whether, given the fact that the infant mortality rate (IMR) correlates well with HALE and LE, it is best to focus on improving mortality data such as the IMR, which is less difficult to collect in many developing countries.[8] As a counterargument, Mathers cited the example of female life expectancies in India and Zimbabwe. Both countries had infant mortality rates close to 63 per 1,000 in 2000, but the life expectancy at birth in Zimbabwe was 46.0 and in India 62.7 years, reflecting the devastating impact of the AIDS epidemic in Zimbabwe.[9]

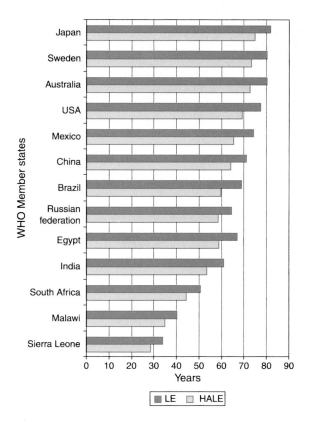

Figure 2-2. Healthy life expectancy at birth, 2002, for selected WHO member states.

Health Gaps

DISABILITY-ADJUSTED LIFE YEARS

Disability-adjusted life years (DALYs) have been used to estimate the global burden of disease by the World Bank and WHO to determine global priorities for health policy and research. In 1992, the World Bank, WHO, and the Harvard School of Public Health under the leadership of Murray and Lopez initiated the Global Burden of Disease (GBD) study to provide detailed estimates of death and disability for eight global regions, by sex and age, for over 100 conditions and 10 risk factors. DALY belongs to the second group of composite indicators, called health gaps, and involves estimates of health-related quality of life attached to specific diseases, rather than to health states (as in QALY). DALYs for a disease or health condition are calculated as the sum of the *years of life lost* (YLL) due to premature mortality for each disease and the *years lost to disability* (YLD) based on the incidence of cases of the health condition. DALY = YLL + YLD. YLL = N × L, where N is the number of deaths, and L is standard life expectancy at age of death in years. YLD = I × DW × L, where I is the number of incident cases, DW is disability weight, and L is the average duration of the case until remission or death in years.

The age-specific and sex-specific prevalence for each of the 483 diagnoses was estimated for the year 1990 using the best available data, or expert opinion if data were lacking. Data were tabulated for eight country groups defined by the World Bank as being demographically and economically similar (established market economies, former socialist economies of Europe, sub-Saharan Africa, Latin America and the Caribbean, Middle Eastern crescent, China, India, and other Asia and islands). All diseases and health outcomes were categorized into the following three groups:

I. Communicable, maternal, perinatal, and nutritional

II. Noncommunicable

III. Accidents and injuries

In the original study, severity scores for disability or disability preference weights for 22 sample diagnoses or indicator conditions were determined by an international panel of health professionals. An iterative "person trade-off" approach was used—participants chose whether it was more desirable to treat a given number of people with one condition than to treat a given number with another condition. For example, informants were asked whether they would prefer to purchase an intervention that provided 1 year of health for 1,000 fully healthy people or for 2,000 people with paraplegia. After each round of scoring for each condition, the policy consequences of the ratings were fed back to inform changes in scores made for the next round. Scores for the remainder of the 483 diagnoses were estimated by comparison and extrapolation with these 22 sample diagnoses, also by an expert panel. Diagnoses were then divided into seven classes of disability according to their scores. Weights of 1 are equated with full disability or death, and 0 with no disability or full health on the DALY scale (Table 2-3). These disability weights are thought to be equal or universal across countries and cultures.

DALY architects made two additional adjustments. The first of these is an age weighting that gives greater value to years lived in young adulthood and less to years lived at the beginning and end of life. The value of a healthy person's life peaks around age 25 by this calculation. The final adjustment to the DALY formula is to discount time in the future at a rate of 3%. The idea is that a future benefit is worth less than one you get now. A treatment that extends a person's lifespan from 65 to 75 is more cost-effective if provided to a 65-year-old than to a 50-year-old who sees no benefit

Table 2-3. Ten sample health conditions and their disability weights from the original Global Burden of Disease (GBD) study.

Health condition	Rank order GBD study	Average severity weights
Quadriplegia	1	0.895
Dementia	2	0.762
Severe migraines	3	0.738
Active psychosis	4	0.722
Paraplegia	5	0.671
Blindness	6	0.624
Major depression	7	0.619
Down syndrome without cardiac malformation	8	0.407
Recto-vaginal fistula	9	0.373
Mild mental retardation	10	0.361
Total deafness	11	0.333
Below the knee amputation	12	0.281

From Table 1.3 of the Global Burden of Disease study. Murray CJ, Lopez AD, (eds). The Global Burden of Disease. Geneva: WHO, 1996.

for another 15 years. With nonuniform age weights and 3% discounting, a death in infancy corresponds to 33 DALYs, and death at ages 5 to 20 to around 36 DALYs.[10] It is important to keep in mind that DALY measures are designed to look at whole populations; in order to measure a burden, a society must make value choices.

DALYs are different from QALYs in their population perspective. From the work of the Global Burden of Disease study, DALYs allow global comparisons of major diseases and risk factors. DALYs are additive in the sense that they can be additively decomposed with respect to causes and are a more sensitive measure of changes in burden. However, disability states in DALYs do not take account of comorbid conditions. There is no way to capture the burden of diabetes, hypertension, and coronary artery disease within the same individual. DALYs take 82.5 years for women and 80 years for men as their standard life expectancy at birth, based on the average life expectancy of Japanese people, who presently have the longest overall life expectancy in the world. This will lead to overestimation of years of life lost in high-mortality countries. Through these assumptions about social value of people at different ages and uniform life expectancy in all different countries, Murray and Lopez tried to uphold a moral and political notion of equity and comparability for this population health measure.

Tables 2-4a and 2-4b show that as you move from a less developed country to the more developed ones, group I and group III causes of death and DALYs tend to decrease in importance, whereas group II causes tend to increase. However, group II causes are already of significant importance in most countries. The importance of neuropsychiatric causes of DALYs is obvious.

HEALTHY LIFE YEAR

DALYs provide a better measurement of the health burden associated with specific causes than do health expectancies and are additive across disease categories. Moreover, DALYs are a more sensitive indicator of changes in burden through disease elimination than gains in health expectancies. Healthy life years (HeaLYs), the newest population health indicator, also measures the gap between the current situation in a country with that of a certain ideal in which people live into old age free of disease and without disability. It is an evolution of the seminal work on days of life lost by the Ghana Health Assessment Team two decades ago. HeaLYs offer health ministries in developing countries a simplified way to estimate a summary measure of health using the same data requirements as for DALYs. More important, the measure focuses on the pathogenesis and natural history of diseases to assess morbidity, mortality, and health interventions (Figure 2-3).

The HeaLY approach has unlinked some value choices—age weighting and discounting—from the calculations; however, the extent of disability is based on the disability severity scale developed by expert opinion and a group consensus process by the Ghana Health Assessment team. Life lived at any age is valued equally, and the expectation of life lost due to mortality and the duration of disability is discounted at a rate of 3% per annum. Discounting is done separately rather than being integrated into the formula. Because diseases that afflict the young receive more weight in the DALY formulation than in the HeaLY approach, this leads to a greater loss of DALYs in the young per 1,000 per year. Likewise, the total DALYs are more than total HeaLYs because the HeaLY formulation uses expectation of life from disease

Table 2-4(a). Deaths and death rates of four selected countries by groups I, II, and III.

	Burkina Faso		Indonesia		United States		Canada	
	Deaths	Death rate	Deaths	Death rate	Deaths	Death rate	Deaths	Death rate
All causes	248.9	1979.6	1626.1	748.9	2420.6	831.7	222.4	711.1
Group I: Communicable, maternal, and perinatal	194.3	1538.7	476.7	219.5	148.2	50.9	10.5	33.7
Infectious and parasitic	119.3	942.5	264.8	122.0	64.4	22.1	3.4	10.7
HIV/AIDS	31.9	252.5	1.7	0.8	13.1	4.5	0.5	1.5
Maternal	5.6	44.1	10.4	4.8	0.5	0.2	0.0	0.0
Perinatal	13.7	108.3	73.3	33.7	15.9	5.5	0.9	2.8
Nutritional deficiency	4.6	36.5	21.9	10.1	7.4	2.5	0.5	1.7
Group II: Noncommunicable	40.0	317	985.6	453.9	2119.7	728.3	199.0	636.4
Neoplasms	7.2	56.9	188.1	86.6	558.6	191.9	65.1	208.1
Diabetes	1.3	10.7	46.3	21.3	76.8	26.4	7.2	23.0
Neuropsychiatric	1.5	12.2	35.3	16.3	154.3	53.0	17.0	54.5
Cardiovascular	18.8	148.7	468.7	215.9	922.7	317.0	76.6	245.1
Group III: Injuries	15.6	123.9	163.8	75.4	106.5	52.5	12.8	41.1

Deaths in thousands; death rate is per 100,000 population. Data from the World Health Organization, 2002.

Table 2-4(b). DALYs for four selected countries by causes.

	Burkina Faso		Indonesia		United States		Canada	
	DALYs	**DALY rate**	**DALYs**	**DALY rate**	**DALYs**	**DALY rate**	**DALYs**	**DALY rate**
All causes	8709	68,990	46,385	21,363	41,521	14,266	3693	11,808
Group I: Communicable, maternal, and perinatal	**6881**	**54,506**	**14,372**	**6619**	**2738**	**941**	**183**	**585**
Infectious and parasitic	4083	32,341	7689	3541	1058	364	63	201
HIV/AIDS	953	7552	107	49	380	131	16	50
Maternal	268	2123	865	398	194	67	10	33
Perinatal	520	4118	3029	1395	723	249	40	129
Nutritional deficiency	261	2068	1375	633	438	150	44	140
Group II: Noncommunicable	**1108**	**8780**	**25,959**	**11,955**	**34,747**	**11,939**	**3207**	**10,256**
Neoplasms	83	658	2302	1060	5077	1744	581	1859
Diabetes	18	146	899	414	1280	440	130	417
Neuropsychiatric	311	2465	5827	2684	12,288	4222	1197	3837
Cardiovascular	194	1535	5191	2391	6156	2115	460	1472
Group III: Injuries	**720**	**5704**	**6054**	**2788**	**4036**	**1387**	**302**	**967**

DALYs in thousands; DALY rate is per 100,000 population. Data from the World Health Organization, 2002.

onset in conjunction with the pattern of healthy life lost (disability and fatality) for a particular disease or condition (see Figure 2-3). In addition, the years of life lost component in DALYs is based on mortality in the current year regardless of when the onset of disease occurred. Hence, the true burden of a disease with rising incidence could be underestimated. Table 2-5 offers a comparison of essential features of the various summary measures.

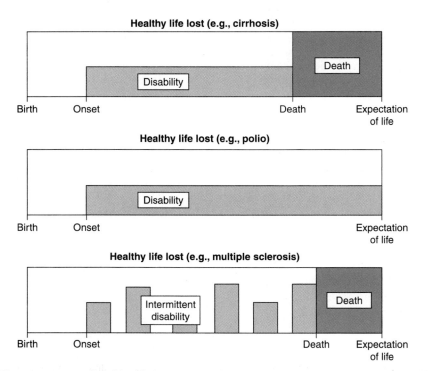

Figure 2-3. Different patterns of healthy life lost. From Hyder AA, Rotlant G, Morrow RH. Measuring the burden of disease: healthy life years. *Am J Public Health* 1998;88:196–202. (Reproduced with permission.)

Example: Burden of Road Traffic Injuries Hyder estimated the burden of road traffic injuries among children and adolescents in urban South Asia and found mortality due to road traffic injuries to be 17 deaths per 100,000 urban persons aged 0 to 19 in South Asia.[11] The burden of disease was calculated to be 16 HeaLYs per 1,000 general population lost from road traffic mortality alone, and 27.7 HeaLYs with disability data added.

Example: Burden of Neonatal Mortality Neonatal mortality, defined as death of an infant during the first 28 days of life, contributes substantially toward under-five and infant mortality. Data on neonatal mortality were gathered from peer-reviewed literature, reports of the Demographic and Health Surveys, and websites of country-based organizations.[12] Lack of valid data is noted for sub-Saharan Africa (SSA), and this study did not evaluate the impact of neonatal morbidity or disability. Sri Lanka has the lowest rates (17 per 1,000 live births). The mean regional neonatal mortality rate for SSA (39 per 1,000 live births) was lower than South Asia's (46 per 1,000 live births) in 1995. However, this represents a loss of roughly 39 HeaLYs per 1,000 population in South Asia and 157 HeaLYs per 1,000 population for SSA from neonatal deaths, reflecting the very high burden relative to the population in SSA (differences in expectation of life at age of onset or death).

ESTIMATION OF ATTRIBUTABLE BURDEN FOR SELECTED CONDITIONS AND RISK FACTORS

One increasing interest in summary measures is their use to identify the relative magnitude of different risk factors. Cause attribution for disease and injuries can be assessed using either categorical attribution or counterfactuals.[13] In categorical attribution, death or the onset of a particular health state can be attributed categorically to one single cause according to a defined set of rules. For example, in WHO's tenth International Classification of Diseases (ICD-10), deaths from tuberculosis in HIV-positive individuals are assigned to HIV. This method becomes more problematic with multicausal events, such as stroke in a person with diabetes and hypertension, or liver cancer resulting from chronic hepatitis C. In counterfactual analysis, the contribution of a disease, injury, or risk factor can be estimated by comparing the current or future burden with the hypothetical level that would prevail if the cause were reduced or eliminated. The Global Burden of Disease 2000 study developed a framework in which the contribution of certain risk factors to the global burden of

Table 2-5. Comparison of summary population health measures.

Features	QALYs	Health expectancies (e.g., HALE)	DALYs	HeaLYs
Organizations	Academia, research, North America and Europe	REVES, EU, OECD, WHO	WHO, World Bank, etc.	WHO, others
Type	Health expectancy	Health expectancy	Health gap	Health gap
Health status instrument	Yes	Yes	No	No
Disability weights	Yes	Generic disability or handicap severity classes	Derived for each health state linked to specific conditions	Yes
Disability measures	Yes	Self-report of disability	Expert consensus and epidemiologic data	Expert consensus and epidemiologic data
Estimating burden	No	Overall health status; hard to relate health expectancy back to disease and risk factors	Yes; more sensitive measure of changes in burden than gains in health expectancies through disease elimination	Yes
Causes additive	No	No	Yes	Yes
Prevalence vs. incidence	Variable	Prevalent disability	Incidence based	Incidence based
Multicausality or comorbidities	Yes	Potential	No	No

QALYs, quality-adjusted life years; HALE, health-adjusted life expectancy; DALYs, disability-adjusted life years; HeaLYs, healthy life years; REVES, Reseau Esperance de Vie en Sante; EU, European Union; OECD, Organization for Economic Cooperation and Development; WHO, World Health Organization.

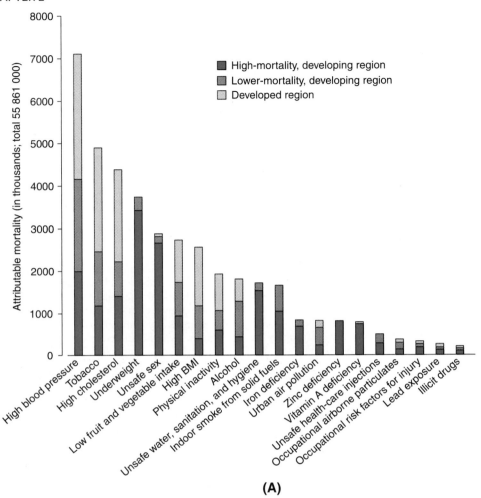

(A)

Figure 2-4A. Mortality (A) and burden of disease (B) due to leading global risk factors. From Ezzati M, et al. Selected major risk factors and global and regional burden of disease. *Lancet* 2002;360:1347–1360. Copyright 2002. (Reproduced with permission from Elsevier.)

disease is based on a counterfactual exposure distribution. This study set up the Comparative Risk Assessment (CRA) project to provide conceptual and methodological consistency in measuring the impacts of various risk factors on population health.

Figure 2-4 presents mortality and burden of disease due to leading global risk factors from the GBD 2000 study. Malnutrition (underweight and micronutrient deficiency) has remained the single leading global cause of health loss. The other top risk factors to attributable DALYs include unsafe sex, high blood pressure, tobacco, alcohol, unsafe water, and poor sanitation and hygiene.[14]

Diabetes is an example of a disease whose total burden includes its directly attributable burden and its role as a risk factor for death and disability from other diseases.

According to *The World Health Report 2003*, diabetes accounted for only 987,000 deaths for the year 2002. Roglic estimated that the total number of deaths attributed to diabetes was 2.9 million in 2000 by incorporating higher risks of cardiovascular disease among diabetic people.[15] Routinely reported death statistics can underestimate mortality from diabetes because individuals with diabetes most often die of ischemic heart disease and renal disease and not from a cause uniquely related to diabetes, such as ketoacidosis or hypoglycemia.

Diseases and injuries are often caused by multiple risk factors. Ezzati and the CRA Collaborating Group analyzed the potential health effects of these risks on healthy life expectancy (HALE) and the benefits of simultaneous reductions in multiple risks.[16] Table 2-6 shows the individual

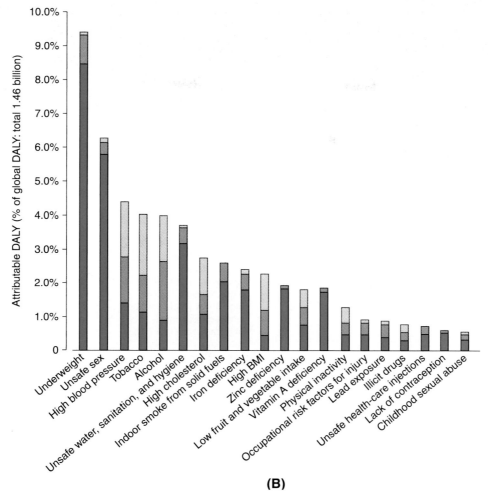

(B)

Figure 2-4B. *(Continued).*

and joint contributions of the selected risk factors for the ten leading diseases in the world. Exposure to these 20 risk factors is responsible for a large proportion of cases of lower respiratory tract infection, diarrhea, lung cancer, ischemic heart disease, and stroke. Removal of these risks would increase global healthy life expectancy by 9.3 years. The current estimates take into account only the primary health benefits of preventive measures, not benefits from the prevention of major diseases. There is obvious uncertainty in these combined risk factor estimates due to complex and multifactor causation effects.

Some critics caution that we should not place too much emphasis on the relative rankings of the different risk factors. The ranking awarded to a risk factor will partially reflect the choice of minimum exposure, such as a zero level of tobacco, below a certain level of physical activity, or some ideal cholesterol level. Quantitative risk assessment is affected by uncertainty in causal relations, degree

of bias in measurement, and magnitude of hazard. The hazard estimates are highly dependent on the quality of the studies that underlie them. Obesity is a good example: its long-term sequelae may be underestimated because the full harm from current exposure may not be completely manifested in current mortality levels.

Example: Burden of Unsafe Water and Poor Sanitation A group of researchers estimated the disease burden from water, sanitation, and hygiene at the global level by taking into account disease outcomes such as infectious diarrhea, schistosomiasis, trachoma, ascariasis, trichuriasis, and hookworm disease using relative risk information obtained mainly from intervention studies.[17] In 2000, they found that the disease burden from diarrheal disease is about 5.7% of total global DALYs, a drop from 6.8% in 1990. The recent decrease in the burden of disease due to poor water and sanitation is due to a decline in mortality associated with global diarrheal disease,

Table 2-6. Individual and joint contributions of 20 selected risks to ten leading diseases, and total burden of disease (expressed in DALYs) in the world.

	%GBD (total 1.46 billion DALY)	%global mortality (total 55.9 million deaths)	Contributing risk factors (individual PAF for disease burden)	Joint PAF[a] (disease burden)	Joint PAF[a] (mortality)
Lower respiratory infections	6.1%	6.8%	Underweight (childhood) (40%); zinc deficiency (16%); indoor smoke from solid fuels (36%); tobacco (2%)[b]	55–62%	40–45%
HIV/AIDS	5.5%	4.6%	Unsafe sex (94%); unsafe health care injections (5%); illicit drugs (3%).	96%	96%
Unipolar depressive disorders	4.5%	0.0%	Alcohol (2%); childhood sexual abuse (6%)	7%	N/A[c]
Diarrheal diseases	4.2%	3.5%	Underweight (childhood) (45%); vitamin A deficiency (18%); zinc deficiency (10%); unsafe water, sanitation, and hygiene (88%)	92–94%	92–94%
Ischemic heart disease	4.0%	12.6%	High blood pressure (49%); high cholesterol (56%); high BMI (21%); low fruit and vegetable intake (31%); physical inactivity (22%); tobacco (12%); alcohol (2%)	83–89%	78–85%
Low birth weight	3.5%	2.5%	Underweight (maternal) (10%); iron deficiency (19%); alcohol (0.2%)	29%	31%
Stroke	3.1%	9.6%	High blood pressure (62%); high cholesterol (18%); high BMI (13%); low fruit and vegetable intake (11%); physical inactivity (7%); tobacco (12%); alcohol (4%)	70–76%	65–73%
Malaria	2.9%	2.0%	Underweight (childhood) (45%); vitamin A deficiency (16%); zinc deficiency (18%)	56–59%	60–62%
Road traffic accidents	2.6%	2.2%	Alcohol (20%); illicit drugs (2%); occupational risk factors for injuries (6%)	28%	29%
Tuberculosis	2.5%	2.9%	Tobacco (10%)[b]	10%	12%
Communicable, maternal, perinatal, and nutritional conditions	42.0%	32.6%	Multiple risks	49–50%	50–51%
Noncommunicable diseases	45.7%	58.3%	Multiple risks	35–36%	49–52%
Injuries	12.3%	9.1%	Multiple risks	22%	25%
All causes	100%	100%	All 20 selected risks	39–40%	47–49%

PAF, the population-attributable fraction, is defined as the proportional reduction in population disease or mortality that would occur if exposure to the risk factor were reduced to an alternative exposure distribution.

In all regions, the risk factors also contribute to other diseases that are not in the leading ten.

[a]The first number is the PAF for the adjusted scenario, and the second for the unadjusted scenario in cases where adjustment for mediated effects and effect modification applied (see Methods).

[b]Affected by tobacco in the category other respiratory diseases or selected other medical causes. The PAF has large uncertainty.

[c]The number of deaths coded to hearing loss, unipolar depressive disorders, osteoarthritis, and Alzheimer and other dementias is zero or very small in the GBD database, making the mortality PAF for these diseases undefined or unstable.

From Ezzati M, et al. Estimates of global and regional potential health gains from reducing multiple major risk factors. *Lancet* 2003;362:271–380. Copyright 2003. Reprinted with permission from Elsevier.

a result of improved case-management intervention, particularly oral rehydration therapy.

Example: Difficulties in Estimating the Global Burden of Disease for Hepatitis C   The WHO estimates that hepatitis C affects about 180 million people worldwide and 3 to 4 million people annually. High prevalence estimates (in the 10% range) are found in many countries in Africa, Latin America, and Central and Southeastern Asia. The compiled evidence for the burden of hepatitis C relies on many assumptions because the acute disease is usually not recognizable, the incubation period is long, and there are significant regional differences in transmission patterns. Most prevalence data derived from blood donors likely represent underestimation of the true prevalence. On the other hand, the burden of hepatitis C virus (HCV) infection can also be overestimated because of comorbid conditions such as chemical dependency and mental illness that are often present in individuals with HCV.[18] Acknowledging that critical data are lacking to make accurate estimates on a global scale, a working group was created to assist the WHO in estimating the GBD associated with HCV infection in the year 2000. They adopted estimates of 25% for rate of acute hepatitis, 75% for chronic infection, 20% for cirrhosis after 20-plus years of infection, and 1.6% for the annual rate of hepatocellular carcinoma among patients with cirrhosis. However, better estimates of HCV prevalence and better characterization of the morbidity, natural history parameters, and prevalence of HIV infection among injection drug users are all needed to allow precise estimation of DALYs for hepatitis C.[19]

Example: Burden of Unsafe Injection   Unsafe injection practices are still prevalent in many parts of the developing world. Hauri, Armstrong, and Hutin estimated the global burden of disease attributable to contaminated injections given in health care settings in 2000. Their model is based on theoretical cohorts of infected individuals followed for background mortality and disability and infection-associated deaths from acute hepatitis, hepatocellular carcinoma, end state liver disease, and AIDS. They estimated 3.4 injections per person per year, with 39.3% of these injections given with reused equipment. Contaminated injections caused an estimated 21 million hepatitis B virus infections, 2 million HCV infections, and 260,000 HIV infections, for a burden of 9 million DALYs between 2000 and 2030.[20]

CRITICISMS OF SUMMARY MEASURES OF POPULATION HEALTH

Burden of disease studies are data intensive, expensive, and time consuming and place added demand on staff and resources, especially in developing countries. They often rely on extrapolations and expert guesses and therefore lack

validation by locally measured epidemiologic data in regions such as sub-Saharan Africa. Infant mortality rate and life expectancy may suffice as surrogate markers for assessing health in many parts of the world.

Implicit in the DALY calculation is the attempt to capture different social roles and economic productivity at different ages. Applying the DALY principle that implies that a disabled person is valued less than a fully healthy person and that the elderly are less preferable than young adults, a young adult should be higher on a kidney transplant list than a very young or older patient or one with a preexisting condition or disability!

Disability advocates and social scientists have criticized the disability weight of the DALY for not accounting for the importance of social, cultural, and environmental context as a determinant of the severity and impact of those health states. A person with paraplegia in sub-Saharan Africa is compared with one who lives in the United States, for example. The former person may be stigmatized by family and villagers, lack support from the community, and be without any mobility-assistive device. This person would probably have a very poor quality of life, and hence the disability weight associated with paraplegia in this case would be high, close to 1. The person with paraplegia living in a developed country, who has access to rehabilitation and wheelchair or easy access to buildings and public places because of building codes and ordinances, can lead a very independent existence with less perceived disability. It appears likely that a fixed-context disability weight will underestimate the burden of disease in populations that lack social infrastructure and overestimate the burden in well-resourced populations.[21]

The egalitarian principle design of the DALY may inadvertently prevent equitable allocation of resources. Many researchers have argued that allocating resources by aggregate DALY minimization has been shown to be inequitable. Scarce resources should not always be allocated simply to maximize population health. Studies have shown that health care providers and individuals do not favor or apply strict economic analysis when deciding on health care options or interventions.

Williams argues for a reappraisal of the global burden of disease calculations.[22] He favors redirecting the resources devoted to the GBD project into measuring the cost-effectiveness of particular interventions and health technology. According to Williams, the discount rate of 3%, the adoption of 82.5 years as the standard life expectancy, and the age weights introduce too many idiosyncratic elements into the DALY calculations, resulting in older people in richer countries given more weight under certain scenarios. To measure health status, he favors using some simple generic measure of health-related quality of life in any survey of a representative sample of the general population, without the need to compile comprehensive aggregates on a global basis.

WHO PROJECTIONS FOR 2030

Using the most pessimistic assumptions about income growth and advances in health technology, based on the Global Burden of Disease estimates for the year 2002, the WHO projects large declines in mortality between 2002 and 2030 for all of the principal group I (communicable, perinatal, and maternal) causes, with the exception of HIV/AIDS. The burdens attributable to groups II (noncommunicable) and III (injuries) are expected to rise compared with group I conditions over the next 30 years (Figure 2-5). The impact of infectious diseases over the next 20 years will ultimately depend on control of microbial resistance, development of new antibiotics and vaccines, and national and global disease surveillance and response.

The four leading causes of death in 2030 are projected to be ischemic heart disease, stroke, HIV/AIDS, and chronic obstructive pulmonary disease (Table 2-7). Deaths from infectious diseases, maternal and perinatal conditions, and nutritional deficiencies are expected to fall slightly (from 15.5 million in 2002 to 10.2 million in 2030), with the exception of HIV/AIDS. This is due in part to the relative contraction of the world's young population. This phenomenon of increase in life expectancy, aging populations, and changes in the mortality profile to chronic diseases is often referred to as the demographic-epidemiologic transition (see Chapter 11). Cardiovascular disease, diabetes, neuropsychiatric disorders, and cancers have traditionally been associated with rich countries, but according to data from the WHO's *World Health Report 2002*, they are becoming significant problems in poorer regions of the world, reflecting the convergence of morbidity and mortality patterns for developing and developed countries.

The three leading causes of disease burden in 2002—perinatal conditions, lower respiratory infections, and HIV/AIDS—will be replaced in 2030 by HIV/AIDS, depression, and ischemic heart disease (Table 2-8). Chronic obstructive pulmonary disease and perinatal conditions

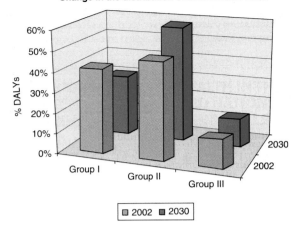

Change in the distribution of DALYs 2002–2030

Figure 2-5. Projections in the burden of group I, II, and III conditions.

follow as leading causes of DALYs. The global DALYs per population rate will actually decrease because the increasing number of deaths is shifted to older ages, associated with fewer lost years of life. Nevertheless, life expectancy at birth is projected to increase in all WHO regions in 2020.

A separate model was used for HIV/AIDS mortality by the Joint United Nations Program on HIV/AIDS (UNAIDS) and WHO. The most likely or baseline scenario estimates that antiretroviral (ARV) coverage will be around 80% by 2012, remaining constant beyond that year, and that there will be no changes to current transmission rates due to increased prevention efforts. Global HIV/AIDS deaths are projected to rise to 6.5 million in 2030 by this model. Figure 2-6 illustrates the death rates for the pessimistic and most optimistic scenarios. ARV coverage results in temporary postponement of deaths

Table 2-7. Causes of death worldwide, 2002–2030.

Rank	Death or injury	% total deaths, 2002	Rank	Death or injury	% total deaths, 2030
1	Ischemic heart disease	12.6	1	Ischemic heart disease	13.1
2	Cerebrovascular disease	0.7	2	Cerebrovascular disease	10.3
3	Lower respiratory infections	6.9	3	HIV/AIDS	8.7
4	HIV/AIDS	4.8	4	COPD	7.9
5	COPD	4.8	5	Lower respiratory infections	3.5
6	Perinatal conditions	4.3	6	Diabetes mellitus	3.1
7	Diarrheal diseases	3.3	7	Lung cancers	3.0
8	Tuberculosis	2.7	8	Road traffic accidents	2.8
9	Lung cancers	2.2	9	Tuberculosis	2.4
10	Road traffic accidents	2.1	10	Perinatal conditions	2.1

HIV/AIDS, human immunodeficiency virus/acquired immunodeficiency syndrome; COPD, chronic obstructive pulmonary disease.
From World Health Organization Statistical Information System. Working paper and summary tables for projections. http://www3.who.int/whosis/menu.cfm?path=evidence,burden,burden_proj,burden_proj_results&language=english.

Table 2-8. Leading causes of DALYs, 2002 and 2030.

2000			Projection 2030		
Rank	**Cause**	**% total**	**Rank**	**Cause**	**% total**
1	Perinatal conditions	6.6	1	HIV/AIDS	10.3
2	Lower respiratory infections	6.3	2	Unipolar major depression	5.3
3	HIV/AIDS	5.7	3	Ischemic heart disease	4.4
4	Unipolar major depression	4.5	4	Chronic obstructive pulmonary disease	3.8
5	Diarrheal diseases	4.3	5	Perinatal conditions	3.8
6	Ischemic heart disease	4.0	6	Cerebrovascular disease	3.7
7	Cerebrovascular disease	3.3	7	Road traffic accidents	3.6
8	Road traffic accidents	2.6	8	Cataract	2.9
9	Malaria	2.3	9	Lower respiratory infections	2.8
10	Tuberculosis	2.3	10	Tuberculosis	2.5

HIV/AIDS, human immunodeficiency virus/acquired immunodeficiency syndrome; COPD, chronic obstructive pulmonary disease.
From World Health Organization Statistical Information System. Working paper and summary tables for projections. http://www3.who.int/whosis/menu.cfm?path=evidence,burden,burden_proj,burden_proj_results&language=english.

until they rise again, reflecting the underlying disease history and trends in incidence rates. Only with the most intense scale-up in treatment and prevention could HIV/AIDS deaths start to decline around 2018.[23]

The GBD study also projects that by 2030, tobacco is expected to kill 10 million people—more people than any single disease, surpassing even the HIV epidemic. Seventy percent of tobacco-attributable deaths will be in developing countries; 2 million deaths are expected in China alone. One-third of all China's young men will eventually be killed by tobacco if current smoking patterns persist.[24] Cardiovascular diseases, lung cancer, and chronic obstructive pulmonary disease are the leading causes of death from smoking globally. A majority of smoking-attributable deaths were among men, with the exception of North America, where women have smoked for several decades and female deaths accounted for 45% of total smoking-attributable deaths. Tobacco consumes a significant percentage of household expenditures, especially in low- and middle-income countries, diverting resources from education, food, and health care. Indeed, the link between tobacco and poverty is often ignored. More than ever, cost-effective tobacco control measures such as advertising controls, price and tax increases, smoke-free area legislation, and other trade regulations are absolutely critical to decrease tobacco consumption worldwide.

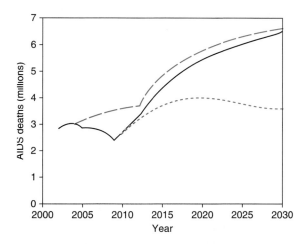

Figure 2-6. Projections of global AIDS deaths (millions) from 2002 to 2030, for three scenarios: baseline (solid lines), optimistic (dotted lines), and pessimistic (dashed lines). From Mathers CD, Loncar D. Updated *Projections of Global Mortality and Burden of Disease, 2002–2030.* World Health Organization, Evidence and Information for Policy Working Paper. October 2005. http://www.who.int/healthinfo/statistics/bodprojectionspaper.pdf. (Reproduced with permission.)

POVERTY AND THE GLOBAL BURDEN OF DISEASE

Low- to middle-income countries account for 85% of the world's population and 92% of the global burden of disease. The Global Forum for Health Research refers to the 10/90 gap to indicate that only 10% of worldwide expenditure on health research and development is devoted to the problems that primarily affect the poorest 90% of the world's population as measured by DALYs or similar indicators.[25] Socioeconomically disadvantaged communities and individuals are often exposed to higher levels of risk factors for poor health than their less disadvantaged counterparts, and they also bear a disproportionately higher health burden. Evaluation of the global patterns of healthy life expectancy in 2002 suggests that people living in poor countries not only face lower life expectancies than those in richer countries but also live a greater proportion of their lives in poor health.[26] Some scholars and public health activists criticize the 10/90 gap concept as misleading because many illnesses in developing countries (such as malaria, pneumonia, and diarrhea) are treatable or preventable with existing medicines or interventions.[27] According to this viewpoint, ineffective governments, poor health care infrastructure, and poverty are responsible for the burden of disease in low- and middle-income countries.

Public health officials have long recognized that human health is the foundation of economic growth and development. In the projections by the GBD study, "diseases of poverty" such as malaria, tuberculosis, and AIDS will still affect developing countries disproportionally more than affluent countries. This will perpetuate the never-ending cycle that starts with poor health status, underdevelopment of the workforce, and lack of economic growth and results in poverty and worsening of overall health status.

Researchers have long been interested in estimating the potential health benefits of eradicating poverty, with the belief that poverty is a major underlying determinant of health. In reality, the association of any specified socioeconomic factor with risk factors for disease or health is likely to be confounded by other variables such as education, age, and ethnicity, by contextual factors related to government and infrastructure development, and by time lags (i.e., the time it takes for income improvement to manifest as change in risk factor exposure).

Example: The Burden of Poverty To quantify the disease burden of socioeconomic position, Blakely, Hales, and Woodward used the "population-attributable risk" to estimate the impact of income poverty amelioration on child malnutrition as a health risk factor in Pakistan.[28] Based on the assumption that the relative risks of disease states are often comparable for different socioeconomic factors, they estimated that 60% of the population lives on US $1 to $2 per day. The counterfactual scenario requires that those people living on less than US $2 per day adopt the risk factor profile of those living on more than US $2 per day. The impact fractions or the population-attributable risk is then 50%. That is, 50% of childhood malnutrition is attributable to poverty by this calculation, reinforcing the importance of income poverty as a determinant of risk factor prevalence (and as a proxy for health). The authors acknowledge that this may be an overestimate. Other studies suggest that both poverty eradication and public health programs targeted at poor communities are required to improve health and to reduce socioeconomic inequalities in health.

GLOBAL HEALTH DISPARITIES

The World Health Organization is interested in measuring health inequalities separately from measuring the average levels of health as indications of a country's performance on health. The achievement of health equalities translates to equality of healthy lifespans and equality of

health risks that involve unavoidable factors and individual choices. Gakidou, Murray, and Frenk propose a framework to study health inequality as the distribution of health expectancy across individuals in the population.[29] Interest in health risk inequality will focus attention on the role of occupational and environmental exposures and on the significant inequality in adult male mortality risk compared with child or adult female mortality risks in many developed countries. A summary measure of health inequality has yet to be formalized at the time of this publication.

The burden of disease in the United States among racial or ethnic minorities mirrors that in developing countries and resembles global inequities in health. In 1996, there were 2.3 million deaths in the United States, which contributed to over 33 million DALYs. Ischemic heart disease was the leading source of DALYs for both men and women. HIV/AIDS and violent injuries were the leading sources of DALYs for black males. HIV/AIDS was the third leading cause among Hispanic men and black women. Perinatal conditions accounted for over 3% of the DALYs among blacks in the United States, much higher than the proportion of DALYs attributed to these conditions in other developed regions.[30]

The World Health Report 2002 drew attention to how much of the world's disease burden is the result of undernutrition among the poor and of overnutrition among those who are better off. According to the report, at the same time that there are 170 million children in poor countries who are underweight, more than 1 billion adults worldwide are overweight, an alarming statistic. In contrast to the long-established killers due to poverty, the killer due to overconsumption—obesity—was thought to be responsible for over 500,000 deaths in North America and western Europe in 2000. Blood pressure, cholesterol, tobacco, alcohol, obesity, and the diseases linked to them are no longer common only in industrialized countries. These are all compelling reasons for governments and health ministries to tackle risk reduction strategies and to place more emphasis on preventing the actual causes of diseases as well as (or more than) treating the diseases themselves.

The poorest and most vulnerable people in the world are still affected by infectious diseases that are largely treatable and preventable. Lower respiratory tract infections, tuberculosis, diarrheal diseases, HIV, and malaria remain leading causes of death and burden of disease in low- and middle-income countries. At the same time, chronic diseases have become much more prominent due to social and economic development and the associated consumption of tobacco, alcohol, and high-sugar, high-fat foods. Such diseases further strain health care resources and infrastructure in these countries, which now have to deal with a double burden of disease. The prospect of a triple burden of disease is also looming with the rising incidence of injuries, particularly from road traffic accidents. Avian influenza and influenza pandemics have the potential to inflict catastrophic mortality and economic costs worldwide, especially in the poorest countries that have limited resources for surveillance coupled with poor health care and health status.

We are at the critical junction in global health at which efforts to reform health systems and to control risk factors will require the commitment and coordination of policy makers, researchers, health ministries, the World Health Organization, the World Bank, private donors, and nongovernmental organizations to improve the health of those who survive beyond childhood around the world. Summary measures of population health such as DALYs and HeaLYs still need to prove their value in affecting health policy changes and resource allocation worldwide, especially in the poorest regions in the world. Such summary measures should also be sensitive to changes in the current health status and to changes in risk factors by particular interventions. Nevertheless, most experts believe in and advocate for better health data and disease surveillance as a first step to improving global health status and reducing health inequalities.

STUDY QUESTIONS

1. Try to obtain the latest mortality rates by age and sex of a developing country. How reliable are the data? What are your sources?

2. In 2000, the CDC reported that approximately 440,000 persons die in the United States of an illness attributable to cigarette smoking, resulting in 5.6 million years of potential life lost, $75 billion in direct medical costs, and $82 billion in lost productivity.[31] How were these estimates derived? What are the limitations of these findings?

3. Scientists have tried to estimate the health impacts of climate change. What type of health outcomes or diseases would be associated with climate change?

4. What are the leading risk factors causing the greatest burden of disease among the 2.4 billion people living in low-mortality developing countries? What are the implications for public policy?

5. How valid are the future projections in the GBD study? The study's authors believe that four factors are responsible for the projected changes: aging of the population, impact of HIV, rise in tobacco-related mortality and disability, and decline in deaths caused by group I conditions. What other major determinants of the total burden of disease would be important to consider?

REFERENCES

1. Murray CJL, Salomon J, Mathers C. A critical examination of summary measures of population health. http://www.whoint/healthinfo/paper02.pdf.

2. Field MJ, Gold M, Institute of Medicine Committee on Summary Measures of Population Health. *Summarizing Population Health: Directions for the Development and Application of Population Metrics.* Washington, DC: National Academy Press,1998.

3. Centers for Disease Control and Prevention. Alcohol-attributable deaths and years of potential life lost—United States, 2001. *MMWR* 2004;53(37):866–870.

4. Freedberg KA, et al. The cost effectiveness of combination antiretroviral therapy for HIV disease. *N Engl J Med* 2001; 344(11):824–831.

5. Kim WR, et al. Cost-effectiveness of 6 and 12 months of interferon-alpha therapy for chronic hepatitis C. *Ann Intern Med* 1997;127(10):866–874.

6. World Health Organization. *World Health Survey.* http://www.who.int/healthinfo/survey/en/index.html.

7. Mathers CD. Alternative methods to measure burden of disease. June 1999. http://www.skyaid.org/Skyaid%20Org/Medical/BurdenOfDiseaseMethods.htm.

8. Reidpath DD, Allotey P. Infant mortality rate as an indicator of population health. *J Epidemiol Community Health* 2003; 57(5):344–346.

9. Mathers CD, Salomon JA, Murray CJ. Infant mortality is not an adequate summary measure of population health. *J Epidemiol Community Health* 2003;57(5):319.

10. World Health Organization. Disability adjusted life years (DALY). http://www.who.int/healthinfo/boddaly/en/index.html.

11. Hyder AA, et al. Estimating the burden of road traffic injuries among children and adolescents in urban South Asia. *Health Policy* 2006;77(2):129–139.

12. Hyder AA, Wali SA, McGuckin J. The burden of disease from neonatal mortality: a review of South Asia and sub-Saharan Africa. *BJOG* 2003;110(10):894–901.

13. Mathers CD, Essati M, Lopez AD, Murray CJL, Rodgers AD. Causal decomposition of summary measures of population's health. In: Murray CJL, Salomon J, Mathers CD, Lopez AD, eds. *Summary Measures of Population Health.* Geneva: World Health Organization, 2002.

14. Ezzati M, et al. Selected major risk factors and global and regional burden of disease. *Lancet* 2002;360(9343):1347–1360.

15. Roglic G, et al. The burden of mortality attributable to diabetes: realistic estimates for the year 2000. *Diabetes Care* 2005; 28(9):2130–2135.

16 Ezzati M, et al. Estimates of global and regional potential health gains from reducing multiple major risk factors. *Lancet* 2003;362(9380):271–280.

17. Pruss A, et al. Estimating the burden of disease from water, sanitation, and hygiene at a global level. *Environ Health Perspect* 2002;110(5):537–542.

18. Ray Kim W. Global epidemiology and burden of hepatitis C. *Microbes Infect* 2002;4(12):1219–1225.

19. The Global Burden of Hepatitis C Working Group. Global burden of disease (GBD) for hepatitis C. *J Clin Pharmacol* 2004;44(1):20–29.

20. Hauri AM, Armstrong GL, Hutin YJ. The global burden of disease attributable to contaminated injections given in health care settings. *Int J STD AIDS* 2004;15(1):7–16.

21. Reidpath DD, et al. Measuring health in a vacuum: examining the disability weight of the DALY. *Health Policy Plan* 2003; 18(4):351–356.

22. Williams A. Calculating the global burden of disease: time for a strategic reappraisal? *Health Econ* 1999;8(1):1–8.

23. Mathers CD, Loncar D. *Updated Projections of Global Mortality and Burden of Disease, 2002–2030.* World Health Organization, Evidence and Information for Policy Working Paper. October 2005; http://www.who.int/healthinfo/statistics/bodprojectionspaper.pdf.

24. Niu SR, et al. Emerging tobacco hazards in China: 2. Early mortality results from a prospective study. *BMJ* 1998; 317(7170): 1423–1424.

25. Global Forum for Health Research. *The 10/90 Report on Health Research 2003–2004.* Geneva: Global Forum for Health Research, 2004. http://www.globalforumhealth.org/Site/002__What%20we%20do/005__Publications/001__10%2090%20reports.php.

26. Mathers CD, et al. Global patterns of healthy life expectancy in the year 2002. *BMC Public Health* 2004;4:66.

27. Stevens P. *Diseases of Poverty and the 10/90 Gap.* London: International Policy Network, 2004. http://www.fightingdiseases.org/pdf/Diseases_of_Poverty_FINAL.pdf.

28. Blakely T, Hales S, Woodward A. *Poverty: Assessing the Distribution of Health Risks by Socioeconomic Position at National and Local Levels.* Geneva: World Health Organization, 2004. http://www.who.int/quantifying_ehimpacts/publications/ebd0.pdf.

29. Gakidou EE, Murray CJ, Frenk J. Defining and measuring health inequality: an approach based on the distribution of health expectancy. *Bull World Health Organ* 2000;78(1):42–54.

30. McKenna MT, et al. Assessing the burden of disease in the United States using disability-adjusted life years. *Am J Prev Med* 2005;28(5):415–423.

31. Centers for Disease Control and Prevention. Cigarette smoking-attributable morbidity—United States, 2000. *MMWR* 2003; 52(35):842–844.

APPENDIX

Table 2A-1. Calculation of health expectancy from age x_i: France, 1991, females, simplified calculation.

Age x_i(1)	I_{x_i}(2)	L_i(3)	$1 - \pi_i$(4)	$(1 - \pi_i)L_i$(5)	Time spent free of disability after age x_i(6)	$DFLE_x$ (7)
0	100,000	496,892	0.990	491,930	7,010,958	70.1
5	99,244	496,003	0.976	483,872	6,519,028	65.7
...	...	...	...	...	...	...
...	...	...	...	...	...	...
...	...	...	...	...	...	...
65	89,367	436,589	0.804	350,877	1,097,520	12.3
70	84,968	408,793	0.714	291,942	746,643	8.8
75	78,012	364,013	0.630	229,175	454,701	5.8
80	66,625	290,533	0.487	141,559	225,526	3.4
85	48,532	289,068	0.710	83,967	83,967	1.7

Researchers are interested in measuring the potential gains in disability-free life expectancy (DFLE) resulting from the elimination of a disease or injury. The Sullivan method is often used to estimate cause-deleted health expectancies using the cause-deleted prevalences in the cause-elimination life tables. The key is to estimate the contribution of specific diseases to the prevalence of disability, assuming independence among causes of death and disability. The method also requires information on the duration or age of onset of the disability.

$$DFLE_k = \frac{1}{I_k} \sum_{i=x}^{w} (1 - \pi_i)\, L_i \quad k = 0, \ldots, w$$

This calculation is reproduced in Table 2A-1.

The different columns of Table 2A-1 are as follows.

- **Column 1:** Ages. Here, $x_i = 0, 5, 10, \ldots, 80, 85$ for $i = 0, 1, 2 \ldots 17$. The different age groups are as follows: [0,5], [5,10], [...], [85 and older].
- **Columns 2 and 3:** I_{x_i} and L_i—respectively, number of survivors at age x_i and number of years lived between age x_i and age $x_i + 1$ by people living at age x_i. The values are taken from an ordinary complete life table calculated with deaths registered during the year of the health survey (here, the French life table for 1991).
- **Column 4:** Nondisabled prevalences (percentage of persons free of disability in the different age groups). These rates derive from a health survey on a sample of the whole population (here, the French health survey of 1991).
- **Column 5:** approximation of the time spent free of disability between $x_i + 1$ and x_i by the I_{x_i} persons. We have calculated the products between figures of column 3 and those of column 4.
- **Column 6:** Approximation of the time spent free of disability after age x_i. It is the sum of values of column 5 from x_i to the end of the column.
- **Column 7:** Expectancy of time to be spent free of disability. It is the result of the division of column 6 by column 2.

Adapted from Hauet E. *Practical Guide on Health Expectancy Calculation: Sullivan Calculation.* June 1996. http://sauvy.ined.fr/euroreves/methods/cookdef/cookdef.html.

Epidemiology, Biostatistics, and Surveillance

3

Christopher Martin

LEARNING OBJECTIVES

- To understand the important contributions of chance, bias, and confounding as potential sources of false epidemiologic associations
- To understand the measures of morbidity and mortality as they are used in the global setting
- To be able to describe the various types of epidemiologic study designs and the measures of association they provide
- To understand how to interpret tests and how they apply to global health

THE EPIDEMIOLOGIC APPROACH

Epidemiology is concerned with the identification, measurement, and analysis of factors that may be associated with differences in the health status of populations. The goal of such investigations is to modify these factors to improve the health status of individuals. Accordingly, some familiarity with epidemiologic methods is essential to the understanding of public and global health. The approach is illustrated by the epidemiologic triad as applied to malaria (Figure 3-1).

According to this model, disease arises through interactions between a host, environment, and agent. In the case of many infectious diseases, a vector through which the agent is transmitted is also relevant. This model allows opportunities for the interruption of disease transmission to be clarified. For example, in the case of malaria, opportunities might include the use of insecticide-treated bednets for the host, reduced areas of standing water in the environment, destruction of the *Anopheles* mosquito

vector through pesticides, and chemoprophylaxis targeted at the plasmodium.

Although the distinction between epidemiology and biostatistics is not always apparent, biostatistics has a relatively greater emphasis on data gathering and analysis. Accordingly, this field provides a variety of measures used to quantify both disease outcomes (morbidity) and death (mortality). Further, biostatistics offers methods to examine the relationships between variables, especially whether such relationships could have arisen purely as a result of chance, a procedure known as *statistical inference*.

Chance, Bias, and Confounding

It is important to appreciate the distinction between an association and a causal relationship. An *association* refers to a relationship in which a change in the frequency of one variable is associated with a change in the frequency of another. For example, x and y may be described as associated if an increase in x also results in an increase in y. *Causation* is a special type of association in which one condition precedes the other and must be present in order for the outcome to occur.

Although all causal relationships are forms of associations, the converse is not true; that is, there are many additional reasons that might account for any observed association. To illustrate the difference, epidemiologists classically refer to the example of storks and babies. It can be shown that for many parts of the world, birth rates are higher in those regions with higher populations of storks. However, while these two variables may be positively associated, this is clearly not a causal relationship.

This distinction is important because statistics and epidemiology only provide insight into associations. Determining whether the association is causal depends on the application of nonepidemiologic principles. The most widely used are what have now come to be known as the Bradford Hill criteria.[1] The most important of these are listed in Table 3-1.

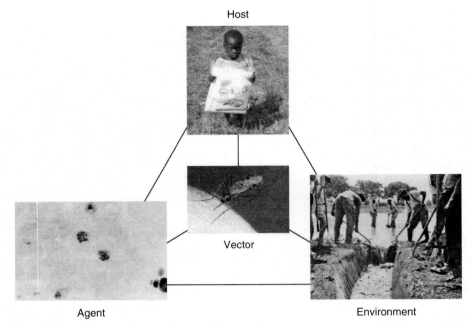

Figure 3-1. Epidemiologic triad for malaria.

Table 3-1. Bradford Hill criteria.

Strength	Greater associations (large relative risks or odds ratios, generally above 1.5) are observed. In such instances, other influences, such as bias and confounding, are less likely to account for an association.
Consistency	The same association is observed repeatedly. Note that this criterion is only useful when different populations are studied using different experimental designs.
Specificity	One detailed association rather than claims of multiple outcomes for any one intervention. By this criterion, we often dismiss so-called cure-alls that are advocated for a plethora of ailments.
Temporality	The cause must precede the effect. This is the only mandatory criterion for causality.
Biological gradient	A dose-response relationship is observed in which the association becomes stronger with increases in the amount of the causal factor.
Plausibility	A mechanism can be advanced to explain the association.
Experimental evidence	Other types of investigations, such as animal studies, are supportive of the association.

From Bradford Hill A. *A Short Textbook of Medical Statistics.* 11th ed. 1977 London: Hodder and Stoughton. (Reproduced with permission.)

Other than causality, the three most important potential sources for a false association are chance, bias, and confounding. To critically interpret epidemiologic studies, it is essential to address the potential contribution of each of these three factors. If chance, bias, and confounding are not felt to account for an association, the findings are considered *valid*.

Chance refers to a fluke association. Whenever data are collected in an experiment, unusual results can be obtained in a random manner. For example, a coin may be flipped four times and yield heads on all occasions. Clearly, such unusual associations are more likely to occur when the sample size of an experiment is small. The role of chance is well handled by biostatistics, which provides information on the likelihood that any observed association could have arisen by chance through tests of statistical significance. Generally, when the probability of an association occurring by chance is calculated to be less than 0.05 (5%), chance is rejected as an explanation for the association.

Even when study results are reported as statistically significant, we must still determine whether the association is real. In some studies, a very large number of independent associations are explored. Often, these associations were not specified *a priori* as hypotheses under study. If 20 such comparisons were made, on average 1 will appear to be statistically significant with the use of a 5% or 1-in-20 threshold for significance. Such findings are best described as *hypothesis generating* since they require further study to determine if the specified associations are real.

Table 3-2. Types of error.

	H_0 is true	H_0 is false
Do not reject H_0 (*not* statistically significant)	Correct!	Type II error (beta)
Reject H_0 (statistically significant)	Type I error (alpha)	Correct! Statistical power

On the other hand, a *negative study* refers to no association being observed in the study. Two potential explanations must be considered in such a scenario. The first factor is insufficient sample size. A sample size justification should be included in the study that makes explicit the assumptions underlying the methods by which the number of participants was chosen. This sample size calculation depends on the magnitude of the effect under study (smaller effects require larger sample sizes) as well as information about the frequency of exposure and outcome in the study.

When a study is performed, investigators propose the so-called null hypothesis, denoted as H_0, which states that there is no association between the risk factor and the outcome under study. After the data are collected and analyzed, the null hypothesis will either be accepted (the findings are not statistically significant) or rejected (the findings are statistically significant). Therefore, four situations can arise, as depicted in Table 3-2. If the null hypothesis is accepted when it is true, a correct decision has been made. If the null hypothesis is accepted when in fact it is false, a type II error, denoted by beta, is committed. Beta is conventionally set at 20% in calculating an appropriate sample size.

Conversely, if one rejects the null hypothesis and concludes that there is a statistically significant relationship between two variables when in fact the null hypothesis is true, one commits a type I error, denoted by alpha. Alpha is 5% conventionally and corresponds to the threshold used for *p* values. Finally, if the null hypothesis is rejected when it is in fact false, a correct decision has been made.

Note that type I and type II errors are trade-offs, because these are opposite actions. Therefore, a decrease in the likelihood of one increases the likelihood of the other. Because it is generally felt that errors involving incorrect rejection of the null hypothesis are worse, alpha is set at a lower level than that of beta.

What do these values of alpha and beta really mean? They provide distributions reflective of the values of statistical tests if there is no relationship between the two variables. The process of *statistical inference* involves the calculation of parameters such as *z, t,* or chi-square statistics, which all involve a difference between the observed results and those expected if there was no association in the numerator and some measure of variability in the denominator. Accordingly, as observed results become more extreme from those predicted under the null hypothesis or the variability in the results decreases, the likelihood of achieving statistical significance increases. The calculated statistic is then compared with the distribution of the values that occur given no relationship between the variables for specified values of alpha and beta. A *p* value can be obtained. Lower *p* values correspond to test statistics that fall near one end of this distribution and therefore to findings that are unlikely to have arisen by chance.

Confounding occurs when there is a third variable that is independently linked to both the risk factor and the disease outcome under study. For example, epidemiologic studies published a number of years ago suggested an association between consumption of coffee and the development of certain types of cancer. However, it was subsequently shown that the findings were confounded by failure to control for cigarette smoking. Those individuals who drink coffee are more likely to also smoke more, and smoking is an independent risk factor for cancer. Although the investigators thought they were comparing groups who differed in the amount of coffee consumed, in reality they were comparing groups with differing amounts of cigarettes consumed, and it was this latter risk factor that resulted in the observed difference in cancer between the groups.

Confounding can be handled using a variety of approaches, listed in Table 3-3. However, it is obvious that in order to control a confounder, one must be aware of it. The only method available to control for unknown confounders is *randomization* in a clinical trial. With appropriate randomization, groups will be the same with respect to every variable, including both known and unknown confounders, and differ only with respect to the intervention under study.

Finally, *bias* is a systematic error that affects one group preferentially in comparison with another. For example, *recall bias* refers to the observation that sick people tend to recall more of any exposures, even those that have nothing to do with disease. Many types of bias exist; some of the more common forms are listed in Table 3-4. Because bias is difficult to quantify or measure, it is not easily handled using statistical methods. Accordingly, efforts are targeted at minimizing bias in study design through assessment tools that are objective and standardized. A clinical trial offers one of the most powerful methods to reduce bias through *blinding*. As the name suggests, with this technique, a person (the study subject or investigator) is unaware of the intervention (if any) being received.

If chance, bias, and confounding are not felt to account for an association, the findings are considered *valid*. However, many other factors must be considered before one can conclude that valid results are causal and relevant. These factors are discussed in "Study Design," later in this chapter. Valid results may not apply to populations other than those included in the study. This consideration relates to the *generalizability* of the findings.

Table 3-3. Methods to control confounding.

Method	Example	Limitation
Matching	For each case with disease, a control is selected with the same level of confounder	Does not allow any measurement of the strength of the confounder
Stratification	Divide subjects into different levels of the confounder	Only practical for a small number of confounders
Randomization	Randomly allocate subjects to receive the intervention under study	Requires control of the intervention on the part of investigators
Multivariate analysis	Control influence of other variables using statistical software to isolate and examine the effect of one	Methods are complex
Restriction	A study of cardiovascular disease only enrolls men	Reduces the generalizability of the study findings

Table 3-4. Forms of bias.

Type of bias	Definition
Selection bias	Error in how subjects are enrolled in a study.
The healthy worker effect	Working populations appear to be healthier when compared with the general population due to outmigration of sick people from the workforce.
Volunteer bias	Subjects who agree to participate in a study differ from those who refuse, generally by being healthier.
Berkson's bias	Patients receiving medical treatment are different from those in the general population. For example, patients with comorbid conditions may be more likely to seek treatment than those with a single diagnosis, leading to false associations between the two diseases if only treated populations are studied.
Information or observer bias	Error in how data are gathered about exposure or disease.
Recall bias	Subjects who are sick recall more past exposures, independent of any causal role.
Interviewer bias	Investigators may preferentially elicit information about exposure or outcomes if aware of the subject's status in a study.
Systematic or differential misclassification	Errors in how exposure or outcome status is determined.
Loss to follow-up	Error introduced if loss to follow-up in a study is related to outcome under investigation.

BASIC HEALTH INDICATORS

To study the causes of disease, it is necessary to begin by examining basic health indicators, which include measures of mortality and morbidity. In spite of the widespread use of such indicators, particularly to compare the health status of different countries, it is important to recognize that health is a much more complex notion than is reflected by such statistics. In 1948, the World Health Organization (WHO) defined health as "a state of complete physical, mental and social well being and not merely the absence of disease or infirmity." The WHO provides basic health indicators together with additional health statistics for all member states in the World Health Report, produced annually since 1995 and available online at http://www.who.int/whr/en/.

Measuring Morbidity

The two key measures of disease frequency are prevalence and incidence. Whereas *prevalence* refers to the number of existing cases at one time, *incidence* is restricted to the number of new cases occurring over a defined period of time.

There are two types of prevalence: point and period prevalence. The *point prevalence* is calculated as the number of existing cases divided by the population at risk at that same time. However, obtaining such instantaneous information is commonly quite difficult, especially for larger populations. In practice, it might require a prolonged period of time simply to assess the population for the number of cases. Suppose a survey was carried out in the year 2005 in a province of Indonesia to ascertain the number of cases of tuberculosis. The number of cases, divided usually by the mid-2005 population of the province, is a *period prevalence*. Note that for either type of prevalence, there are no units of time. Therefore, prevalence is not a rate.

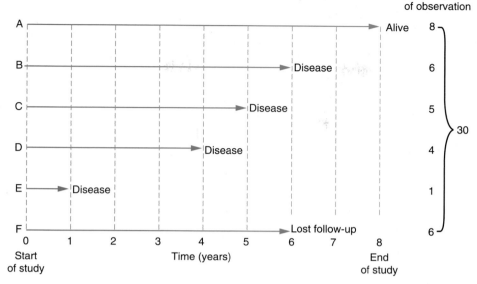

Figure 3-2. Calculation of incidence rate or density in an 8-year study of six persons (A through F).

The significant limitation of prevalence is that it does not reflect differences in whether a case was recently diagnosed or diagnosed quite some time in the past. Clearly, in terms of understanding trends in disease, this distinction is important. For this reason, it is usually preferable to examine the number of new cases by determining the incidence rather than the prevalence.

The denominator for incidence is usually expressed as *person-years*. This is a common metric that allows data from separate observations to be pooled when there is variable follow-up of each individual. If all individuals are considered to have been followed for the same, defined period of time, a *cumulative incidence* is calculated. For example, 10 new cases of disease diagnosed in 100 people over a year represent a cumulative incidence of 0.1 case per person-year.

For smaller populations, each subject may be considered separately rather than assuming that follow-up is uniform. In such situations, an *incidence rate* or *incidence density* is used when there is variable follow-up between subjects. Consider the example shown in Figure 3-2. Only subject A is followed for the entire duration of the study, contributing 8 person-years of disease-free time. However, each of the others can be added, for a total of 30 person-years. The incidence rate or incidence density is then calculated as 4 cases divided by 30 person-years, or 0.13 case per person-year.

There is a clear relationship between incidence and prevalence, namely, prevalence equals incidence times duration. Therefore, factors that increase the duration of disease will increase the prevalence, independent of

any change in incidence. The many factors that can influence prevalence and incidence other than changes in the frequency of new cases are shown in Table 3-5.

Measures of Mortality

Measures of mortality offer the obvious practical advantage of being based on an objective, easily recognized outcome. Three generic measures—rates, ratios, and proportions—are generally used (Figure 3-3). However, incorrect usage of these terms (especially *rate*) is very common in the health literature.

Table 3-5. Factors that may increase incidence and prevalence independent of changes in the number of new cases.

Factors increasing both incidence and prevalence	Factors increasing prevalence only
Greater case ascertainment	Improved (noncurative) treatment
Enhanced diagnostic methods	Out-migration of healthy people from population.
More liberal criteria in disease definition (examples: AIDS; body mass index thresholds for obesity in the United States)	In-migration of people with disease into population

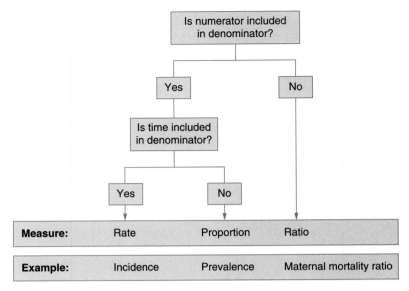

Figure 3-3. Distinguishing between rates, proportions, and ratios.

The most simple death measure is what is usually referred to as the *crude death rate,* which, since it contains no unit of time, is not actually a rate. Because the calculated number is usually very small, the figure is conventionally expressed per 1,000 people. For example, the WHO reported that the crude death rate for Botswana was 28 per 1,000 in 2004. In contrast, the corresponding figure for Brazil was reported to be 7 per 1,000.

Obviously, these figures cannot be directly compared because many other differences between these two countries may independently influence mortality. Perhaps most important, Brazil has an older population than Botswana, a confounder that precludes a meaningful direct comparison of rates. In other words, comparing crude death rates may actually *underestimate* the true difference in health status of these two populations. A variety of approaches can be used to address this limitation. One is to compare age-specific death rates (such as deaths in those aged 25 to 30 years) or cause-specific death rates (such as deaths from pneumonia).

Another method is *standardization*, which can be done either directly or indirectly. Both types involve the same calculation but are performed in different directions, as illustrated using hypothetical data in Table 3-6. Note that the crude death rate of town A is lower than that of town B. However, closer inspection of the rate within each age stratum shows that all are higher in town A than B. The explanation for this paradox lies in the differing age structure of the two towns: more people are in the older age groups in town B. With direct

standardization, the death rate from town A is multiplied by the number of people in that age stratum in town B. The number that arises is the number of deaths given town A's death rate for each age stratum but using town B's overall population structure. This is the directly standardized death rate for town A using town B as a standard. This figure is calculated as follows:

$$(4/1,000) \times 400 = 1.6 \text{ deaths}$$
$$(4/1,000) \times 300 = 1.2 \text{ deaths}$$
$$(6/1,000) \times 1,000 = 6 \text{ deaths}$$
$$(10/1,000) \times 2,000 = 20 \text{ deaths}$$
$$(40/1,000) \times 2,000 = 80 \text{ deaths}$$
$$(150/1,000) \times 400 = 60 \text{ deaths}$$

Total of 168.8 deaths per 6,100 = 27.7 deaths per 1,000 persons

This figure is now higher than the rate of 23.8 in town B. The conclusion is that, when corrected for age, the mortality is higher in town A than B. This disappearance or reversal of an observed difference when data are stratified and standardized by different levels of a confounder illustrates a concept epidemiologists refer to as *Simpson's paradox.*

An alternative approach is to take the death rates of town B and apply them to the age structure of town A. The deaths for each stratum can then be added to yield the number of "expected" deaths if people in town A were dying at the same frequency as those in town B. The observed number of deaths divided by the expected

Table 3-6. Data for standardization example. (see text)

Age	Town A			Town B		
	Population	**Deaths**	**Death rate per 1,000**	**Population**	**Deaths**	**Death rate per 1,000**
0–14	500	2	4	400	1	2.5
15–29	2,000	8	4	300	1	3.3
30–44	2,000	12	6	1,000	5	5
45–59	1,000	10	10	2,000	18	9
60–74	500	20	40	2,000	70	35
75+	100	15	150	400	50	125
Total	6,100	67	11.0	6,100	145	23.8

From Bradford Hill A. *A Short Textbook of Medical Statistics.* 11th ed. London: Hodder and Stoughton. (Modified with permission.)

number of deaths yields the *standardized mortality ratio* (SMR). In this case, the calculation is as follows:

$$(2.5/1,000) \times 500 = 1.25$$
$$(3.3/1,000) \times 2000 = 6.6$$
$$(5/1,000) \times 2000 = 10$$
$$(9/1,000) \times 1000 = 9$$
$$(35/1,000) \times 500 = 17.5$$
$$(125/1,000) \times 100 = 12.5$$
$$\text{Total} = 56.9$$
$$\text{SMR} = 67/56.9 = 1.18$$

The SMR of 1.18 (sometimes multiplied by 100 and expressed as 118) is an indirectly standardized ratio for town A using town B as a standard. Since this figure is greater than 1 (or 100), it provides the same result as the directly standardized rates: the mortality appears to be greater in town A than B. In general, indirect standardization is used when study populations are smaller. Moreover, the SMR provides an intuitive comparison within one figure, rather than two contrasting rates.

Because it is often uncertain what the population at risk for any observed outcome is, it is generally more difficult to obtain information about the denominator than the numerator in calculating measures of mortality. Returning to the crude adult death rate of 770 per 1,000 in 2004 for females in Botswana, it is clear that it is much easier to collect data on the number of females who died in Botswana that year than to know the population at risk, since the number of adult females will vary throughout the year and accurate census data may be difficult to obtain.

Accordingly, the *proportional mortality ratio* (PMR) is frequently used because it only requires more readily available death data. The PMR is calculated as the number of deaths from a specific cause divided by the total number of deaths. If there are 4,000 total deaths in a population and

200 of these are as the result of injury, the PMR is 0.05, or 5%. The obvious disadvantage of this measurement is that a decline in one significant cause of death must elevate the PMR of another, which can lead to misleading impressions. For example, a successful campaign to reduce injury rates might increase the PMR for cancer only because many individuals who previously might have died at a young age from injuries might now be living long enough to develop an alternative cause of death.

It is also useful to know the *case-fatality rate*, which is the number of people diagnosed with a disease who die from it. A number of reproductive and perinatal case-fatality rates are used in global health because these indicators are quite sensitive to significant disruptions affecting the health status of populations and have an enormous public health impact. Figure 3-4 illustrates the eight overlapping fetal and infant periods used to calculate these death rates. Note that for practical reasons, the denominator used is the total number of live births, not the number of pregnancies. Therefore, a woman who dies during the delivery of live-born twins would constitute a maternal mortality ratio of 50%.

Survival Analysis

The concept of case-fatality rate is really only meaningful for shorter periods of observation, that is, for acute diseases. In other situations, it is important to have a more refined measurement that factors in how long each person lived prior to dying. The technique used is referred to as *survival analysis,* which involves following a group of individuals over a period of time.

In the largest sense, this can be done from birth to death. However, such data would be very difficult to obtain because of the length and effort of follow-up required. As a surrogate, populations at any one time are divided into smaller age groups to create a *life table.*

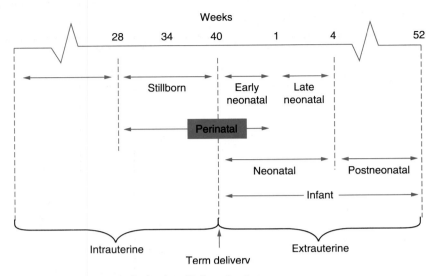

Figure 3-4. Overlapping time periods for fetal and infant deaths.

The life table for the United States has been presented in Chapter 2 (Table 2-2). In this type of survival analysis, the population is divided into smaller units during the first years of life because of increased mortality in this group, and subsequently is divided into 5-year intervals.

The column e_x is the life expectancy—the most frequently cited number from a life table. Someone born in the United States in the year 2002 can expect, on average, to live for 77.3 years. This figure is clearly a hypothetical number, because it is drawn from a cross section of people all born at different times and assumes that conditions affecting mortality will be stable during a person's entire lifetime. Note further that within each age stratum, there is always an additional period of life expectancy. For example, the life expectancy of a 50-year-old American (e_{50}) is 80.3 years (50 + 30.3 years). This life expectancy is greater than that at birth because those causes of death that might affect younger populations, such as perinatal causes, no longer apply to a 50-year-old.

Rather than dividing a large population into arbitrary time intervals and examining how many people survived to the beginning of each interval, one can examine a smaller population and determine the exact duration of survival for each member of the group. The procedure is much the same as that used to calculate an incidence rate or density, shown earlier. Instead of birth, the starting point can be the time at diagnosis of a disease or the time when a treatment was administered. Outcomes other than death can also be considered, in which case the term *time to event analysis* is used. For example, following treatment of breast cancer with mastectomy, time to event analysis may be used with an endpoint of tumor recurrence.

Whenever a group is followed in survival analysis, there will always be those who are lost to follow-up, which might occur whether they die prior to the end of the study or whether they are still alive at the conclusion of the study. In either instance, we do not know the status of such individuals when they are no longer under observation. In survival analysis, such individuals are referred to as being *censored*. However, the refinement of survival analysis is that the contribution of survival time prior to censoring is preserved for each subject.

In the example in Table 3-7, 20 subjects are followed for 10 days. On day 4, one subject dies, on day 6 one subject is lost to follow-up, on day 7 there are two more deaths, on day 8 another is lost to follow-up, on day 9 there are three deaths, and on day 10 four more deaths occur. We can generate a Kaplan-Meier curve (Figure 3-5) showing the successive probability of survival for each of these time spans. According to this analysis, an individual's cumulative probability of survival is 46%. This is a much more refined estimate that retains data provided by those lost to follow-up.

STUDY DESIGN

Recognition of study design is an important precondition for critical interpretation of findings. Although the randomized, double-blind clinical trial is clearly the most superior, application of this study design may be constrained by practical limitations or ethical concerns. Perhaps more so than other fields, global health uses a wide variety of additional epidemiologic study designs to provide essential information.

Table 3-7. Survival data using the Kaplan-Meier method.

Day	Outcomes	Number at risk at start of day	Probability of dying that day (%)	Probability of surviving that day (%)	Cumulative probability of survival (%)
1	None	20	0	100	100
2	None	20	0	100	100
3	None	20	0	100	100
4	1 death	20	5	95	95
5	None	19	0	100	95
6	1 censored	19	0	100	95
7	2 deaths	18	11	89	85
8	1 censored	16	0	100	85
9	3 deaths	15	20	80	68
10	4 deaths	12	33	67	46

Studies have found that different countries show marked variation in the prevalence of disease. One of the greatest differences has been observed for cancer of the esophagus, which has a much higher prevalence in Iran than in other parts of the world.[2] These types of studies are referred to as *descriptive studies* because they are simply initial attempts to describe the general characteristics of disease. They do not involve an explicit hypothesis, because the investigators do not test specifically why one country might have more disease than another.

The findings from descriptive studies need to be investigated further using more rigorous, *analytical study* designs that articulate and explore a specific relationship between disease and exposure. In the previous example, suppose there was a suspicion that consumption of very hot tea was a potential reason for the high prevalence of esophageal cancer in Iran. A variety of different analytical study designs could be applied that involve comparing differences in cancer of the esophagus among individuals with different levels of consumption of hot tea.

Descriptive Epidemiologic Studies

CASE REPORTS AND CASE SERIES

A *case report* is a description of one case of the disease, whereas a *case series* consists of more than one case of the same disease. This type of study is simply a careful description of the disease and the circumstances in which it occurred. Case reports or case series can be drawn from clinical experience or from routine surveillance.

It is worth remembering that some of the first evidence of the HIV pandemic arose from a case series reported by a clinician and through surveillance data.[3] Therefore, although definitive conclusions can seldom

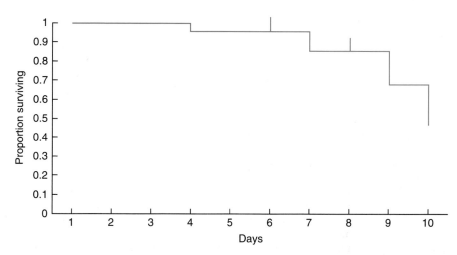

Figure 3-5. Kaplan-Meier curve using data from Table 3-7.

be drawn by this type of study design, it may be the first indication of a new disease. Frequently, when control groups for comparison are logistically difficult, such as for surgical interventions, the only available studies may be case series.

CORRELATIONAL STUDIES

Correlational studies compare disease frequency with respect to another demographic factor, such as place or time. The example provided earlier of a study noting a much higher prevalence of cancer of the esophagus in northern Iran is an example of a correlational or ecological study.

These studies are inexpensive and can be performed rapidly, without the need to examine or follow individuals. Correlational studies have provided the first evidence of important new disease risk factors. However, the results must be interpreted with caution. Because the data are aggregate and at a population level, we do not know what is occurring at the level of individuals within the study population. The reason northern Iranians seem to experience more esophageal cancer may be as a result of genetic or environmental factors or both. Moreover, these findings do not preclude the possibility that there may be smaller subpopulations in northern Iran who have a much lower risk of esophageal cancer. The essential point is that associations observed for populations do not necessarily hold true for individuals. When such incorrect inferences are made, one is said to commit *the ecological fallacy.*

CROSS-SECTIONAL STUDIES

In a *cross-sectional study* design, the cross section is through time, with exposure and disease status (prevalence) in a population ascertained simultaneously. Frequently, this is accomplished through surveys of large numbers of individuals.

Cross-sectional studies are the most important type of study design for understanding the magnitude of a public health problem and planning interventions. One of the most well-known cross-sectional studies is the National Health and Nutritional Examination Survey (NHANES) in the United States. NHANES provides current statistical data on "the amount, distribution and effects of illness and disability in the United States" through a sample of 5,000 people taken over 12 months. The sample includes a home interview and a health exam, including investigations and examination by a physician.

Successive cross-sectional studies performed at intervals on the same population may demonstrate what is known in epidemiology as a *cohort* or *generation effect* (not to be confused with cohort studies, discussed later). Consider the data shown in Figure 3-6 for mortality from gastric ulcer, duodenal ulcer, and ulcerative colitis in the United Kingdom, which show that mortality for gastric ulcer peaked for those born around 1880.[4] Some shared environmental exposure at birth was predictive of

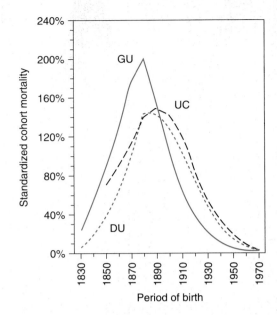

Figure 3-6. Birth cohort effects for gastric ulcer (GU), ulcerative colitis (UC), and duodenal ulcer (DU). From Sonnenberg A, Cucino C, Bauerfeind P. Commentary: the unresolved mystery of birth-cohort phenomena in gastroenterology. *Int J Epidemiol* 2002;31(1):23–26. (Reproduced with permission.)

death many years later. This finding was observed in the 1960s, long before any knowledge of the important contribution of *Helicobacter pylori*. Although the explanation for these observations remains incompletely understood, these studies were the first to draw attention to environmental risk factors for these diseases.

The obvious limitation of cross-sectional studies is a chicken or egg dilemma. Because exposure and disease are studied at the same time, it is not necessarily clear which came first. Additionally, because of the large number of individuals included, cross-sectional studies may become expensive and are inefficient because they are usually performed without regard for disease or exposure status. For this reason, the assessment methods are often limited to simple, inexpensive measurement tools such as questionnaires.

Analytical Epidemiology

Analytical studies are needed to definitively test hypotheses that may have been generated by descriptive approaches. In *observational analytical studies,* the investigator has no control over which group in the study population received the exposure under study. In contrast, *interventional analytical studies* (clinical trials) involve the deliberate administration of an exposure to study subjects. There are two types of observational analytical studies: the case-control study and cohort study.

CASE-CONTROL STUDIES

In case-control studies, as the name suggests, subjects are selected on the basis of having the disease under study (cases) or not having the disease under study (controls). The investigators then look back in time to determine whether there are any differences in previous exposures between the two groups.

It is important that a clear definition of a case be provided and consistently applied. Inclusion criteria must be described in detail and should generally be very strict to avoid misclassifications of controls as cases. Exclusion criteria may also be needed; these should be explicit and applied both in the selection of cases and controls. Cases can be derived from disease registries, clinic or hospital populations, or from the general population. Selection of controls is an important consideration to reduce bias and confounding. The general rule is that controls should resemble cases in every way other than having the disease under study.

If the disease under study is rare, more controls than cases may be enrolled as a way to increase the statistical power of the study. The greatest gain occurs at a ratio of four controls per case; beyond this, the additional costs usually do not justify the modest gain in statistical power.

The results of a study investigating an exposure and a particular disease are depicted in Table 3-8. If this is a case-control study, it is meaningless to calculate a prevalence from this data. The apparent prevalence is artificial because it depends entirely on the ratio of cases to controls selected by the investigators. Instead, the measure of association used in case-control studies is the odds ratio (OR). Most people have some familiarity with odds from gambling, although the concept is used in a slightly different way than in epidemiology. If the odds for a horse are given as 4-1, this means that if you wagered $1 on the horse and it won the race, you would receive $4. Note that, as stated, this was because the horse was felt to be four times more likely not to win the race than to win it. Therefore, the odds in gambling represent the likelihood of an event not happening to the likelihood that it will happen. In terms of probability (p), this type of odds can be expressed as $(1 - p):p$. Thus, the horse has a 20% probability of winning the race, since 80%:20% = 4:1.

Table 3-8. Results of a study investigating disease and exposure.

	Disease present	Disease absent
Exposure present	a	b
Exposure absent	c	d

In a case-control study, instead of connecting a horse to winning, investigators use the OR to connect disease to exposure. Second, instead of the odds expressing the likelihood of the event not happening to the likelihood of it happening, the ratio is calculated the other way around: epidemiologists calculate the odds that an individual will have exposure relative to not having exposure. This is done separately for cases and controls, and the results are compared as a ratio.

Using Table 3-8, the odds of exposure for cases are simply a/c and for controls, b/d. The ratio is therefore

$$\frac{a/c}{b/d} = \frac{ad}{bc}$$

An OR greater than 1 means that the exposure increases the risk of disease, a value equal to 1 means that there is no association, and a value less than 1 indicates that exposure reduces the risk of disease. The calculation of a measure of association such as an OR should not be confused with the concept of statistical inference or significance, discussed later. Even if one observes a greatly elevated OR, it does not necessarily mean that the findings are significant.

Case-control studies are chosen for diseases that have lengthy induction periods between a causative exposure and the onset of disease, such as cancer or cardiovascular disease. Because investigators enroll people who currently have the disease, they do not need to wait until disease develops, and future follow-up is not required. By similar reasoning, this type of study design is most suitable for rare diseases. Multiple different exposures can be studied for any one disease. Case-control studies are also less expensive than other analytical studies.

The major disadvantage of a case-control study is the potential for bias, both on the part of participants and investigators, since disease status is known prior to the determination of exposure status.

COHORT STUDIES

In cohort studies, individuals are selected who are free of the disease under study at the time that observation begins. Their exposure status is then established and they are followed forward in time to determine their subsequent disease status. Cohort studies can either be prospective or retrospective in nature.

In a prospective cohort study, subjects are currently free of the disease under study and are followed into the future to determine who later develops disease. A well-known prospective cohort study is the Framingham Heart Study, which was initiated in 1948 with the enrollment of 5,209 adult residents of Framingham, Massachusetts. To be eligible to participate, these individuals had to have been free of cardiovascular disease in 1948.

Ever since, each of them has undergone a standardized, biannual cardiovascular examination. Daily surveillance of hospital admissions, deaths, and information from other health care providers is performed to determine disease status. A wealth of important information, including much of our current insight about standard coronary risk factors, arose from this study.[5]

The very obvious practical limitation of this study is that years, or in most instances decades, elapsed before sufficient numbers of subjects developed cardiovascular disease to provide a large enough sample size for statistical analysis. One solution to this problem is to apply a retrospective cohort study design. In this case, some of the study subjects have developed disease at the present time. However, the investigators perform the steps in the same order by taking advantage of historical information to avoid the need for future follow-up. A cohort of disease-free individuals are identified from past records and subsequently followed forward in time for a defined period to determine who later developed disease. However, all of these events have occurred in the past relative to the time of the study.

For example, investigators in China were interested in learning whether the use of chimneys to provide ventilation of coal stoves would reduce the incidence of chronic obstructive pulmonary disease. They examined historical data on individuals from 1976 until 1992 who had switched from an unvented to a vented stove and identified a reduction in the incidence of chronic obstructive pulmonary disease. Because the development of disease occurred prior to the onset of the study, this cohort study is retrospective in nature.[6]

Returning to Table 3-8, if these results are from a cohort study, the incidence can be directly calculated because all individuals are disease-free at enrollment. The measure of association from a cohort study, known as the *relative risk*, is simply the incidence of disease in those exposed divided by the incidence of disease in those who are unexposed:

$$\frac{a/(a+b)}{c/(c+d)}$$

In many ways, cohort studies represent a mirror image of case-control studies. The unexposed and exposed people should resemble each other in every way other than having the exposure under study. Cohort studies are good for rare exposures, and many diseases can be studied for any one exposure. Because exposure status is determined prior to disease status, bias is less of a concern than in a case-control study.

However, cohort studies are obviously not suitable for rare disease outcomes. Prospective studies are more expensive and prolonged because future follow-up is required. For retrospective cohort studies, data quality when the cohort is assembled from historical sources may be a concern. Finally, subjects may always be lost to follow-up, which may influence the findings.

CLINICAL TRIALS

An intervention study or clinical trial is the gold standard study design in epidemiology. Because the investigators determine who receives the exposure under study, there is a greater degree of experimental control than in any other epidemiologic study.

Broadly speaking, the two goals of any clinical trial are to determine the efficacy and the safety of the intervention under study. As with a cohort study, a homogenous group without the outcome under study is first assembled. Clearly defined exclusion criteria must exist, and written informed consent must be obtained from all participants.

If the clinical trial involves a pharmaceutical agent, the studies occur in four phases (Table 3-9). Although the distinction between phases is not always clear, there is a relatively greater emphasis on efficacy and less on safety in progressing from phase I to IV. Approval of a pharmaceutical for clinical use usually occurs following satisfactory phase III study outcomes.

Before subjects receive the intervention, several considerations are important. Because subjects will receive a deliberately applied intervention, there are considerable ethical issues involved in a clinical trial; appropriate oversight must be in place, and informed written consent must be obtained from all participants. It is essential that a clinical trial include a sample size justification to ensure it is of appropriate statistical power. This justification should be explicit about the assumptions made in choosing a particular number of participants. Finally, since the investigators can determine who receives the exposure of interest, it allows them to apply two very powerful tools: randomization and blinding.

The importance of *blinding* was first appreciated by Benjamin Franklin in 1784. He recognized that if individuals had an expectation of improvement, beneficial effects could falsely be ascribed to ineffective interventions, a phenomenon now referred to as the *placebo effect*. Accordingly, an essential feature of any clinical trial is an appropriate control group for comparison. The control group may receive standard therapy when it would be unethical for any participant to remain untreated during the study. If the control group receives an inactive intervention, this is referred to as a *placebo* for a pharmaceutical agent or a *sham treatment* for a procedural intervention.

In single blinding, study subjects are not aware of whether they are being allocated treatment or placebo or sham intervention. If the investigators are similarly unaware, the study is described as double blind. Triple blinding includes those individuals performing analysis of data. Clearly, blinding is the ultimate method to deal with bias in study designs.

Table 3-9. Phases of a clinical trial of a pharmaceutical agent.

Phase	Number of subjects	Type of subjects	Goals
I	<100	Healthy volunteers or end stage disease patients in inpatient setting	Determine safety, investigate pharmacokinetics, determine appropriate dosage
II	Hundreds	Healthy volunteers; patients with less severe disease	Further investigate safety, begin to determine preliminary efficacy
III	Hundreds to thousands	Patients	Compare new pharmaceutical with existing therapy
IV	Hundreds to tens of thousands	Patients in long-term studies	Investigate other indications for treatment, explore longer-term and rarer adverse effects

Randomization in clinical trials offers the great benefit that study subjects differ only with respect to receiving the intervention under study. Therefore, randomization is the most desirable method to deal with the problem of confounders, since all such variables will equal out between groups of sufficient size who are appropriately randomized.

Three general designs are used in an intervention study: simple or parallel (Figure 3-7A), cross-over (Figure 3-7B) or factorial (Figure 3-7C). In a *cross-over study*, each subject serves as his or her own control, and the variation between those in the intervention and control arms is eliminated. Accordingly, this design is the most efficient and requires the smallest sample size.

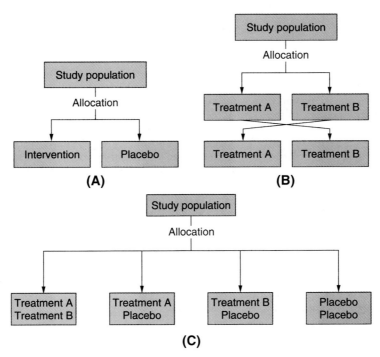

Figure 3-7. Three general designs of intervention studies. (A) Simple or parallel intervention study. (B) Cross-over intervention study. (C) Factorial intervention study of two treatments.

Similarly, it is also the most robust design, since the results are affected to a lesser extent when subjects are lost to follow-up. Obviously, the main disadvantage of a cross-over design is a *carry-over effect* in which a residual influence may persist after subjects have crossed over. Such an effect can obscure the differences between the two treatments studied in a cross-over study.

Further reflection will indicate that a carry-over effect may also occur in simple or parallel studies, since clinical trials are frequently performed on individuals receiving some sort of treatment prior to enrollment in the study. One method to deal with this problem is to include a *wash-out period* before or in between study treatments, during which subjects receive placebo only.

The *factorial design* allows interactions between two treatments to be studied, which may be either synergistic or antagonistic in nature. In either instance, this is important additional information. A well-known example of a factorial study design is the Physicians' Health Study. The first Physicians' Health Study, which ended in 1995, examined the use of aspirin and beta-carotene to prevent cardiovascular disease and cancer. The Physicians' Health Study II, scheduled for completion in December 2007, is a clinical trial of vitamins C and E, beta-carotene, and multivitamin supplementation in a factorial design with 16 different study groups.[7]

Noncompliance and Drops-Outs Once a study group of appropriate size is assembled and randomized, and blinding is applied to participants and investigators, the only remaining threats to validity are noncompliance and drop-outs.

A variety of methods are available to deal with noncompliance. A run-in period may be included prior to randomization during which all participants receive a placebo. Only those subjects who comply with instructions are randomized and included in the study. Obviously, such an approach cannot be used for treatments that must be given acutely. Furthermore, this method will influence the generalizability of the findings, since a selected group showing greater compliance than the general population has been enrolled in the study. Where possible, compliance can be monitored using pill counts or direct measurement of the pharmaceutical agent in subjects. High-risk subjects, who will presumably be more motivated to comply with the study protocol, can be selected for enrollment. Financial incentives and regular contact with the participants can also be used to maintain compliance throughout the study.

Subjects who are lost to follow-up while the study is under way represent another dilemma. Suppose, for example, that a woman enrolled in the drug arm of a study comparing this drug with a placebo is killed in a car collision while the study is under way. Although it may seem intuitive to exclude her death from the study, according to a widely used approach known as *intention to treat analysis,* her death is attributed to the drug. This approach requires all subjects in each group to be followed up and analyzed according to their assignment at the beginning of the study even if they do not complete or comply with the assigned therapy.

Intention to treat analysis guards against conscious or unconscious attempts to influence the results of the study by excluding odd outcomes such as the death of the woman in the car collision. In reality, we do not know the reason for her death. It is conceivable that a side effect of the drug may lead to impaired driving ability, in which case it would be important to retain her death as one due to the drug.

What about outcomes, such as homicide, for which there is absolutely no possibility of a connection with the study protocol? Again, applying intention to treat analysis, those deaths are counted toward the arm of the study in which they occurred. Since such odd outcomes occur randomly, they are equally likely to occur in all arms of the study and therefore should not create false differences between them.

Ultimately, intention to treat analysis is necessary to preserve the baseline homogeneity achieved at the outset of the study through randomization. Consider a study of advanced cancer patients in which chemotherapy is compared with surgery. How would a death that occurred prior to the patient reaching the operating room be handled for a patient randomized to receive surgery? Intention to treat analysis tells us that this death would be ascribed to the surgery. If all patients who died prior to reaching the operating room were excluded, the benefit of randomization would be lost. Rather than comparing two groups that differ only in the treatment received, we would be comparing a group of those with less aggressive disease in the surgical arm, since these individuals had to have survived long enough to reach the operating room.

Intention to treat analysis also provides a greater reflection of how a treatment will perform in the general population by ignoring adherence when the data are analyzed. This relates to a distinction made by epidemiologists between effectiveness and efficacy. *Efficacy* refers to a treatment working under the idealized conditions of the randomized clinical trial. The ability of a treatment to work in the real world is referred to as *effectiveness*. Intention to treat analysis therefore provides a closer approximation of effectiveness.

Number Needed to Treat To complete what has been termed "the three E's" of an intervention, one needs to consider the *efficiency*, or the cost versus benefit, of a particular treatment. One way to measure efficiency is the *number needed to treat* (NNT), a very useful concept in global health given scarce resources. To understand the NNT, it is essential to appreciate the distinction between absolute and relative risk (see the example given later). A very dramatic relative risk reduction cannot be interpreted without some knowledge of baseline risk. For example, a twofold relative risk reduction is consistent both with a change in prevalence from 2 in a million to 1 in a million, or 20% to 10%. Clearly, in terms of the efficiency of a therapy, there is a great difference between these two situations.

The NNT refers to the number of people who would need to receive a given treatment for a defined period of time in order to prevent the specific outcome in one of those individuals. The calculation is simply the reciprocal of the absolute risk reduction.

In a randomized, double-blind study of 84 measles patients during an epidemic in Guinea-Bissau, prophylactic administration of a 7-day course of sulfamethoxazole-trimethoprim was compared with placebo in the prevention of complications.[8] One of 46 participants (2%) who received the antibiotic developed pneumonia, compared with 6 of 38 participants (16%) in the placebo group. Whereas the relative risk reduction is 16%/2%, or 8%, the absolute reduction in risk is 16% − 2% = 14%. The NNT is 1/0.14, or 7. Prophylaxis with sulfamethoxazole-trimethoprim of 7 patients with measles will prevent a complication of pneumonia in 1 of them. Table 3-10 lists the NNTs for a variety of interventions used in different countries.

Finally, criteria need to be considered for stopping a clinical trial. Because blinding is frequently involved, an independent data monitoring group is needed to continuously follow the results while the study is under way. Termination prior to the end of the study may be required if there has been a clear demonstration of benefit or an unacceptably high level of adverse effects.

Because of the great advantages offered by randomization and blinding, there are no inherent disadvantages to a clinical trial. The use of this design is limited by practical constraints or ethical concerns. For example, in the study of a surgical treatment, it may not be possible to appropriately blind the control subjects. Blinding these subjects might mean subjecting them to invasive procedures that, even though they are sham therapies, may nevertheless be painful or otherwise risky.

META-ANALYSIS

Meta-analysis is a method in which many smaller studies are pooled together and handled statistically as if all the subjects were in one larger study. The steps include identification of studies, a critique of the quality of each study, and the performance of summary statistical analysis on the aggregate data.

The search strategy used should be explicit. In addition to electronic databases such as MedLine, it may also be important to search so-called fugitive literature such as dissertations, unpublished manuscripts, or abstract presentations. Therefore, a meta-analysis may also include expert consultations, hand searches, and articles identified through reference lists.

However, published studies may provide a distorted view of the true measure of an association. This effect

Table 3-10. Number needed to treat (NNT) for a variety of interventions.

Intervention	Number needed to treat	Reference
Biweekly phone calls to promote adherence with asthma therapy in Brazil	4.5	Chatkin JM, Blanco DC, Scaglia N, Wagner MB, Fritscher CC. Impact of a low-cost and simple intervention in enhancing treatment adherence in a Brazilian asthma sample. *J Asthma* 2006;43(4):263–266.
Lifestyle modification to prevent type 2 diabetes among those with impaired glucose tolerance in India	6.4	Ramachandran A, Snehalatha C, Mary S, et al. The Indian Diabetes Prevention Programme shows that lifestyle modification and metformin prevent type 2 diabetes in Asian Indian subjects with impaired glucose tolerance (IDPP-1). *Diabetologia* 2006;49(2):289–297.
Prophylactic sulfamethoxazole-trimethoprim in measles patients to prevent pneumonia in Guinea-Bissau	7	Garly ML, Bale C, Martins CL, et al. Prophylactic antibiotics to prevent pneumonia and other complications after measles: community based randomised double blind placebo controlled trial in Guinea-Bissau. *BMJ* 2006;333 (7581):1245.
Telephone counseling of parents who smoke and have children younger than 5 years in Hong Kong	13	Abdullah AS, Mak YW, Loke AY, Lam TH. Smoking cessation intervention in parents of young children: a randomised controlled trial. *Addiction* 2005;100(11):1731–1740.
Sulfamethoxazole-trimethoprim to prevent tuberculosis in HIV-positive adults in South Africa	24	Grimwade K, Sturm AW, Nunn AJ, et al. Effectiveness of cotrimoxazole prophylaxis on mortality in adults with tuberculosis in rural South Africa. *AIDS* 2005;19(2):163–168.

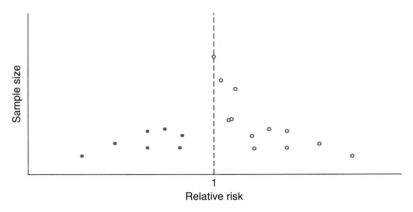

Figure 3-8. Funnel plot.

arises because published articles are more likely to contain positive rather than negative findings, a phenomenon known as *publication bias*.

To determine if publication bias is present in a meta-analysis, it is useful to examine a funnel plot. In the absence of publication bias, a funnel plot should have a pyramid-type distribution. Smaller studies have more variable results; as the sample size of the study increases, the estimate of effect should narrow down closer to the true value. However, with publication bias, there may be asymmetry to the pyramid, with an absence of smaller negative studies. In Figure 3-8, the results of published studies are shown with the ○ symbol. Note that as the sample size of each study increases, the results move closer to a relative risk of 1, suggestive of no difference. However, the plot suggests that there are many small studies showing a reduction in relative risk that were not published. To correct for this observation, a number of such hypothetical studies have been added and denoted with the ● symbol, simply as a mirror image of the smaller positive studies. Failure to correct for publication bias can lead to misleading results if the meta-analysis relies solely on the results of published studies. In this case, publication bias would have resulted in the false conclusion of an elevated relative risk.

Each of the studies must be evaluated both for quality as well as suitability for inclusion in the meta-analysis using a standardized approach. Table 3-11 provides some of the criteria.

Finally, statistical analysis must be performed on the data to summarize the results. There are three components to this analysis. The first is the calculation of a summary measure of effect, which may be a relative risk, an odds ratio, or some change in an important widely used parameter, such as blood pressure. The results of a meta-analysis on two tests used for visceral leishmaniasis are shown in Figure 3-9 as a ladder plot. Sensitivity is shown on the left and specificity on the right. These two concepts will be discussed in a later section. For each individual study, the

sample size is reflected in the size of the box used to denote the point estimate. The 95% confidence interval is the solid line extending out horizontally. Note that as the sample size of the study increases, the 95% confidence interval becomes narrower. The summary measure of effect is shown at the bottom as a diamond.

Second, statistical tests, known as *tests of homogeneity*, are applied to determine if the individual studies are similar enough to be pooled together. Finally, a *sensitivity analysis* should be performed to determine to what extent alterations in important assumptions influence the final results. The results of a meta-analysis are more likely to be valid if similar findings are found, even when assumptions are modified.

EPIDEMIOLOGY OF INFECTIOUS DISEASE

When considering an infectious disease, many of the same epidemiologic principles already discussed apply. In addition, there are unique considerations because of the presence of an infectious agent. Several definitions are provided in Table 3-12.

Table 3-11. Criteria for the evaluation of a meta-analysis.

Study design: clinical trials generally preferred
Year of publication
Language
Sample size
Adequacy of follow-up
Similarity of exposure or treatment
Similarity of outcome measures
Completeness of data
Multiple publication bias: the results of one study may be published in more than one paper

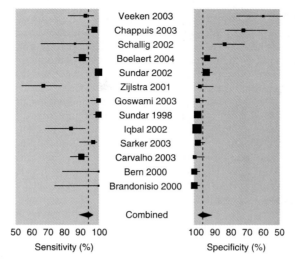

Figure 3-9. Ladder plot showing the results of a meta-analysis. From Chappuis F, Rijal S, Soto A, Menten J, Boelaert M. A meta-analysis of the diagnostic performance of the direct agglutination test and rK39 dipstick for visceral leishmaniasis. *BMJ* 2006;333(7571):723. (Reproduced with permission.)

Reservoirs

Infectious diseases are present in *reservoirs* and are transmitted to hosts in a variety of ways. For any given infectious agent, both the number of reservoirs and routes of transmission are quite limited, because the microbe has evolved to replicate and be transmitted under highly specific conditions. Nevertheless, because of rapid reproduction, the ability of these microorganisms to alter and adapt to new hosts and new modes of transmission is well recognized. The reservoir may be an inanimate object (fomite, contaminated food or water), a symptomatic human, an asymptomatic human (carrier), or another species (zoonosis or vector).

Methods of Transmission

A foodborne infection, such as salmonella, results from ingestion of the microorganism and subsequent establishment in the host. In such cases, illness occurs beginning approximately 24 hours after ingestion of the contaminated food and is accompanied by constitutional

---

Table 3-12. Definitions used in infectious disease epidemiology.

Infection: Presence of a microbe in a host to the benefit of the microbe, with some detectable response on the part of the host either clinically or serologically.

Colonization: Presence of microbe in a host without a response by the host. Example: GI flora.

Latent infection: Persistence of a microbe in the host with the possibility of clinical disease in the future *without* shedding of the microbe in the interval. Example: shingles from *Varicella zoster*.

Inapparent infection: Persistence of a microbe in a host without clinical disease *with* shedding of the microbe. Example: typhoid fever carrier.

Infectivity: The ability of the microbe to cause infection in those exposed. Calculated as the number of people with infection (clinically or serologically) divided by the number exposed.

Pathogenicity: The ability of the microbe to cause clinically apparent disease, generally used without regard for the severity of that disease. Calculated as the number of cases with clinical signs and symptoms divided by the number of those infected.

Virulence: The degree of severity of disease in diagnosed cases of an infectious disease. Calculated as the number of fatalities divided by the number of diagnosed cases.

Epidemic: A sudden increase in the frequency of infection in a particular population or region.

Pandemic: An epidemic that affects populations in large regions—continents or the entire globe.

Endemic: An infection that occurs at a stable, elevated rate in a particular population or region.

---

signs and symptoms such as fever. Conversely, other microorganisms, such as staphylococci, produce a toxin while growing on food products that causes a more rapid illness (after about 6 hours) without constitutional symptoms. Strictly speaking, this is not an infection but rather what is commonly called food poisoning.

Infections may be spread by respiratory tract secretions containing the microorganism, which becomes airborne as a result of sneezing, coughing, or even talking. With evaporation of water, small respirable residual particles, known as *droplet nuclei*, may be formed, which can remain suspended in air for many hours. Droplet nuclei spread some diseases such as tuberculosis over great distances from the source.

A *zoonosis* is an infection normally present in other vertebrate animals but which, under some circumstances, can spread and cause disease in humans. Because the infectious agent has evolved to infect, reproduce, and spread in a nonhuman host, transmission to humans generally requires extensive exposure. Person-to-person spread is rare, and disease in otherwise healthy humans is usually mild.

A *nosocomial infection* is one acquired in a hospital. In such cases, clinical disease usually only occurs in immunocompromised hosts, and bacterial pathogens may be resistant to one or more antibiotic therapies.

Infectious Disease Control

It is important to recognize that there are different time courses with respect to the ability of a host to spread an infectious disease (infectiousness) and the associated clinical course of the same infectious disease. The time between infection and the development of symptomatic disease is referred to as the *incubation period*. The time between infection and the ability of a host to spread the infectious agent to others is defined as the *latent period*. For the vast majority of infectious diseases, the infectious period precedes the symptomatic period. Therefore, efforts to control the spread of an infectious disease based on the identification of clinically affected individuals are usually unsuccessful.

BASIC REPRODUCTIVE RATE

The basic reproductive rate (R_0) is an essential calculation for understanding how infectious diseases spread through a population. R_0 is the average number of persons in a totally susceptible population infected by one case during that case's entire infectious period. R_0 will be influenced by the number of contacts that an infectious person has per unit of time, the probability of transmission with each contact, and the duration of infectiousness in units of time.

For example, R_0 for measles may have a value of 8, meaning that one person with measles introduced into a nonimmune population will produce eight new

secondary infections of measles before that individual recovers or dies. Subsequent infections (known as waves or generations) are not included in the calculation of R_0. Instead, reproductive rates are formulated for each subsequent wave and denoted as R_1, R_2, R_3, and so on.

Note that R_0 is a dynamic number; it will change over time and with changes in circumstances. Of particular importance is a sufficient pool of susceptible hosts. Typically, as an infectious disease spreads, the number of susceptible hosts declines due to death or the development of immunity until R_0 falls below 1 and the epidemic dies out. When R_0 is high, epidemics tend to have explosive increases but, for the same reason, deplete the reservoir of susceptible individuals just as rapidly and have proportionately precipitous declines. Conversely, when R_0 is low, outbreaks are more prolonged.

EPIDEMIC INVESTIGATION

The first step in any investigation of an infectious disease outbreak is to define a case. Two approaches may then be taken. The first is based on seeking a common exposure variable in an outbreak. In such instances, the difference in attack rates is calculated between those who were and those who were not exposed. This method is commonly used in the investigation of foodborne illness to determine what specific food is the source of illness.

If it is not clear how the disease is spreading, it may be useful to generate an epidemic curve by plotting the number of cases on a y axis against time on the x axis to guide preventive efforts. Several different types of epidemic curves are recognized. The first is a *point source outbreak* (Figure 3-10A), which typically occurs when there is one common source of infection without person-to-person transmission. In a *propagated epidemic* (Figure 3-10B), person-to-person transmission occurs, with successive peaks in the number of cases observed. The time between these peaks corresponds roughly to the mean incubation period for the infectious agent. Finally, *continuous,* also referred to as *intermittent* or *common epidemic*, curves (Figure 3-10C) consist of a relatively stable number of elevated cases over time. By definition, this corresponds to the typical pattern seen for an endemic.

HERD IMMUNITY

R_0 provides useful insight into how to control an infectious disease. It is not necessary to completely halt transmission of the agent (reduce R_0 to zero), merely to maintain an R_0 level less than 1 for a sufficient period of time to halt the spread of the agent.

To appreciate the role of control measures, it is important to understand the significance of *herd immunity* (Figure 3-11). In the population to the left, a person with infection is introduced into a population with a low level of immunity. So long as each infected person has a reasonably high likelihood of coming into contact with a susceptible host, the disease can spread.

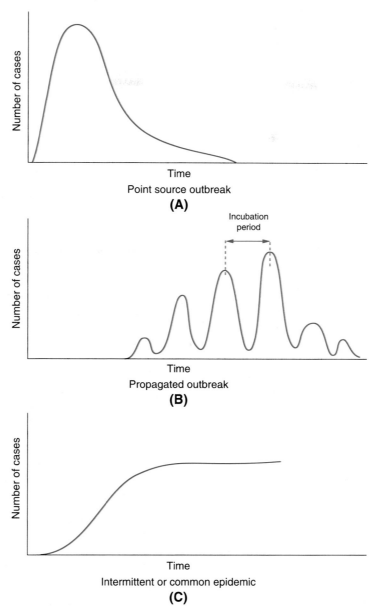

Figure 3-10. Types of epidemic curves. (A) Point source epidemic curve. (B) Propagated epidemic curve. (C) Continuous epidemic curve.

Conversely, in the population to the right, because of a sufficiently high prevalence of immunity, the probability of contact with a susceptible person is so low that the disease cannot propagate. Many susceptible individuals in this population are protected from infection by the preponderance of immune members.

Herd immunity tells us that an entire population can be protected from an infectious disease if a sufficiently high number of members of that population have immunity. It

is therefore not necessary to vaccinate 100% of a population, but rather a sufficiently high number to achieve herd immunity.

Ring treatment is a method of infection control based on herd immunity. Using this approach, when a case is identified, aggressive efforts are made to immunize all those individuals who may come into contact with the case. In effect, a ring of immunity is created to prevent the infection from spreading to susceptible individuals.

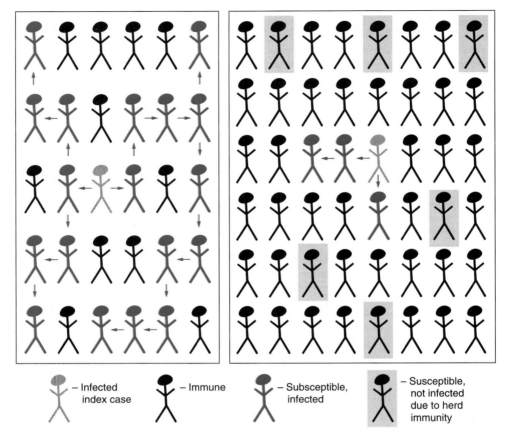

Figure 3-11. Herd immunity.

Ring treatment was successfully used in the final stages of the smallpox eradication effort.

CONTROL MEASURES

There are two basic strategies targeted to the host to control an infectious disease. The first is *quarantine*, which refers to the restriction of the activities of healthy people on the basis of exposure. In addition, quarantine frequently includes measures for the early detection of the infectious disease, such as periodic measurements of temperature. Quarantine can follow a spectrum from *absolute quarantine* with complete restriction of activities to a *modified quarantine,* which might involve confining individuals to their homes. The latter approach was used by public health authorities in Toronto during the severe acute respiratory syndrome (SARS) outbreak, which involved a modified quarantine with over 15,000 people confined to their homes.

In contrast, *isolation* refers to the restriction of activities of an individual on the basis of having infection for the duration of the infectious period. Isolation may be complete or specific to the mode of transmission of the infectious agent (respiratory isolation, enteric precautions, etc.).

Disease Eradication

Eradication means a permanent reduction to zero incidence for a disease. Since treatment and preventive measures will never be needed in the future, eradication is of tremendous long-term benefit relative to cost. It is intuitive that the only diseases that can be eradicated are those due to an infectious cause. Other types of diseases, such as silicosis, can be reduced to the lowest feasible levels, a condition the WHO refers to as *elimination*.

Disease eradication efforts involve nonsustainable campaigns, with enormous amounts of resources dedicated for a defined period of time in the hope of permanent control. The only infectious disease eradicated in its wild form to date is smallpox, following the fifth WHO eradication campaign. Previous efforts targeting yaws and malaria were unsuccessful.

A variety of considerations must be taken into account in selecting an infectious disease for eradication:

- The disease should be easily recognized on the basis of signs and symptoms.
- A control intervention conferring long-term protection and suitable for application in the field must be available.
- All populations experiencing or at risk for the infectious disease must be accessible.
- There must be no nonhuman reservoir for the disease.

The WHO is currently attempting to eradicate polio and has successfully done so in Europe, the Americas, and the western Pacific. Northern Nigeria and neighboring countries remain a reservoir for this condition. The only other disease currently targeted by the World Health Assembly for eradication is dracunculiasis, with efforts centered around the use of filters and a larvacide for drinking water. In this case, the reservoir of disease is Sudan, and the WHO has estimated that 3 to 4 years of intense activity in this country is required to eradicate dracunculiasis.

EPIDEMIOLOGY OF TESTS

Correct interpretation of any medical test requires an understanding of both the properties of the test and the setting in which the test is applied.

Test Properties

The *accuracy* of a test is defined as how close the measured value is to the true value of the parameter under measurement. *Reliability* or *reproducibility* refers to consistency in test results when repeated measurements are made on the same sample. This property should not be confused with *precision*, which relates to the lowest amount that can be measured by a technique. To illustrate this concept, in measuring distance, a set of calipers may be able to measure much shorter lengths (down to 0.01 mm) than a ruler (1 mm). Therefore, the calipers would be described as more precise than the ruler. *Validity* refers to the extent to which a test really measures what it purports to measure. For example, it is possible to measure a variety of metals in hair. However, because it is difficult to wash off metals that may be sources of external contamination, this is generally not considered a valid measure of human exposure.

In evaluating a test, it is important to consider how it compares with a given gold standard. Although there may be limitations, the gold standard represents the closest one can come to the truth for a particular test. For practical purposes, results are usually dichotomized as either positive or negative, generating the contingency table depicted in Table 3-13. Those individuals in cell *a* are true positives, in cell *b* false positives, in cell *c* false negatives, and in cell *d* true negatives. Four essential calculations can

Table 3-13. Contingency table.

	Gold standard positive	Gold standard negative
Test positive	a	b
Test negative	c	d

then be obtained: sensitivity, specificity, positive predictive value, and negative predictive value.

Sensitivity is calculated as $a/(a + c)$ and refers to the ability of the test to correctly identify those with disease. Specificity is calculated as $d/(b + d)$ and refers to the ability to correctly rule out disease, or to identify those who are healthy. Although it is obvious that both properties should be maximized in a test, an increase in one means a decrease in the other and vice versa.

Consider the extreme example of a new test used to diagnose death. Because the developers did not want to ever miss a case of death, the sensitivity was maximized to 100% by having the test always indicate that a person was dead. Examination of the table indicates that because the test is always positive, the value of cell *c* is zero, and the sensitivity ($a/[a + c]$) becomes a/a, or 100%. The test will never fail in identifying a dead person. However, the value of cell *d* is also zero, so the sensitivity is 0%, meaning that the test will never be able to correctly identify a living person.

Sensitivity and specificity are fixed properties of the test and do not change when the same test is applied in different settings. Suppose the test just discussed was used in a typical outpatient clinic and then brought to a morgue. In either location, the test always indicates that a person is dead and therefore will never fail in correctly identifying death yet will always mistakenly classify live people as dead (100% sensitivity, 0% specificity, respectively). However, although the test always provides wrong answers in the clinic, it is always correct in the morgue, even though the test itself has not changed.

The change in the performance of the test is a result of the prevalence or *pretest likelihood* of the outcome in the population being tested. In this case, when the prevalence increases from 0% to 100%, the test went from generating only false positive results in the office to generating only true positive results. This property of the test is known as the *positive predictive value* and is calculated as $a/(a + b)$.

As the example shows, the positive predictive value will increase as the prevalence of disease in the population tested increases, a phenomenon of enormous clinical significance. Tests must be carefully selected to be used on individuals for whom a clinical assessment identifies a sufficiently high likelihood of disease such that positive test results are more likely to be true rather than false positives. Conversely, as the prevalence of disease increases, the negative predictive value declines.

Applications of Tests

A medical test can be performed in three different contexts: diagnosis, screening, and surveillance. In this section, only screening and surveillance are considered.

SCREENING

The object of any screening test is to identify disease at an earlier point in time than when signs and symptoms develop. Screening is targeted at individuals with the aim of improving clinical outcomes (secondary prevention).

The amount of time by which knowledge of disease status is advanced by a screening test is known as the *lead time*. In other words, the lead time is the difference between the period of time when disease is detected on clinical grounds and when the disease is detected through a positive screening test. Individuals identified by a screening test usually undergo additional tests to either confirm that they have the disease or identify false positive test results (Figure 3-12). Therefore, screening tests should have high sensitivity, even at the expense of specificity. In clinical practice, this means that most positive screening tests are found to be false positive results upon additional investigation. A variety of practical considerations are important before screening tests are applied. These include the following:

- High sensitivity
- Low cost
- Acceptable test
- Suitable for outpatient or community application
- Screened disease has significant adverse impact
- Early identification leads to improved outcomes in screened individual or prevents further spread of disease to others

In terms of validity, there are two types of bias specific to screening tests: lead time bias and length bias. These are both sources of error that may result in screened populations falsely appearing to have improved survival when compared with unscreened populations.

By definition, for any individual who screens positively, we will have knowledge of his or her disease status earlier than an unscreened individual. Part of this time is simply the lead time. Therefore, a demonstration that a screened population survives for a longer period of time than an unscreened population *from the time of diagnosis* does not mean that the screening was necessarily useful when the starting point for the screened population is the positive screening test and, for the unscreened population, the development of symptoms. Such comparisons must show that the increased survival is beyond that which arises solely because of the lead time.

Length bias arises because not all cases of the same disease follow the same natural history; some are more aggressive, and some milder. Because the time between development of symptoms and death may vary between diseases, so too the preclinical phase can vary proportionately. Because the preclinical phase represents the window of opportunity for an individual to screen positive on a test, it follows that those individuals screening positive are more likely to have milder courses of disease. The most extreme form of length bias is overdiagnosis. This identifies individuals who would have never known they had the disease if not for screening positively on a test.

SURVEILLANCE

Surveillance involves performing tests on populations to identify outbreaks of disease. Therefore, surveillance targets populations. The aim of surveillance is the prompt identification of shared exposures in order to prevent

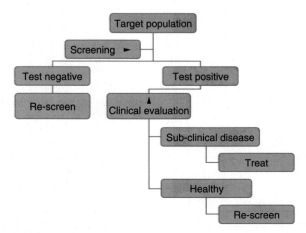

Figure 3-12. Application of a screening test.

additional cases of disease. Ultimately, surveillance is a form of primary prevention; the goal is to prevent new cases of disease.

There are four essential components to any surveillance program:

1. Case reporting
2. Data analysis
3. Communication of results
4. Application of findings

Case Reporting *Passive surveillance* systems rely on the reporting of cases by health care providers. Most jurisdictions have specified lists of conditions that must be reported to public health authorities. These lists are mostly, but not exclusively, infectious diseases. Other potentially reportable conditions include diseases resulting from overexposure to toxic substances, such as lead poisoning, or certain types of cancer. Although reporting of these conditions is required by law and failure to comply is punishable by fines, compliance is generally very poor.

Accordingly, *active surveillance* seeks to improve ascertainment through supplemental measures to prompt case reporting. Public health authorities may contact health care providers to encourage reporting, or large-scale surveys may be undertaken. Although case ascertainment is superior using active surveillance, such programs are more time consuming and costly.

Data Analysis Data must be continuously compiled and analyzed by a central agency to ensure that important trends are promptly recognized. For infectious diseases, this is an essential precondition for effective containment measures. In some cases, such as Ebola virus, even a single case is noteworthy. However, in the case of diseases such as influenza that occur at a regular background rate, the key determination is whether the number of cases is greater than expected, a parameter known as the *epidemic threshold*.

Communication of Results The results of the analysis of surveillance data must be both rapidly and widely disseminated to all who need to know. Therefore, a properly functioning surveillance system involves a bidirectional flow of information: case reporting to a central public health agency and reporting of results from the agency back to health care providers and others. In the United States, an important vehicle for communicating the results of surveillance is the *Morbidity and Mortality Weekly Report* from the Centers for Disease Control and Prevention, which is circulated both electronically and in hardcopy formats.

Application of Findings Surveillance systems have a variety of uses, including the following[9]:

- Triggering rapid interventions as appropriate
- Measuring the burden of disease

- Guiding control measures
- Evaluating health-related policy
- Prioritizing resource allocation
- Characterizing the natural history of disease
- Initiating further research

SUMMARY

Epidemiology is often described as the basic science of public health, and some familiarity with this field is essential to the understanding of causes of disease in global health. Biostatistics provides important measures of morbidity and mortality that serve as indicators of the overall health status of populations and countries. However, a variety of different techniques are needed, such as stratification and survival analysis, to provide greater insight when comparisons are made.

Several study designs are available, each with advantages, disadvantages, and practical limitations. When a disease association is reported by a study, it is important to first address the roles of chance, bias, and confounding as potential explanations. If these three factors are not felt to account for the association, in whole or in part, the association is considered valid. Additional criteria are applied to determine if the association is causal.

Epidemiology has important applications in the management of infectious disease and the early detection of disease through screening and surveillance. Because primary prevention of disease is always preferred, epidemiology and biostatistics provide very powerful tools in global health.

STUDY QUESTIONS

1. A disease has an annual incidence rate of 50 cases per year, mortality of 10 cases per year, and prevalence of 200 cases (all per 1,000,000 people). What is the average duration of the disease?

2. You are working in a hospital in Africa that admits approximately 50 patients a day. There is a concern that deaths from malaria have risen sharply in the past year, and you are asked to analyze data to explore this suspicion. You are told that fairly good-quality mortality data have been kept for several years, which include age and gender of the decedent. However, morbidity data are extremely limited. Moreover, a census has not been carried out in the country in over 25 years. Under these circumstances, what measure of mortality for malaria would you recommend be calculated? What is the limitation of this measure?

3. The minister of health of a Central American country is concerned that a great many citizens have a poor diet and is wondering about spending

additional funds in next year's budget on a community-based dietary education effort that has been shown to be very successful in other parts of Central America. He is well aware of the known adverse health effects of a poor diet but really wants to know how much money will be needed. What is the best choice of study design you could recommend to assist the minister in such circumstances?

4. A medical student unfamiliar with epidemiology proposes to do a case-control study involving in-person interviews with chemotherapy patients (cases) and patients with nonmalignant chronic disease (controls). You point out that some of the signs of chemotherapy, such as hair loss, are very obvious. Thus, determining exposure status in this way may introduce what threat to the validity of the findings?

5. A study is performed examining the relationship between vitamin A consumption and measles. One hundred forty children are enrolled at birth, and the mothers are interviewed. Based on this interview, each child's diet is categorized as either vitamin A adequate or vitamin A deficient. The children are then followed until age 5, and the number of cases of measles is recorded. What is the risk of measles as a result of a vitamin A–deficient diet?

	Measles	No measles
Vitamin A–deficient diet	20	20
Vitamin A–appropriate diet	40	60

6. Three hours following a picnic, 30 of 100 people develop vomiting and diarrhea without fever. All food is immediately disposed of. What type of epidemic curve would be seen for this outbreak?

7. Investigators are studying the use of a new rapid field test to identify patients with cysticercosis. The accompanying table summarizes the results of initial research involving 200 subjects.

	Cysticercosis present	Cysticercosis absent	Total
Test result positive	60	40	100
Test result negative	20	80	100
Total	80	120	200

What is the sensitivity of this test for cysticercosis?

REFERENCES

1. Bradford Hill A. *A Short Textbook of Medical Statistics.* 11th ed. London: Hodder and Stoughton. 1977.

2. Kmet J, Mahboubi E. Esophageal cancer in the Caspian littoral of Iran: initial studies. Science 1972;175(4024):846–853.

3. Centers for Disease Control and Prevention. *Pneumocystis pneumonia—Los Angeles. MMWR* 1981;30(21):1–3.

4. Sonnenberg A, Cucino C, Bauerfeind P. Commentary: the unresolved mystery of birth-cohort phenomena in gastroenterology. *Int J Epidemiol* 2002;31(1):23–26.

5. Centers for Disease Control and Prevention, National Center for Health Statistics. *National Health and Nutrition Examination Survey Data.* Hyattsville, MD: U.S. Department of Health and Human Services, Centers for Disease Control and Prevention. http://www.cdc.gov/nchs/about/major/nhanes/DataAccomp.htm.

6. Chapman RS, Hex, Blair AE, Lan Q. Improvement in household stoves and risk of chronic obstructive pulmonary disease in Xuanwei, China: retrospective cohort study. *BMJ* 2005;331(7524): 1050.

7. Christen WG, Gaziano JM, Hennekens CH. Design of Physicians' Health Study II—a randomized trial of beta-carotene, vitamins E and C, and multivitamins, in prevention of cancer, cardiovascular disease, and eye disease, and review of results of completed trials [abstract]. *Ann Epidemiol* 2000;10(2):125–134.

8. Garly ML, Bale C, Martins CL, et al. Prophylactic antibiotics to prevent pneumonia and other complications after measles: community based randomised double blind placebo controlled trial in Guinea-Bissau. *BMJ* 2006;333(7581):1245.

9. Centers for Disease Control and Prevention. Updated guidelines for evaluating surveillance systems. *MMWR* 2001;50 (RR13):1–35.

The Health of Women/Mothers and Children

4

Judy Lewis and Monika Doshi

LEARNING OBJECTIVES

- *Describe the social and economic context of maternal and child health*
- *Understand the basic terms and definitions of indicators*
- *Understand the main causes of mortality and morbidity*
- *Distinguish maternal health issues and interventions from other women's health issues and describe the relationships among them*
- *Identify low-cost, effective, community-based approaches to intervention*

INTRODUCTION

Global Context

Maternal and child health (MCH) refers to the health status and health services provided to women and children. The emphasis has been on women in their roles as mothers (childbearing and child rearing) and on children, primarily focusing on the healthy survival of infants and young children. Maternal and child health indicators are often used to measure the social, economic, and educational status of women as well as community-level access to primary care. Maternal and child health was the mainstay of international health and development programs until the human immunodeficiency virus/acquired immunodeficiency syndrome (HIV/AIDS) became an epidemic in many parts of the world.

Remarkable achievements have been made in reducing child and maternal mortality and morbidity. However, there is still a large disparity between high- and low-income countries. The highest levels of mother and child health can be found in the Scandinavian countries and Japan. Infant mortality rates of 3/1,000 in Sweden and Japan, child mortality rates of 3/1,000 in Sweden, and maternal mortality rates of 2/100,000 in Sweden represent the best current outcomes. These statistics compare with very poor health indicators in lower-income countries. The highest maternal mortality rate in 2000 was 2,000/100,000 in Sierra Leone. Eighteen countries had maternal mortality rates higher than 1,000/100,000; most of these were in sub-Saharan Africa or in countries experiencing war and conflict, or both.[1] The regions with the highest maternal deaths are Africa and Asia (Table 4-1), with 99% of maternal deaths occurring in low-income countries.[2] Infant mortality disparities show the same trend, although not to the same extreme level. The highest infant mortality rates are found in the same countries with high maternal mortality, with the highest reported in 2003 in Sierra Leone at 166/1,000, comparable to Afghanistan with 165/1,000. Twenty-four countries had infant mortality rates higher than 100/1,000.[1]

The means to improve MCH outcomes have been well demonstrated in high-income countries. It is not just a matter of technology; the health of mothers and children is inexorably linked to the status of women, women's education, and the general socioeconomic well-being of communities. This chapter explores some of the reasons for these differences, with an emphasis on interventions that have made a difference.

A Basic Primer of Maternal and Child Health Indicators and Terms

Prior to an exploration of the issues, it is important to have a basic understanding of some of the terms and indicators used in maternal and child health.

- **Maternal mortality rate (MMR):** The number of maternal deaths per 100,000 births. The formal definition

Table 4-1. Maternal mortality estimates by United Nations Millennium Development Goal regions, 2000.

Region	Maternal mortality ratio (maternal deaths per 100,000 live births)	Number of maternal deaths	Lifetime risk of maternal death, 1 in:
World total	**400**	**529,000**	**74**
Developed regions[a]	**20**	**2,500**	**2,800**
Europe	24	1,700	2,400
Developing regions	**440**	**527,000**	**61**
Africa	830	251,000	20
Northern Africa[b]	130	4,600	210
Sub-Saharan Africa	920	247,000	16
Asia	330	253,000	94
Eastern Asia	55	11,000	840
South-central Asia	520	207,000	46
Southeastern Asia	210	25,000	140
Western Asia	190	9,800	120
Latin America and the Caribbean	190	22,000	160
Oceania	240	530	83

[a]Includes, in addition to Europe, Canada, the United States of America, Japan, Australia, and New Zealand, which are excluded from the regional totals.
[b]Excludes Sudan, which is included in sub-Saharan Africa.
From World Health Organization. *Maternal Mortality in 2000: Estimates Developed by WHO, UNICEF, UNFPA.* Geneva: World Health Organization, 2004. (Reproduced with permission.)[2]

of maternal mortality is death while pregnant or within 42 days of the termination of pregnancy, regardless of the duration or site of the pregnancy. Death may be from any cause related to or aggravated by the pregnancy or its management, but not from accidental or incidental causes.

- **Infant mortality rate (IMR):** The number of infant deaths per 1,000 births. This is defined as a death of a child after birth and during the first year of life.
- **Perinatal mortality rate (PNMR):** The number of perinatal deaths per 1,000 births. Perinatal deaths are defined as occurring during late pregnancy (at 22 completed weeks' gestation and over), during childbirth, and for up to 7 completed days of life.
- **Neonatal mortality rate (NMR):** The number of deaths during the first month of life per 1,000 births.
- **Postneonatal mortality rate (PNNMR):** The number of postnatal deaths (1 month through 12 months) per 1,000 births.
- **Child mortality rate (CMR):** The number of deaths among children younger than 5 years per 1,000 births. This is also referenced as the under-five mortality rate (U5MR).
- **Preterm birth:** Birth at gestational age of less than 37 weeks.
- **Low birth weight (LBW):** Less than 2,500 grams, as defined by the World Health Organization (WHO); may be due to preterm delivery or smallness for

gestational age (intrauterine growth retardation), or to a combination of both.

- **Very low birth weight (VLBW):** Less than 1,500 grams; these infants are too small and undeveloped to survive in most developing country situations.
- **Total fertility rate (TFR):** The number of children that would be born to each woman if she were to live to the end of her childbearing years and bear children at each age at the same rate as the existing age-specific fertility rate. TFR is used to estimate population growth rates.
- **Contraceptive prevalence rate (CPR):** The percentage of married women of reproductive age (15–49) who are using or whose partners are using contraception.
- **Traditional birth attendant (TBA):** A person who assists the mother during childbirth and delivery. This person, who may be male or female, depending on the country and culture, is usually trained through apprenticeship. *Trained TBA* refers to a TBA who has had some formal training in hygienic delivery, often through the provision of WHO birthing kits.
- **Skilled birth attendance:** Delivery by a nurse, nurse midwife, or doctor who is licensed to practice and has undergone specific training.

A warning about mortality and morbidity data: Measurement issues are often a problem; many countries' vital statistics are not reliable or consistently collected. In these situations, there are two approaches to estimating mortality: very large sample sizes and interviews to determine maternal or child deaths, and methods that use smaller sample sizes, such as the Sisterhood Method that was developed in the 1980s for MMR estimation and has been used in many parts of the world to provide data.[3] Obviously, if mortality data can be difficult to estimate, morbidity data have even greater potential for being unreliable.

HISTORICAL PERSPECTIVE

Maternal and child health has always been used as an indicator of the overall health of a society. MCH really began to improve around the beginning of the 20th century in developed countries, when general public health improvements reduced the spread of infectious diseases and economic development increased access to food and better housing. This overview focuses on the period after World War II, when global efforts were initiated after the founding of the United Nations.

Prior to World War II, the health care systems of developed and developing countries were more or less similar. A gradual increase in the standard of living among developed countries led to the betterment of health services, including those that revolved around maternal and child health. After World War II, the health care systems of many developing countries emphasized tertiary care, modeled after the systems that existed in industrialized nations. This resulted in increasing medical specialization and a hierarchy in health care systems in which most of the resources went to tertiary care and technology. The major emphasis for international development agencies during this time was on the eradication of specific diseases such as smallpox, tuberculosis, and malaria. Although there were some successes with this approach, it did not do much to improve health care access at the community level, and MCH health indicators did not greatly improve. Furthermore, the overall disease burden of the poor was not being addressed. The limitations of vertical disease programs were recognized and by 1978, in the Declaration of Alma-Ata, the importance of a holistic approach to health (complete physical, mental, and social well-being) and the role of economic and social development, individual and government responsibility, and primary health care were incorporated in the goal of Health for All by 2000.[4] Unfortunately, this laudable goal was not accomplished, but the striving continues.

Two notable examples of comprehensive, community-based initiatives to provide basic health services to the whole population occurred in China and Cuba. The following discussion provides a specific emphasis on the impact of the comprehensive, bottom-up approach to life expectancy and maternal and infant mortality. For both countries, the foundation for improving population health rested on the commitment to social equity in health services.

China

Despite being a poor nation in the late 1950s, China's highly autocratic government developed an innovative system of medical care. The system was centralized, and the government owned, funded, and ran all hospitals both in the urban and rural areas. The comprehensive approach emphasized medical care for the rural population through capacity development by grassroots recruitment of "barefoot doctors," who were farmers who received basic medical training focused on anatomy, bacteriology, diagnosing disease, acupuncture, prescribing traditional and Western medicines, birth control, and maternal and infant care. They continued to be involved in farmwork, and as a result the rural farmers perceived them as peers and respected their advice. Furthermore, their proximity made them readily available to help those in need of medical attention.

The barefoot doctors were integrated into a three-tier system in which they represented the first tier. Township health centers constituted the next tier. These centers functioned primarily as outpatient clinics and were staffed by assistant doctors. These two lower tiers made up the "rural collective health system" that provided most of the country's medical care. The third and final tier was composed of the county hospitals, which were staffed by senior doctors. For illnesses beyond their training, barefoot doctors referred patients to physicians at the township health centers. The urban model was similar to the rural model. In the urban setting, paramedical personnel were assigned to factories and neighborhood health stations. If the patient required more professional care, then he or she was referred to the district hospital. The final tier in the urban referral system was the municipal hospital.

Barefoot doctors delivered preventive and basic health services to more than 90% of the population. Through preventive care measures, health education, health promotion, and basic health services, the barefoot doctors' work began to improve China's overall health. Between 1952 and 1982, China reduced the rate of infant mortality from 250 to 40 deaths per 1,000 live births, decreased the prevalence of malaria from 5.5% to 0.3% of the population, and increased life expectancy from 35 to 68 years.[5] Maternal mortality fell from over 1,500/100,000 in 1950 to 50/100,000 in 1995.[6]

The success in China led the WHO and leaders in some developing countries to consider the program as an alternate model to health care centered on tertiary care. The model provided an inexpensive way to deliver health care specifically to rural populations. Additionally, a centralized public health focus led to the eradication of many infectious diseases. By the beginning of the 1980s,

China was undergoing an epidemiologic transition in which infectious diseases were giving way to chronic diseases (e.g., heart disease, cancer, and stroke) as the leading causes of illness and death.[7]

The barefoot doctors program ended in the late 1980s and early 1990s. The government provided less financial support for the program, and the barefoot doctors began charging fees for services. The WHO recently ranked China as fourth worst out of 190 countries for equality of health care.

Cuba

Despite poverty and exclusion from mainstream globalization, Cuba has produced excellent health outcomes. The health system in Cuba guarantees universal access to and equity of care for its population. The system is decentralized and delivers everything from basic preventive and primary care to expensive, sophisticated tertiary care. Similar to China, there are three tiers or levels: national, provincial, and municipal. The Ministry of Pubic Health, the central health authority, controls, coordinates, regulates, and operates health care services.[8] For the most part, health services are free of charge to Cuban citizens.

The primary health care system in Cuba focuses on maternal and child health, vaccines, and disease surveillance programs. An intricate public health system monitors the spread of communicable and noncommunicable diseases. Cuba's leading causes of death are now heart disease, cancer, cerebrovascular disease, influenza, pneumonia, and accidents.[8]

The Family Doctor program, created in 1984, is the point of entry to the health system. A physician and nurse team is provided for every 120 to 150 families. The teams live in the community, make home visits, and provide 97% of the national health coverage.[8] The charge of the team is to identify problems and make referrals as needed. The team keeps a census on each family and all medical conditions for each individual within the family, neglecting no one. As a result of this active surveillance and the quality of public health care, in 2001 Cuba had the lowest rates in infant mortality (7.2/1,000), and maternal mortality (34.4/100,000) among Caribbean countries.[8] An increase in life expectancy to 76.3 years has also been observed.[8] These rates are comparable to what is being achieved in developed countries such as the United States and Canada.

Cuba's successes serve as lessons for other nations. The key factors for this achievement include a focus on primary health care as well as 100% population coverage. However, due to a strict US embargo, the scientific and public policy communities are scarcely able to learn what they should from this experience. There has been very little research evaluating how Cuba's successes have been achieved as well as sustained during a period of heavy embargo.

Given this historical background on integrated primary care and MCH service, the rest of the chapter focuses on current health issues and interventions. The success of community-based and community participatory programs is the focus of the last section of this chapter.

MATERNAL AND CHILD HEALTH IN THE 21ST CENTURY: THE UNITED NATIONS MILLENNIUM DEVELOPMENT GOALS

The Millennium Development Goals (MDGs) were developed in the late 1990s using data from 1990 as a baseline to set goals for global development for 2015. Of note, two of the eight goals are specific to MCH, two others are related to women's status and access to education, and two are related to critical issues for women and children: the elimination of extreme poverty and hunger and the reduction of infectious diseases such as HIV and malaria. The remaining two are also of importance, but are more general, addressing environmental and global development partnerships. The eight MDGs are as follows:

1. Eradicate extreme poverty and hunger.
2. Achieve universal primary education.
3. Promote gender equality and empower women.
4. Reduce child mortality.
5. Improve maternal health.
6. Combat HIV, malaria, and other infectious diseases.
7. Ensure environmental sustainability.
8. Develop global partnerships for development.

It is unlikely that these goals and their specific objectives, such as reducing by 50% the proportion of people whose income is less than $1 a day and reducing the under-five mortality rate by two-thirds by 2015, will be realized.[9]

BACKGROUND FACTORS IN GENDER EQUITY

Women's Roles and Health Status

EARLY AGE AT MARRIAGE

A woman's age at first marriage is an important indicator of her social, educational, and economic status and has significant implications for her reproductive health, specifically with respect to childbearing. A woman's exposure to childbearing follows the start of marriage very closely. In many developing countries, between 50% and 75% of all births to married women occur less than 2 years after the women enter their first union.[10] Early marriage, therefore, coincides with childbearing at a young age. A great number of health risks are associated with early pregnancy for a young woman and for her infant, if she carries the pregnancy to term. Moreover, for women who marry young, motherhood often becomes the sole focus, and opportunities for education, employment, and personal growth are lost. Early age at first marriage is often associated with a higher probability of divorce and separation. With the dissolution of marriage, women face economic and social challenges because they usually assume full responsibility for dependent family members.

Prevalence of Early Marriage   Although the situation varies greatly by country and region, marriage during the teenage years is common in developing countries. Women are most likely to marry at a young age in sub-Saharan Africa, as documented by Singh and Samara, who found that 60% to 92% of all women aged 20 to 24 had entered their first union by age 20 in this region.[10] A high prevalence of early marriage was also found in a few countries in other regions. In Bangladesh, Guatemala, India, and Yemen, 60% to 82% of all women aged 20 to 24 had married by age 20.[10] Compared with sub-Saharan Africa, marriage during the teenage years is less common in Latin America, Asia, North Africa, and the Middle East. Twenty percent to 33% of 20- to 24-year-olds in those regions had entered their first marriage by age 18, and 33% to 50% had married by age 20.[10] Even in France and the United States, 11% of all 20- to 24-year-olds had begun their first marriage or were cohabiting by age 18, and 32% had done so by age 20.[10] The only exception to such high rates of marriage during adolescence can be found in Japan, where only 2% of 20- to 24-year-olds had married by age 20.

There are a few developing countries in which marriage before age 18 is uncommon. The proportions of women married by age 18 (10%–14%) in Botswana, Namibia, the Philippines, Sri Lanka, and Tunisia are similar to those in France and the United States. Although most countries have declared 18 as the minimum legal age of marriage, child marriages remain common in rural areas and among groups with the least economic resources. For example, in Ethiopia and some areas of West Africa, some girls are married by age 7, and in Bangladesh, 45% of young women between 25 and 29 were married by age 15. Despite the sanctions on child marriage, more than 100 million young girls are expected to marry in the next decade.[11] Child marriages are most common in sub-Saharan Africa and South Asia.[11] In other parts of Asia, the Middle East and North Africa, marriage at, or shortly after puberty is common among some groups. Figure 4-1 displays averages for young women (aged 15–24) who were married before the age of 18.[11] The regional averages have been segregated further to demonstrate the wide variations that exist among countries in the region.

In some countries, more than half of all girls under 18 are married. Specifically, the percentage of girls (aged 15–19) married by age 18 was as follows[11]:

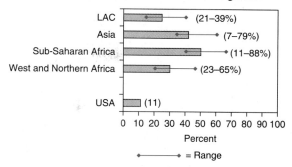

Figure 4-1. Child marriage: substantial variation within countries. LAC, Latin American and the Caribbean. From United Nations Population Fund. Reproductive health and family planning. In: United Nations Population Fund. *State of world population 2005: child marriage fact sheet.* http://www.unfpa.org/swp/2005/presskit/factsheets/facts_child_marriage.htm

- 76% in Niger
- 74% in the Democratic Republic of Congo
- 54% in Afghanistan
- 50% in India

Child Marriage   Child marriage brings additional dimensions that further exacerbate the health status of women. Because it curtails educational opportunities, many girls may be unfamiliar with basic reproductive health issues. Social isolation, limited social support, and powerlessness pose additional reproductive health risks. Lack of autonomy in movement and decision making among young wives can aggravate the risks of maternal mortality and morbidity for pregnant adolescents who already face high-risk pregnancies. There is a strong correlation between the age of the mother and maternal mortality and morbidity. Girls aged 10 to 14 are five times more likely to die in pregnancy or childbirth than women aged 20 to 24.[11] Girls aged 15 to 19 are twice as likely to die (Figure 4-2).[11] The ability to negotiate sexual relations, contraception, and childbearing, as well as other aspects of domestic life, diminishes as the age at first marriage decreases. Furthermore, women who marry younger are more likely to be victims of domestic violence, and more likely to believe that the violence is justified.[11]

Determinants of Early Marriage   The prevalence data clearly indicate that there are variations in the timing of marriage within and between regions. Three factors, however, are thought to be closely correlated and relevant to a women's age at first marriage: female labor

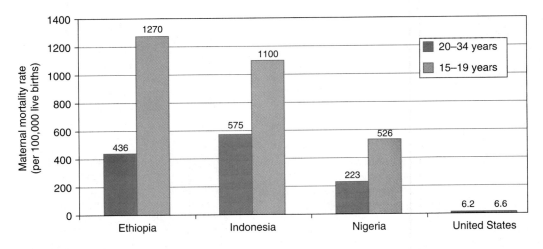

Figure 4-2. Child marriage and maternal mortality: maternal mortality by age. From United Nations Population Fund. Reproductive health and family planning. In: United Nations Population Fund. *State of world population 2005: child marriage fact sheet. http://www.unfpa.org/swp/2005/presskit/factsheets/facts_ child_marriage.htm*

force participation, women's acquisition of formal education, and urbanization. A woman's participation in the formal work sector often exposes her to new ideas and norms that discourage early marriage. Furthermore, economic stability and/or independence as a result of participation in the labor force may enhance a woman's ability to postpone marriage. Moreover, there is an economic incentive for parents to encourage their daughters to remain single and continue working. Therefore, the family pressure to get married often subsides or disappears.

Education is another key variable that is relevant to a woman's age at first marriage. Exposure to formal schooling helps shape values and ideas, often resulting in the adoption of Western values and behavior. Additionally, exposure to and attainment of education often leads to better jobs and higher wages, which, in turn, increase economic stability and reduce motivation for early marriage. Furthermore, with access to higher education and with knowledge in areas such as reproduction, women often have increased ability to regulate their own fertility.

Urbanization is the third factor that influences a woman's age at first marriage. Research shows that there are significant differences in the age at marriage between women who live in urban settings compared with those who live in rural settings. Women living in urban areas marry at a later age. Possible explanations for this include a greater sense of independence gained from greater access to the labor force, increased accessibility to higher education, a greater distance from community-and kinship-based social control, and greater exposure to modern values and beliefs.

OVERVIEW OF MAJOR MATERNAL AND CHILD HEALTH ISSUES

This section addresses the major health problems in MCH, presenting information about epidemiology, causation, health care delivery, and basic treatment or interventions. These topics are organized around a life cycle approach that begins with family planning. The other major issues that affect both mothers and children are anemia, pregnancy, childbirth, and perinatal, infant, child, and adolescent health.

Access to Family Planning

Reproductive choice is a basic human right. The aim of family planning programs is to enable individuals to decide freely and responsibly the number and spacing of their children; to have the information and means to do so; to ensure informed choices; and to make available a full range of safe and effective methods of contraception.[12] However, access to relevant information and high-quality services is limited in many regions of the world. Most family planning programs have been targeted at women; therefore, this section concentrates on them.

During the 1994 International Conference on Population and Development (ICPD), 180 nations adopted a program of action that included, among its major goals, improving reproductive health and making family planning services universally available. However, there are approximately 137 million reproductive-age women, 122.7 million of them in the developing countries and the former Soviet republics, who are not using contraception in spite of an expressed desire to space or limit the numbers of their births.[11,13] These women are considered to have an "unmet need for family planning."

Women between 15 and 49 years are considered to be of reproductive age. Before examining the global estimates as well as the impact of unmet need on MCH, it is beneficial to understand how the unmet need for family planning is estimated. It has conventionally been estimated from representative population-based surveys of currently married women as the sum of the currently pregnant women who report that their pregnancy is unintended (those who wish to limit their births) and the number of currently nonpregnant women who are not using contraception and would not like to have any more children or, at least, none in the next 2 years (those who wish to space their births).[14] This method to estimate unmet need has been criticized because it is thought to underestimate the actual numbers. Furthermore, it excludes both currently married women who are not pregnant and who are using ineffective or unsatisfactory methods of contraception and sexually active women who are not currently married and who do not wish to become pregnant, at least in the next 2 years.

The debate about expanding the definition of unmet need continues. Ross and Winfrey used an expanded definition to offer an updated estimate of unmet need in the developing world and the former Soviet republics.[13] Under their definition, the group includes all fecund women, married or living in union, who are not using any method of contraception and who either do not want to have any more children or who want to postpone their next birth for at least 2 more years. The group also includes all pregnant married women and women who have recently given birth and are still amenorrheic. They are included if their pregnancies or births are unwanted or mistimed because they were not using contraception. This approach may still underestimate the number of women with unmet need because the group does not include users of traditional methods who may have an unmet need for modern methods. Their inclusion would result in considerably larger estimates, especially in regions where the use of traditional methods is popular.

Table 4-2 shows the number and percentage of women with an unmet need for contraception in various regions.[13] The number of women in the reproductive-age group varies by region, with 58% of the total for the developing world in Asia, which contains 61 million married women with unmet need. It is important to keep in mind that Asia contains several countries with very large populations (India, Indonesia, Pakistan, and Bangladesh). With the inclusion of populous countries such as Nigeria, Ethiopia, South Africa, and the Democratic Republic of the Congo, sub-Saharan Africa contains

24 million married women with unmet need (22% of the total). Latin America contributes 11 million married women with unmet need (11%), nearly half of whom live in Mexico and Brazil. North Africa and the Middle East account for only about 8 million (8%). The Central Asian republics, which have smaller populations, have a total of 1.1 million (1%).

Regional variations in the prevalence among women who wish to space or limit births are evident. Ross and Winfrey found that in sub-Saharan Africa, 65% of unmet need is for spacing, in contrast to Latin America, where it is only 42%. In other regions, such as Asia, spacing and limiting needs are nearly equal. Unmarried women add to unmet need, accounting for 7% of the developing world total.[13] The proportion varies by region, ranging from 4% in Asia to 16% in sub-Saharan Africa. These differences in demand affect the kinds of contraceptive supplies needed as well as budgetary allocations.

There are a number of proven benefits associated with family planning, including maternal health, child survival, gender equality, and HIV prevention. Additionally, family planning can improve family well-being, raise female economic productivity, and lower fertility, thereby reducing poverty and promoting economic growth.[11] Despite these outcomes, the unmet need for family planning still persists. The causes for unmet need include lack of accessible services; shortages of equipment, commodities, and personnel; lack of method choices appropriate to the situation of the woman and her family; lack of knowledge about the safety, effectiveness, and availability of choices; lack of community or spousal support (social opposition); misinformation and rumors; health concerns about possible side effects; and financial constraints.[11,15]

A number of social, cultural, and gender-related obstacles can prevent a woman from realizing her childbearing preferences. At the policy level, for example, decision makers may not place high priority on funding contraceptive services because they view them as "women's programs." Laws may require the woman to seek her husband's approval to use some methods.[16] At the health facilities level, service providers' bias may limit options for contraception.[16] At the community level, contraceptives may be considered as contributing to female promiscuity.[16] Furthermore, men often have a greater decision-making power to determine family size. Additionally, social norms regarding fertility and virility, and the overall low status of women, keep many women and men from seeking family planning.[16]

Over the years, the WHO and the United States Agency for International Development (USAID) have made varying recommendations on birth spacing. These recommendations, which have traditionally been based on pregnancy outcomes, have caused confusion due to the differences in the time interval recommended between births by each agency. A 2006 WHO

Table 4-2. Number and percentage of women with an unmet need for contraception, by region, according to marital status, and, for married women, reason for needing contraception, 2000.

Region	Number (thousands)					Percentage				
		Married women					Married women			
	All women	All	Spacing	Limiting	Unmarried women	All women	All	Spacing	Limiting	Unmarried women
Developing world	**113,647**	**105,205**	**55,402**	**49,803**	**8,842**	**13.0**	**17.1**	**9.0**	**8.1**	**3.2**
Asia (except China)	63,650	61,142	31,658	29,484	2,508	12.9	16.4	8.5	7.9	2.0
Sub-Saharan Africa	27,997	23,550	15,269	8,281	4,447	19.4	24.2	15.7	8.5	9.5
Latin America/ Caribbean	11,837	11,088	4,615	6,473	749	8.5	13.7	5.7	8.0	1.3
North Africa/ Middle-East	8,925	8,306	3,345	4,961	619	10.6	15.6	6.3	9.3	2.0
Central Asia	1,238	1,119	515	604	119	8.5	11.4	5.2	6.2	2.6
Other regions	**9,050**	u	u	u	u	u	u	u	u	u
Russia	4,604	u	u	u	u	14.5	u	u	u	u
Eastern Europe	3,594	u	u	u	u	10.7	u	u	u	u
Caucasus	633	u	u	u	u	14.3	u	u	u	u
Baltic republics	219	u	u	u	u	11.5	u	u	u	u

Currently married women include those in consensual unions. u=unavailable.
From Ross JA, Winfrey W. Unmet need for contraception in the developing world and former Soviet Union: an updated estimate. *Int Fam Plann Perspect* 2002;28(3):138–143.
(Reproduced with permission.)

report, supported by USAID, recommends an interval of at least 24 months following a live birth to the next pregnancy in order to reduce the risk of adverse maternal, perinatal, and infant outcomes. An interval of at least 6 months to the next pregnancy is recommended following a miscarriage or induced abortion.

The unmet need for spacing has multiple consequences on maternal and child health. First, maternal depletion, defined as a broad pattern of maternal malnutrition resulting from the combined effects of dietary inadequacy, heavy workloads, and energy costs of repeated pregnancy, can result in increased maternal morbidity and mortality. There is, however, limited empirical evidence to support the theory of maternal depletion. The consequences for infants born after a short birth interval can include poor intrauterine growth and an increased risk of preterm birth.[17] Second, close birth spacing may further burden already limited family resources. Third, a child born before a short birth interval can also suffer from nutritional deficits as the mother interrupts breastfeeding to focus on the newborn. Fourth, the likelihood of transmission of infectious diseases is increased as a result of overcrowding and the presence of children of similar ages.

As with the unmet need for spacing, a number of consequences are associated with the unmet need to limit births. The WHO estimates that approximately 38% of all pregnancies occurring around the world every year are unintended. Moreover, about six of ten such unplanned pregnancies result in induced abortion. Unintended pregnancies increase the lifetime risk of maternal mortality. They can also lead to unsafe abortion, poor infant health, and lower investment in the child.

Table 4-3. Cut-offs for the World Health Organization's definition of anemia.

	Hemoglobin below (g/dL)	Hematocrit below (%)
Children 6–60 months	11.0	33
Children 5–11 years	11.5	34
Children 12–15 years	12.0	36
Nonpregnant women	12.0	36
Pregnant women	11.0	33
Men	13.0	39

From UNICEF. *Prevention and Control of Iron Deficiency Anaemia in Women and Children: Report of the UNICEF/WHO Regional Consultation.* Geneva: UNICEF and World Health Organization, 1999.[18]

Anemia

Iron deficiency, specifically iron deficiency anemia, remains one of the most severe and important nutritional deficiencies in the world today. Anemia is characterized by a hemoglobin concentration below the established cut-off levels (Table 4-3).[18] Although the greatest burden is felt in the developing world, anemia and iron deficiency anemia exist in every country of the world. It is important to differentiate between anemia, iron deficiency, and iron deficiency anemia (see Box 4-1).[19] Dietary iron deficiency is the most common cause of anemia; however, it is not the sole contributor to the etiology of anemia. Other causes include malaria, other parasitic diseases

---

BOX 4-1. DEFINITIONS AND DISTINCTIONS: ANEMIA, IRON DEFICIENCY, AND IRON DEFICIENCY ANEMIA

- **Anemia:** Abnormally low hemoglobin level due to pathological condition(s). Iron deficiency is one of the most common causes, but not the only cause, of anemia. Other causes of anemia include chronic infections, particularly malaria; hereditary hemoglobinopathies; and other micronutrient deficiencies, particularly folic acid deficiency. It is worth noting that multiple causes of anemia can coexist in an individual or in a population and contribute to the severity of the anemia.

- **Iron deficiency:** Functional tissue iron deficiency and the absence of iron stores, with or without anemia. Iron deficiency is defined by abnormal iron biochemistry with or without the presence of anemia. Iron deficiency is usually the result of inadequate bioavailable dietary iron, increased iron requirement during a period of rapid growth (pregnancy and infancy),

and/or increased blood loss, such as gastrointestinal bleeding due to hookworm or urinary blood loss due to schistosomiasis.

- **Iron deficiency anemia:** Iron deficiency, when sufficiently severe, causes anemia. Although some functional consequences may be observed in individuals who have iron deficiency without anemia, cognitive impairment, decreased physical capacity, and reduced immunity are commonly associated with iron deficiency anemia. In severe iron deficiency anemia, capacity to maintain body temperature may also be reduced. Severe anemia is life threatening.

Source: Yip R, Lynch S. Definitions of anemia, iron deficiency, and iron deficiency anemia. Presented at: Technical Workshop, UNICEF; October 7–9, 1998; New York, NY.[19]

(hookworm, schistosomiasis), folate deficiency, HIV infection, and hemoglobinopathies.

The WHO estimates that there are 2 billion anemic people worldwide and that approximately 50% of all cases can be attributed to iron deficiency. Women of reproductive age, especially during pregnancy, infants older than 6 months of age, and young children are among the most affected.[20]

PREVALENCE

Anemia is more prevalent in women than men, in younger than older individuals, and in the poor than the better-off.[21] Estimates of prevalence rates of iron deficiency anemia often use rates of anemia as a proxy. The prevalence of anemia differs from region to region, and its links to poverty are apparent. It ranges from 5% to 16% in industrialized countries.[18] The lowest rates are found in western Europe (5% anemic) and North America (10% anemic); the highest rate in an industrialized area is eastern Europe (16% anemic).[18] In nonindustrialized countries, 30% to 60% of nonpregnant women are anemic, with the highest rates occurring in Africa and Asia.[18] The main cause of anemia in industrialized countries is iron deficiency. However, in nonindustrialized countries, factors such as malaria and parasitic infections (hookworm) often play a role.

The population most affected differs between industrialized and nonindustrialized countries. In industrialized countries, the most affected groups are pregnant women (18% anemic), school children (17% anemic), and nonpregnant women and the elderly (both 12% anemic).[18] In contrast, in the nonindustrialized countries, the most affected population groups are pregnant women and school-aged children (both 53% anemic), nonpregnant women (44% anemic), preschool children (42% anemic), and the elderly (51% anemic).[18]

HEALTH CONSEQUENCES

The consequences of iron deficiency anemia in the general population include increased morbidity from infectious diseases because anemia adversely affects the immune system. It also reduces the body's ability to monitor and regulate body temperature when exposed to cold. Furthermore, cognitive performance is impaired at all stages of life, and physical work capacity is significantly reduced as a result of iron deficiency.

Women, in particular, are at risk of anemia due to periodic menstrual blood loss and an increase in red blood cell mass and expansion of plasma volume during pregnancy.[21] Anemia affects nearly half of the pregnant women in the world—52% in nonindustrialized countries compared with 23% in industrialized countries.[22] For example, in India, up to 88% of pregnant women are affected, and in Africa, about 50% of pregnant women

are affected.[20] In Latin America and the Caribbean, the prevalence of anemia in pregnancy is about 40%. The highest levels, reaching 60% in pregnant women, are found on some Caribbean islands. In most industrialized countries, the prevalence of anemia among pregnant women is around 20%, and it is more likely to be adequately treated.[20]

Iron deficiency anemia during pregnancy has serious clinical consequences. It is associated with multiple adverse outcomes for both mother and infant, including intrauterine growth retardation, an increased risk of hemorrhage, sepsis, maternal mortality, infant mortality, perinatal mortality, increased stillbirths, low birth weight, and prematurity. Forty percent of all maternal perinatal deaths are linked to anemia.[20] Favorable pregnancy outcomes occur 30% to 45% less often in anemic mothers, and their infants have less than one-half of normal iron reserves.[20] Pregnant women who are severely anemic are less able to withstand blood loss and may require blood transfusion. The availability and safety of blood poses a dilemma in poorer countries, which usually have a higher prevalence and a more complex etiology of anemia.

PREVENTION AND CONTROL

A range of strategies is used to control and prevent anemia. These strategies include food-based approaches, food fortification, and iron supplementation. Food-based approaches center on dietary improvement by increasing the micronutrient intake. They ensure year-round availability and accessibility to micronutrient-rich foods, especially for those at risk, such as women of reproductive age. Building and strengthening food-based approaches centered on the activities and needs of women is essential because women play multiple roles as food providers and primary caregivers. Enrichment of food, or food fortification, is another alternative. However, due to its technical, operational, and financial feasibility, this alternative may not be sustainable in resource-poor settings. When food fortification does not prove to be a sustainable alternative, iron supplementation is the strategy of choice to control iron deficiency in resource-poor countries. Traditionally, target groups for supplementation programs have been pregnant women and infants.[20]

Pregnancy and Childbirth

Pregnancy and childbirth are a natural part of the human life cycle. However, pregnancy and delivery can be very dangerous for women with complications who do not have access to emergency care. Delivery and the immediate newborn period is a similarly dangerous period for infants. Two factors that play major roles in both maternal and neonatal birth outcomes are where and by whom a woman is delivered. Whereas hospital delivery with a doctor in attendance is the norm for high-income countries, most women, especially in the lowest-income countries, deliver at home with assistance from unskilled caregivers.

PRENATAL CARE

The relationship between early and frequent provision of prenatal care and better MCH outcomes has been well documented. The WHO recommends a minimum of four antenatal visits with skilled health professionals (nurses, nurse midwives, or doctors).[23] The purpose of these visits is to provide early contact with health care, immunization, maternal monitoring, screening, treatment, and referral. Early and more frequent contact with health care provides the opportunity to increase health knowledge and improve health behaviors, as well as access to the following services:

- Maternal monitoring, including monitoring of nutrition and weight gain, and the identification of problems such as anemia and hypertension. In some programs prenatal care includes food supplementation for pregnant women.
- Screening and treatment for sexually transmitted infections (STIs) and HIV, and preparing HIV-positive pregnant women for antiretroviral treatment to prevent mother-to-child transmission.
- Treatment of malaria, tuberculosis, and other diseases that may cause additional problems for a pregnant woman and her fetus.

Prenatal care allows for the identification of women at high risk based on obstetric history, complications, and general health status. It is important to note that 40% of all pregnant women experience some type of complication and 15% have a serious complication requiring immediate obstetric attention. In most cases this risk cannot be predicted, which means that all women require skilled care to prevent maternal and neonatal deaths.

THE ROLE OF TRADITIONAL BIRTH ATTENDANTS

Traditional birth attendants (TBAs) are usually apprenticed with an experienced TBA to learn the skills of delivering babies. In some countries, training in more sanitary delivery techniques, such as the use of new razors, and in the recognition of danger signs and when to refer, has been provided to TBAs, who are then called trained TBAs. The WHO has provided home delivery kits (soap, new razors, gauze, and other materials for delivery) to many programs, which provide soap, new razors, gauze, and other materials for delivery. These kits can also be assembled locally. TBAs provide accessible community-based care that incorporates local beliefs and traditions. Many women prefer to deliver at home with their family, where they can follow traditional practices regarding care of the mother and baby and disposition of the placenta.

TBAs typically do not provide prenatal care, although this has been incorporated in TBA training so that they can identify women at risk. However, there has been considerable controversy about the role of TBAs and whether it is possible to improve maternal and prenatal outcomes during home deliveries by TBAs.[24,25] A major issue is that even trained TBAs observing best practices are unable to refer and transport mothers and babies to higher-level intervention when emergencies occur.[26] As a result, the WHO recommended that women be delivered by skilled health personnel (an accredited health professional, midwife, doctor, or nurse who has been educated and trained to manage normal pregnancies and deliveries and to refer complications). These goals were incorporated in the Millennium Development Goals. The MDGs set the objective of 80% of all births assisted by skilled attendants by 2005; however, this goal has not been reached, nor is it likely that the goal of 95% will be reached by 2015.[9] Currently, only 58% of women in developing countries deliver with skilled attendance, but this does not reflect the situation in countries such as Haiti and regions such as sub-Saharan African, where 80% to 90% of deliveries occur at home with TBAs. The MDGs also set the goal of reducing maternal mortality by 75% between 1990 and 2015.

LIMITED ACCESS TO PRIMARY CARE AND HOSPITAL SERVICES

Related to the issue of home delivery by TBAs is access to primary care and hospital services. Prenatal care, especially tetanus immunization and iron supplementation, has been demonstrated to improve pregnancy outcomes, but it requires that women have access to basic primary care services. The recommendation is that women have a minimum of four prenatal visits. At least 35% of women in developing countries receive no antenatal care during pregnancy, almost 50% give birth without a skilled attendant, and 70% receive no postpartum care in the 6 weeks following delivery (Figure 4-3).[27] This lack of care is most life threatening during childbirth and the days immediately after delivery, because these are the times when sudden, life-threatening complications are most likely to arise.

DELIVERY CARE

As mentioned previously, the majority of maternal complications occur within 24 hours of delivery, requiring access to appropriate care. Although the percentage of births with skilled attendance has increased in all regions of the world, there is still a large gap between high-income and low-income countries (Figure 4-4).

Delivery Sites and Personnel It is important that delivery sites have the appropriate medications and technology, as well as well-trained staff. They should be affordable and accessible, and emergency transport

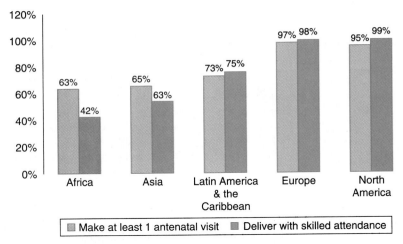

Figure 4-3. Maternity care. From World Health Organization. *Coverage of Maternity Care: A Listing of Available Information.* 4th ed. Geneva: World Health Organization, 1997. (Reproduced with permission.)[27]

should be provided for women who do not live near the facilities. One approach has been the development of maternal waiting homes, where women who are having problems during pregnancy, and those who are very young or very old, can stay near a hospital, receiving treatment and good nutrition.

An intermediate intervention when skilled attendance at a hospital or clinic is not available has been to train TBAs to provide better services during delivery and to recognize complications and refer. This has been the subject

of considerable controversy because some research found no difference between trained and untrained TBAs.[24,25] Even skilled attendance is not necessarily enough to make a difference and is contingent on other systemic factors.[26]

Where skilled delivery is available in sterile clinic sites, midwives and nurses as well as doctors are able to provide more appropriate interventions, such as active management of the third stage of labor. This includes both physiologic and drug management to limit labor time and reduce maternal and infant complications

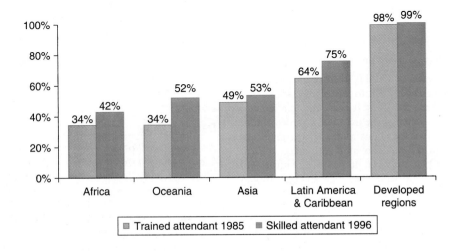

Figure 4-4. Changes in attendance at delivery, 1985–1996. From http://www.safemotherhood.org/ facts_and_figures/maternal_health.htm. (Reproduced with permission.)

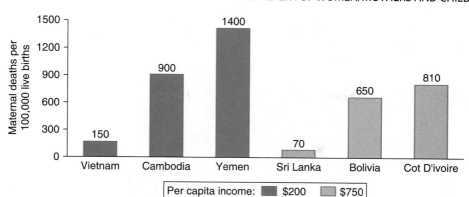

Figure 4-5. Maternal mortality by income levels, selected countries. From Tinker A. Safe motherhood as an economic and social investment. Presented at: Safe Motherhood Technical Consultation; October 18–23, 1997; Sri Lanka; and World Health Organization and United Nations Children Fund. *Revised 1990 Estimates of Maternal Mortality: A New Approach by WHO and UNICEF.* Geneva: World Health Organization, 1996. (Reproduced with permission.)[29]

such as postpartum hemorrhage and infant death. This can be done with relatively inexpensive medications (oxytocics) and simple physical maneuvers in a hospital setting and does not require extensive equipment or training.

Financial resources are not the only answer to reducing maternal mortality (Figure 4-5). Countries with a per capita gross national product (GNP) of $1,000 or less have maternal mortality ratios ranging from as low as 70 to as high as 1,400.[28] This suggests that there are many ways to improve maternal mortality in resource-poor settings.

Consequences for the Mother Thirty million women developed complications from pregnancy and childbirth in 2004. The most common causes of maternal morbidity and mortality were as follows:[22]

- Hemorrhage (25% of deaths, often associated with anemia as a result of poor nutrition or malaria)
- Infections (15% of deaths, mainly sepsis)
- Unsafe abortion (13% of deaths due to a variety of severe complications, including sepsis, hemorrhage, uterine trauma, and poisoning due to ingestion of toxic substances)
- High blood pressure (12% of deaths due to eclampsia during pregnancy)
- Obstructed labor (8% of deaths and a cause of many long-term complications for the mother, as well as newborn death and disability)

These five conditions account for over 70% of the MMR. Inadequate health care, poor health status, and inadequate nutrition are the major underlying causes.[2,29]

With limited resources and deficient health care systems, many preventable emergencies occur because of lack of treatment or a delay in care.[30] The "three delays

model" was developed by Thaddeus and Maine to describe the complex issues preventing pregnant women from receiving adequate care.[31] Phase 1 involves delay in seeking care (unawareness of complications, acceptance of maternal death, and sociocultural factors such as beliefs, practices, and women's decision-making ability), phase 2 involves delay in reaching care (due to poor roads, geographic barriers, and poor service organization), and phase 3 involves delay in the decision to seek care (because of health care system problems, including lack of facilities and personnel and lack of a family's ability to pay for services). This complex array of causes leads to the causes of maternal death listed previously, resulting in 529,000 maternal deaths in 2004.[2]

This section addresses the major causes of maternal death and morbidity. Figure 4-6 illustrates the proportion of deaths attributable to these causes and interventions that have been developed to prevent or treat them.

- **Hemorrhage:** Severe bleeding has been identified as the most important cause of maternal death. Over half of maternal deaths occur within 24 hours of delivery, and most of these are from hemorrhage. Anemia is a major contributor to maternal deaths from hemorrhage. Because risk for hemorrhage cannot be predicted with high accuracy, skilled attendance and access to hospital services are recommended for all women. Women should be monitored for complications of hemorrhage during the immediate postpartum period. If severe bleeding occurs, women should be stabilized and referred to the next level of care.[32]

- **Infection:** Postpartum endometritis, puerperal sepsis, and urinary tract infection are the most common infections following childbirth. These infections can be prevented by good prenatal, delivery, and postpartum care,

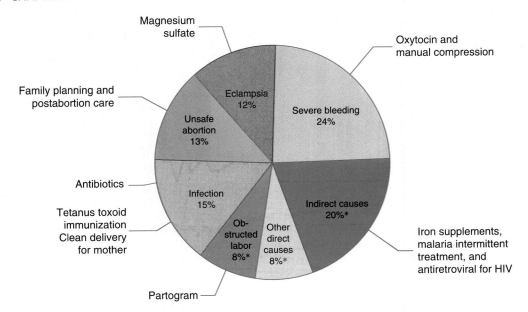

Figure 4-6. Proportion of deaths attributable to major causes of maternal death and morbidity and the interventions that have been developed to prevent or treat them. *Other direct causes include ectopic pregnancy, embolism, and those related to anesthesia. Indirect causes include anemia, malaria, and heart disease. From USAID. Maternal and child health: technical areas. Postpartum and newborn care. 2005. http://www.usaid.gov/our_work/ global_health/mch/ mh/techareas/maternal_mortality.html.

especially by maintaining sterile delivery techniques. Infections must be treated immediately after occurrence to prevent chronic problems, including infertility and death from generalized sepsis.[33]

- **Unsafe abortion:** 68,000 maternal deaths each year can be attributed to unsafe abortion, and essentially all of these occur in developing countries.[34] Unsafe abortion is a procedure for terminating an unwanted pregnancy by persons lacking the necessary skills or in an environment lacking the minimal medical standards, or both.[35] The risks are determined by the health of the woman, the method used, and the hygiene of the instruments and the setting. Severe complications such as infection, hemorrhage, perforated uterus, and poisoning due to ingestion of harmful substances may result in death or permanent disability.[36]

- **Obstetric fistula:** *Fistula* refers to any abnormal connection between two bodily organs. There are two types of obstetric fistula: vesicovaginal and rectovaginal. A vesicovaginal fistula is a hole between the wall of the vagina and the bladder, resulting in urinary incontinence. A rectovaginal fistula is a hole between the wall of the vagina and the rectum, resulting in fecal incontinence. Both types of obstetric fistula are caused by abnormal pressure of the fetal

head during obstructed labor, which interrupts the flow of blood to nearby tissues in the mother's pelvis. Early childhood marriage is the most common cause of obstructed labor resulting in fistula. Very young women are not physically developed enough to allow the easy passage of a baby. The result is that the child dies in childbirth and the mother suffers a lifetime of ostracism and neglect due to chronic infections, poor hygiene, and social stigma. Another contributing factor is female genital cutting or mutilation, when the cutting of the vaginal wall goes too deep.

- **Eclampsia:** Eclampsia and preeclampsia are hypertensive disorders of pregnancy. Eclampsia is a seizure activity or coma in a pregnant woman with preeclampsia. Preeclampsia is characterized by high blood pressure and proteinuria. Preeclampsia occurs in 5% to 8% of pregnancies; symptoms include swelling, sudden weight gain, headaches, and changes in vision, although some women may be asymptomatic. The specific cause of these conditions is not well understood.[37] Two major collaborative research projects in the past 12 years examined the effectiveness of treatment. The first project, the Collaborative Eclampsia Trial, found that magnesium sulfate was the most effective treatment for controlling eclamptic convulsions.[38] More recently, the Magpie Trial conducted a randomized controlled trial of magnesium sulfate versus placebo in 33 countries and found a 50% reduction in eclampsia in response to magnesium sulfate.[39] A *Lancet* commentary in the same issue as the report of that study made a call for global implementation of magnesium sulfate treatment for women with preeclampsia, stating that it is safe, effective, and relatively inexpensive, costing no more than US $5 per patient.[40]

In addition to the loss of women's lives, maternal deaths directly affect child health and well-being. According to a 2004 WHO report, an estimated 1 million children die as a result of their mother's death every year. Large numbers of orphans become the responsibility of extended families and communities, which often lack resources to provide proper care.[2]

On the continuum of maternity care, antenatal and perinatal care take precedence over postpartum/postnatal care. Many maternal and neonatal deaths occur in the 48 hours after labor and birth; therefore, care of the mother and child should not stop after delivery. Postpartum/postnatal care and follow-up are essential for the health of the mother and her child. There must be collaboration between parents, families, caregivers (trained or traditional), health professionals, health planners, health care administrators, and other related sectors such as community groups, policy makers, and politicians.[41] Basic postpartum/postnatal care includes warmth and cleanliness of the newborn, treatment for complications such as birth asphyxia, hygienic cord care, antibiotics for infection, immunizations, exclusive breastfeeding, maternal nutrition (including micronutrient supplementation) and counseling, birth spacing and other family planning services, and interventions for the prevention of mother-to-child transmission.[42]

Perinatal and Neonatal Mortality

Perinatal deaths occur during childbirth and the first week of life; *neonatal mortality* occurs during the first 28 days of life and includes perinatal mortality. These periods are also referred to as early and late neonatal mortality. The causes of death in the first week and the first month are similar, although the role of infectious diseases increases with age in the first month.

PERINATAL DEATHS

There were more than 6.3 million perinatal deaths in 2000.[43] Almost 98% of deaths occurred in developing countries, with 27% of these in the least developed countries. Africa had the highest regional perinatal death rate (62/1,000), followed by Asia (50/1,000), Oceania (42/1,000), the Caribbean (31/1,000), and Latin America (20/1,000).[43]

However, in reality the situation is even worse. In developing countries, many infants who die in the womb or soon after birth are not reported.[44] Underregistration of perinatal mortality has been estimated to be as high as 20% of perinatal deaths.[44,45]

The most common causes of perinatal mortality are unexplained intrauterine death in pregnancy, intrauterine death due to maternal complications, intrapartum death due to obstetrical complications, inadequate management of birth, birth asphyxia, preterm birth, sepsis, congenital anomalies, and low birth weight. Deaths in the early neonatal period (during the first week of life) are largely the result of inadequate or inappropriate care during pregnancy, childbirth, or the first critical hours after birth.[44,46]

Perinatal mortality is generally high in most developing countries because of low socioeconomic conditions and lack of emergency obstetric and neonatal services.[46] The perinatal mortality rate is used as an indicator of the quality of antenatal and perinatal care and of the general health status of pregnant women, new mothers, and newborns.[45] This indicator is a major marker of maternal care and of maternal health and nutrition as well; it is also affected by the availability and quality of in-hospital care for neonates.[43]

Perinatal mortality varies by country and region. Some developing countries have reduced the perinatal mortality rate by regular mortality review and auditing of practice.[46] Effective technical and community interventions are important to reduce the incidence and severity of major complications associated with pregnancy and childbirth, including perinatal mortality.[2]

Other serious newborn morbidity results from neonatal tetanus, disturbance in thermoregulation, jaundice, ophthalmia neonatorum, neonatal herpes infection, hepatitis B, and HIV; the last two result from vertical transmission.[41]

Figure 4-7 illustrates the relative proportion of neonatal deaths by cause, and interventions that have been proven effective in preventing or treating these conditions.

Maternal health factors play a role in neonatal death, including access to family planning and prenatal care (syphilis screening, folate and nutrition supplementation, vaccination against tetanus, malaria treatment, and promotion of exclusive breastfeeding). Access to health interventions such as safe delivery practices, eye care, kangaroo care (discussed later in this chapter), and treatment of infections is also critical for the newborn. Some of the most important recent developments in MCH address these issues in a comprehensive way.

POSTNEONATAL AND INFANT MORTALITY

Postneonatal mortality refers to infant deaths during the period of ages 1 month to 12 months. Deaths in this age group are primarily due to infection, malnutrition, and dehydration. These conditions are similar to those

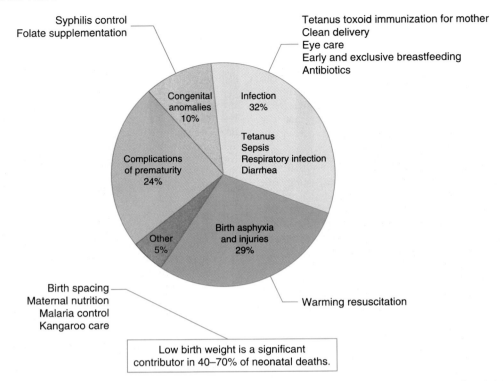

Figure 4-7. Evidence-based interventions for major causes of neonatal death. From USAID. Maternal and child health: technical areas. Postpartum and newborn care. 2005. http://www.usaid.gov/our_work/global_health/mch/mh/techareas/neonatal_death.html.

of early childhood and are addressed in the following section. It is important to note that in the first year of life the severity of these conditions is often greater and more likely to result in death. Nutrition is critical during the first year of life, both in terms of the promotion of exclusive breastfeeding in the first 6 months and the transition to other foods, which is often a time of decreasing growth for infants due to the poor quality of weaning foods. These issues are addressed more fully in Chapter 6.

Infant mortality refers to all deaths of children younger than 1 year of age and thus is the sum of neonatal and postneonatal mortality.

Early Childhood

Although the risk of death during the neonatal period is greater, much of the attention and data on child health concentrates on children younger than 5 years of age.

Malnutrition (undernutrition) is the underlying cause of 53% of deaths among children younger than 5 years (Figure 4-8).[47] The nutritional status of a woman during adolescence, pregnancy, and lactation has a direct impact on her child's health as well as her own health. In many developing countries, the nutritional status of large segments of the population, especially women, is inadequate. Undernutrition of women can be attributed to discrimination in terms of food allocation, to the heavy burden of physical labor, and to reproduction.[41] Nutritional indicators such as low birth weight, wasting, stunting, and underweight are discussed in Chapter 6. Micronutrient malnutrition also has public health significance. The four main vitamin and mineral nutritional deficiencies are vitamin A, iron, zinc, and iodine (see Chapter 6). Ensuring proper nutrition for both mother and child is essential. With respect to infant feeding practice, the WHO and UNICEF recommend exclusive breastfeeding for 6 months. Thereafter, infants should receive complementary foods with continued breastfeeding up to 2 years of age or beyond. Breastfeeding promotes sensory and cognitive development. Furthermore, infants who are exclusively breastfed are likely to suffer only one-fourth as many episodes of diarrhea and respiratory infections as babies who are not breastfed.[48] Breastfeeding contributes to the health and well-being of mothers as well. It helps to space children and reduces the risk of ovarian cancer and breast cancer.

About 20% of all deaths in children younger than 5 years are due to acute respiratory infection (ARI). A

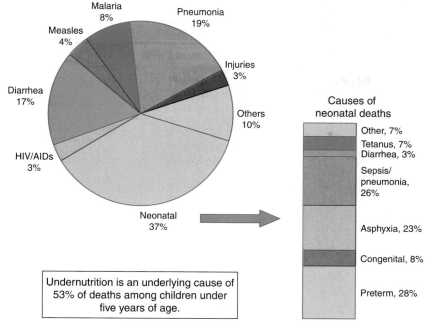

Figure 4-8. Major causes of death among children younger than 5 years and neonates in the world, 2000–2003. From World Health Organization, Department of Child and Adolescent Health and Development. Overview of CAH: major causes of death among children under five years of age and neonates in the world, 2000–2003. http://www.who.int/child-adolescent-health/Overview/Child_Health/map_00-03_world.jpg.[47]

subgroup of ARI is acute lower respiratory infection (ALRI), which includes pneumonia, bronchiolitis, and bronchitis. Ninety percent of ARI deaths are due to pneumonia.[49] The risk of getting pneumonia increases if the child is of low birth weight, malnourished, and non-breastfed. The risk is also increased among children living in overcrowded conditions. These children are at higher risk of death from pneumonia as well. The spread of ARI is worldwide; however, the burden is most felt in developing countries. Whereas 1% to 3% of the deaths in children under 5 in industrialized countries are due to pneumonia, the disease causes 10% to 25% of these deaths in developing countries.[50] Treatment is possible through inexpensive pneumonia medications; however, accessibility and affordability of health care becomes an issue in many developing countries.

Diarrhea is the second leading cause of child deaths and kills 1.9 million young children every year, mostly from dehydration. As with ARI, the greatest burden of diarrheal diseases is in the developing world. Dehydration from diarrhea can be prevented by giving extra fluids at home or can be treated simply, effectively, and cheaply in all age groups.[51] With the exception of severe cases, diarrhea can be treated with administration (by mouth) of an adequate glucose-electrolyte solution. Oral rehydration therapy (ORT), that is, giving fluids

to prevent or treat dehydration, combined with guidance on appropriate feeding practices, is the main strategy recommended by the WHO to achieve a reduction in diarrhea-related mortality and malnutrition in children. ORT can be delivered by village health workers and practiced in the home by mothers with some guidance. In 2006, the WHO and UNICEF announced a new formula for the manufacture of oral rehydration salts, which will better combat acute diarrheal diseases and advance the MDG of reducing child mortality by two-thirds before 2015.

Malaria is another leading cause of mortality among children younger than 5 years. Ninety percent of the over 1 million deaths due to malaria each year occur in sub-Saharan Africa, mostly among young children.[52] Pregnant women and their unborn children are particularly vulnerable to malaria, which is a major cause of perinatal mortality, low birth weight, and maternal anemia. The tragedy is that, through effective, low-cost strategies, this is a preventable, treatable, and controllable disease. Prevention of malaria in pregnant women through measures such as intermittent preventive treatment and the use of insecticide-treated nets results in improvement in maternal health, infant health, and child survival. Prompt access to antimalarial drug combination therapy saves lives. However, the rapid spread of resistance to antimalarial drugs, coupled with widespread poverty and a weak health infrastructure, means that mortality from malaria continues to rise in developing countries.

Measles remains a leading cause of death among children younger than 5 years in developing countries, despite the availability of a safe and effective vaccine. In 2004, an estimated 454,000 people died from measles, a majority of them children. Severe measles is particularly likely in poorly nourished young children, especially those who are vitamin A deficient or whose immune systems have been weakened by HIV/AIDS or other diseases. Suffering, complications, and death caused by measles can be easily prevented through immunization. Immunizations are important in reducing child mortality and morbidity. The target diseases, beside measles, include tuberculosis, diphtheria, tetanus, pertussis, poliomyelitis, and hepatitis B. There are immunization schedules that one should follow during the prenatal and postnatal period. However, in the developing world, there are many obstacles to realizing these schedules.

Middle Years and Adolescence

The uses and meanings of the terms *young people, youth,* and *adolescents* vary according to region, depending on the political, economic and sociocultural contexts. The following definitions are most commonly accepted[53]:

- **Adolescents:** 10- to 19-year-olds (early adolescence, 10–14; late adolescence, 15–19)
- **Youth:** 15- to 24-year-olds
- **Young people:** 10- to 24-year-olds

According to the WHO, adolescents constitute 20% of the world's population. Of 1.2 billion adolescents worldwide, about 85% live in developing countries.[54] Table 4-4 presents the current and projected populations of young people aged 10 to 24, by region.

Generally speaking, adolescents are thought to be healthy because they have survived the diseases of early childhood and have many years before the onset of health problems associated with aging. Yet, an estimated 1.7 million young men and women between ages 10 and 19 lose their lives every year.[54] Trends in adolescent morbidity and mortality have shifted over the past decade from predominately infectious to social etiologies.[55]

SOCIAL TRENDS

A global increase in child survival has led to a growth in the youth population. The distribution of youth has begun to drift toward developing countries, with the greatest concentration in sub-Saharan Africa and Asia. A demographic shift, resulting from both rural-to-urban and cross-national migration, has also been evident over the last 20 years. Youth migration is a major cause of rural-to-urban migration and predisposes to

Table 4-4. Population of young people aged 10 to 24 years by region.

Region	Population aged 10 to 24 years (in millions)	
	2006	**2025**
The World	1,773	1,845
Africa	305	424
Asia	1,087	1,063
North America	71	74
Latin America	162	165
Europe	140	111
Western Pacific	8	8

Source: The World's Youth Data Sheet: Population Reference Bureau, 2006.

significant behavioral health risks that stem from unemployment and poverty, such as violence, prostitution, STIs/HIV, and substance abuse.[55]

Other trends that have a major impact on the health of adolescents include marriage, education, and globalization. The prevalence and consequences of early marriage and education have already been addressed. The cultural aspects of globalization have a large influence on adolescents' values and lifestyles. As a result of rapid globalization over the last decade or so, new patterns of disease have emerged in the world. For example, tobacco-related morbidities have risen, largely owing to multinational cigarette companies targeting adolescents in developing countries, where fewer restrictions are placed on marketing and distribution.[55] The increasing prevalence of obesity worldwide, partially stemming from the greater availability of cheap vegetable oils and fat, is another impact that globalization has had on adolescent health.[55] One of the most detrimental effects of globalization has been the AIDS epidemic, which has spread to every part of the world through travel and migration.

CAUSES OF MORTALITY

Table 4-5 depicts the five leading causes of death for young adults aged 15 to 29, both globally and by regions. These include unintentional injury, HIV/AIDS and other infectious diseases, homicide, war, and interpersonal violence.[55] Unintentional injury is the leading cause of death among young people in industrialized countries and an increasing concern in developing countries. The most prevalent unintentional injuries are traffic related. Beyond traffic-related injuries, recreational and sports accidents in developed countries, burns and poisonings in developing countries, and falls and drowning in every region also represent major risks (see Chapter 10).[55]

The second leading cause of death among young people worldwide, specifically in the developing world, is

Table 4-5. Five leading causes of mortality in 15- to 29-year-olds.

World regions	Leading causes of death[a]				
	Unintentional injuries	**AIDS**	**Other infectious causes**	**Homicide/war/other intentional injuries**	**Suicide/self-inflicted injuries**
All world regions	1 (531,000)	2 (326,000)	3 (229,000)	4 (227,000)	5 (124,000)
South America/Caribbean	2 (64,000)	5 (11,000)	4 (12,000)	1 (72,000)	3 (14,000)
Africa	4 (56,000)	1 (225,000)	2 (104,000)	3 (66,000)	5 (6,000)
Southeast Asia	1 (178,000)	3 (72,000)	2 (81,000)	5 (33,000)	4 (37,000)
Western Pacific	1 (119,000)	5 (8,000)	3 (19,000)	4 (17,000)	2 (32,000)
Eastern Mediterranean	1 (40,000)	4 (7,000)	2 (21,000)	3 (15,000)	5 (5,000)
Europe	1 (74,000)	5 (2,000)	4 (10,000)	3 (23,000)	2 (30,000)
North America[b]	1	6	5	3	2

[a]Data on maternal mortality among 15- to 29-year-olds not available.
[b]In North America, cancer is the fourth leading cause of death in the adolescent/young adult years.
From Blum RW, Nelson-Mmari K. The health of young people in a global context. *J Adolesc Health* 2004;35:402–418. (Reproduced with permission.)

HIV/AIDS. However, in Africa, it is the number one killer of young adults between ages 15 and 29 years. In most industrialized countries, suicide ranks after injuries as the second leading cause of death among adolescents. Globally, however, suicide ranks fifth. Other infectious diseases represent the third leading cause of death among young people, particularly in the developing world. Injuries resulting from violence are also among the chief causes of mortality for young people, particularly for adolescent males (see Chapter 10). Maternal mortality is a prominent cause of mortality among women, particularly in developing countries.

CAUSES OF MORBIDITY

For adolescents, causes of morbidity center on reproductive health issues (pregnancy and early childbearing, abortion, STIs, and various traditional reproductive practices such as female genital mutilation), violence (sexual coercion and abuse), mental health, and tobacco/substance abuse (tobacco use, alcohol and drug use). Pregnancy and early childbirth were addressed earlier in this chapter, as was abortion. According to WHO estimates, 1 in 20 adolescents worldwide acquires an STI each year. However, in the wake of the HIV and AIDS epidemic, very little attention has been focused on STIs, even though they can lead to serious reproductive morbidity and mortality. Since STIs frequently go undetected and untreated, they are considerably underreported. The actual prevalence among adolescents worldwide is not known.

A reproductive health issue that specifically affects adolescents is the traditional practice of female genital mutilation (FGM), which is common in many developing countries. FGM involves cutting away parts of the female external genitalia as a rite of passage for young girls to womanhood and marriage. It is estimated that more than 130 million girls and women worldwide have undergone FGM, and nearly 2 million more girls are at risk each year.[55] Razor blades, kitchen knives, sharp rocks, scissors, scalpels, and glass are used to perform FGM. During these procedures, infections such as tetanus occur. Long-term consequences include damage to the urinary system, painful intercourse, and scarring of the tissue, which often seals the edges of the wound together and shrinks the genital passage.[55] Other long-term consequences include infibulation, obstructed labor, repeated urinary tract infections, reproductive tract infections, and lowered fertility and sterility. Beyond the physical damage, psychological trauma often results.

Sexual violence (sexual coercion and abuse), which is particularly sensitive among youth, has not been well studied due to the nature of the topic. Although girls are more likely to be victims of sexual abuse or coercion, several studies show that large numbers of boys also suffer from sexual abuse. Sexual abuse and coercion can lead to a wide variety of negative health consequences, including behavioral and psychological problems, sexual dysfunction, low self-esteem, relationship problems, thoughts of suicide, alcohol and substance abuse, and sexual risk taking.[55] In addition, sexual violence has been linked to many serious physical health problems, such as injury, chronic pain syndromes, and gastrointestinal disorder.[55]

Up to 20% of children and adolescents worldwide suffer from a disabling mental illness.[55] According to WHO estimates, by the year 2020 adolescent psychiatric disorders will increase more than 50% worldwide to become one of the five leading causes of disability among adolescents.[55] Depression is one of the most common mental disorders affecting adolescents and young people worldwide. The primary concern with depression among adolescents is that it is often combined with substance abuse, which puts adolescents at even greater risk for suicide.[55]

Tobacco and substance abuse (alcohol and drug abuse) is quite prevalent among adolescents, particularly among males. Recent trends show an even earlier age of initiation and rising smoking prevalence rates among children and adolescents.[55] Worldwide, 300 million young people are smokers, and 150 million will die of smoking-related causes later in life.[56] According to the Global Burden of Disease 2000 study, alcohol is the number one killer of young men in Europe. Marijuana appears to be the most widely used illicit substance worldwide.[55] Studies have also shown that, similar to tobacco and alcohol use, more boys than girls engage in illicit drug use.[55]

INNOVATIVE COMMUNITY-BASED APPROACHES TO MATERNAL AND CHILD HEALTH

Although clearly many facility-based interventions could contribute to improved MCH outcomes, this section focuses on community-based approaches that are closely linked to facility-based care. These approaches have the potential for the greatest impact on a population basis. Technology and training in clinic- and hospital-based facilities also have to be improved to reduce mortality and morbidity for women and children.

Integrated Management of Childhood Illnesses

The Integrated Management of Childhood Illnesses (IMCI) strategy is designed to reduce mortality among children younger than 5 years. It was initially developed during the mid-1990s by the WHO, UNICEF, and their technical partners. IMCI was a response to the vertical, disease-specific child health programs that had evolved over time to separately address the major causes of child death. Although IMCI focuses on curative care, it also addresses aspects of nutrition, immunization, and other important elements of disease prevention and health promotion. The objectives of the strategy are to reduce death and the frequency and severity of illness and disability, and to contribute to improved growth and development.[57] Currently this approach is being adapted to the neonatal period.

The IMCI strategy has three main components (Figure 4-9):

- Ensuring health system support for child health (including drug and vaccine supply, supervision, and health information systems)
- Improving the performance of health workers in first-level facilities through a training course addressing leading causes of infant and child mortality
- Strengthening family practices needed to prevent disease, to stimulate appropriate utilization of health services, and to improve home care for sick children

The IMCI case-management guidelines are designed to address major causes of child mortality— pneumonia, diarrhea, malaria, measles, and malnutrition—in countries with a mortality of 40 (or greater) per 1,000 live births. The guidelines are based on underlying principles (Box 4-2) that should be adapted to a country's situation.

Since its introduction at the country level in 1996, more than 100 countries have adopted the IMCI strategy. The global planning guidelines recommend three stages for implementing IMCI: the introduction, early

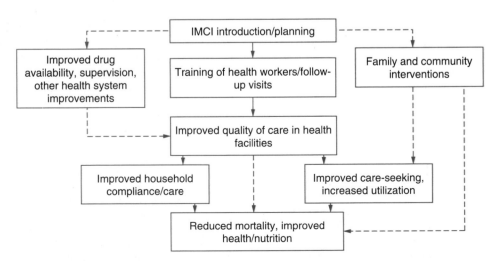

Figure 4-9. IMCI model. From World Health Organization. *IMCI: Model Chapter for Textbooks.* Geneva: World Health Organization, 2001. WHO/FCH/CAH/00.40.

BOX 4-2. PRINCIPLES OF INTEGRATED CARE

- All sick children must be examined for "general danger signs" that indicate the need for immediate referral or admission to a hospital.

- All sick children must be routinely assessed for major symptoms (for children aged 2 months up to 5 years, cough or difficult breathing, diarrhea, fever, ear problems; for young infants aged 1 week up to 2 months, bacterial infection and diarrhea). They must also be routinely assessed for nutritional and immunization status, feeding problems, and other potential problems.

- Only a limited number of carefully selected clinical signs are used, based on evidence of their sensitivity and specificity to detect disease. These signs were selected considering the conditions and realities of first-level health facilities.

- A combination of individual signs leads to a child's classification rather than a diagnosis. Classifications indicate the severity of conditions. They call for specific actions based on whether the child (a) should be urgently referred to another level of care, (b) requires specific treatments (such as antibiotics or antimalarial treatment), or (c) may be safely managed at home. The classifications are color coded: pink suggests hospital referral or admission, yellow indicates initiation of treatment, and green calls for home treatment.

- The IMCI guidelines address most, but not all, of the major reasons a sick child is brought to a clinic. A child returning with chronic problems or less common illnesses may require special care. The guidelines do not describe the management of trauma or other acute emergencies due to accidents or injuries.

- IMCI management procedures use a limited number of essential drugs and encourage active participation of caretakers in the treatment of children.

- An essential component of the IMCI guidelines is the counseling of caretakers about home care, including counseling about feeding, fluids, and when to return to a health facility.

Source: World Health Organization. *IMCI: Model Chapter for Textbooks.* Geneva: World Health Organization, 2001. WHO/FCH/CAH/00.40.

---

implementation, and expansion phases. In the introductory phase, countries conduct orientation meetings, train key decision makers in IMCI, define a management structure for IMCI planning and early implementation, and build government commitment to move forward with the IMCI strategy.[58] In the early implementation phase, countries gain experience while implementing IMCI in limited geographic areas. They develop their national strategy and plan, adapt the IMCI guidelines to their national context, develop management and training capacity in a limited number of districts, and start implementing and monitoring IMCI.[58] The end of this phase is marked by a review meeting with the objective of synthesizing early implementation experience and planning for expansion. In the expansion phase, countries increase both the range of IMCI interventions and IMCI coverage.[58]

In 1997, Bryce and associates launched a multicountry evaluation of IMCI effectiveness, cost, and impact.[58] Preliminary data from this evaluation show that

- IMCI training for health workers managing children in first-level health facilities can lead to rapid and sustained improvement in health workers' performance.

- Ministries of health and their partners in some countries, however, have not been able to maintain and expand training coverage beyond a few pilot districts.

- Scaling up IMCI to the national scale will require stronger management, increased funding, coordination with other child health programs, elimination of conflicting regulations, improvement of supervision, and reduction of staff turnover.

- Implementation of IMCI at the household and community levels is essential for improving care-seeking practices, but efforts to implement have been insufficient for achieving even minimal coverage.

An ongoing assessment by Cesar Victora and colleagues of how well the IMCI strategy has reached the poor shows that it is being implemented least energetically in the most needed areas.[59] Ironically, this new approach for improving the overall health and well-being of a child is contributing further to inequalities in child health care, creating the greatest burden for those most in need.

Enhancing the Role of Men in Maternal and Child Health

MCH services have traditionally focused on women and children to the exclusion of men as partners and fathers. This focus occurred because maternity care during pregnancy appropriately focuses on the health and risks of the woman, and because women are the primary caregivers for infant and child health. Another reason, especially in reproductive health services, was to provide women some degree of self-determination in male-dominant societies. Although this may have been important to establish the importance of women's roles in their own health and that of their children, this approach ignored the role of men in families and the fact that they are often the decision makers about when, where, and what health services the family members access. These facts were recognized at the 1994 International Conference on Population and Development in Cairo in the Program of Action, and at the 1995 Conference on Women in Beijing. Both action plans had sections on male responsibilities in reproductive health, parenthood, and maternal and child care.

Although outcome research on programs involving men in MCH services is currently taking place, there is evidence of effectiveness in several countries. The Men in Maternity study was conducted in India and South Africa to examine the effectiveness of involving the male partners of women in their care during the antenatal and postpartum periods. These two sites offered different challenges in male participation. In India, women were married and their husbands (and their husbands' mothers) were the key decision makers determining their access to health services. In the South African communities, women were unlikely to be married or have live-in partners, and men often had several female partners, so women were more likely to access health care independently, with little involvement by their partners. Both programs focused on involving the men in prenatal care, delivery, postnatal care, and family planning.

Differential levels of success were achieved, due in part to local culture and male roles and also to the type of service integration. Both interventions provided valuable insights into incorporating men in maternity care and family planning. In Delhi, India, the clinic sites were linked to men's places of work, and men frequently accompanied their wives to initial prenatal visits; therefore, it was easier to recruit them. In KwaZulu, South Africa, there was little precedence for men's involvement in their partner's care, and their employers were not committed to the program. In India, the results showed that couples in the program group were more likely to communicate about family planning, engage in joint decision making, and continue use of family planning 6 months postpartum. This program is expanding to 34 clinics and five hospitals in Delhi. In KwaZulu, men have traditionally not played any role in prenatal care and delivery because of the cultural view that this exposure makes them weak. Initially, involving men was also strongly opposed by health providers. In spite of these barriers, about one-third of the male partners in the intervention group participated in the counseling sessions. Men felt that they learned something useful from the counseling, and women felt that the main benefit was that their partner became more helpful and supportive. Communication about STIs, sexual relations, immunization, and breastfeeding increased.[60,61]

Other examples of involving men in MCH are through the formation of Fathers' Clubs (to parallel Mothers' Clubs) at the Haitian Health Foundation in Jeremie, Haiti[62]; a study of gender and family dynamics in El Alto, Bolivia[63]; and a major National Institutes of Health study of men's sexual health in relation to women's health in Mumbai, India.[64]

Home Based Life Saving Skills

Home Based Life Saving Skills (HBLSS) is a training and intervention program developed by the American College of Nurse-Midwives (ACNM) to address the needs of mothers and newborns in situations where skilled attendance at birth is not immediately available. Although the standard for maternal delivery is skilled attendance for all deliveries, the reality for much of the developing world is that women deliver at home by themselves, or with family members and traditional birth attendants. Although the goal is to improve the quality of referral facilities and upgrade the training in emergency obstetrical care (EMOC) as well as to increase access to hospital and clinic delivery by skilled health professionals, this will take years to achieve in many countries. HBLSS is a community-based approach to complement EMOC, also called essential life saving skills (LSS), at the facility level. It was designed to provide education, motivation, and mobilization of pregnant women, families, and communities. It is a community- and competency-based program focused on reducing maternal and newborn mortality by increasing access to basic life-saving methods in the home and community and decreasing delays in reaching facility-based care in an emergency.

The concept for this program emerged in the mid-1990s and was developed by ACNM staff and consultants with extensive field experience in developing countries. They worked for several years to create the materials and conduct baseline studies. The materials were pretested in India and Ethiopia in 2001 and are currently in use in several countries, including a USAID-funded Child Survival project focused on reducing maternal and newborn mortality in rural Haiti.

HBLSS consists of 12 topic modules organized into three domains: core topics (introduction, mother and baby problems, preventing problems and referral), maternal problems (too much bleeding, birth delay, sickness and pain with fever, pregnancy swelling and fits, too many children), and newborn problems (trouble breathing at birth, born too small, baby is sick). The program is based on a Training of Trainers model, with selection of TBAs and other health providers who work through all the modules with ACNM-certified trainers and then practice by teaching the modules to others in the community with ACNM supervision. The initial emphasis of training was on the birth team at the home level: mother, family members, and TBA. The continued expansion of HBLSS implementation has resulted in some other models, such as community-level training of the population through mothers' groups and other representative groups in communities as well as community health workers and TBAs. Each module uses a stepwise process of problem identification, problem solving, negotiation, and practice and incorporates a respectful discussion of existing community practices and how to apply new strategies. The modules are accompanied by picture "Take Action" cards for the steps appropriate to each problem. The materials are well suited to communities with low literacy and include a pregnancy and birth tracking system that can be completed by TBAs or other community residents.

Preliminary research in Ethiopia demonstrated increased management of postpartum hemorrhage, but less impact on management of newborn infections. This approach is being implemented in several countries, and further research will enhance understanding of the program operation and outcomes in other field sites.[65,66]

Kangaroo Mother Care

Kangaroo mother care is care of preterm infants carried skin-to-skin with the mother to prevent hypothermia (low body temperature and poor temperature regulation) and promote breastfeeding, mother-infant bonding, and infant health.[67] Preterm and low-birth-weight (LBW) infants are at greater risk for hypothermia, malnutrition, and infection. Health consequences of hypothermia include hypoxia, cardiorespiratory complications, and acidosis. These can progress to neurologic complications, hyperbilirubinemia, clotting disorders, and death.[68]

In developed countries, the treatment is placing the infant in an incubator in the hospital nursery; although this approach is effective, it has been criticized for disrupting mother-infant attachment. The kangaroo care method was first developed in a hospital in Bogota, Colombia, in 1979, primarily because the hospital had limited resources and a high mortality for premature infants. This approach demonstrated reduced mortality and morbidity.[69] Since the early 1980s, research and implementation of this approach has demonstrated its effectiveness in thermal control, breastfeeding, and bonding for all newborns.[70]

In developing countries, kangaroo care has been implemented by trained community health workers in home settings. For some infants this provides adequate treatment; for those at higher risk, it can be used to stabilize them until they can be transferred to a hospital facility. Kangaroo care has also been expanded from "mother care" to include fathers and grandmothers.

CONCLUSION

The health outcomes for mothers and children continue to be poor in many parts of the world. The interconnectedness of MCH with women's roles, education, and poverty makes single-focus disease or health promotion initiatives of limited value. The inclusion of maternal and child mortality as the focus of two MDGs as well as the integration of MCH into the goals of reducing poverty, increasing access to primary education, and improving nutrition is a first step. The MDGs provide evidence that a holistic approach to MCH is critical for global health and development.

Maternal mortality and morbidity and maternal health services pertain to all aspects of women's health related to her role as a mother, including pregnancy and after delivery, breastfeeding, and child care. Child health services have primarily focused on infants and children younger than 5, although there is increasing awareness of the health needs of neonates, older children, and adolescents. The focus on women as mothers is a strength because it helps to target primary health care services on improving the quality of life of the next generation as well as saving the lives of women in their reproductive roles. However, it can be criticized for neglecting the health of women in roles other than that of a mother. The emphasis on women as baby carriers and baby/child caregivers results in a lack of attention to other important health issues of women, including preconceptual health, infectious diseases other than STIs or those that might have an effect on the child, violence against women, and health of women past the age of childbearing. Because many of the determinants of a pregnant woman's health begin well before childbearing, attention to the nutrition, education, development, and treatment of illnesses of girls must become a priority for MCH in addition to the traditional services.

The health and well-being of women and children also depends on the involvement of families and communities. The inclusion of men in MCH is often neglected; however, their role as decision makers often supersedes that of women. The challenge is how to involve men in MCH without undermining the goal of gender equity. Community-based interventions provide the opportunity for a gender-inclusive participatory approach.

STUDY QUESTIONS

1. Why is it difficult to reduce maternal mortality in low-income countries?

2. How do maternal factors influence child health?

3. What are the determinants of marriage at an early age? What are the consequences?

4. How can men be more effectively engaged in MCH?

5. Describe and discuss several low-cost interventions that reduce maternal and child mortality. Focus on sustainability as well as impact.

REFERENCES

1. United Nations Statistics Division. Maternal mortality ratio per 100,000 live births (WHO, UNICEF and UNFPA/MDG) [code 1000]. http://unstats.un.org/unsd/cdb/cdb_series_xrxx.asp?series_code=1000; United Nations Statistics Division. Infant mortality rate per 1,000 live births (UN Pop. Div. quinquennial estimates and projections) [code 13620]. http://unstats.un.org/unsd/cdb/cdb_series_xrxx.asp?series_code=13620.

2. World Health Organization. *Maternal Mortality in 2000: Estimates Developed by WHO, UNICEF, UNFPA.* Geneva: World Health Organization, 2004.

3. World Health Organization. *The Sisterhood Method for Estimating Maternal Mortality: Guidance Notes for Potential Users.* Geneva: World Health Organization, 1997. WHO/RHT/97.28.

4. International Conference on Primary Health Care. Declaration of Alma-Ata. Paper presented at: International Conference on Primary Health Care; September 6–12, 1978; Alma-Ata, USSR. http://www.who.int/hpr/NPH/docs/declaration_almaata.pdf.

5. Hsiao WCL, Liu Y. Economic reform and health: lessons from China. *N Engl J Med* 1996;335(6):430–432.

6. Hesketh T, Zhu WX. Health in China: maternal and child health in China. *BMJ* 1997;314:1898.

7. Blumenthal D, Hsiao W. Privatization and its discontents: the evolving Chinese health care system. *N Engl J Med* 2005; 353(11):1165–1170.

8. Burkle FM. Lessons learned in complex emergencies: could this happen in the struggle for a democratic transition in Cuba? Paper presented at: USAID seminar, Humanitarian Aid for a Cuba in Transition; January 16, 2004; Washington, DC.

9. United Nations. *The Millennium Development Goals Report 2006.* New York: United Nations, 2006.

10. Singh S, Samara R. Early marriage among women in developing countries. *Int Fam Plann Perspect* 1996;22:148–157, 175.

11. United Nations Population Fund. State of world population 2005: child marriage fact sheet. http://www.unfpa.org/swp/2005/presskit/factsheets/facts_child_marriage.htm.

12. United Nations Population Fund. Summary of the ICPD programme of action. March 1995. http://www.unfpa.org/icpd/summary.htm.

13. Ross JA, Winfrey W. Unmet need for contraception in the developing world and former Soviet Union: an updated estimate. *Int Fam Plann Perspect* 2002;28(3):138–143.

14. World Health Organization. *Measuring Access to Reproductive Health Services: Report of WHO/UNFPA Technical Consultation 2–3 December 2003.* Geneva: World Health Organization, 2005. WHO/RHR/04.11.

15. Casterline JB, Sinding SW. Unmet need for family planning in developing countries and implications for population policy. *Popul Develop Rev* 2000;26(4):691–723.

16. United Nations Population Fund. Reproductive health: a measure of equity. In: United Nations Population Fund. *State of World Population 2005. The Promise of Equality: Gender Equity, Reproductive Health, and the Millennium Development Goals.* New York: UNFPA, 2005. http://www.unfpa.org/swp/2005/english/ch4/chap4_page2.htm.

17. Rawlings JS, Rawlings VB, Read JA. Prevalence of low birth weight and preterm delivery in relation to the interval between pregnancies among white and black women. *N Engl J Med* 1995;332(2):69–74.

18. UNICEF. *Prevention and Control of Iron Deficiency Anaemia in Women and Children: Report of the UNICEF/WHO Regional Consultation.* Geneva: UNICEF and World Health Organization, 1999.

19. Yip R, Lynch S. Definitions of anemia, iron deficiency, and iron deficiency anemia. Presented at: Technical Workshop, UNICEF; October 7–9, 1998; New York, NY.

20. World Health Organization, UNICEF, and the United Nations University. *Iron Deficiency Anaemia: Assessment, Prevention and Control. A Guide for Programme Managers.* Geneva: World Health Organization, 2001. WHO/NHD/01.3.

21. Scholl TO, Hediger ML. Anemia and iron-deficiency anemia: compilation of data on pregnancy outcome. *Am J Clin Nutr* 1994;59(suppl):492s–501s.

22. World Health Organization. *The World Health Report 2005: Make Every Mother and Child Count.* Geneva: World Health Organization, 2005.

23. World Health Organization. *Antenatal Care.* Geneva: World Health Organization, 1996. WHO/FRH/MSM/96.8.

24. Bergström S, Goodburn E. The role of traditional birth attendants in the reduction of maternal mortality. In: De Brouwere V, Van Lerberghe W, eds. *Safe Motherhood Strategies: A Review of the Evidence.* Antwerp: ITG Press, 2001.

25. Ray AM, Salihu HM. The impact of maternal mortality interventions using traditional birth attendants and village midwives. *J Obstet Gynaecol* 2004;24(1):5–11.

26. Graham W, et al. Can skilled attendance at delivery reduce maternal mortality in developing countries? In: De Brouwere V, Van Lerberghe W, eds. *Safe Motherhood Strategies: A Review of the Evidence.* Antwerp: ITG Press, 2001.

27. World Health Organization. *Coverage of Maternity Care: A Listing of Available Information.* 4th ed. Geneva: World Health Organization, 1997.

28. Tinker A. Safe motherhood as an economic and social investment. Presented at: Safe Motherhood Technical Consultation; October 18–23, 1997; Sri Lanka; and World Health Organization and UNICEF. *Revised 1990 Estimates of Maternal Mortality: A New Approach by WHO and UNICEF.* Geneva: World Health Organization, 1996.

29. Pan American Health Organization. *Health in the Americas, 2002 Edition.* Vol. 1. Washington, DC: Pan American Health Organization, 2002.

30. Barnes-Josiah D, Myntti C, Augustin A. The three delays as a framework for examining maternal mortality in Haiti. *Soc Sci Med* 1998;46(8):981–993.

31. Thaddeus S, Maine D. Too far to walk: maternal mortality in context. *Soc Sci Med* 1996;38:1091–1110.

32. Foundation for Women's Health Research and Development. Definitions of vesicovaginal fistula (VVF) and rectovaginal fistula (RVF). http://www.forwarduk.org.uk/key-issues/fistula/definitions.

33. World Health Organization. Management of STIs/RTIs. 2005. http://www.who.int/reproductive-health/publications/rtis_gep/infection_childbirth.htm.

34. World Health Organization. Preventing unsafe abortion. http://www.who.int/reproductive-health/unsafe_abortion/map.html.

35. World Health Organization. *The Prevention and Management of Unsafe Abortion.* Geneva: World Health Organization, 1992. WHO/MSM/92.5.

36. World Health Organization. *Unsafe abortion: Global and Regional Estimates of Incidence of Mortality due to Unsafe Abortion with a Listing of Available Country Data.* 3rd ed. Geneva: World Health Organization, 1997. WHO/RHT/MSM/97.16.

37. Castro LC. Hypertensive disorders of pregnancy. In: Hacker N, Moore JG, eds. *Essentials of Obstetrics and Gynecology*. 3rd ed. Philadelphia: WB Saunders, 1998:196–207.

38. The Eclampsia Trial Collaborative Group. Which anticonvulsant for women with eclampsia? Evidence from the Collaborative Eclampsia Trial. *Lancet* 1995;345(8963):1455–1463.

39. The Magpie Trial Collaborative Group. Do women with pre-eclampsia, and their babies, benefit from magnesium sulphate? The Magpie Trial: a randomised placebo-controlled trial. *Lancet* 2002;359(9321):1877–1890.

40. Sheth SS, Chalmers I. Magnesium for preventing and treating eclampsia: time for international action. *Lancet* 2002;359(9321):1872–1873.

41. World Health Organization. *Postpartum Care of the Mother and Newborn: A Practical Guide*. Geneva: World Health Organization, 1998. WHO/RHT/MSM/98.3.

42. USAID. Maternal and child health: technical areas. Postpartum and newborn care. 2005. http://www.usaid.gov/our_work/global_health/mch/mh/techareas/post.html.

43. World Health Organization, Regional Office for South-East Asia. http://www.searo.who.int/EN/Section13/Section36/Section129/Section396_1445htm.

44. Zupan J. Perinatal mortality and morbidity in developing countries: a global view. *La Medicina Tropical* 2003; 63: 366–368.

45. Richardus JH, Graafmans WC, Verloove-Vanhorick SP, Mackenbach JP. The perinatal mortality rate as an indicator of quality of care in international comparisons. *Med Care* 1998;36(1):54–56.

46. Kuit OO, Orji EO, Ogunlola IO. Analysis of perinatal mortality in a Nigerian teaching hospital. *J Obstet Gynaecol* 2003;23(5):512–514.

47. World Health Organization, Department of Child and Adolescent Health and Development. Overview of CAH: major causes of death among children under five years of age and neonates in the world, 2000–2003. http://www.who.int/child-adolescent-health/Overview/Child_Health/map_00-03_world.jpg.

48. World Health Organization. *Essential Antenatal, Perinatal and Postpartum Care. Training Modules*. Geneva: World Health Organization, 2003. EUR/03/5035043.

49. World Health Organization, Department of Child and Adolescent Health and Development. Acute respiratory infections in children. http://www.who.int/child-adolescent-health/Emergencies/ARI_in_children.htm.

50. Benguigui Y, et al., eds. *Respiratory Infections in Children*. Washington, DC: Pan American Health Organization, 1999.

51. World Health Organization and UNICEF. *Oral Rehydration Salts: Production of the New ORS*. Geneva: World Health Organization, 2006.

52. Roll Back Malaria. What is malaria? http://rbm.who.int/cmc_upload/0/000/015/372/RBMInfosheet_1.htm.

53. United Nations Population Fund. About adolescents. http://www.unfpa.org/adolescents/about.htm.

54. World Health Organization, Department of Child and Adolescent Health and Development. Overview of CAH: adolescent health and development. http://www.who.int/child-adolescent-health/OVERVIEW/AHD/adh_over.htm.

55. Blum RW, Nelson-Mmari K. The health of young people in a global context. *J Adolesc Health* 2004;35:402–418.

56. World Health Organization, Department of Child and Adolescent Health and Development. Prevention and care of illness: adolescents and substance use. http://www.who.int/child-adolescent-health/PREVENTION/Adolescents_substance.htm.

57. World Health Organization. *IMCI: Model Chapter for Textbooks*. Geneva: World Health Organization, 2001. WHO/FCH/CAH/00.40.

58. Bryce J, Victora CG, Habicht JP, Black RE, Scherpbier RW. Programmatic pathways to child survival: results of a multi-country evaluation of Integrated Management of Childhood Illness. *Health Policy Plan* 2005;20(suppl):5s–17s.

59. Gwatkin DR. IMCI: what can we learn from an innovation that didn't reach the poor? *Bull World Health Org* 2006; 84(10).

60. Population Council. Mixed success involving men in maternal care worldwide. *Population Briefs* 2005;11(1).

61. Mullick S, Kunene B, Wanjiru M. Involving men in maternity care: health service delivery issues. *Agenda: Special Focus on Gender, Culture and Rights* 2005;(special issue):124–134. http://www.popcouncil.org/pdfs/frontiers/journals/Agenda_Mullick05.pdf.

62. Gebrian B, Tobing S, Lowney M, Anderson F, Bourdeau R. Madonna Project. Innovations in maternal-newborn and child health. Unpublished manuscript, 2002.

63. Population Council. Bolivia: the involvement of men in perinatal health in El Alto. 2006. http://www.popcouncil.org/genfam/menbolivia.html.

64. Schensul SL, Sharma S, Maitra S, Pinto N. *Gender Concepts, Marital Relationships and Sexual Risk Behavior in Mumbai, India*. September 2003. http://www.jhuccp.org/igwg/presentations/Monday/Plen2/GenderConcepts.pdf.

65. Sibley L, Buffington S, Haileyesus D. The American College of Nurse-Midwives' home-based lifesaving skills program: a review of the Ethiopia field test. *J Midwifery Women's Health* 2004;49(4):320–328.

66. Sibley L, Buffington S, Beck D, Armbruster D. Home based life saving skills: promoting safe motherhood through innovative community-based interventions. *J Midwifery Women's Health* 2001;46(4):258–266.

67. World Health Organization. *Kangaroo Mother Care: A Practical Guide*. Geneva: World Health Organization, 2003.

68. Hackman PS. Recognizing and understanding the cold stressed term infant. *Neonatal Network* 2001;20(8):35–41.

69. Bosque EM, Affonso DD, and Wahlberg V. Physiologic measures of kangaroo versus incubator care in a tertiary-level nursery. *J Obstet Gynecol Neonatal Nurs* 1995;24(3):219–226.

70. World Health Organization. *Thermal Control of the Newborn: A Practical Guide*. Geneva: World Health Organization, 1993. WHO/FHE/MSM/93.2.

Environmental Health in the Global Context

5

Jeffrey K. Griffiths and Edward Winant

LEARNING OBJECTIVES

- *Understand the major ways in which environmental pollutants such as industrial chemicals make their way into humans*
- *Learn appropriate methods of personal drinking water treatment and sanitation for traveling and living in the developing world*
- *Learn to recognize health problems caused by contaminated drinking water or inadequate wastewater treatment and the benefits enjoyed by populations with good drinking water and sanitation*
- *Gain a basic understanding of appropriate methods of treating community drinking water and wastewater in the developing world*
- *Understand the magnitude of and health effects associated with air pollution*

Environmental factors profoundly influence human health. A recent report by the World Health Organization (WHO) estimates that 24% of the world's burden of disease, and about one-third of the burden in children, is due to preventable environmental factors.[1] By *preventable,* it is meant that these risks can be altered or mitigated. This burden of avoidable disease is disproportionately felt by the residents of poor countries, with attributable disease burdens often tenfold higher or more than that seen in wealthier nations.[2] Reasons for the disproportionate effects felt in developing countries include a lack of modern technology, weak protective environmental laws and regulations, a lack of awareness,

and poverty.[3] Nonetheless, residents of wealthy countries are also affected by air pollution, poorly designed urban environments, flooding, and lead poisoning, among other risks, and thus environmental health is truly of global concern.

Unclean water and poor sanitation remain the most potent environmental causes of illness worldwide. Industrial chemical contaminants affect health everywhere. Of the more than 30,000 chemicals commonly used today, fewer than 1% have been studied in detail as to their health effects and toxicity,[4] and our understanding of the effects of simultaneous low-level exposure to hundreds or thousands of chemicals is rudimentary at best. Air pollution has been found to be a top-ranked problem in nearly every country undergoing economic transition. This chapter outlines a number of the global environmental challenges to health.

BIOLOGICAL, PHYSICAL, AND CHEMICAL ENVIRONMENTAL RISKS AND THEIR AVOIDANCE

Environmental hazards include biological, physical, and chemical ones, along with the human behaviors that promote or allow exposure. Some environmental contaminants are difficult to avoid (the breathing of polluted air, the drinking of chemically contaminated public drinking water, noise in open public spaces); in these circumstances, exposure is largely involuntary. Amelioration or elimination of these factors may require societal action, such as public awareness and public health measures. In many countries, the fact that some environmental hazards are difficult to avoid at the individual level is felt to be more morally egregious than those hazards that can be avoided. Having no choice but to drink water contaminated with very high levels of arsenic, as is the situation in Bangladesh, or being forced to passively inhale tobacco smoke in restaurants, outrages people more than the personal choice of whether an individual smokes tobacco. These factors are important when one considers how change (risk reduction) happens.

It should be noted that environmental health hazards often affect political elites as well as the poor in many countries. Although there are usually higher risks for the poor than the rich, principally because the rich enjoy improved disinfection of drinking water and sanitation, other hazards, such as air pollution or chemical and heavy metal contamination of foodstuffs, can affect all sectors of society, assisting in the development of a political consensus for change.

Some environmental hazards are associated with specific individual human behaviors, which in principle can be changed. In the absence of clean water and sanitation, simple handwashing with soap has been shown to dramatically decrease the rates of infectious diseases such as diarrhea, pneumonia, and impetigo.[5] Occupational exposures to pesticides, fertilizers, and microbial pathogens can be minimized by the use of protective gear, careful application techniques, and the provision of water and soap for decontamination. Irrigation not only improves crop production but also provides a conducive environment for the expansion and transmission of waterborne diseases such as schistosomiasis. In this case, reducing body contact with water will decrease rates of disease.

The handling of environmental hazards to human health must be tailored to the contaminant(s) and to the associated behaviors. It usually involves an assessment of the health burden, the routes of exposure, and identification of the stakeholders. Economic factors are often critical. Because the burden of disease may fall on people who do not share in the economic or social benefits of an environmental hazard, community action or political negotiations are often involved in the amelioration of environmental risks.

Biological Hazards

The term *biological hazards* usually refers to diseases caused by pathogens such as viruses, bacteria, prions, fungi, and parasites. It should be noted that the product of an infection can cause disease as well as the live pathogen. For example, in Ghana and other countries where foodstuffs may be stored in a damp state, fungal infections of tubers or maize (corn) produce aflatoxins, proteins that are potent carcinogens that especially affect the liver.

An astounding 94% of the disability-adjusted life years (DALYs) of disease burden due to diarrhea, principally caused by viruses and bacteria, is environmental in origin.[1] Approximately 1.5 million deaths a year, mostly in young children, are caused by poor sanitation, contaminated water, and lack of hygiene (a complex behavioral and socioeconomic component). When feces and urine are not disposed of carefully, and when hygiene (the ability to wash hands with soap) is absent, human pathogens contaminate food, surface and groundwater, and hands. Lifespan in the United States increased in the period from 1900 to 2000 by more than three decades, and a good two-thirds of this increase has been attributed to clean water, clean food, and sanitation.[6] One reason that some countries with limited budgets for health, such as Cuba and Costa Rica, have recently achieved major increases in lifespan and major decreases in childhood mortality and adult morbidity is that they have focused on water and sanitation risks.[7] If the reader is to take a single point away from this chapter, it is the crucial importance of keeping human and animal feces out of water and food.

Pathogens found in human feces are exquisitely adapted to causing human disease, and it should be obvious that breaking the cycle of transmission through basic sanitation and the provision of clean water should be an extraordinarily high societal priority.[8] The major pathogens causing illness and death through these transmission pathways include rotavirus, enteroviruses (a group that includes polio), *Salmonella, Shigella, Escherichia coli, Cryptosporidium, Campylobacter,* and hepatitis A and E viruses. Some of these are shared with domestic or peridomestic animals of economic importance, such as *Salmonella, Campylobacter, E. coli,* and *Cryptosporidium.* Typhoid (*Salmonella typhi*), in contrast to most of these pathogens, is a disease only of humans, and one way to judge the adequacy of water treatment and sanitation is to look at decreases in typhoid incidence.

WATER SUPPLY

The issues of water supply and sanitation in the developing world are of great importance. As the saying goes, "An ounce of prevention is worth a pound of cure." More to the point is the fact that public health engineers have saved many more lives than doctors over the course of human history. Safe, clean drinking water and adequate sanitation are critical needs for the developing world. However, projects to improve these conditions must include appropriate technology, cultural sensitivity, and long-term management procedures or they will quickly fail.

Water supply starts at the source, either surface water or groundwater. Surface water (i.e., streams, lakes, rivers, or ponds) is easily found and used. Large rivers and lakes provide year-round sources of water, whereas small streams and ponds may fail in dry seasons. Impoundments (dams) may be used to store stream flow from the wet season to supply community needs during the dry season. However, all surface water sources are unprotected. That is, they are very susceptible to pollution and should not be used without treatment.

Groundwater falls into two sources, shallow and deep. Shallow groundwater comes from water infiltrating the soil and trickling down until it is caught on top of the bedrock. This upper aquifer, or water table, fluctuates in depth depending on the season, dropping in dry seasons and rising in wet weather. Although the soil can filter out many pollutants, shallow groundwater is susceptible to pollution and should be used with care.

Shallow groundwater is tapped through wells or springs. Shallow wells are typically hand dug down to the water table and use a hand pump or bucket to bring water up. Springs are natural points where the water table meets the ground surface and water seeps out. Typically these occur at the toes of slopes or on hillsides.

Shallow wells and springs are very common water sources for developing countries. Although they are not pristine sources of water, the method of getting water from them can add considerable pollution to the water, and the solutions are usually easy and inexpensive to employ. For wells, a small wall around the top of the well made of stone, brick, or concrete serves to keep animals and small children from falling in and diverts rainwater runoff from entering the well. A cover also serves to protect the well from trash and pollution, while providing a bucket and rope, with a windlass to gather the rope when out of use, solely for the well helps keep these items clean and keeps dirt out of the well (Figure 5-1).

Hand pumps provide the best protection for a shallow well, since the well remains covered while the water is withdrawn. Further, using a bucket and rope will introduce some contamination because buckets are frequently set on the ground, and ropes pass through the unwashed hands of the users. Many types of hand pumps are available in developing countries, and their use is limited only by cost. They typically cost more than submersible electric pumps in the United States, but have the advantage of working without power (Figure 5-2).

If an event occurs to contaminate a well, perhaps an animal drowning in the bottom, it is possible to "shock" the well to cleanse it. This will remove the existing pollution but will not guard against recontamination. The procedure is to add chlorine, typically in the form of bleach, to the well and then draw out all of the chlorinated water and dispose of it. This prevents people from drinking overchlorinated, and dangerous, water and removes the source of contamination. The bleach should be added to a bucket of water, mixed well, and then lowered into the well to mix with all of the water at the bottom. It is necessary to get an idea of how much water is in the bottom of the well so that the proper amount can be withdrawn. Without too much math, the volume is the area of the well times the water depth. A typical circular well, 1 meter in diameter (3.28 feet) with a water depth of 2 meters (6.56 feet), holds

$$h \times (\pi\, d^2/4)$$
$$2 \times (3.14 \times 1^2/4) = 1.6 \text{ cubic meters or } 1{,}600 \text{ liters}$$
$$(410 \text{ gallons})$$

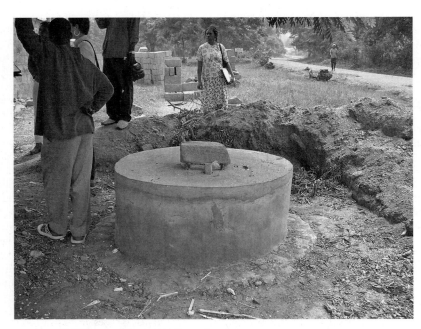

Figure 5-1. Protected well. (Photo by Edward H. Winant.)

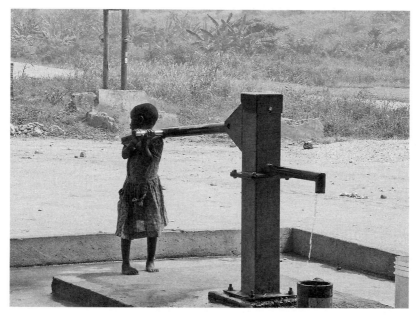

Figure 5-2. **Hand pump.** (Photo by Edward H. Winant.)

For a spring, a spring box or house helps gather the water from the ground and stores it in a protected place until needed. Typically, a pipe drains the box and allows users to fill their buckets under the pipe, keeping buckets and dirt out of the spring. Also, washing and bathing activities then take place downstream of the spring and do not affect the water quality at the source.

Deep wells, or boreholes, tap a water source (aquifer) that is much deeper and more protected than shallow wells. These deeper aquifers are contained in water-bearing rock layers under layers of impermeable rock. Thus, their waters are safe from most forms of pollution but are also more of a finite resource, because they are so hard to recharge.

Reaching these deep aquifers can be quite a challenge. They need to be drilled or bored into the rock with specialized machinery. Further, the hole has to be cased through the upper soil levels to keep potentially dirty waters out of the well. Finally, an electric, submersible pump is extended into the hole to access the deep waters, thus requiring modern machinery and electricity for use.

A final source of drinking water is collecting rainwater. This is most commonly done on the roofs of houses, with gutters to collect and carry the rain to a storage basin, the prototypical American rain barrel. Gutters are fairly easy to install, but sizing the storage basin can be a problem. Ideally, it would be large enough to store all the water needed by the inhabitants of the building from one rainfall until the next. The difficulty arises because so many locations on Earth have wet seasons and dry seasons, and the time between rainfalls may last weeks or even months. Storing enough rainfall from a rainy season to last through a dry season requires large and expensive storage tanks (Figure 5-3).

The other aspect of rainwater collection is that roofs are typically quite dirty, with leaves, sticks, and bird droppings. There are two solutions to the problem of a dirty roof: foul flush tanks and filters. The foul flush tank diverts and stores the initial rainfall, which is assumed to rinse the roof clean. After a short time, the rest of the rain is collected in the main storage tank. Filters are usually sand columns that are placed on top of the storage tank to remove contamination. Filtration is discussed in more detail later in the chapter.

WATER DELIVERY

Once the water source has been identified and developed, some thought must be given to getting it to the users. The most common and low-tech method is to have users come to the water source and carry their daily supply home in buckets or jars. This requires a lot of human effort and also serves to reduce daily consumption. People are not inclined to take long baths or to waste water when they have to tote it a long way. In these cases, water use is usually restricted to cooking, cleaning, drinking, and occasionally bathing. Washing clothes and bathing may take place nearer to the source. This reduces the need for transporting water, but usually leads to further contamination of the

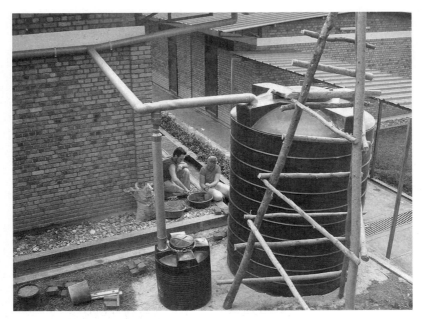

Figure 5-3. Rain water. (Photo by Edward H. Winant.)

source water unless protective steps are taken as outlined previously.

Another method of water delivery is the commercial water cart. Here, larger supplies of water are brought to homes by cart, and the water is sold to the homeowner. Carts can vary from small pushcarts carrying 50 gallons or so to animal-drawn carts with a few hundred gallons, or to tanker trucks capable of delivering thousands of gallons (Figure 5-4).

The "modern," or preferred, method of water delivery is through pipes. Laying pipes in the ground is an expensive investment in community infrastructure, which is the main drawback to its universal adoption. When using pipes, it is also necessary to provide pressure to force the water through them. This is typically done by pumps, which require a power source. Water towers are usually included in the system, because the demand for water varies through the day and can exceed the pumping rate. Thus towers store water at night, when demand is low, and assist the pumps in the morning and evening, when demand is highest. In some places pressure may be provided by gravity, if the water source is sufficiently elevated above the users. When relying on gravity, storage tanks are sometimes required to maintain a sufficient supply of water.

A commonly adopted system is to pipe water into a community center from a remote source and then require users to carry their daily supply from the tap to their homes. This reduces individual treks to find water from miles of walking to more reasonable distances, but

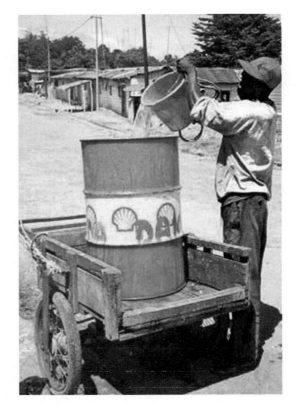

Figure 5-4. Water cart. (Photo from "Water in Africa" US Peace Corps Photograph Archive.)

also saves money on laying pipes throughout the community to every home.

WATER QUANTITY

What options exist for poor, rural people in the developing world? It must be recognized that in many places, an adequate *quantity* of water is more important than *quality*. Water may have to be carried, sometimes for miles, which consumes a huge amount of time, principally for women and children. In developed countries, the basic assumption is that each person uses 50 to 70 gallons per day (195–275 liters per day). Of course, this covers various uses such as watering the lawn, washing cars, laundry, automatic dishwashers, and teenagers taking long showers. The World Health Organization suggests that the minimum amount in the developing world, where people must carry their own water, is 2.5 gallons per day (10 liters per day). An adult in the setting of drought needs at least 5 liters of water per day for basic food and hydration needs, without even considering the needs for basic hygiene (washing hands, etc.).[9] Actual use will fall somewhere in this range and will tend to increase if water is piped directly into each house. Thus, efforts to decrease the environmental risks of unclean water must often address both quantity and quality.

- Feces should be kept out of water supplies with the use of basic or improved pit latrines.
- Water can be boiled if there is sufficient fuel in the area.
- Simple filtration (e.g., through cloth, such as a sari) will remove some pathogens, as has been amply demonstrated in Bangladesh and India.[10]
- It is being increasingly recognized that simply letting water settle after collection will carry many pathogens down with the sediment.
- Relatively simple methods for treatment at the household point of use—such as chlorinating water with the use of household bleach, or storing water in translucent or transparent vessels that allow ultraviolet (sunlight) sterilization to occur—are being tested.
- Communities can organize themselves to build simple water distribution systems, using PVC or similar pipes, where the source water is upstream of the community and therefore unlikely to be fecally contaminated.

WATER QUALITY

With water provided to homes, the next thought is treating it to improve the water quality and reduce incidents of sickness. Treatment may occur on many levels, from small doses for the individual, to a household system for all occupants, to community-wide treatment systems. However, the basic steps and methods of treatment are similar at all levels.

Water treatment consists of three basic steps, though not every method includes all the steps.

1. Primary, or physical, treatment consists of settling out particles in the water.
2. Secondary, or biological, treatment involves filtering the water through a benign biological layer to reduce organic contamination. The biological layer is typically fixed or suspended in some type of filter medium, such as sand. Modern plants in the developed world sometimes use plastic shapes or grids for the same purpose.
3. Tertiary, or chemical, treatment (also known as disinfection) is aimed at killing and removing harmful pathogens in the water. The most common chemical for disinfection is chlorine.

Personal water treatment, mostly used in travel situations, consists of either portable filters (backpacking water filters) or chemical tablets. Backpacking filters use a hand pump to force water through extremely small pores in a filter medium and remove particles, organic materials, and possibly pathogens, depending on the pore size. Tablets, either chlorine or iodine, disinfect the water, killing pathogens but not removing any silt, particles, or organic material. These tablets will not remove color or existing bad taste from the water.

Household treatment accounts for daily water use for several people. The simplest method is to store water in large covered barrels. This form of primary treatment will settle out particles in the water that lead to bad taste and color. Secondary treatment, or filtration, can be achieved with a range of commercially bought units that use porcelain candles or fabric bags to strain out contaminants. In general, the pore sizes on these filters are not small enough to remove pathogens, so a disinfection step is also required. Forcing water through a pore size small enough to remove pathogens requires pressure, and this complication would make most home-sized filters too complex (Figure 5-5).

The most accepted method of disinfection for a household is boiling. Water temperatures higher than 140°F (60°C) will kill pathogens. Of course, without a thermometer it is hard to judge 140°F, so bringing the water to boiling temperature is a nice visual indication of the proper amount of heat. Some authorities recommend boiling water for 30 minutes to ensure complete disinfection. This can be quite wasteful of fuel, however, and boiling water for 5 minutes or less will typically give good results. The water should be boiled in a covered pot for protection and be allowed to cool. When sufficiently cool, it may be poured into the filter or other storage container.

Household filters can also be constructed using local materials. Typically the container is an oil drum or other large barrel. Gravel is placed at the bottom around the outlet pipe, which needs to be punched through the barrel wall. The gravel should be small enough, such as pea gravel, so that the sand does not settle into the pore spaces. Over the gravel, at least 24 inches (0.60 m) of

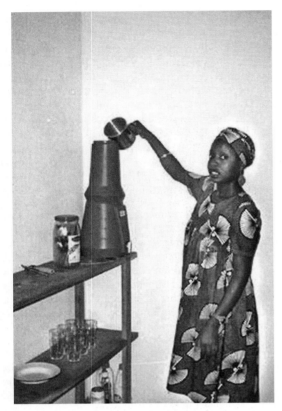

Figure 5-5. Home water. (Photo from "Water in Africa" US Peace Corps Photograph Archive.)

Community water treatment is generally an extension of the procedures just mentioned. Settling basins are used to remove solid particles suspended in the water. Filters are then used to further purify the water, and then it is disinfected and stored.

Historically, the first community filters were slow sand filters. These were large beds of sand through which water slowly percolated. The slow rate of application kept the sand from getting clogged too often. When the sand had trapped enough contamination to clog the filter and reduce the percolation, the filter was cleaned by manually raking the sand and removing the top layer. As demand for water in cities grew, these slow filters soon became too large, and rapid sand filters were introduced. As the name implies, the water is applied much more quickly to a rapid sand filter, and the filter tends to clog much sooner. The cleaning method is to apply a backwash periodically to the filter. Backwashing means forcing water through the filter in the reverse direction, which expands the sand, cleans out the clogging material, and readies the filter for continued operation. In developing countries with available land, especially for small communities, slow sand filters are preferred for their low cost and easily understood maintenance. Where land is not available, rapid sand filters should be considered.

For disinfection, the most commonly used chemical is chlorine. It comes in three forms: gas, liquid, and solid tablet. The gas form can be somewhat tricky, so for small systems, a liquid drip is the preferred method. This drip is introduced by a small feed pump into the water line so that the concentration of chlorine in the water is roughly constant. Chlorine is a dangerous chemical, both for the operator and for the end user if the concentration is too high. However, it is well understood, relatively inexpensive, and leaves a residual in the water line that continues to protect the quality of the water throughout transmission.

People living in the developed world as well as the developing world have the need to maintain rigorous water treatment and sanitation practices. The methods used for water treatment—halogenation, usually with chlorine or chloramines, and then filtration—were devised over a century ago, and although effective when optimally implemented, suffer the deficiencies of old technology. Chlorination is highly effective against bacterial and viral infections, and when first instituted it uniformly leads to major decreases in the burden of disease due to these infections. However, it is ineffective against a number of emerging pathogens that are chlorine resistant. Many of these resistant pathogens are most active where especially susceptible populations exist, such as people with acquired immunodeficiency syndrome (AIDS) or pregnant women.

An epidemic of waterborne toxoplasmosis was detected in Vancouver, Canada, stemming from the use of water from a reservoir that was chlorinated but not

sand should be placed. This should leave enough room at the top of the barrel for water to stay while it filters through the sand. The outlet pipe should also be equipped with a tap, so that water may be withdrawn without problem. Of course, this means the filter needs to be raised enough to get a container under the tap.

Another good household disinfection method is using clay filters treated with colloidal silver, such as those made by Potters for Peace.[11] These filters, which can be made locally in almost any village, are inexpensive and do a fair job of destroying pathogens. The silver impregnation lasts for about a year of normal use before replacement is needed.

Of all these household treatment methods, the single most important is boiling, because this does an effective job of removing pathogens, and every household has a way of heating water. Thus, teaching villagers to boil water is the single most effective way of getting them to improve their water quality. It can be difficult to convince them of the need, however, since the fuel cost of boiling all drinking water can be excessive. However, this simple step can reduce the incidence of sickness dramatically, especially for infants, young children, and the aged.

filtered. Astute clinicians noted an increase in the number of cases of in utero (congenital) *Toxoplasma* infections, as well as retinal disease in the general population. An epidemiologic investigation revealed that cougar feces in the watershed contained *Toxoplasma* oocysts. Presumably, the infectious oocysts were washed by rainfall into the reservoir and (unaffected by the chlorination) then directly entered the drinking water supply.[12] To globalize this incident, one only needs to reflect on the absence of filtration in many countries where basic chlorination is provided. Estimates from Central America and Africa suggest that the majority of cases of toxoplasmosis are the result of infection with the oocyst form of the parasite, which is only excreted by felines. In the United States and Europe, most toxoplasmosis is the result of eating undercooked meat that contains *Toxoplasma* cysts.[13] The addition of filtration to water treatment, even simple sand filtration, is believed to decrease the risk of infection from pathogens such as *Giardia, Cryptosporidium* (and, one supposes, *Toxoplasma*) by about 100-fold.[14]

Filtration is not a perfect defense, even though it may remove the vast majority of pathogens (99.00% to 99.99% of pathogens is typical for modern conventional treatment plants).[14] Unfortunately, the infectious dose needed to infect 50% of people for *Cryptosporidium* is under ten oocysts for some strains,[15] suggesting that even the rare organism that slips through the filtration system can cause illness. The largest outbreak of waterborne disease in the history of the United States occurred in Milwaukee in 1993 when more than 400,000 people became clinically ill with cryptosporidiosis when one of the two filtration plants in Milwaukee failed.[16] Of note, infection rates in households with tap water filters were approximately 80% lower than in households without them. In 1994, an epidemic of cryptosporidiosis in Las Vegas in people with AIDS was epidemiologically linked to the municipal water supply, even though it met all relevant chlorination and filtration standards.[17] It must be emphasized that the two major causes of persistent diarrhea in people with HIV/AIDS in the developing world are cryptosporidiosis and microsporidiosis.[18] These pathogens cause chronic diarrhea and malabsorption with wasting. Neither of these diseases has reliably effective drug treatment, and thus prevention (through paired drinking water treatment and sanitation) is the only real option against these scourges.

The use of halogens in treating water introduces variable levels of these elements into water. Halogens have been linked (at higher levels) to bladder cancer, fetal congenital defects, and miscarriages.[19] The balance between a halogen level sufficient to kill pathogens and low enough to minimize other risks is a delicate but necessary one.[20] Failures of chlorination have led to outbreaks of dysentery and diarrhea in Canada[21] and typhoid in Central Asia,[22] proving the point that water

treatment systems cannot be allowed to fail, no matter the location. One of the ironies of water treatment practices is that source water protection (e.g., not letting fecal material enter source water for drinking purposes) has been ignored in many communities, under the assumption that water treatment will invariably render the water completely safe.

A safer, though somewhat more expensive, method of disinfection is ultraviolet (UV) light. This involves passing the water past UV light bulbs, where the radiation kills off the pathogens. UV disinfection requires relatively "clean" water, meaning that most of the suspended solids have been removed.

Of course, the application of water treatment depends heavily on the source water available. Surface waters, being unprotected, are usually suspected of being highly contaminated with organic material and pathogens. Further, many rivers and streams carry a high silt load, so settling basins (primary treatment) are almost always required when treating surface waters. Springs and shallow wells may be contaminated, depending on what is "upstream" of them in a groundwater sense. Mountaintop springs, which basically are fed by pure rainwater, can be of very high quality. Springs situated below farms or houses are likely to be quite contaminated. Still, groundwater does not carry the silt loads that surface waters do, so in many cases disinfection is all that is required of spring or well water. Deep wells, if properly constructed and drawing from a quality source, may not require any treatment to be safe for drinking.

SANITATION

Sanitation deals with treating the waste products of human society and making them safe for the environment and for public health. This section discusses human waste (feces and urine) and solid waste (garbage).

As with water treatment, wastewater treatment falls into the same three levels: primary (physical), secondary (biological), and tertiary (disinfection and polishing). Further, these apply to all wastewater treatment, from individual house systems up to the largest municipal plants.

Sanitation provides benefits beyond those of decreasing diarrheal disease. For example, intestinal nematode infections from *Ascaris, Trichuris,* and hookworm are all transmitted after fecal contamination of soil. The first two nematodes are ingested (either in soil or in contaminated uncooked food), and hookworm larvae penetrate the skin of people without shoes. All three of these cause diseases that contribute to malnutrition and to anemia but which can be completely prevented by the implementation of adequate disposal of feces. In the United States, rural poor farmers residing in the southern areas of the country were once regarded as lazy, before it was understood that most of them were severely anemic from hookworm infections. After World War I, the Rockefeller Foundation devoted enormous resources to convincing people to spend scarce resources on shoes and sanitation facilities.[23] Schistosomiasis, a trematode infection, affects hundreds of millions of people, and the infectious eggs are all excreted in urine or feces. Again, simple sanitation would abolish this disease over time in affected regions.

The most common form of sanitation in developing countries is the latrine or outhouse. These may be provided for individual houses or combined into a community facility. The latrine is a simple pit, covered with a durable slab, where users go to relieve themselves. Concrete slabs, at least 6 inches (15 cm) thick and reinforced with iron bars, make the best latrine floors. They are easy to clean, last a long time, and are very sturdy. A less expensive floor may make use of wooden planks or even logs.

Because no water is used to transport the waste, there is no need for wastewater treatment. The pit holds the solids, allowing for some biological degradation, but in general serves only for storage. Eventually the pit will reach capacity, leading to removal of the solids or digging a new pit. Ash or lime is sometimes added to the pit to help control odors.

The pit is usually left unlined if it is dug in a stable soil such as clay. Where sandy soils predominate, some reinforcement of the pit may be required. Although there is no effluent to treat, the urine will seep out the pit floor and walls into the surrounding soil. This is normal, even beneficial, but some care must be taken to separate the pit from the surrounding groundwater.

Two feet (0.61 m) of soil separation is sufficient to protect the groundwater. Thus, the pit should not be dug deeper than 2 feet above the water table. The water table may be determined roughly by the water depth of nearby shallow wells. Remember, however, that the water table will fluctuate according to wet and dry seasons; the latrine should be sited using the wet season water levels. If the groundwater level reaches the bottom of the pit, it will become contaminated and threaten nearby shallow wells and springs.

Where there are high groundwater tables, it may be necessary to construct vault latrines. This variation includes a lining for the pit of concrete, brick, or stonework to prevent groundwater contamination. Obviously, this method is more expensive, and so it is used only when absolutely required to protect the groundwater (Figure 5-6).

An implementation that many groups prefer is the ventilated, improved pit latrine (VIP latrine). This involves building solid walls that do not allow light through, a tight roof covering, and a screened ventilation pipe running to the top of the roof. The doorway must be set away from the prevailing winds, so that the wind draws air out of the latrine rather than forcing it in. Further, with no light in the latrine, the only light available to the pit comes from the pipe, which draws the flies up to the screen. Unable to escape, they die (Figure 5-7).

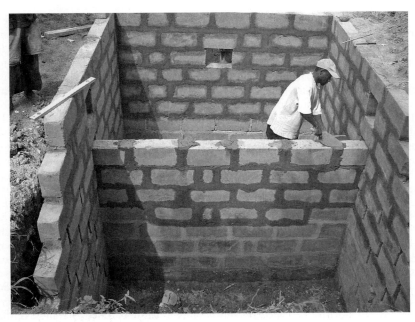

Figure 5-6. Vault latrine. (Photo by Edward H. Winant.)

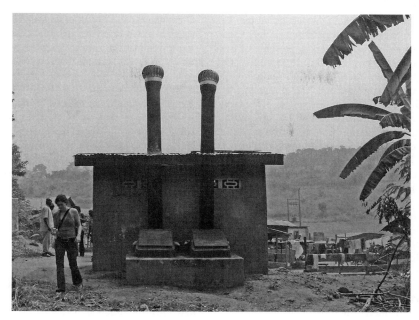

Figure 5-7. VIP latrine. (Photo by Edward H. Winant.)

Culturally, VIPs are unacceptable to some people. Because they are so used to latrines, they consider it improper to relieve oneself inside. Adding a roof to a latrine makes it a building, and thus not suitable. Many latrines are thus simple affairs with walls of plaited leaves or sheet metal for privacy, or situated so they are screened naturally by trees.

Another improvement on the common latrine is the composting latrine. This involves improvements to the pit so that air and heat are available to promote the composting process. Additionally, access is needed because the pile needs to be turned. This is usually done manually with a pitchfork to stir the accumulated waste. A carbon source is also needed and can be provided by sprinkling sawdust or throwing paper waste down the latrine hole after every use.

Once water is provided to individual homes, flush toilets can be installed, at which point wastewater becomes a much larger problem. The first step toward treatment is usually to pipe wastewater to the latrine pit, thus making it into a cesspool. However, this pit now has to deal with a great quantity of polluted water in addition to the solids it was storing. The water will leach out the sides of the pit; given the amounts of water used and the organic contamination, this will eventually clog the soil around the pit and back up into the house.

Septic systems, in which the solids settle into a tank and the effluent passes to a field of perforated pipes to soak into the ground, are much more effective in the long term. They require additional investment and a larger area for application, however. In areas of low housing density, they are undoubtedly the best method for wastewater treatment.

For areas of greater housing density, sewers are the preferred method. These large pipes, laid so gravity will convey the sewage, collect wastewater and convey it to a central treatment location. This treatment plant usually consists of settling tanks (primary treatment); biological treatment, such as filters or aeration tanks (secondary treatment); perhaps some polishing or additional filtration, and then disinfection (tertiary treatment). The treated effluent is then discharged to a nearby surface water body; the removed solids, now called sludge, will be deposited in a land fill, incinerated, or used as a soil amendment or crop fertilizer.

Biological treatment for community wastewater may be in several forms. The least technological is lagoons, or sewage ponds, where the sewage is contained for long periods of time to allow proper treatment. Lagoons do occupy large areas of land, but they do not require much maintenance. Sand filters are also frequently used to treat wastewater, as are aerobic tanks and wetlands. Aerobic tanks introduce air into the sewage to promote the growth of aerobic bacteria, which are very efficient at consuming organic waste. Filters work much the same as for water treatment, supporting a layer of bacteria that consume the organic waste, as well as physically straining the water to remove solids.

Constructed wetlands combine both methods of treatment. Here, the effluent flows through a gravel bed, which performs the tasks of a filter. Water-loving plants, such as reeds or cat-tails, grow in the gravel, and their roots provide oxygen for treatment, take up some of the effluent for their water needs, and also remove nitrogen and phosphorus from the waste as plant nutrients.

Proper sanitation also includes solid waste, or garbage. Sadly, this is commonly overlooked, and many villages have no way of dealing with their accumulating garbage. It is frequently piled in heaps or scattered about carelessly. Both conditions are unsightly, smelly, and can support rodents, insects, and other disease vectors.

When garbage is collected in central locations around the community, it is common to periodically set fire to the collected waste and burn off the combustibles. Although incineration is certainly an accepted method of reducing the volume of solid waste, it is helpful to attempt it in controlled conditions. Certain materials, notably plastics and tires, give off noxious fumes when burned. In general, the smoke from trash fires can be hazardous and is certainly annoying to nearby residents. Finally, some materials will not burn and will remain after the attempted incineration.

Another method of solid waste treatment is land filling. This requires a suitable area of land set aside to receive the solid waste, preferably away from most residents. It also requires soil to be placed over layers of garbage to contain the odors and disease vectors. The soil cover, with accompanying ditches and landscaping to control runoff, is important to keep water contaminated by the waste (termed *leachate*) away from other sources of water that serve the community. If possible, the floor of the landfill should be a heavy clay soil, compacted by machinery to further contain the leachate.

Given that landfills and dumps should not be too close to communities, a garbage collection and transport method should be established. Although it is certainly possible for each resident to make a trip to the town dump, it is more convenient to have local community collection points throughout the town and have the garbage picked up and taken to the landfill using community resources.

RECREATIONAL WATER EXPOSURE

Recreational water exposure has also been recognized as a potent source of fecal-oral contamination. Indeed, the US Centers for Disease Control and Prevention defined swimming in pools and other recreational waters as "communal bathing" and has published studies on the average mass of feces carried by swimmers into pools. In the United States, epidemics of disease caused by *Giardia, Shigella,* and *Cryptosporidium* occur every year because of fecal contamination of recreational swimming sites such as pools, lakes, rivers, and beaches.[24] Recreational waters in some countries are contaminated not only by diarrheal fecal pathogens but also by parasitic pathogens such as schistosomes and by viruses such as polio, other

enteroviruses, and hepatitis A. Historically, polio was frequently waterborne in the now-developed world, and swimming in rivers, ponds, or lakes (which are obviously not chlorinated) was a recognized risk for the disease.

MANAGEMENT OF WATER AND SANITATION SYSTEMS

Use of community resources brings up an important point: management. In many cases, it is not the technology or even the resources that are a barrier to project implementation; it is the continued management of the project that causes failure. Any village in the world can dig latrines and shallow wells and provide for trash collection. What is lacking is the community management needed to marshal the community resources to accomplish these tasks and see to their continued operation and maintenance.

For instance, tales of broken and unrepaired pumps, caved-in wells, or dilapidated spring boxes are common throughout the developing world. Many of these projects are installed by well-meaning and dedicated volunteers and nonprofit organizations. The projects work well and are much appreciated for several years. But something eventually breaks and there is no money to fix it. The impressive and helpful project goes to waste, and the residents return to their previous ways of getting water or eliminating waste.

It is important to involve local residents in project planning and implementation. This means more than just asking the opinions of the village elders. In many cases the elders, usually men, want a project that will bring prestige or honor to their village. However, the women and children who must make use of the new infrastructure have other ideas. For instance, when it is the children's job to get water, it is no good installing a hand pump that requires great strength to use. It is also sometimes the case that women who walk a good way to gather water at a remote spring cherish the communal time they have together and resent the piping of this spring into the village to relieve them of some of their hard work.

Thus, project planning should involve representatives of all groups in a community. It should also deal with requirements for upkeep and use of the installed equipment. The minimum level of management should be the creation of a community committee charged with overseeing and maintaining the project. This committee should have a maintenance budget and a way to collect money from the users. For example, a hand pump costing $1,500 and expected to last 20 years should have $75 collected each year in a replacement fund ($6.25 each month). If this pump serves 25 homes, then each family would be expected to contribute $0.25 each month.

What happens, in many cases, is that some people do not pay, even when they have the best of intentions. Perhaps the harvest failed, or a child was sick and they needed the money for medicine. If they fail to pay and yet can still use the community resource (pump or spring box or latrine), they have less incentive to pay in the future. Neighbors, seeing this, are also less inclined to pay. Sadly, it is very common for no one to pay into community repair funds. Then, 15 or 20 years down the road, when the pump breaks or the latrine is full, there is no money to fix it.

It is helpful, therefore, to have some enforcement capacity for the committee. At the very least, peer pressure can be exerted on noncontributing families to encourage their participation. The most effective management, of course, is the utility model, where users pay for the amount of water or sanitation services that they use and can be cut off for nonpayment. This provides an enforcement action to ensure continued participation.

DISTURBANCE OF THE NATURAL ENVIRONMENT AND RISKS FOR INFECTIOUS DISEASES

Some ecosystems support *Anopheles, Culex,* or *Aedes* mosquitoes, which transmit diseases such as malaria, filariasis, dengue, and yellow fever. Brackish water, as found in coastal mangrove swamps, is a reservoir for *Vibrio cholerae,* the agent of cholera. Perhaps by convention or out of reverence for the natural environment, we do not usually consider a pristine swamp an environmental hazard. However, it is clear that our forebearers did, for they industriously drained swamps to provide more arable land and to decrease the risks of diseases such as malaria. One of the greatest accomplishments of the fascist Italian dictator Mussolini was the drainage of the swamps near Rome and the eradication of malaria from the region. When the Tennessee Valley Authority in the United States built dams in the 1930s and 1940s to provide electricity to Appalachian areas, studious care was taken to periodically alter the water levels in dams and rivers in order to disrupt the hatching of mosquito eggs. This had, at times, devastating effects on the aquatic habitat of the affected rivers, but the incidence of malaria was dampened by these tactics.

A counterexample demonstrating the importance of intact ecosystems to human health is that of the Naivasha Lake region in the Rift Valley of Kenya. The town of Naivasha does not treat its sewage, which flows into a lake that is used for both drinking water purposes and fishing. Fortunately, the Kenya Wildlife Service maintains a game preserve where the contaminated water from the town flows into wetlands. The wetlands detoxify and decontaminate the wastes before they enter the lake. Indeed, the use of artificial wetlands in tropical countries is being promoted globally as a way to treat wastewater without the capital expense of a modern treatment plant.[25]

There is substantial evidence that the destruction of ecosystems increases the hazards of infectious diseases. Malaria epidemics often follow the construction of roads and houses in forested areas because new water pools (breeding sites for mosquitoes) are unintentionally left without adequate drainage near the construction. Indeed, deforestation of tropical forests, and the concomitant construction of crude logging roads to remove the trees, results in predictable increases in mosquito-borne infections. As an example, yellow fever is maintained in a high forest canopy (sylvan) cycle between primates and mosquitoes in South America that does not involve humans. When trees are felled by loggers, however, the yellow fever-infected mosquitoes then bite the workers, who carry the infection to cities, where the cycle is maintained in humans via *Aedes aegypti* mosquitoes (the urban cycle).

Other examples are plentiful. The damming of the Nile River at Aswan in Egypt led to an explosion in the incidence of schistosomiasis, as did the damming of the Volta River in Ghana. Schistosomes have difficulty penetrating the skin of human hosts in rapidly flowing waters, but the damming led to placid waters and greatly increased transmission. The introduction of irrigation in Puerto Rico for sugar cane production led to extremely high rates of schistosomiasis at the turn of the last century.[26] The several decades long increase in the incidence of Lyme disease in the densely populated northeastern United States is considered by most biologists to be the result of an exploding deer population (after elimination of their natural predators) and the desire of humans to live in suburban or semirural areas. Both of these factors increase the likelihood of exposure to the tick vector, which normally feeds on deer and mice. Thus, environmental risks for acquiring infectious diseases often are linked to both disturbed or changed ecosystems and increasing human presence in the involved area.

As delineated by the WHO, three approaches to the environmental management of mosquito-borne diseases such as malaria, Japanese encephalitis, and dengue are as follows:[1]

1. Modification of the environment to reduce vector habitats
2. Manipulation of the environment on some periodic basis
3. Modification of human behavior or habitation

Draining swamps, leveling land, filling in pools, modifying river boundaries, lining irrigation canals to prevent water loss, and avoiding stagnant waters are examples of the first approach. In urban environments, these methods include the construction of drains, improving house design so that water does not pool in gutters, and providing wastewater and sanitation facilities to remove mosquito breeding sites.

The second approach is represented by efforts such as changing the levels of reservoirs. The third includes simple methods such as fine screens in household windows to decrease contact with mosquitoes, and the use of bednets. Bednets are an interesting tool because they incorporate both an environmental barrier between the vector and humans, and, if insecticide treated, a chemical defense as well. Treated bednets have been found to reduce overall mortality in children younger than 5 living in malaria-endemic regions by as much as 40%.[27]

CLIMATE, THE ENVIRONMENT, AND HUMAN HEALTH

The linkage between climate, alterations in the environment, and specific diseases is regarded as well founded. The incidence of cholera in western South America and of diseases such as Oroya fever in the Andes has been linked to the sea temperature of the Humboldt Current, especially during El Niño phenomena.[28] The details and mechanistic explanations for these relationships are still being delineated, but it is not hard to imagine that sea temperature affects land conditions, which in turn affect vegetation and humidity, and in turn the density of insect vectors of disease. By way of example, my colleagues and I have shown that cases of *Salmonella* and *Campylobacter* infection reported to the Massachusetts Department of Public Health are tightly linked to the ambient temperature, whereas reported cases of *Cryptosporidium, Shigella,* and *Giardia* infections peak some weeks after the peak in summer temperature.[29] *Salmonella* and *Campylobacter* are known to reproduce in foodstuffs, and the coinciding peaks of temperature and infection with these two bacterial pathogens probably represent the product of maximal bacterial growth during the hottest days of the year. In contrast, it can be argued that the triad of *Cryptosporidium, Shigella,* and *Giardia* infections in Massachusetts represents transmission via recreational water exposure. Surface waters used for recreational purposes (ponds, rivers, outdoor pools) achieve their highest temperatures some weeks after ambient air temperatures peak, explaining the lag period, since people are most likely to swim when the water is warmest.

Environmental factors also include rainfall. In many cities and towns in the United States, surface water runoff is drained into the sewage treatment system, because separate runoff and sewage treatment systems are more expensive than a combined system. However, heavy rainfall can overwhelm the capacity of sewage systems, leading to the discharge of untreated sewage into rivers or lakes. Indeed, Curriero and colleagues have shown that waterborne disease epidemics in the United States tend to follow periods of very heavy rainfall.[30] In the developing world, it has been noted that epidemics of diseases such as cryptosporidiosis tend to occur at the beginning of the rainy season, when rainfall is likely to sweep human and animal wastes into waters eventually used for drinking and cleaning.[31]

Infectious disease is also the final mechanism by which other physical environmental factors cause human disease. For example, air pollution both decreases lung function and increases the risk of pneumonia.

Physical Hazards

Physical environmental hazards include not only catastrophic events such as hurricanes, drought, earthquakes, cyclones, and floods, but also the hazards of the human-constructed, or human-altered, environment. One way the constructed environment interacts with catastrophic environmental events is the building of towns in floodplains. Another way is extensive deforestation above towns, which promotes increased flash flooding and mudslides after heavy rains. The rainwater is no longer retained in the sponge of forest vegetation. In addition to the risk of catastrophic loss of life and property, even periodic minor flooding can be dangerous. It has been shown in Brazil that periodic flooding of lower-lying neighborhoods is strongly associated with hemorrhagic fever due to leptospirosis.[32]

Global warming is another physical hazard. Scientific consensus concludes that higher overall global temperatures have led to both higher and lower rainfall for different areas, higher sea levels, and at times drastic changes in climate and vegetation. Whereas climate determines the geographic range of infectious diseases, extreme weather related to climate variability (and manifested in our physical environment through rain, heat, cold, etc.) affects the timing and intensity of infectious disease outbreaks.[33]

The linkage between a changing climate, the environment, and human health may prove dramatic or subtle. Drought, which can be the result of both climate change and of deforestation, can lead to such severe economic shocks that the risk of civil war increases.[34] Catastrophic environmental events often lead to displaced populations and refugee communities. These catastrophes can be rapid (a flood, a drought) or slow (desertification near the Sahel, slow sea-level rises) but are, in either case, severe. For example, should the sea level rise by a meter in the next 50 years, a substantial minority of the population of Bangladesh will lose their low-lying land. How will they survive? Will they die of starvation as they lose their subsistence farmland, or will they attempt to immigrate into neighboring countries that are unlikely to welcome them (e.g., India, Myanmar)? Some Pacific island nations may become submerged. One can argue that this form of slowly advancing catastrophe is no less profound than a dramatic, immediate one.

THE BUILT ENVIRONMENT

There is a growing recognition that the *built environment* (of towns, cities, and roads) can contribute to, or be deleterious to, health. Urban environments often provide social, economic, and cultural opportunities that more rural areas do not, and in so doing, provide a mixture of environmental benefits and risks. For example, water treatment systems and sewerage (with their major benefits) are often more available in urban environments than in rural ones, because cities have the ability to raise the capital for water and sewerage projects. Other aspects of urban life are negative: for example, some wealthy towns have eliminated sidewalks in residential areas and isolated commercial areas so they can only be reached by automobiles. This practice promotes the use of (polluting) automobiles even for minor errands and, through discouraging exercise, indirectly promotes obesity, diabetes, and cardiovascular disease.[35,36] High levels of noise are common in urban areas and in some occupations. It has been estimated that 16% of all deafness can be attributed to such occupational exposures.[1,37]

Pedestrian and traffic deaths are also a major concern. In northern Europe, roadway designs have been developed over the past 50 years that minimize pedestrian deaths from traffic accidents. Traffic speed is limited by "traffic calming" through roadway bumps, one-way streets, road narrowing, traffic circles, and other measures that decrease speed and increase the likelihood of pedestrian survival. These intelligent designs are uncommon; thus, increased deaths from traffic accidents (as well as air pollution) commonly accompany urbanization. In many parts of the world, improvements in roadways are not accompanied by segregated bicycle lanes, parallel walking paths with roadside barriers, or designated pedestrian crossways. Pedestrian deaths then occur when people walk on roadways. Other contributing factors include a lack of street lighting and signage, narrow roads, and poor road maintenance. Traffic accident death rates in many countries are an order of magnitude higher than they are in developed countries such as the United States.[38] (Unbelievably, most motor vehicles imported into India are not currently equipped with seat belts as a "cost saving" measure.) Traffic accidents are believed to account for 2.6% of DALYs worldwide.[1] The leading cause of tourist death is traffic accidents, not infectious diseases.

Chemical Hazards

NATURALLY OCCURRING CHEMICAL RISKS

The natural physical environment can be a source of naturally occurring chemical and radiological risks, such as heavy metals (arsenic) or radionuclides (uranium, radium, thorium, actinium, radon, etc.). For example, the US Environmental Protection Agency (EPA) estimated that approximately 420,000 and 620,000 US residents are potentially exposed to elevated levels of radium-228 and uranium, respectively, from drinking water.[39] Radon is the decay product of radium, which in turn is the decay product of uranium. It is a risk factor for lung cancer and is usually present as a dissolved gas in groundwater. It is released into household basements from the surrounding ground or when groundwater with dissolved radon is aerosolized (e.g., in the shower). The EPA estimates that approximately 1 in

15 households in the United States is at risk of exposure to elevated levels of radon. The global burden of risk is unknown.[40] Uranium miners are at a very increased risk of cancer because of their occupational exposures to this potent carcinogen. In Europe this risk was recognized as early as 1879, yet little protection was afforded to miners in the United States before 1962, again demonstrating the need for adequate health regulations and standards for environmental exposures.[41]

Heavy metals exposure is common. Lead is ubiquitous: it is used in batteries and in industrial processes, is added to paint and gasoline, and is found in water distribution pipes and fittings. Lead exposure leads to mental retardation, anemia, and hypertension, among other conditions. Acutely high lead levels lead to anemia and seizures, but even chronically low levels are a cause for concern. In 2002, the WHO estimated that lead-associated mental retardation represented about 0.75% of all DALYs.[37] These risks existed even in ancient times; for example, the Romans ate and drank from lead cups and plates, and added lead to foodstuffs. This practice is thought to have led to an epidemic of infertility. Leaded gasoline is still frequently used globally, and lead poisoning is common where its use in paint and gasoline has not been banned. The extent of this burden has been poorly studied.

Globally, more than 100 million people are believed to be exposed to high levels of arsenic from drinking water.[42] The digging of deep tube wells to provide potable water in Bangladesh has sharply decreased deaths due to fecally contaminated water but has sharply increased the incidence of skin disease, renal impairment, hypertension, and cancer because of arsenic contamination of the groundwater.[43] Estimates exist that one-third of the Bangladeshi population is drinking water with an unacceptably high level of arsenic. In one study from the Matlab region of Bangladesh, 54% of people consumed water containing more than 50 μg/L of arsenic.[44] The US National Academy of Sciences has concluded that there is no safe level of arsenic in water.[45] In contrast to the situation in Bangladesh, arsenic exposure in other areas is secondary to industrial processes or mining. For example, exposure to high levels of arsenic (via water contamination) in the western United States is usually due to abandoned mine wastes (tailings) entering the water supply. In the eastern United States, high levels of arsenic are naturally found in some groundwater or in waters contaminated by industry over the past 150 years.[46]

Occupations such as sandblasting place workers at risk of the scarring lung disease known as silicosis. Occupational exposures to hazardous physical environments are common and are a major opportunity for decreasing the human disease burden. Occupational risks can include exposure to industrial chemicals and solvents, including carcinogens such as benzene as well as heavy metals such as mercury. Mercury is used to isolate gold from ore; in informal gold mines in South America, mercury poisoning affects not only the miners but also their families because they bring contaminated clothing home. In the rivers where the mercurial wastes are dumped, the mercury is concentrated in fish, which are then consumed by the population, further distributing the ill effects of mercury.[47] As described later in this chapter in the section "Air Pollution," the combustion of coal for power generation is another significant source of mercury exposure.

SYNTHETIC CHEMICALS

As the world has industrialized, risks from nonnatural, synthetic chemicals associated with manufacturing and agriculture have risen sharply. The manifestations of exposure to these chemicals depend on the class of chemical. Suffice it to say these manifestations may include damage to fetuses; malignancies; damage to specific organs such as the nervous system, kidneys, or liver; metabolic syndromes; and damage to fertility. Exposure to these chemicals can occur occupationally; through contamination of food, water, or air; and through dermal contact. It is not possible in the space of this chapter to review all of these, and indeed the global burden of disease from synthetic chemicals is unknown.

Pesticides and herbicides have achieved a level of notoriety related to their overuse and application without safety precautions. Many examples exist of neurologic effects due to acute exposures.[48] Chronic exposures to these agents can lead to unexpected results. For example, the pesticide 1,2-dibromo-3-chloropropane (DBCP) was developed in the 1950s to kill banana root nematode parasites. In the mid-1970s a group of 35 workers in California were found to be sterile after applying DBCP, and its use was banned in 1979. However, it continued to be exported and used in countries such as Ecuador, Guatemala, Nicaragua, Honduras, the Philippines, and Costa Rica. It is believed that many thousands of workers became sterile after using DBCP without proper equipment. Pesticides and other noxious chemicals that are otherwise useful may be casually stored at the household level in unmarked, leaky containers. These containers can be opened by children, allowing accidental poisonings and exposures. Better packaging and storage could eliminate these frequent events.[49] Ingestion of a pesticide is also a frequently used method of suicide.[50]

Air Pollution

Studies over the past 30 years have identified air pollution as one of the most, if not the most, important environmental hazards to humans. Air pollution has been linked to respiratory disease (infections, asthma, and chronic obstructive pulmonary disease); cardiovascular diseases, including myocardial infarction; cancer; impaired lung development in adolescents; and intrauterine growth retardation and congenital anomalies.[51-55] Rapidly growing societies, such as modern China, are characterized by severe air pollution in nearly all major cities. The principal causes of outdoor air pollution include exhaust products of internal combustion engines and power generation, as well as industrial releases. Air pollutants are a complex mixture of gases (carbon monoxide, nitrogenous compounds, ozone, etc.) and particulates, which vary in size. The gases may have effects in isolation, but also undergo chemical reactions once produced, resulting in smog that may contain sulfuric acid and other respiratory irritants. Particulates (soot) can act as inanimate vectors that deliver carcinogenic polyaromatic hydrocarbons into the lungs when inhaled.

Buses and trucks in some cities are the major sources of air pollution, and reducing air pollution may require mandatory modifications to their engines. Interestingly, in studies done in the Andean countries of South America, the modifications made to reduce pollutants usually led to increased engine energy efficiency, decreased costs for fuel, and a net increase in profits for the operators of the buses and trucks.[56] This point is made to remind the reader that the benefits of remediating environmental risks may easily outweigh the costs when fully examined. Cost-benefit analyses in the United States and the European Union have strongly suggested that the control of air pollution leads to major improvements in human health.

Air pollution can occur very locally, such as in the household from heating or cooking, or across a large swath of land. Power generating plants and incineration facilities tend to release pollutants from high chimney stacks, and thus the pollutants are dispersed much higher in the atmosphere than those from houses or automobiles. In the United States, approximately 48 tons of mercury are released into the environment every year from coal-burning plants. This amount is about 40% of the annual release of around 120 tons of mercury. Half of this amount is deposited locally, and the other half distantly.[57] The global burden of mercury release has been estimated to be between 4,400 and 7,500 tons per year.

Indoor air pollution, from the use of biofuels such as wood and from tobacco smoke exposure, is now understood to be a major contributor to respiratory infections. Lower respiratory infection (LRI), especially pneumonia, remains the leading cause of death in children younger than 5 years, and 36% of all LRIs have been attributed to the use of biofuels for cooking and heating.[58,59] This percentage translates into approximately 1 million deaths a year in children younger than 5. Environmental exposure to tobacco smoke leads to recurrent otitis media in children[60,61] and to lung cancer and chronic obstructive lung disease, even in people who are not active smokers.[62,63] Fuels such as natural gas and propane gas burn more cleanly and efficiently than biofuels, and their use reduces household pollution levels. Innovative cooking stoves that use biofuels are being devised that are both more fuel efficient and ventilate outside the household, so that indoor pollution levels are minimized. Volatile organic compounds, nitrogen dioxide, carbon monoxide, and biological allergens are other forms of indoor air pollution. These contribute to a total of perhaps 1.5 to 2.0 million deaths yearly from indoor air pollution.[64]

Increased rates of tuberculosis have been linked to both indoor air pollution and environmental tobacco smoke, but the degree of this association is not well understood.[1]

SUMMARY

This brief overview has used a definition of environmental health that tries to encompass the biological, physical, and chemical risks to humans that are mediated through the environment. Major improvements to human health could be accomplished by increased attention to these risks, since they represent a large proportion of the total global disease burden. It is important to emphasize that this burden of disease disproportionately falls upon developing and transitional countries. Indeed, it is difficult to see how progress toward meeting the Millennium Development Goals[65,66] can be achieved without attention to these factors. Reducing child mortality and improving maternal health (goals 4 and 5), combating the major infectious and noncommunicable diseases (goal 6), ensuring environmental sustainability (goal 7), and promoting responsible development (goal 8) all require addressing environmental issues. Even the developed, richer countries are by no means immune to environmental risks, given the increased use of chemicals in agriculture and industry, heavy reliance on road transportation, and air pollution.

Despite the enormity of the challenge, there is room for hope. Environmental issues are being addressed, and many of the risks are well understood and easily avoided. Complex technology is not needed to remove lead from the environment, clean water and sanitation are not new processes, and there are now many examples of the successful control of air pollution. In addition, there are now many societies that have successfully tackled these problems and improved the lives of their citizens. From the global perspective, these instances of success should be models for others.

STUDY QUESTIONS

1. Name three leading pollutants that influence human health and describe their health consequences, delineating both their magnitude and how these health effects can be prevented.

2. There are three levels of water treatment: physical, biological, and chemical. What are the effects of each type of treatment? Are they always necessary? How can they be combined or avoided?

3. In a situation in which raw sewage disposal is contaminating a water supply, what problem should be addressed first, treating the sewage or the drinking water? What are the advantages or disadvantages to doing one project before the other?

SELECTED BIBLIOGRAPHY ON WATER AND SANITATION

Brush RE. *Wells Construction: Hand Dug and Hand Drilled*. Washington, DC: Peace Corps, 1979. Information Collection and Exchange Manual M-9.

Cairncross S, Feachem R. *Small Water Supplies*. London: Ross Institute of Tropical Hygiene, 1986.

Elder JR. *Manual of Small Public Water Supply Systems*. Washington, DC: US Environmental Protection Agency, 1991.

Hutton LG. *Field Testing of Water in Developing Countries*. Marlow, UK: Water Research Center, 1983.

Manja KS, et al. A simple field test for the detection of faecal pollution in drinking water. *Bull World Health Organ* 1982;60(5):797–901.

Mara D. *Sewage Treatment in Hot Climates*. New York: John Wiley and Sons, 1976.

Pickford J, et al. *The Worth of Water: Technical Briefs on Health, Water and Sanitation*. London: Intermediate Technology Publications, 1991.

Ross Institute of Tropical Hygiene. *The Preservation of Personal Health in Warm Climates*. London: Ross Institute of Tropical Hygiene, 1985.

Talbert DE. *Water/Sanitation Case Studies and Analysis*. Washington, DC: Peace Corps, 1984.

US Environmental Protection Agency. *Onsite Wastewater Treatment Systems Manual*. Washington, DC: US Environmental Protection Agency, 2002. EPA/625/R-00/008.

Viessman W, Hammer MJ. *Water Supply and Pollution Control*. 4th ed. New York: Harper and Row, 1985.

Wilkie W. *Jordan's Tropical Hygiene and Sanitation*. London: Bailliere, Tindall and Cox, 1965.

Winblad U, Kilama W. *Sanitation Without Water*. London: MacMillan, 1985.

USEFUL INTERNET SITES

American Waterworks Association: http://www.awwa.org

London School of Hygiene and Tropical Medicine, University of London, United Kingdom: http://www.lshtm.ac.uk

National Small Flows Clearinghouse and National Drinking Water Clearinghouse, West Virginia University: http://www.nesc.wvu.edu

US Army Water Supply Program: http://www.apgea.army.mil/dwater

Water Engineering and Development Centre (WEDC), Loughborough University, United Kingdom: http://www.info.lboro.ac.uk/departments/cv/wedc/index.html

REFERENCES

1. Prüss-Üstün A, Corvalán C. *Preventing Disease Through Healthy Environments. Towards an Estimate of the Environmental Burden of Disease*. Geneva: World Health Organization, 2006.

2. Ezzati M, Lopez AD, Rodgers A, et al. Selected major risk factors and global and regional burden of disease. *Lancet* 2002;360:1347–1360.

3. Briggs D. Environmental pollution and the global burden of disease. *Br Med Bull* 2003;68:1–24.

4. Royal Commission on Environmental Pollution. *Chemicals in Products: Safeguarding the Environment and Human Health.* London: Royal Commission on Environmental Health, 2003.

5. Luby SP, Agboatwalla M, Feikin DR, et al. Effect of handwashing on child health: a randomised controlled trial. *Lancet* 2005;366(9491):185–187.

6. Esrey SA, Habicht JP. Epidemiologic evidence for health benefits from improved water and sanitation in developing countries. *Epidemiol Rev* 1986;8:117–128.

7. World Health Organization. *Evaluation of the Costs and Benefits of Water and Sanitation Improvements at the Global Level.* Geneva: World Health Organization, 2004.

8. World Health Organization and UNICEF. *Water for Life: Making It Happen.* Geneva: World Health Organization, 2005.

9. Howard G, Bartram J. *Domestic Water Quantity, Service Level and Health.* Geneva: World Health Organization, 2003. http://www.who.int/water_sanitation_health/diseases/WSH03.02.pdf.

10. Huo A, Xu B, Chowdhury MA, et al. A simple filtration method to remove plankton-associated *Vibrio cholerae* in raw water supplies in developing countries. *Appl Environ Microbiol* 1996;62:2508–2512.

11. Potters for Peace. Filters. http://www.pottersforpeace.org/.

12. Bowie WR, King AS, Werker DH, et al. Outbreak of toxoplasmosis associated with municipal drinking water. *Lancet* 1997;350:173–177.

13. Griffiths JK. Exotic and trendy cuisine. In: Schlossberg D, ed. *Infections of Leisure.* Washington, DC: American Society for Microbiology Press, 2004.

14. US Environmental Protection Agency. National primary drinking water regulations: long term 2 enhanced surface water treatment rule. *Federal Register* 2006;71:653–702.

15. Teunis PF, Chappell CL, Okhuysen PC. *Cryptosporidium* dose response studies: variation between isolates. *Risk Analysis* 2002;22:175–183.

16. MacKenzie WR, Hoxie NJ, Proctor ME, et al. A massive outbreak in Milwaukee of *Cryptosporidium* infection transmitted through the public water supply. *N Engl J Med* 1994;331(3):161–167.

17. Goldstein ST, Juranek DD, Ravenholt O, et al. Cryptosporidiosis: an outbreak associated with drinking water despite state-of-the-art water treatment. *Ann Intern Med* 1996;124(5):459–468.

18. Franzen C, Muller A. Cryptosporidia and microsporidia-waterborne diseases in the immunocompromised host. *Diagn Microbiol Infect Dis* 1999;34(3):245–262.

19. US Environmental Protection Agency. National primary drinking water regulations: long term enhanced surface water treatment rule. Final rule. *Federal Register* 2002;67(9):1811–1844.

20. Nieuwenhuijsen MJ, Toledano MB, Eaton NE, Fawell J, Elliott P. Chlorination disinfection byproducts in water and their association with adverse reproductive outcomes: a review. *Occup Environ Med* 2000;57(2):73–85.

21. Waterborne outbreak of gastroenteritis associated with a contaminated municipal water supply, Walkerton, Ontario, May–June 2000. *Can Commun Dis Rep* 2000;26(20):170–173.

22. Mermin JH, Villar R, Carpenter J, et al. A massive epidemic of multidrug-resistant typhoid fever in Tajikistan associated with consumption of municipal water [see comment]. *J Infect Dis* 1999;179(6):1416–1422.

23. Ettling J. *The Germ of Laziness: Rockefeller Philanthropy and Public Health in the New South.* Cambridge, MA: Harvard University Press, 1981.

24. Dziuban EJ, Liang JL, Craun GF, et al. Surveillance for waterborne disease and outbreaks associated with recreational water—United States, 2003–2004. *MMWR CDC Surveill Summ* 2006;55(12):1–30.

25. Stottmeister U, Wiessner A, Kuschk P, et al. Effects of plants and microorganisms in constructed wetlands for wastewater treatment. *Biotechnol Adv* 2003;22(1–2):93–117.

26. Hillyer GV. The rise and fall of Bilharzia in Puerto Rico: its centennial 1904–2004. *P R Health Sci J* 2005;24(3):225–235.

27. D'Alessandro U, Olaleye BO, McGuire W, et al. Mortality and morbidity from malaria in Gambian children after introduction of an impregnated bednet programme. *Lancet* 1995;345(8948):479–483.

28. Chinga-Alayo E, Huarcaya E, Nasarre C, del Aguila R, Llanos-Cuentas A. The influence of climate on the epidemiology of bartonellosis in Ancash, Peru. *Trans R Soc Trop Med Hyg* 2004;98(2):116–124.

29. Naumova EN, Jagai JS, Matyas B, et al. Seasonality in six enterically transmitted diseases and ambient temperature [serial online]. *Epidemiol Infect* June 19, 2006.

30. Curriero FC, Patz JA, Rose JB, Lele S. The association between extreme precipitation and waterborne disease outbreaks in the United States, 1948-1994. *Am J Public Health* 2001;91(8):1194–1199.

31. Gatei W, Wamae CN, Mbae C, et al. 2006. Cryptosporidiosis: prevalence, genotype analysis, and symptoms associated with infections in children in Kenya. *Am J Trop Med Hyg* 2006;75(1):78–82.

32. McBride AJ, Athanazio DA, Reis MG, Ko AI. Leptospirosis. *Curr Opin Infect Dis* 2005;18(5):376–386.

33. Epstein PR. Climate change and emerging infectious diseases. *Microbes Infect* 2001;3(9):747–754.

34. Miguel E, Satyanath S, Sergenti E. Economic shocks and civil conflict: an instrumental variables approach. *J Political Economy* 2004;112:725–753.

35. Frank L, Andresen M, Schmid T. Obesity relationships with community design, physical activity, and time spent in cars. *Am J Prevent Med* 2004;27:87–96.

36. Ewing R. Can the physical environment determine physical activity levels? *Exerc Sports Sci Rev* 2005;33:69–75.

37. World Health Organization. *World Health Report 2002: Reducing Risks, Promoting Healthy Life.* Geneva: World Health Organization, 2002.

38. Nordberg E. Injuries as a public health problem in sub-Saharan Africa: epidemiology and prospects for control. *East Afr Med J* 2000;77(suppl 12):S1–S43.

39. US Environmental Protection Agency. National primary drinking water regulations; radionuclides; final rule. *Federal Register* 2000;65(236):76708–76753.

40. US Environmental Protection Agency. Radon information. http://www.epa.gov/radiation/radionuclides/radon.htm.

41. Brugge D, Goble R. The history of uranium mining and the Navajo people. *Am J Public Health* 2002;92:1410–1419.

42. Alaerts G, Khouri N, Kabir B. Strategies to mitigate arsenic contamination of water supply. In: *Arsenic in Drinking Water. United Nations Synthesis Report on Arsenic in Drinking Water.* 2001. http://www.who.int/water_sanitation_health/dwq/ arsenicun8.pdf.

43. Rahman MM, Chowdhury UK, Mukherjee SC, et al. Chronic arsenic toxicity in Bangladesh and West Bengal, India—a review and commentary. *J Toxicol Clin Toxicol* 2001;39(7):683–700.

44. Parvez F, Chen Y, Argos M, et al. Prevalence of arsenic exposure from drinking water and awareness of its health risks in a Bangladeshi population: results from a large population based study. *Environ Health Perspect* 2006;114:355–359.

45. National Research Council. *Arsenic in Drinking Water: 2001 Update.* Washington, DC: National Academies Press, 2001.

46. Durant JL, Ivushkina T, MacLaughlin K, et al. Elevated levels of arsenic in the sediments of an urban pond: sources, distribution and water quality impacts. *Water Res* 2004;38(13):2989–3000.

47. Tarras-Wahlberg NH, Flachier A, Lane SN, Sangfors O. Environmental impacts and metal exposure of aquatic ecosystems in rivers contaminated by small scale gold mining: the Puyango River basin, southern Ecuador. *Sci Total Environ* 2001;278(1–3):239–261.

48. Jamal GA. Neurological syndromes of organophosphorus compounds. *Adverse Drug React Toxicol Rev* 1997;16(3):133–170.

49. McGuigan MA. Common culprits in childhood poisoning: epidemiology, treatment and parental advice for prevention. *Paediatr Drugs* 1999;1(4):313–324.

50. Gunnell D, Eddleston M. Suicide by ingestion of pesticides: a continuing tragedy in developing countries. *Int J Epidemiol* 2003;32:902–909.

51. Pope CA III, Burnett RT, Thun MJ, et al. Lung cancer, cardiopulmonary mortality, and long-term exposure to fine particle air pollution. *JAMA* 2002;287:1132–1141.

52. Kaur S, Cohen A, Dolor R, Coffman CJ, Bastian LA. The impact of environmental tobacco smoke on women's risk of dying from heart disease: a meta-analysis. *J Womens Health* 2004;13:888–897.

53. Gauderman WJ, Avol E, Gilliland F, et al. The effect of air pollution on lung development from 10 to 18 years of age. *N Engl J Med* 2004;351:1057–1067.

54. Ritz B, Yu F. The effect of ambient carbon monoxide on low birth weight among children born in southern California between 1989 and 1993. *Environ Health Perspect* 1999;107(1):17–25.

55. Ritz B, Yu F, Fruin S, Chapa G, Shaw GM, Harris JA. Ambient air pollution and risk of birth defects in Southern California. *Am J Epidemiol* 2002;155(1):17–25.

56. Environment and Sustainable Development Project. Enhancing competitiveness while protecting the environment. Center for International Development, Harvard University. http://www.cid.harvard.edu/esd/programs/urbanmgt/envcost.html.

57. Stockstad E. Toxic air pollutants. Inspector general blasts EPA mercury analysis. *Science* 2005;307:829–830.

58. Smith KR, Smet JM, Romieu I, Bruce N. Indoor air pollution in developing countries and acute lower respiratory infections in children. *Thorax* 2000;55(6):518–532.

59. Smith KR, Mehta S, Maeusezahl-Feuz M. Indoor air pollution from solid household fuels. In: Ezzati M, Lopez AD, Rodgers A, Murray CJL, eds. *Comparative Quantification of Health Risks.* Geneva: World Health Organization, 2004.

60. Sternstrom R, Bernard PA, Ben-Simhon H. Exposure to environmental tobacco smoke as a risk factor for recurrent acute otitis media in children under the age of five years. *Int J Pediatr Otorhinolaryngol* 1993;27(2):127–136.

61. Etzel RA, Pattishall EN, Haley NJ, Fletcher RH, Henderson FW. Passive smoking and middle ear effusion among children in day care. Pediatrics 1992;90(2 pt 1):228–232.

62. Taylor R, Cumming R, Woodward A, Black M. Passive smoking and lung cancer: a cumulative meta-analysis. *Austr N Z J Public Health* 2001;25(3):203–211.

63. Vineis P, Airoldi L, Veglia P, et al. Environmental tobacco smoke and risk of respiratory cancer and chronic obstructive pulmonary disease in former smoker and never smokers in the EPIC prospective study. *BMJ* 2005;330(7486):265–266.

64. Viegi G, Simoni M, Scognamiglio A, et al. Indoor air pollution and airway disease. *Int J Tuberc Lung Dis* 2004;8:1401–1415.

65. United Nations. UN Millennium Development Goals. http://www.un.org/millenniumgoals/.

66. United Nations. *The Millennium Development Goals Report 2006.* New York: United Nations. http://mdgs.un.org/unsd/mdg/Resources/Static/Products/Progress2006/MDGReport2006.pdf.

Nutrition

Clydette Powell

6

LEARNING OBJECTIVES

- *Describe nutrition problems around the world: their extent, causes, and manifestations*
- *Identify the signs and symptoms of micronutrient deficiencies and understand approaches to addressing these deficiencies*
- *Describe key interventions for malnutrition in various settings: in developing countries, during complex humanitarian emergencies, and in the context of HIV/AIDS and tuberculosis*
- *Identify some tools for measuring malnutrition and distinguish between growth monitoring and rapid emergency assessment*

THE GLOBAL CONTEXT

In a century characterized by modern approaches to identifying and solving global health problems, malnutrition prevails in the world's children, one-third of whom are wasted or stunted in growth.[1] Moreover, malnutrition continues to claim the lives of half the world's children, according to the World Health Organization (WHO) (Figure 6-1).[2] In addition, one-third of the developing world suffers from micronutrient deficiencies—deficiencies that accompany poor nutrition and are silent until their effects are advanced and, in some instances, irreversible. In tropical settings, infections, such as human immunodeficiency virus (HIV), tuberculosis (TB), and parasites, intensify the impact of malnutrition.

Malnutrition has many direct and indirect causes. The two primary direct causes are inadequate food intake (in amount or quality) and illness. The indirect causes of malnutrition are many: poverty, the low status of women, unsanitary health conditions, wars and conflict, low national income growth, and poor governance in countries. Underlying poor health services are human, economic, and organizational resources and their control. This is one reason that malnutrition can be seen in conflict-affected areas or in areas where a local governing authority does not have the will, the commitment, or the effectiveness to carry out services for a population. Political ideologies, ethnic discrimination, and marginalization of the poor can create pockets of malnutrition in countries where abundant nutritional sources are inequitably allocated. However, not all malnutrition is seen in developing countries or in complex humanitarian emergencies. Consider inner cities, where food is accessible but not affordable or where lack of knowledge about good nutritional choices leads to poor selection of foods and poor eating habits.

Where in the developing world does malnutrition remain a problem for 21st century populations? The countries of South Asia (India, Bangladesh, Afghanistan, and Pakistan) have both high numbers and high rates of malnourished children, with Pakistan leading the list. In fact, although malnutrition is decreasing in Asia overall, the prevalence of undernutrition in South Asia (38%–51%) is much higher than that in sub-Saharan Africa (26%) (Figure 6-2).[3]

In sub-Saharan Africa (SSA), undernutrition accounts for 60% of child deaths, with perinatal causes, pneumonia, diarrhea, and other infections accounting for the rest.[4] Malnutrition in SSA is to some degree fueled by HIV/AIDS. In absolute terms, the number of underweight children has increased from 19.8 million to 34.5 million. Almost half (48.6%) of the burden of disease, disability, and death in SSA is attributable to malnutrition.

Populations, and children in particular, are vulnerable to malnutrition because of poor access to health services, poor sanitation, and ignorance of basic health care practices. Poverty and lack of education exacerbate and prolong malnutrition. Poor feeding practices and lack of adequate nutrition result in poorly nourished children. However, these factors are not just at work after

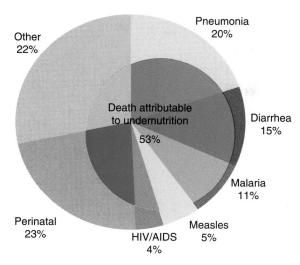

Figure 6-1. Leading causes of death in children younger than 5 years in developing countries and the contribution of undernutrition. Data from World Health Organization. *World Health Report 2003: Shaping the Future.* Geneva: World Health Organization, 2003; and Caulfield LE, de Onis M, Blossner M, Black RE. Undernutrition as an underlying cause of child deaths associated with diarrhea, pneumonia, malaria and measles. *Am J Clin Nutr* 2004;80:193–198.

a child is born. Stunted mothers can give birth to low-birth-weight babies. Malnutrition in the mother can result in major damage to a child's health and well-being, much of which is irreversible, manifesting as less physical capacity, lowered intelligence, and more frequent illnesses. Those factors may result in irregular school attendance or diminished ability to learn, and ultimately in lower likelihood of employment, lowered productivity, and inability to meet the daily economic demands of life. Because this can be a generational phenomenon in households and communities, it is a difficult cycle to break. These children and adolescents rarely escape the cycle of poverty and despair into which they are born.

Graphs of malnutrition (weight-for-age by region) show that malnutrition happens early in life (Figure 6-3).[5] Studies demonstrate that for younger children, the risk of dying increases exponentially with degree of undernutrition (Figure 6-4).[6] As children get older, however, the degree of undernutrition drops off; in other words, younger children are more represented in the data showing undernutrition.

The nutrition literature debates the relationship between malnutrition and mortality.[7] It is generally thought that the rates of acute malnutrition and mortality increase exponentially rather than linearly and that they do not increase in parallel. This means that food insecurity can

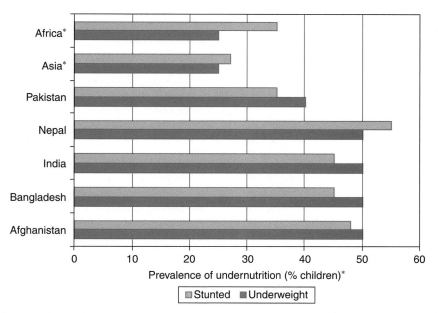

Figure 6-2. The prevalence of undernutrition in South Asian countries is much higher than in Africa. From World Bank. *Repositioning Nutrition as Central to Development: A Strategy for Large-Scale Action.* Washington, DC: World Bank, 2006. (Reproduced with permission.)
*Estimates are based on WHO regions.

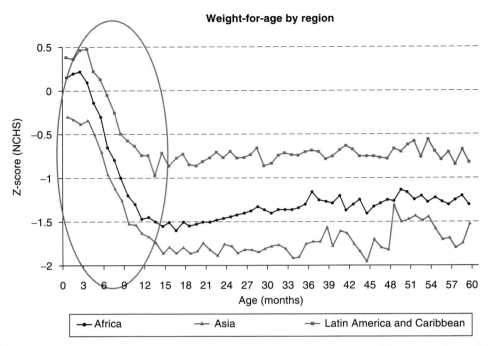

Figure 6-3. Malnutrition happens early. From Shrimpton R, Cesar G, et al. The worldwide timing of growth failure; implications for nutritional interventions. *Pediatrics* 2001;107(5):e75. (Reproduced with permission.) Circled area represents a window of opportunity.

increasingly lead to deaths as famine is approached. Where low rates of malnutrition exist, high mortality rates in children of refugee populations can be explained by acute illnesses such as acute diarrhea and dehydration.

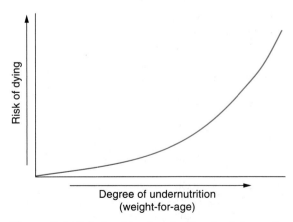

Figure 6-4. Relationship of under-five death to nutrition. From Pelletier DL. The relationship between child anthropometry and mortality in developing countries: implications for policy, programs and future research. *J Nutr* 1994;124(suppl):2047S–2081S. (Reproduced with permission.)

More stable populations, where public health services and stable home environments exist, can weather higher rates of malnutrition when severe food insecurity and famine occur. Although high mortality rates can mask deteriorating nutrition status, high death rates can occur for reasons other than malnutrition. This is only true when under-five death rates are very high—more than 10 per 10,000 per day. Some nongovernmental organizations (NGOs) have developed models to characterize whether a situation is a food crisis, a health crisis, or a combination of both (emergencies out of control).

One solution to malnutrition begins with preventing and treating malnutrition in pregnant women and in children up to 2 years of age. Providing health and nutrition education along with micronutrient fortification and supplementation is also very important. Contrary to popular perception, school feeding programs do not intervene soon enough, although they may draw children into school and keep them there.

Malnutrition is not limited to developing countries. Its presence, as overweight and obesity, is apparent in poor urban slums and underserved rural areas of the developed world. Sedentary lifestyle, dietary excesses, high fat content in food, and consumption of the empty calories in processed and fast foods lead to overnutrition and obesity. These diets can also be marginal in certain nutrients; stunted growth coupled with excess body fat can be the result. The increasing stress levels of modern life have also resulted in rising morbidity and mortality. Data from the Centers for Disease Control and Prevention (CDC) indicate that nearly two-thirds of the US population is overweight. This finding is accompanied by increases in deaths due to noncommunicable chronic disease, such as cardiovascular disease, diabetes, stroke, cancer, and liver cirrhosis, all of which are linked to excess calories, saturated fat, salt (sodium), cholesterol, sugars, and alcohol, along with inadequate fiber intake. Dietary factors also are linked to higher risks for hypertension, dental and renal disease, and osteoporosis.

Paradoxically, overnourished populations have the greatest access to information and approaches that would increase their health and well-being. To counter food advertising and the convenience of fast foods, public health messages promote awareness of better food choices and lifestyle. Package labeling, media campaigns, and social marketing have led to some increased nutrition awareness among the public as well as among health care providers. However, food availability and affordability, ethnic preferences, and levels of education and income still negatively influence these choices.

Many low- and middle-income countries are caught in a situation referred to as *nutritional transition*. These countries face simultaneous public health challenges: malnutrition in some populations and obesity in others, along with diet-related noncommunicable diseases, such as cardiovascular disease, cancers, and diabetes. This phenomenon can be very costly for countries because it presents competing priorities for limited health budgets and health personnel, who may still be grappling with programs to combat traditional communicable diseases.[3] Over- and undernutrition can coexist not only in the same country but also in the same household. In Mauritania, more than 40% of mothers are overweight, while at the same time more than 30% of children are underweight. As many as 60% of households with an overweight person also had an underweight person.[3]

It is important to note two disturbing trends in eating disorders in children, most of which are seen in developed countries, and in particular in the United States: obesity and bulimia/anorexia nervosa. Obesity is defined using body mass index (BMI) as a surrogate for maladaptive fat storage. BMI is calculated as body weight in kilograms divided by height in meters squared. Acceptable BMI varies by age and gender. Some 10% of children between 2 and 5 years old are considered obese.[8] The rates have doubled for teens aged 12 to 19 years.[9] They have tripled for children aged 6 to 11 years. In 2005, the Institute of Medicine called these trends a "harmful upward trajectory."[10] Many factors are strong predictors of childhood obesity: genetics (having overweight parents), childhood characteristics (having

been overweight in middle childhood), psychosocial factors (such as depression), and behavior (such as eating while watching TV and lack of regular exercise).

In contrast to obesity, anorexia nervosa is an eating disorder in which a person voluntarily restricts caloric intake, resulting in weight loss. This disorder is accompanied by an obsession to be thinner and a delusion of being fat. Bulimia is associated with binge eating and subsequent purging. Some 0.5% to 5% of teenaged females are affected by these disorders, and white adolescents are more commonly affected. These conditions are best managed with medical, psychological, and nutrition counseling and interventions.

PROTEIN-ENERGY MALNUTRITION

Malnutrition is sometimes referred to as protein-energy malnutrition (PEM). When the body's basic maintenance needs for the energy found in protein and calories exceeds its dietary intake of them, undernutrition is the result. Children develop PEM for many reasons, such as inadequate food intake, poor composition of the diet, and unclean environments (poor hygiene), diarrhea, and infections.

Classically, three types of PEM have been described: kwashiorkor, marasmus, and marasmic kwashiorkor. *Kwashiorkor* comes from the Ghanaian term meaning "the sickness that the older child gets when the next baby is born"; the older child is displaced from breastfeeding by the newborn, who is offered the breast first. The older child is left to forage from the family table or may be given complementary foods for which he or she is not yet ready. Kwashiorkor is accompanied by edema, mostly in the feet and legs, along with flakey skin, sparse, light-colored (even red) hair, apathy or irritability, and poor appetite. Because of the edema, children may look "fat" and appear to be well fed to the untrained observer or to the parent who is not aware of the silent effects of undernutrition in their child. Children with severe kwashiorkor may have hair that falls out easily and skin that looks burned or ulcerated and that peels easily (Figure 6-5).

Marasmus due to prolonged starvation, is characterized by severe wasting of fat and muscle, which results in an old-person, skin-and-bones appearance (Figure 6-6). This is the most common form of PEM seen in nutritional emergencies where food shortages are severe. In contrast to the apathy seen in children with kwashiorkor, children with marasmus are hungry. Marasmus may also be the result of chronic or recurring infections with decreased food intake. Marasmic kwashiorkor has both wasting and edema.

Chronic PEM has both short-term effects, such as lowered resistance to infections, and long-term effects, such as growth retardation, reduced intellectual development

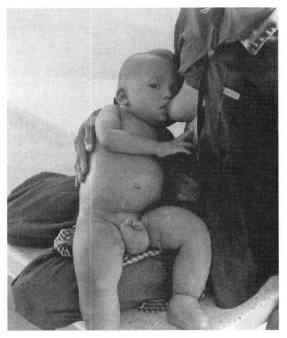

Figure 6-5. Cambodian child with kwashiorkor. (Photo credit: Debra Coats, FNP.)

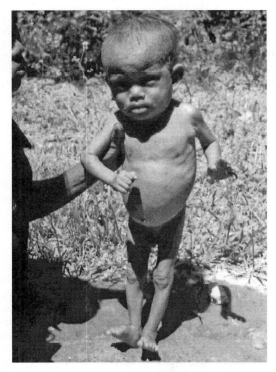

Figure 6-6. Cambodian child with marasmus. (Photo credit: Debra Coats, FNP.)

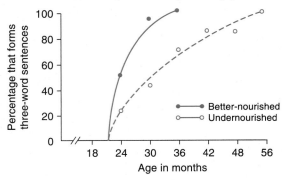

Age at which child constructs first three-word sentence, cumulative percentage, Mexico

Figure 6-7. Reduced intellectual development. From Chavez A, Martinez C. *Growing Up in a Developing Country: A Bio-ecological Study of the Development of Children from Poor Peasant Families in Mexico.* Mexico, DF: Instituto Nacional de la Nutrition, 1982:90. (Reproduced with permission.)

(Figure 6-7), and increased death rates, especially among children 1 to 3 years old, who are more vulnerable to measles and diarrhea. These children are also more vulnerable to TB, which is highly prevalent in many developing countries. Malnutrition is closely associated with TB in developing countries and often is considered a clinical sign of TB.

To quantify the degree of malnutrition, public health specialists and health care providers speak of wasting and stunting in terms of muscle mass (weight) and height, respectively. In children 6 to 59 months old, *wasting* (low weight for height) is defined as more than 2 standard deviations, or Z scores, below the reference values set by the WHO or the National Center for Health Statistics (NCHS); the term excludes edema (Table 6-1). Almost 10% of children younger than 5 years suffer from wasting. This puts them at great risk for death or severe growth impairment and delayed psychological development. Populations in which 10% to 14.9% of children are wasted are said to have a high (serious) risk of death. Usually the crude mortality rates (CMRs) in those populations are 2 to 4.9 deaths per 10,000 per day. Populations that are considered critical have wasting percentages of 15% or higher; CMRs tend to be over 5 deaths per 10,000 per day.

Stunting (low height-for-age) occurs when children fail to reach their linear growth potential. As with wasting, stunting is associated with poverty, poor feeding practices, and risk of illnesses. Its prevalence varies widely: from 5% to 65% around the world. Stunting is a manifestation and long-term consequence of chronic

Table 6-1. Nutritional status, weight-for-height (WFH) Z scores and percentage of median, and MUAC.

Nutritional status	WFH Z score	WFH % of median	MUAC (6–59 months old)
Moderate acute malnutrition	−3.00 to −2.01	Between 70% and 80%	11.0 cm to 12.49 cm; no edema
Severe acute malnutrition (SAM)	< −3.00 and edema	< 70% and edema	< 11.0 cm and edema
Global acute malnutrition (GAM)	< −2.00 and edema	< 80% and edema	< 12.5 cm and edema

MUAC, mid-upper arm circumference. Results expressed by different methods are not directly comparable. From Médicins Sans Frontières. *Nutrition Guidelines.* 1st ed. Paris: Médicins Sans Frontières, 1995:6. (Reproduced with permission.)

malnutrition. Stunted children may never reach their full growth potential, even when nutritional interventions are introduced.

MICRONUTRIENT DEFICIENCIES

Micronutrients are vitamins and minerals that are required in very small quantities (micrograms or milligrams per day) for good health. For example, the average person requires only about one teaspoon of iodine during his or her entire lifetime. Because the human body does not produce most of these micronutrients, they have to be obtained from foods in the daily diet, as supplements added to food (i.e., food fortification), or in the form of capsules, powders, tablets, or injections. Among the many micronutrients, the ones of greatest interest and importance are iron, iodine, and vitamin A, followed by zinc, vitamin D, and folic acid. Micronutrient deficiencies have several causes: poverty, poor diet, lack of clean water and adequate sanitation, illness, and malabsorption. The WHO, UNICEF, and the United Nations University have been researching the efficacy and effectiveness of multiple micronutrient supplementation during pregnancy.[11]

Unlike PEM, micronutrient deficiencies may not be readily apparent. In fact, micronutrient deficiencies may be silent until major signs and symptoms appear. Fortunately, solutions to micronutrient malnutrition are relatively easy, inexpensive, available, and politically feasible.

Of the billions of people in the world, it is estimated that some 2 billion are at risk for iron deficiency, 1.6 billion for iodine deficiency, and 0.8 billion for vitamin A deficiency. Each day some 300 mothers die in childbirth due to iron deficiency, 4,000 children die from the effects of vitamin A deficiency, and 50,000 infants are born with reduced mental capacity due to iodine deficiency.[12]

Iron

Iron deficiency is the most common micronutrient deficiency in the developing world. Often the cause is poor nutritional intake and lack of adequate iron sources in the diet. Early childhood and the childbearing years are the two most vulnerable periods in life for iron deficiency. Iron depletion in the full-term infant occurs by about 6 months of age and may be marked by age 1 year, when anemia is apparent. The consequences of iron deficiency may be anemia, lowered immunity to fight infection, adverse pregnancy outcomes, reduction in work capacity or school performance, and behavioral and learning difficulties in the child.

Correction of iron deficiency can be a targeted intervention in which vulnerable populations are screened and then provided iron supplements, or it can be a universal approach in which everyone is given iron supplements in areas where iron deficiency anemia is prevalent. Routine iron supplementation for pregnant women is a standard practice in most of the world. Hookworm infection can account for a large portion of iron deficiency. In these instances periodic deworming programs, coupled with sanitation and hygiene practices, can decrease the worm burden in the local population. When nutrition education is added to such programs, including at the time of growth monitoring, better food choices and feeding practices can help communities to be self-vigilant and self-monitoring and less reliant on rescue micronutrients from outside providers. Promotion of exclusive breastfeeding, delayed introduction of tea water given to infants, and iron fortification of commonly consumed foods (e.g., flour, cereals) can make a difference in lowering the incidence of iron deficiency in the community.

Iodine

Lack of iodine in the diet of a pregnant mother has several adverse effects on the growing fetus: it may result in stillbirth or infant death or may manifest as mild mental retardation or even cretinism, which includes severe brain damage, deafness, and dwarfism. Iodine deficiency reduces intelligence, education, and productivity. The average reduction in IQ is 13.5 points with iodine deficiency; in cretinism, this reduction is far greater.

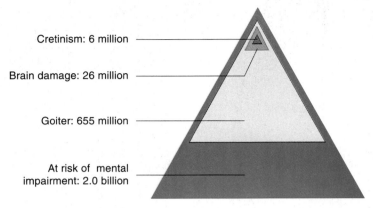

Cretinism: 6 million

Brain damage: 26 million

Goiter: 655 million

At risk of mental
impairment: 2.0 billion

Figure 6-8. Population with iodine deficiency. From Micronutrient Initiative and UNICEF. *Vitamin and Mineral Deficiency: A Global Progress Report.* Ottawa, Canada: Micronutrient Initiative, 2004. http://www.micronutrient.org/reports/reports/Full_e.pdf. (Reproduced with permission.)

Iodine deficiency is the greatest cause of preventable brain damage in fetuses and infants, with over 130 countries and 2 billion people affected worldwide. If the allocation of iodine deficiency were visualized as a pyramid, it would show 2 billion people at risk at the bottom of the pyramid, 655 million with goiter, 26 million with brain damage, and 6 million with cretinism (Figure 6-8).

Iodine deficiency must be corrected before conception. This can be accomplished through food fortification, such as salt iodization. Major advances have been made over the last 15 years. In 1990 only 46 countries had iodized salt programs, whereas in 2007, 120 countries had such programs. Universal iodization of salt is a known, safe way to control iodine deficiency for most of the world. The public health challenge is in getting the job done. Fortification also reduces the short-term effects on children and adults, such as lethargy and motor and mental impairment. Additional economic and social benefits include improved health and work capacity, improved efficiency of education, reduced health care expenditure, and improved quality of life.

Vitamin A

Vitamin A deficiency mostly affects children and women. It is the leading cause of preventable blindness in young children and is increasingly recognized as a contributor to maternal mortality. Over 90 countries around the world and approximately 250 million children are affected by this deficiency, with as many as half a million children becoming blind each year. Of those who develop blindness, half die within 1 year, in part because of their impaired ability to combat infection, particularly measles. Of the 250 million children with vitamin A deficiency, 13.5 million have night blindness,

3.1 million have xerophthalmia, and nearly half a million are blind (Figure 6-9). Clinically, there is dryness of the cornea and conjunctiva (xerophthalmia), with scars and ulceration, Bitot's spots, and ultimately keratomalacia.

Vitamin A deficiency is usually seen in community clusters, meaning that cases of xerophthalmia are surrounded by groups of affected mothers and young children. This phenomenon reflects community dietary practices and shared risks of malnutrition and infection. As children grow older, their tastes change, they are able to search more widely for food on their own, and they are less likely to have vitamin A lacking in their diet.

Diarrhea, liver disease (hepatitis, cirrhosis), and intestinal infections with worms decrease the body's ability to absorb vitamin A. The infection-malnutrition cycle is the downward spiral of decreased food intake, decreased nutrients, and decreased ability to fight infection. This is sometimes seen in cases of measles. Metabolic needs for vitamin A are higher during growth, infection, and pregnancy. Any kind of corneal ulceration, especially when associated with measles, is an indication to provide vitamin A immediately, on the presumption that vitamin A deficiency exists.

Treatment is urgent and not expensive. In the mid-1980s, research in Indonesia—the Aceh Trial—demonstrated that 2 cents' worth of vitamin A decreased child mortality by 34% (Figure 6-10).[13] Studies between 1986 and 1992 from India, Nepal, and Africa confirmed that preschool mortality could be reduced by 25% to 30%. The Nepal Nutrition Intervention Project studied 44,000 rural women, half of whom were pregnant. Results showed that weekly dietary supplement of vitamin A or beta-carotene could reduce maternal mortality by 40% (Figure 6-11).[14]

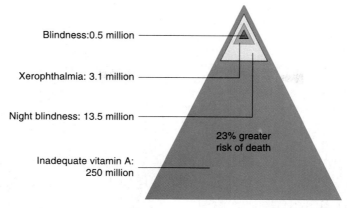

Blindness:0.5 million

Xerophthalmia: 3.1 million

Night blindness: 13.5 million

23% greater risk of death

Inadequate vitamin A: 250 million

Figure 6-9. Children with vitamin A deficiency. From Micronutrient Initiative and UNICEF, Vitamin and Mineral Deficiency: A Global Progress Report. Ottawa, Canada: Micronutrient Initiative, 2004. http://www.miconutrient.org/reports/Full_e.pdf. (Reproduced with permission.)

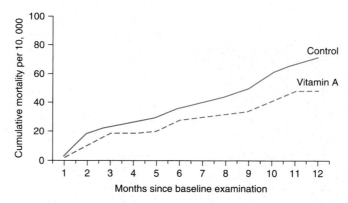

Figure 6-10. Mortality of 1- to 5-year-old children in vitamin A–supplemented versus control villages in Aceh, Indonesia, 1982–1984. From Sommer A, Tarwotjo I, Djunaedi E, et al. Impact of vitamin A supplementation on childhood mortality: a randomized controlled community trial. *Lancet* 1986;1:1169. (Reproduced with permission.)

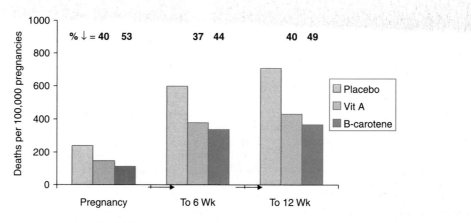

Bold no. = statistically significant % reduction

Figure 6-11. Mortality related to pregnancy in Nepal. From West K, Katz J, Khatry S, et al. Double blind, cluster randomized trial of low dose supplementation of vitamin A or beta-carotene on mortality related to pregnancy in Nepal. *BMJ* 1999;318:570–575. (Reproduced with permission.)

Public health surveys for night blindness and other manifestations of eye problems are one way of determining the prevalence of vitamin A deficiency in populations at risk. Trained interviewers and observers and large samples of children are necessary for such surveys. Among children younger than 5 years in sub-Saharan Africa, about two-fifths are at risk for vitamin A deficiency, and adequate vitamin A programs could avert 645,000 deaths each year. Vitamin A supplements can decrease infant mortality by 25%; reduce HIV-related morbidity, measles, and kwashiorkor mortality in children; and decrease maternal mortality by 40%. Vitamin A is often distributed at the time of immunization campaigns called national immunization days, or NIDs. It should be noted that concerns have been raised regarding increased progression to death for HIV-positive mothers and infants because of universal maternal or neonatal vitamin A supplementation in HIV-endemic areas.[15]

One way to prevent vitamin A deficiency is breastfeeding, because breast milk is a rich source of vitamin A. Exclusive breastfeeding for the first 4 to 6 months is recommended. Dietary counseling is important for mothers of children who are beyond the breastfeeding years. Vitamin A occurs naturally in animal products (dairy, egg yolks, liver) as well as vegetable sources (palm oil, dark green leafy vegetables, colored fruit such as papayas and mangos). Foods such as sugar, cooking oil, and flour can also be fortified with vitamin A. Children and women after childbirth can be given supplements for 6 months: 200,000 IU for children and 300,000 IU for the mother 4 to 8 weeks' postpartum. Finally, dietary diversification can help guarantee that vitamin A is consumed in adequate amounts. UNICEF now supplies between 600 and 800 million 2-cent vitamin A capsules to more than 75 countries around the world, essentially covering some 300 to 400 million children each year.

Zinc

Zinc is an essential element for growth, in both humans and plants, and for proper immune function and mucosal integrity. Lack of zinc in the human diet increases risk for diarrhea, respiratory infection, and developmental delays. In its severe form, zinc deficiency is characterized by acrodermatitis, gastrointestinal discomfort and diarrhea, and slow growth.

Many studies have demonstrated scientifically that daily zinc supplements reduce diarrhea and pneumonia in preschoolers (Figure 6-12).[16] In addition, zinc supplementation (taken as 20 mg tablets) decreases the frequency and the volume output of diarrhea and shortens the time to recovery. The effervescent tablets can be dissolved in breast milk or oral rehydration solution. Zinc supplementation for 10 to 14 days has a preventive effect on childhood illnesses in the 2 to 3 months after treatment.

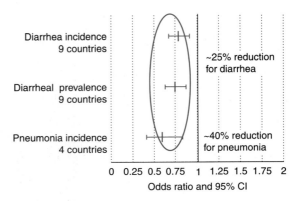

Figure 6-12. Effects of daily zinc supplement use on diarrhea and pneumonia in preschoolers. From Zinc Investigators' Collaborative Group. Prevention of diarrhea and pneumonia by zinc supplementation in children in developing countries: pooled analysis of randomized controlled trials. *J Pediatrics* 1999; 135:689–697. (Reproduced with permission.)

Zinc is found in breast milk, meats, and crustaceans. It is generally low in most vegetables, grains, and fish. Years of overcultivation of the soil and mismanagement of land can deplete zinc in the soil, leading to low zinc levels in plants, crop yields, and seeds, contributing to the deficiency cycle.

Vitamin D

Vitamin D is needed for bone growth. Bone softening and ultimately rickets are the result of defective mineralization of growing bone—an imbalance of calcium and phosphorus. Nutritional rickets typically affects children younger than 2 years, during the period of rapid growth when demands for calcium and phosphorus are high (Figure 6-13). Vitamin D–deficient children will fail to thrive, be short in stature, be developmentally delayed, and have gait abnormalities.

Vitamin D deficiency can be prevented in all breastfed babies by the daily administration of 200 IU of vitamin D for the first 2 months of life. All formulas have at least 400 IU/L. A multivitamin tablet that contains that amount should be given if the formula intake is less than 500 mL per day or if the child does not get regular sunlight exposure. In nutritional rickets caused by vitamin D deficiency, calcium supplementation is essential. It takes about 3 to 6 months for the physical changes to resolve, and some deformities may still require orthopedic correction.

Natural sources of vitamin D include fish liver oils, egg yolks, and fatty fish. Vitamin D precursors are converted in the skin by exposure to sunlight. Living in places where the weather is constantly cloudy, wearing

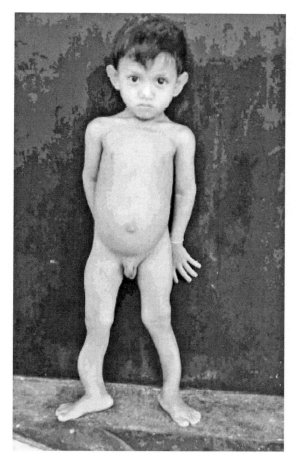

Figure 6-13. Cambodian child with rickets. (Photo credit: Debra Coats, FNP.)

clothing all the time, and residing mostly indoors will diminish exposure to sunlight and therefore can lead to vitamin D deficiency.

Folic Acid

Folic acid, also known as vitamin B_9, is required for the production of DNA and is needed for the development of tissues and organs early and throughout pregnancy.[17] It prevents neural tube defects (NTDs), as well as other birth defects, such as in the lip/palate, the heart, and the limbs. Neural tube defects are serious birth defects of the spine and brain that are the result of incomplete formation or closure of the neural tube. Neural tube defects are the leading cause of infantile paralysis in the United States, with spina bifida as the most frequently occurring permanently disabling birth defect. Because folic acid lowers homocysteine levels, it may also reduce the risk of heart attack and stroke as well as the risk of some cancers, such as colon cancers.

In 1992, the US Public Health Service recommended that all women capable of becoming pregnant should consume 400 micrograms (0.4 mg) of folic acid daily to reduce their risk of a pregnancy resulting in neonatal spina bifida or other NTDs. Research in 1998 demonstrated that the incidence of NTDs in the United States had declined by almost 20% since folic acid fortification began.[18] Preliminary data from Chile show a decline by 31% in NTDs in 2000–2001 following wheat fortification. This implies that fortification with folic acid is effective in preventing NTDs and should be given due consideration in flour fortification programs.[19] The dietary approach to increase consumption of folic acid/folate is to improve overall dietary habits, take daily folic acid supplement, and consume fortified foods.

The reader should consult medical references for the daily allowances for the most important micronutrients and preventive and curative treatments for their deficiencies. Table 6-2 shows risks of vitamin and micronutrient deficiencies when consuming diets high or (low) in certain commodities. Possible solutions are listed.

Nutrition Surveillance and Monitoring Progress

The collection and analysis of nutrition data provides information that can be useful in various settings. For example, as a routine part of maternal and child health programs, nutrition surveillance can monitor population trends in nutrition status. During an emergency situation, the rapid assessment of nutrition status can determine the extent and severity of malnutrition and thereby predict change or the threat of deterioration. Nutrition surveillance can guide public health programs and assist government and nongovernmental organizations in project monitoring and evaluation. These data can indicate the effectiveness of an intervention and track overall trends for preparedness reasons. Donor organizations often require such benchmarks for assessment of the delivery and performance of humanitarian assistance. Demographic and health surveys collect nutrition information on a 5-year basis in developing countries. UNICEF makes use of multi-indicator cluster surveys.

Global efforts at collecting and analyzing nutrition data during complex humanitarian emergencies began in 1993 as the Refugee Nutrition Information System (RNIS). RNIS evolved to become a Geneva-based system called the Nutritional Information in Crisis Situations (NICS). The NICS is the only system that considers all causes of malnutrition, key constraints in delivering humanitarian assistance, and the prevalence of acute malnutrition. Deriving its information from a wide range of voluntary UN and NGO sources, it issues quarterly reports that judge risks and threats to a population's nutrition status. As a warning system, NICS considers a

Table 6-2. Other micronutrients, risks, and food sources.

Commodity	Risk	Possible solutions
Maize	Pellagra (Vitamin B$_3$ [niacin] deficiency or a low-protein diet with no tryptophan)	• Nuts, beans, whole-grain cereals • Meat, fish, eggs, milk • Fortification
Polished rice	Beriberi (Vitamin B$_1$ [thiamine] deficiency)	• Parboiled rice/whole grains • Groundnuts, legumes • Meat, fish, milk, eggs • Fortification
No fresh fruits or vegetables	Scurvy (Vitamin C deficiency)	• Onions, cabbage, peppers • Canned tomato paste • Vitamin C tablets
	Night blindness and xerophthalmia (Vitamin A deficiency)	• Green leaves and bright-colored vegetables/fruits • Butter or red palm oil • Vitamin A capsules
	Anemia (Iron deficiency)	• Greens • Meat/fish • Iron/folic acid supplementation • Fortification

From Médicins Sans Frontières. *Nutrition Guidelines.* 1st ed. Paris: Médicins Sans Frontières, 1995:13. (Reproduced with permission.)

prevalence of 5% to 8% malnutrition to be a concern and 10% to be a serious situation. NICS reports are meant to raise awareness and advocacy for interventions when action or donor responses are insufficient. On the other hand, delays in reporting sometimes result in the lack of timely intervention by donors and key stakeholders.

In the United States, the National Health and Nutrition Examination Surveys (NHANES) collect data from dietary interviews, physical examinations, and biochemical tests on samples of the US population, including minority populations and elderly Americans.

RAPID ASSESSMENT IN EMERGENCY CONTEXTS

The SPHERE Project guidelines, developed by a large consortium of humanitarian NGOs, emphasize the importance of investigating the possible causes of malnutrition before attempting an anthropometric survey.[20] Information on the extent of malnutrition and its underlying causes can help to shape interventions. For humanitarian relief needs, it is important to identify the most affected populations and at-risk geographic areas and then to prioritize them for nutritional interventions. Assessments allow more effective use of limited resources as well as the monitoring of the effectiveness of local aid, in terms of both coordination and the impact on at-risk populations or individuals already affected. Many studies in the literature illustrate the approach to assessing malnutrition in developing countries.[21,22]

Survey assessments may be conducted for different purposes. An organization that delivers food rations in bulk metric tons will have different objectives and population-based indicators compared with an organization that sets up therapeutic feeding programs for affected individuals. Another organization may focus on identification of the underlying causes of malnutrition, with a plan for targeted interventions. Whereas one set of surveys may be for assessing food stores (food security), market activity, land use, livestock, and livelihoods, another may be for conducting anthropometric surveys in targeted populations. A challenge occasionally encountered is that nutrition surveys may not conveniently overlap with surveys of food security and livelihood assessments. Data may be specific to the area surveyed and not readily extrapolated. Broader surveys may miss the smaller, remote pockets of poverty, malnutrition, or mortality.

Surveys also measure the extent of coverage of populations by interventions. Therefore, they have a place in both relief and development settings, that is, in measuring progress toward objectives that are either implicitly or explicitly stated and required by donor agencies or international organizations. Many of the standards for humanitarian assistance have been agreed upon within the international community through the Sphere Humanitarian Charter and Minimum Standards in Disaster Response Project and Standardized monitoring and Assessment of Relief and Transitions (SMART) (see Chapter 9).[23]

Data in emergency settings are sometimes collected by a standard two-stage cluster-sampled survey to estimate the prevalence of acute undernutrition in program areas.[24] Cluster-sampling methodology selects 30 clusters (e.g., villages) and then surveys 30 units (e.g., households) in those 30 villages. Such an approach, though appearing straightforward, can be limited by difficulties in identifying the sampling frame for targeted populations. This limitation is especially seen in settings where refugee communities are closely integrated into host communities, making them hard to disaggregate for study purposes; where populations are highly mobile (nomadic or migrating); and where population density is sparse or households are small. As a result, such surveys can be resource intensive in terms of time, personnel, and costs. Alternative survey methodologies use a stratified design, defining strata from a central systematic area sample method.[25]

Before a new survey is planned, it is useful to see if population-based data already exist, for example, trends in the health of children seen in primary health care clinics, or data from recent surveys. If an assessment still needs to be done, it can be achieved fairly quickly by measuring mid-upper arm circumference (MUAC) among affected children or by sampling high-risk populations and measuring weight-for-height.

MUAC measurement is both easy to teach and to do and is therefore gaining in popularity and use. It can be applied to rapid triage settings, especially where quick assessment of children (6 months to 59 months old) is needed. MUAC measurement uses a tri-colored band around the mid-upper arm (Figure 6-14). Position and placement are critical so that proper correlation can be made with the protein composition and lean tissue mass.

MUAC is more closely correlated with mortality than is weight-for-height, thereby making MUAC a more reliable measure for planning emergency nutrition interventions and predicting mortality rates. Some international organizations also recommend that this measure be used as a criterion for admission to an outpatient therapeutic feeding center.

COMMUNITY-BASED GROWTH MONITORING AND PROMOTION

In contrast to rapid assessment of nutrition status in populations for emergency and food distribution purposes, growth monitoring serves as an ongoing public health activity in nonemergent settings in both developed and developing countries. *Anthropometry* is the scientific term used to describe this process of weighing and measuring. Anthropometry provides both the prevalence and incidence of undernourished children in a community. Moreover, it can serve as an early warning system in both acute and nonurgent settings. In situations where there is a massive influx of refugees or internally displaced persons, anthropometry can serve as a quick triage tool, rapidly identifying those who need acute nutrition interventions. Anthropometry can also serve to monitor ongoing programs where food distribution or onsite preparation and feeding are occurring.

Measurement of a child's weight and height is accompanied by recording those data points in a child's health record, commonly known in developing countries as a "road to health" chart. Such measurement can result in a significant interaction between a health care provider and the child's caretaker, where both look to see if the child's weight and height are progressing on the road to health.

Although this activity may be done privately in a health center, in developing countries it is more often performed in the outdoors or in a public place. Salter scales for weighing an infant or young child hang from a tree in the outdoor setting (Figure 6-15). Mothers gather around to see the measurement of their own child as well as that of the children of their neighbors. Much talk and laughter can accompany this process. The measurement activity also benefits the bystanders who gather to watch the process. The experienced health care provider takes timely advantage of these sessions for community instruction about good nutrition, proper food choices, breastfeeding practices, and even broad health and hygiene messages. He or she can reinforce the importance of good nutrition and can publicly acknowledge mothers who made the appropriate nutrition and feeding choices for their children. Other mothers may learn the reasons for malnutrition or lack of growth in their own offspring. In addition, this activity can be coupled with immunization activities, supplementary feeding activities, family planning discussions, and general monitoring of family health and health needs.

Because anthropometry is easy and simple to apply, relatively untrained staff can effectively assist in the activities. Training should start with careful selection and qualification of community workers who have an interest in the process and are willing to receive instruction. Although they do not necessarily need to be literate or previously trained as health workers, they must be capable of being objective, comfortable with children, and able to work in a team. Role playing often helps to reinforce key teaching points as well as to identify strengths and weaknesses of the candidate trainees. It is useful to have them work in pairs, because this will be the requirement in the field. Trial runs can highlight the steps in the process of child selection, measurement, and recording. It is essential to have a separate session on writing numbers on the records and charts, because the number 7 can look like 1, and sixes, zeros, and eights can be confused. When both height and weight are being measured, height should be done first. Use a separate team for age assessment to keep the teams focused on specific tasks in the growth monitoring process.

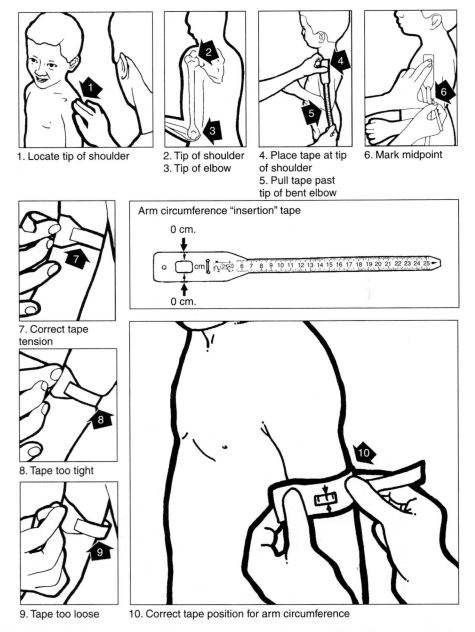

Figure 6-14. Child mid-upper arm circumference measurement. From Coghill B. *Anthropometric Indicators Measurement Guide.* Washington, DC: Food and Nutrition Technical Assistance Project, Academy for Educational Development, 2001. (Reproduced with permission.)

Because it may be difficult to know the exact age of a child, weight-for-height (WFH) rather than weight-for-age (WFA) is often used. In instances where a child's age is needed, age sometimes can be determined by asking questions that relate physical, historical, or seasonal events to the birth of the child: for example, was the child born during the rainy season, when the president came to power, or when the tsunami struck?

Although relatively easy and simple, anthropometry data can be subject to unintentional errors. Errors of

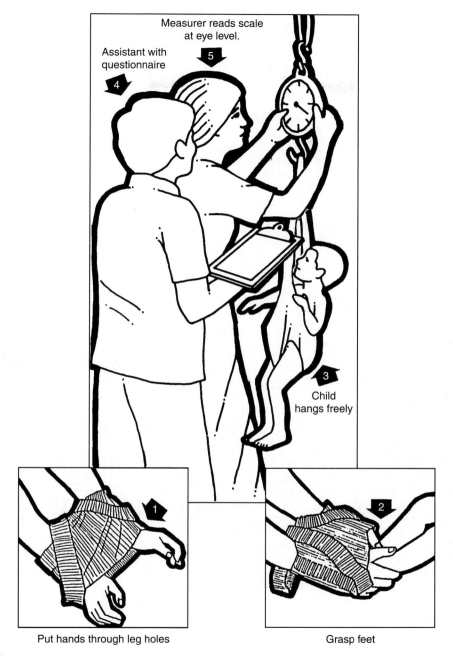

Figure 6-15. Child measurement using Salter scale. From Coghill B. *Anthropometric Indicators Measurement Guide.* Washington, DC: Food and Nutrition Technical Assistance Project, Academy for Educational Development, 2001. (Reproduced with permission.)

weight include those of taring the scales, movement by the child being measured, the degree of undress or cooperation, the presence of edema, parasite and stool load, dehydration status, and reading errors by those not adequately trained to read and record numbers. Health care workers performing the measurements should be sure that the child is not holding onto the scale or onto an anxious parent or caregiver.

Height can be more difficult to measure. An approved height/length board should be used (Figure 6-16). Ideally, the measurement requires three people: one to hold the child's head, one to straighten the knees, and a third to record the measurement called out by the assistants. It is important to ascertain that the child is standing straight, looking straight ahead, not slouching or wearing shoes, nor manifesting clubfoot or other deformities of the spine or legs. Hairdos can sometimes interfere with an accurate measurement and should be noted on the chart. For those

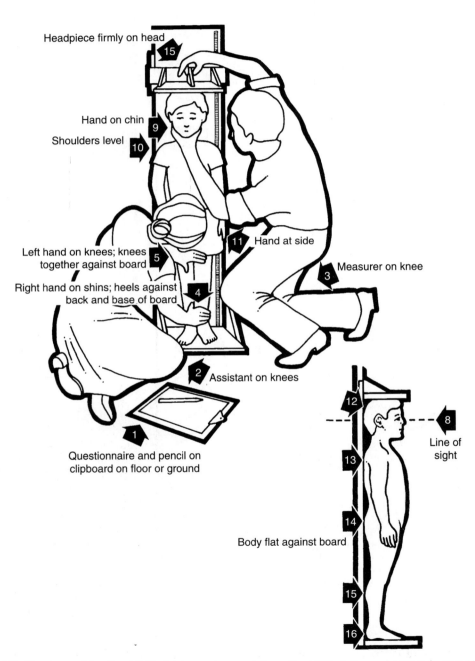

Figure 6-16. Correct position for child height measurement. From Coghill B. *Anthropometric Indicators Measurement Guide.* Washington, DC: Food and Nutrition Technical Assistance Project, Academy for Educational Development, 2001. (Reproduced with permission.)

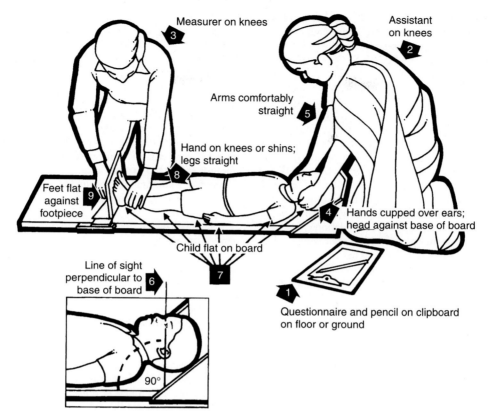

Figure 6-17. Child length measurement. From Coghill B. *Anthropometric Indicators Measurement Guide.* Washington, DC: Food and Nutrition Technical Assistance Project, Academy for Educational Development, 2001. (Reproduced with permission.)

children who are unable to stand or are too young to cooperate, length is measured instead of height (Figure 6-17).

Other measures of nutrition status include measurement of the thickness of fat folds (triceps and subscapular). However, fat folds are usually not measured in developing country settings, and exist primarily for academic purposes. In addition, fat fold measurements do not have good international references, and fat folds stabilize after 1 year, making this measurement less useful in anthropometry of children younger than 5 years. Some training and consistency of application of the calipers are also required to measure fat folds.

Interpreting Weight and Height Measurements

Results are commonly expressed in Z scores, for ease in interpreting anthropometric measurements. The Z score is a standard deviation (SD) score, which is reflective of an individual measurement in relation to a standard reference population (the expected value). The Z score is derived by taking the difference between the observed value of a measurement and the median value in the reference population and dividing that difference by the SD value for the reference population. Z scores can be for height-for-age, weight-for-age, and weight-for-height.

Weight-for-height is preferred because it has two objective measurements and because it is often not possible to know the exact age of a child. Cut-off points for moderate malnutrition are defined as 2 SDs below the median of the reference population, or 80% of the median of the reference population. For severe malnutrition, this is 3 SDs, or 70% of the median (Table 6-1).

When WFA is used, percentages of the standard expected WFA are used. Ninety percent of the standard is roughly at or above the 15th percentile on a standard growth curve (specific for age and gender), 80% is at the 3rd percentile of that growth curve, and 60% is about 3 SDs below the mean. Therefore, for kwashiorkor, the WFH is 60% to 80% of the expected; for marasmus, this is less than 60%, and for nutritional dwarfism, this is also less than 60%. Gender, age, the presence of edema, and sometimes measles immunization status are noted as part of the data collection to assist in the interpretation.

International reference standards are generated by the WHO,[26] the CDC, and the NCHS. In 2006, the WHO announced growth standards that more closely parallel growth trends in developing countries.[27] It will take some time for these growth standards to be disseminated and utilized around the world and to be accepted by the ministries of health responsible for dissemination of the standards.

In contrast to individual measurements, surveys for prevalence of malnutrition in populations use percentages of sampled populations that are below 2 SD for moderate malnutrition and below 3 Z scores for severe malnutrition. This is somewhat akin to the interpretation of individual measurements. Frequency distributions in tables or charts serve to profile the population.

Data need to be interpreted within their context. The public health provider or the researcher must ask several questions to derive a rational perspective. What might be the causes of malnutrition? Is there food insecurity, a lack of adequate health care for a population, or is there an external factor (drought, natural disasters) that has led to poor harvests, displacement of populations, and other adverse conditions? Seasonal trends should be taken into consideration. Some countries experience droughts every 7 to 10 years. Populations can suffer from poor harvests, dying livestock (as food sources), debilitation, and death of those who already have marginal health.

Infectious diseases may lay the groundwork for subsequent malnutrition; conversely, malnutrition can predispose an individual to infectious disease, as well as increase the risk of dying from that cause. When interpreting malnutrition data, it is important to keep in mind that malnutrition can be mimicked by infectious disease, notably TB and HIV/AIDS. Children who are chronically malnourished and do not respond to feeding supplementation are frequently assumed to have active TB. Although this is not a good diagnostic criterion on which to make the diagnosis of childhood TB, it is often the approach in settings where TB prevalence is high in the community and good diagnostic means are lacking.

PREVENTION

Several components make up the package of essential preventive actions against malnutrition: breastfeeding, complementary feeding, maternal nutrition, vitamin A supplementation, management of sick children, and iodized salt. Moreover, larger community issues such as food security and food safety must also be considered in preventing malnutrition among the most vulnerable.

Breastfeeding

Strong evidence supports the advantages of breastfeeding.[28] Practices vary widely over time and continue to change as experts learn more about breast milk, population behavior, and individual preferences. The nutrient content of breast milk is regarded as the best (and uncontaminated) source of protein (including immunoglobulins), carbohydrates, lipids, minerals, and micronutrients (except vitamin K and D) for newborns, including premature infants, and for infants. Vitamin D fortification of the breastfed baby is recommended by the American Academy of Pediatrics and the WHO, beginning within the first 2 months after birth. The WHO has recommended that exclusive breastfeeding occur for up to 4 months of age, and in some instances for up to 6 months.[29] Protective immunoglobulins in breast milk reduce the risk of diarrhea, respiratory illness, and otitis media (Figure 6-18).

Neurobehavioral (bonding) and maternal (faster recovery postpartum) benefits also accrue with breastfeeding. Other benefits include economic benefits, which are especially important to those with limited household income. There is no need to purchase formula, and breastfed infants tend to have fewer medical illnesses. Moreover, the nutrient content of breast milk remains fairly constant and independent of the mother's dietary intake until her own bodily stores are severely depleted.[30]

Original concerns that breastfed infants did not gain as much weight as formula-fed infants were based on comparisons with infant growth curves that did not include adequate numbers of non-formula-fed babies. The curves have been considered inappropriate for human milk–fed infants, and some newer curves reflect better sampling frames. The growth of breastfed infants should be considered the norm.

Although rates of breastfeeding initiation continue to rise in the United States, not all demographic groups have increased breastfeeding practices. Ethnicity, education, employment, age, and multiparity can influence breastfeeding choices. Support and promotion of breastfeeding by many groups, including the Special Supplemental Nutrition Program for Women, Infants, and Children, have helped raise awareness and lower barriers to breastfeeding among eligible populations. In addition, the Healthy People 2010 goals focus on breastfeeding initiation and maintenance and on the elimination of health disparities, including racial and ethnic, as they pertain to breastfeeding.[31]

The HIV status of the mother modifies the choice of breast milk as the first source of nutrition for the newborn. Because HIV is transmitted in the breast milk of infected mothers, exclusive breastfeeding or exclusive use of formula is recommended, because mixed feeds are associated with a higher rate of HIV transmission to the child. The risk of HIV transmission in breast milk varies with the timing of initiation of breastfeeding, the duration, the mother's health (her viral load and her CD4 count), the condition of her breasts, and the integrity of the infant's oral and intestinal mucosae.[32]

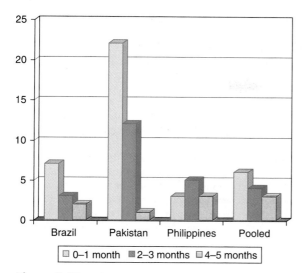

Figure 6-18. Infant mortality due to infectious diseases associated with not breastfeeding, by country and age group. From Hill Z, Kirkwood B, Edmond K. Family and Community Practices that Promote Child Survival, Growth and Devlopment: A Review of the Evidence. Geneva: World Health Organization, 2004:21–26.

Replacement feeding (use of formula) is recommended, where appropriate. If not, the mother should exclusively breastfeed, and then discontinue when the infant reaches 6 months. The design of breastfeeding promotion interventions should consider these recommendations in the context of the local prevalence of HIV and the availability of replacement formula.

Complementary Feeding

Complementary feeding is an important step in the process of transitioning from exclusive breast or formula feeding to solid foods. The WHO has developed guidance that promotes the initiation of complementary feeding at 6 months of age, using prepared energy- and nutrient-rich complementary foods. Appropriate feeding behaviors and activities underlie successful complementary feeding. Breastfeeding can continue up to 2 years of age, and has many benefits to the infant and young child. Complementary feeding can have a significant impact on lowering the incidence of child diarrhea and child mortality, as well as enhancing child growth.

Food Security

Food security can be defined as those conditions in which people have both physical access to affordable food and the economic means to obtain it. Food should be available

in sufficient quality and quantity to meet nutritional needs and to allow for a healthy and productive life. When poverty, policies, or forced migration due to conflict, war, or natural disasters disrupts this access and availability of food for prolonged periods of time, global acute malnutrition (GAM) and severe acute malnutrition (SAM) can ensue. SAM and GAM are often used as health indicators of food insecurity. Médecins Sans Frontières (MSF) uses four stages to describe progressively worsening conditions: food insecurity, food crisis, serious food crisis, and famine. Other organizations may refer to suffering from chronic food insecurity, extended food crisis, prevalence of acute malnutrition, mortality, access to food, coping strategies, livelihood assets, probability of hazards, and civil security.

Food security assessments tend to be qualitative and can be based on rainfall data, crop production, and market prices. Famine Early Warning Systems Network, (FEWSNET) which is supported by the United States Agency for International Development (USAID), publishes monthly or bimonthly reports on a regional basis to track these and other parameters. FEWSNET and other assessments take into account food production, market prices, coping strategies, and population migration. This information may be derived from a variety of local sources. Some surveys are supplemented by dietary diversity information, such as number of types of food available, weekly consumption of selected foods, and main sources of food used by a household. Although these data do not reveal the whole picture, they do reflect local conditions where populations are at increased risk due to ethnic and political marginalization, conflict and violence, or natural disasters such as drought. Demographic and health surveys also complement this information and provide valuable trends assessments.

On a more focused basis, local market surveys and household surveys can complement nutrition assessments. A market survey will indicate whether meats or fish can be bought, for what price, and in what quality or quantity. It is helpful to see if alternate sources of protein are available in the form of legumes and nuts and beans. Much can be learned by visual inspection of a household: the cooking and eating areas, food preparation utensils, food storage areas, hygiene conditions, number of family members eating in one household, gender and ages of those members, sick relatives who are bedridden, and the presence of rats, dogs, and cats, as well as other basic health measures, such as bednets, water storage pots (covered or not), and latrines.

Sometimes in the rush to address food insecurity and to provide emergency food supplies, the "food first" approach by donor agencies and their implementing partners predominates. Such an approach may fail to consider underlying causes of malnutrition that could be tackled directly. In the culture of donors, however, it is easier to quantify and fund food commodities. Such aspects of the humanitarian relief effort carry more visibility, good will, and political impact. Nevertheless, food interventions per se do not address the root causes of malnutrition in maternal and child populations, those populations living with HIV/AIDS, or the elderly who are chronically malnourished.

Food Safety

Food safety—the proper handling of food and its preparation—plays an indirect role in nutrition problems. Although a thorough discussion of food safety is not the purview of this chapter, acute food poisoning as well as periodic contamination of food due to unclean food handling and preparation can have significant public health impact. Pesticides can also contaminate food and provoke serious reactions when ingested. Chronic malnutrition can occur when bacteria, parasites, and even viruses are found in food sources on a regular basis (see Chapter 5).

Foodborne outbreaks can be attributed to poor personal hygiene, improper storage temperatures, contaminated equipment, inadequate cooking, and food from unsafe sources. Primary symptoms are usually gastrointestinal (nausea, abdominal cramps, vomiting, diarrhea), as well as neurologic and systemic manifestations in some instances.

Classically, food handling and preparation by those who have not washed their hands or who have not washed or cleaned the food can lead to illness in any susceptible person. Typical organisms and illnesses such as typhoid, *Salmonella, Shigella*, staphylococcal toxins, botulinum toxins, hepatitis A, cholera, *Escherichia coli, Yersinia, Clostridium perfringens, Bacillus cereus, Giardia*, and amebiasis plague many locals and visitors alike. Parasites, such as tapeworms (in beef, pork, and fish), *Cryptosporidium*, and *Cyclospora*, and toxins in shellfish and bottom-dwellers (e.g., paralytic shellfish poisoning) can be prevalent. It is worth inquiring what pathogens and illnesses predominate in the area. Of interest is that in some communities, the most common cause of epilepsy is neurocysticercosis from the pork tapeworm. Tuberculosis of the gut can be traced back to consumption of unpasteurized cow's milk.

INTERVENTIONS

From time to time, when malnutrition is widespread in a community, the question arises as to whether health providers should start community-based or camp-based nutrition programs. WHO's framework states that malnutrition rates under 10% (10% of children 6 to 59 months old who are either below 2 SDs of the reference median WFH or 80% of the reference WFH) do not require population interventions.[33] Instead, individuals may need attention through regular community services. MUACs can also be used as eligibility criteria for selective feeding programs. MUACs less than 11.0 cm indicate severe malnutrition, and those between 11.0 and 12.49 cm reflect moderate malnutrition (Table 6-1).

For malnutrition rates between 10% and 14%, the WHO recommends starting targeted supplementary feeding programs (SFP) and therapeutic feeding programs (TFP) for those who are severely malnourished. With malnutrition rates of 15% or more, the WHO recommends the distribution of general rations, plus SFP for all members of vulnerable groups (Table 6-3), particularly children and pregnant/lactating mothers, and TFP. These recommendations can be modified when other deteriorating circumstances so indicate—for example, general food rations below the mean energy requirement; crude mortality rates above 1 per 10,000 per day; epidemics of measles or pertussis; severe cold and inadequate shelter; high prevalence of respiratory and diarrheal disease; and severe public health hazards.

The treatment of malnourished children,[34] though beyond the scope of this chapter, includes key steps: the prevention or treatment of hypoglycemia, hypothermia, and dehydration; correction of electrolyte imbalance

Table 6-3. Supplementary food types.

Blended food[a]
Corn-soya blend (CSB)
Wheat-soya blend (WSB)
Corn-soya-milk (CSM)
Wheat-soya-milk (WSM)

Locally produced mixes
1. Base: Cereal
     Rice
     Maize
     Sorghum
2. High-protein source
     Beans
     Groundnuts
     Lentils
     Soya beans
     Dried skim milk
     Oil seeds
3. High-energy source
     Vegetable oil
     Oil seeds
     Butter oil
     Groundnuts
     Sugar

[a]Blended foods may be available through the World Food Programme or directly from donors. They are nutritionally valuable (fortified with vitamins and minerals), easy to transport and store, and can be very useful to initiate a supplementary feeding program when appropriate local foods are lacking.
From Médicins Sans Frontières. *Nutrition Guidelines*. 1st ed. Paris: Médicins Sans Frontières, 1995.

and micronutrient deficiencies; gradual initiation of feeding; rebuilding of wasted tissues (catch-up growth); provision of stimulation, play, and loving care; and preparation for follow-up after discharge.

Premature termination of treatment increases the risk of recurrence of malnutrition. Children should reach the expected weight for their height before discharge from a feeding program. Some children will always remain underweight because they are on the low end of the normal distribution curves of WFH. If they demonstrate continued growth rates and no functional impairments, they can be discharged after 1 month of adequate food intake and weight gain. The parents or caregivers should be instructed in the causes of PEM, the proper use of foods (quality and quantity), personal and environmental hygiene, immunizations, and early management of diarrhea and respiratory infections.

Community-Based Therapeutic Care

First implemented in Ethiopia in 2000, community-based therapeutic care (CTC) is a community-based approach for managing large numbers of acutely malnourished people as a viable alternative to therapeutic feeding centers.[35,36] Although it was primarily designed to meet the needs of children younger than 5 years, it is being considered for treatment of severe and acute malnutrition among adults, particularly those with HIV/AIDS. It can be used in emergency situations or in development settings.[37] CTC uses people's homes, not hospitals, so the focus of assistance is on villages rather than health centers. It works through local people wherever possible rather than through imported experts. It considers the social, economic, and cultural aspects of malnutrition in addition to the medical ones.

Home-based treatment accommodates the fact that women should not spend prolonged periods of time away from their homes. Although malnutrition often is recurrent in households that are chronically vulnerable, the risk of acquiring infection at home is less than at a facility where other sick people are located. This risk would argue for home-based treatment rather than hospitalization for malnutrition.

Protocols for CTC (Figure 6-19) are different from those used by the WHO for managing SAM in facilities. CTC has four components: community mobilization and participation, supplementary feeding programs, outpatient therapeutic care, and stabilization centers.[38]

Most experts recommend that MUAC should be the key criterion for who should participate in CTC activities.[39] MUAC is more closely correlated with muscle mass than is WFH, is a better measure of nutritional status than WFH, and tends to predict the risk of death better than WFH. Because MUAC increases with age, a fixed cut-off point will preferentially select younger children, who have a higher risk of death. The choice of MUAC or

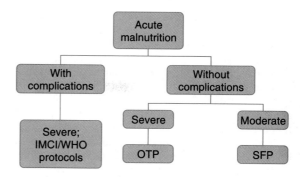

Figure 6-19. Community-based therapeutic care: management of acute malnutrition. IMCI, Integrated Management of Childhood Illnesses; WHO, World Health Organization; OTP, outpatient therapeutic program; SFP, supplementary feeding program. From CTC Research and Development Programme. *Community-Based Therapeutic Care (CTC): A Field Manual.* Oxford, UK: Valid International, 2006. (Reproduced with permission.)

WFH by agencies will depend on whether it is more important to identify the risk for death or the response to treatment, because the latter is better gauged by WFH.

CTC relies on the availability of ready-to-use therapeutic foods (RUTFs),[40] such as Plumpy'nut (Nutriset). RUTFs are a mix of cereals, legumes, oil, water and sugar, vitamins, and minerals, providing a protein source and an energy source. RUTFs often have a peanut base, but not all countries grow peanuts. RUTF can be made at home, does not have to be cooked (no firewood), is easy to store, and can be a vehicle for additives. Plumpy'nut comes as a 92-gram bar that provides 500 calories.

RUTF is easier to prepare than the water-based F100 (a fortified dried milk formula) and does not require high volumes of intake to meet energy requirements, unlike F100. Access to safe water may be limited in disaster and crisis settings. Newer RUTFs do not use milk powder and use only locally produced crops. RUTF can also be considered for replacement feeding of nonbreastfed children older than 6 months, because it is less expensive than infant formula. Because HIV stigma can be associated with the use of infant formula, RUTF may be more acceptable. Some experts think that RUTF should be included in the essential drugs list. Such inclusion would simplify logistics, as RUTF would then be part of the normal package of drugs.

On an emergency scale, RUTFs are imported, regardless of costs, to meet acute needs. As time goes on, it is desirable to encourage local production with locally available ingredients, because the cost of RUTF is tied to the sustainability and success of CTC. CTC provides a market for RUTF; conversely, RUTF is needed for the success of CTC. Other factors that play into the success of CTC are the availability of community volunteers, their motivation, the ability to train and retain them, the availability of training materials, the possibility that volunteers from other development programs could be employed, and whether CTC can be combined with the Integrated Management of Childhood Illnesses (IMCI) strategy.

Two types of indicators can be used to determine whether a nutritional intervention, such as a feeding program, is performing effectively: process indicators, such as the number of staff working at a feeding center; and outcome indicators, such as the percentage of children recovered. The relief and development community debates about other indicators, such as weight gained, or length of stay at a facility. Although donors tend not to use these indicators, international and nongovernmental organizations may use them for internal monitoring. Supplementary feeding programs use indicators such as recovery rate, death rate, and defaulting rate. Therapeutic feeding programs use these three indicators plus weight gain, coverage, and mean length of stay. Organizations such as the World Food Programme, the UN High Commission for Refugees (UNHCR), MSF, and Save the Children (STC) have different thresholds at which "alarming" percentages set into motion other responses.

SPECIAL CIRCUMSTANCES: HIV/AIDS

Over the last 20 years, the story of malnutrition has been made more complicated by the human immunodeficiency virus. Malnutrition and HIV/AIDS have a mutually adverse relationship. By decreasing the natural immune defenses, malnutrition increases susceptibility to HIV and may also contribute to lowered effectiveness of antiretrovirals. HIV/AIDS can be accompanied by gastrointestinal disorders that diminish the body's ability to absorb food and essential micronutrients, further jeopardizing nutritional status. In addition, opportunistic infections, such as TB, increase the body's metabolic demands and burn vital calories, worsening the degree of undernutrition.

PEM negatively affects all aspects of the immune system: cell-mediated immunity, antibody production, acute phase response, and protection of the integument. HIV diminishes the immune system and T cell function. The lack of micronutrients, such as vitamins A, B, C, and E, as well as iron, zinc, and selenium, also affects the immune system, making the body more susceptible to infection. Consequently, PEM and HIV together can be significantly destructive.

HIV-positive women are more likely to deliver low-birth-weight babies, who are more likely to experience slower growth and be at higher risk for malnutrition. Along with the recommendations regarding exclusive breastfeeding and early cessation, periodic vitamin A supplementation lowers morbidity and mortality and improves growth in HIV-positive children. Malnourished HIV-positive adults are known to have an increased risk of opportunistic infections, a shorter survival, and a higher risk of death.

Nutritional needs for people living with HIV/AIDS are different from the noninfected person or child.[41] Moreover, the synergism between infectious disease and malnutrition compounds the problem of morbidity and mortality, especially in low-resource settings.[42] HIV increases resting energy expenditure, reduces food intake, and can be accompanied by malabsorption or loss of key nutrients. Asymptomatic HIV-positive individuals require 10% more energy calories; symptomatic HIV-positive individuals require 20% to 30% more.[43] For HIV-positive children with weight loss, energy requirements increase by 50% to 100%. Given that it would be impossible for children to consume large volumes of food to make up that need, early detection of weight loss and encouragement of feeding is especially important.[44]

The overlap between SAM and HIV/AIDS is considerable. The association of inadequate food intake, malabsorption and diarrhea, and altered metabolism and nutrient storage leads to nutritional deficiencies. These are exacerbated by increased oxidative stress and immune suppression, which in turn allow for more HIV replication, faster disease progression, and increased morbidity and mortality. Special nutritional interventions, therefore, need to be integrated into the medical management of HIV.[45]

The interactions among HIV, livelihood, and food security are complex. People may stay at home to care for sick and dying family members, making them less available for community activities, including food crop production and food sales in the marketplace. This downward spiral further decreases income available for health care and treatment.

The use of home-based care for HIV/AIDS patients shares a number of features with CTC, which can be modified to meet the nutritional needs of people living with HIV/AIDS.[46] CTC can potentially reduce hospitalization rates. It is also seen as a point of entry for voluntary counseling and testing as well as a means for facilitating adherence to antiretroviral therapy. Trust, proximity to home for easier referrals, and the credibility of the CTC work may all increase voluntary counseling and testing in the local population. Just as DOTS (directly observed treatment, short course) programs for TB are enhanced by the supply of food to TB patients to facilitate case management, so too may CTC help with antiretroviral therapy.

Nutritional interventions have a wide range of activities, from good nutrition counseling for positive living to counseling on special food and nutrition needs in conjunction with treatment for opportunistic infections and the use of antiretrovirals, including instances in which antiretrovirals should or should not be taken with food. Antiretrovirals can aggravate nutritional problems and cause metabolic derangements of glucose, fat stores, lipid and cholesterol, and pancreatic enzymes needed for digestion. Good nutrition is essential for response to treatment. Children, pregnant and lactating mothers, and those who lose weight or do not respond to medication may need supplementary feeding; in the case of severe malnutrition, they need therapeutic feeding. Children who are vulnerable or orphaned by parents who died of HIV/AIDS will need special nutrition assistance as well. Palliative care and assistance with coping mechanisms are also important interventions for those doubly affected by malnutrition and HIV/AIDS.

Micronutrients are especially important for people living with HIV/AIDS. Clinical trials have shown that supplementation improves many clinical and laboratory parameters, such as increasing survival times, preventing adverse birth outcomes, and reducing mother-to-child transmission of HIV in nutritionally vulnerable women with advanced disease.

THE INTERNATIONAL POLICY RESPONSE

Economists and others recognize that malnutrition negatively affects a country's economic growth, perpetuates poverty, and results in increased health costs. On a larger scale, where larger proportions of a country's population are affected, the gross national product reflects the result of a long cascade beginning with malnutrition.

To bring global attention and pressure to bear on this situation, the first Millennium Development Goal (MDG) is to halve poverty and hunger in target populations where individual income is less than US $1 per day and where large proportions of children younger than 5 are underweight. MDGs are just a part of the response. It is well known that better incomes and food security are part of the route to solving malnutrition. Yet, these alone are not the answer. Inappropriate feeding and care practices in the face of food-secure environments result in underweight or stunted children. Moreover, poor access to health services, poor sanitation, and ignorance of basic health care exacerbate the problem.

The international community knows that the solutions do not simply lie in investing more money in struggling countries. In addition, other health interventions and poverty reduction strategies will be undercut if the basic problems of hunger and malnutrition are not addressed. Beyond policy analysis, there must be strong linkages between policies and nutrition actions, commitments to forging new partnerships and equipping actors to manage nutrition programs, and the engagement of the business, private, and corporate sectors to act responsibly when it comes to nutrition messaging, food choices, and new markets and products. In the perspective of the World Bank and others, tackling malnutrition is seen as an excellent economic investment.[3] In fact, in May 2004 a consensus of eminent economists (including several Nobel laureates) concluded that the returns on investing in micronutrient programs are second only to the returns on fighting HIV/AIDS among a lengthy list of ways to meet the world's development challenges.[3,47]

Governments will need to show commitment to nutrition programs on a wide scale. This will lay a foundation for the broader agenda of poverty reduction and sustainable growth. Otherwise, malnutrition—the world's largest public health problem and the leading contributor to child mortality—will continue to undermine other worthy public health responses in both the developed and developing world.

STUDY QUESTIONS

1. What factors (in a community, in an individual) predispose to malnutrition? How are these different for communities versus for individuals?

2. What are the advantages of community-based therapeutic care?

3. What are the special considerations for nutrition in HIV-affected and HIV-infected populations?

4. What micronutrient deficiencies require immediate attention?

5. Would you use MUAC or WFH in assessing severe acute malnutrition? Why? What are the advantages and disadvantages of each?

6. What is the cycle of poverty and its link with malnutrition?

7. What areas of research would help inform nutrition interventions for vulnerable populations?

8. How are the nutrition problems different in developing countries versus in the developed world?

9. What is the role of policy formation in influencing ministries of health, the donor community, and nongovernmental organizations in addressing global malnutrition?

SELECTED BIBLIOGRAPHY

Bread for the World Institute. *Frontline Issues in Nutrition Assistance: Hunger Report 2006.* Washington, DC: Bread for the World Institute, 2006.

Emergency Nutrition Network. *Field Exchange,* Issue 27. March 2006.

Epi Info. EpiNut software (for anthropometric data entry and analysis).

Save the Children. *Emergency Nutrition Assessment: Guidelines for Field Workers.* London: Save the Children UK, 2004

Standing Committee on Nutrition. *WHO, UNICEF, and SCN Informal Consultation on Community-Based Management of Severe Malnutrition in Children.* Tokyo: United Nations University Press, 2006. SCN Nutrition Policy Paper 21.

World Food Programme. Vulnerability Assessment and Mapping team reports. http://wfp.org/operations/vam/vam_docustore/index.asp.

Useful Websites

Child and Adolescent Health and Development: http://www.who.int/child-adolescent-health

Emergency Nutrition Network (ENN) Online: http://www.ennonline.net

ENN Online, Infant Feeding in Emergencies: http://www.ennonline.net/ife/index

Famine Early Warning Systems Network: http://www.fews.net/

Food and Nutrition Technical Assistance: http://www.fantaproject.org/

The Sphere Project: http://www.sphereproject.org/

Standardized Monitoring and Assessment of Relief and Transitions: http://www.smartindicators.org/

United Nations System Standing Committee on Nutrition: http://www.unsystem/org/scn/

Valid International: http://www.validinternational.org/pages/

LIST OF ACRONYMS

ART	Antiretroviral Therapy
ARV	Antiretrovirals
BCC	Behavior change and communication
BF	Breastfeeding
BMI	Body mass index
CTC	Community Therapeutic Care
DOTS	Directly observed treatment, short course
FEWSNET	Famine Early Warning System
GAM	Global Acute Malnutrition
GNP	Gross national product
HIV	Human immunodeficiency virus
IMCI	Integrated management of childhood illness
MCH	Maternal and Child Health
MDG	Millennium Development Goals
MTCT	Mother-to-child transmission (HIV)
MUAC	Mid-Upper Arm Circumference
NCHS	National Center for Health Statistics
NGOs	Non-governmental organizations
NHANES	National Health and Nutrition Examination surveys
NICS	Nutritional Information in Crisis Situations
NIDS	National Immunization Days
NTDS	Neural Tube Defects
PEM	Protein Energy Malnutrition
PLWHA	People living with HIV/AIDS
RNIS	Refugee Nutrition Information System
RUTF	Ready-To-Use-Therapeutic-Foods
SAM	Severe Acute Malnutrition
SD	Standard Deviation
SF	Supplementary Feeding
SFP	Supplementary Feeding Program
SSA	Sub-Saharan Africa
TB	Tuberculosis
TF	Therapeutic Feeding
TF	Therapeutic Feeding Program
VCT	Voluntary Counseling and Testing

WFA	Weight-for-Age
WFH	Weight for Height
WFP	World Food Program
WHO	World Health Organization
UNHCR	UN High Commissioner for Refugees
USAID	United States Agency for International Development

REFERENCES

1. UNICEF. *Progress for Children: A Report Card on Nutrition.* New York: UNICEF. Progress for Children no. 4, May 2006.

2. United Nations Standing Committee on Nutrition. *Fifth Report on the World Nutrition Situation: Nutrition for Improved Development Outcomes.* Geneva: Standing Committee on Nutrition, 2004.

3. World Bank. *Repositioning Nutrition as Central to Development: A Strategy for Large-Scale Action.* Washington, DC: World Bank, 2006.

4. World Health Organization. *World Health Report: Reducing Risks, Promoting Healthy Life.* Geneva: World Health Organization, 2002.

5. Shrimpton R, Cesar G, et al. The worldwide timing of growth failure; implications for nutritional interventions. *Pediatrics* 2001;107(5):e75.

6. Pelletier DL. The relationship between child anthropometry and mortality in developing countries: implications for policy, programs and future research. *J Nutr* 1994;124(suppl):2074S–2081S.

7. Pelletier DL, Frongillo EA. Changes in child survival are strongly associated with changes in malnutrition in developing countries. *J Nutr* 2003;133:107–119.

8. Ogden C, Flegal K, et al. Prevalence and trends in overweight among US children and adolescents, 1999–2000. *JAMA* 2002;288:1728–1732.

9. American Academy of Pediatrics, Committee on Nutrition. Pediatric obesity. In Kleinman RE, ed. *Pediatric Nutrition Handbook.* 5th ed. Elk Grove Village, IL: American Academy of Pediatrics, 2004:551–592.

10. Institute of Medicine, Committee on Prevention of Obesity in Children and Youth. *Preventing Childhood Obesity: Health in the Balance.* Washington, DC: National Academies Press, 2005.

11. UNICEF/UNO/WHO Study Team. *Multiple Micronutrient Supplementation During Pregnancy (MMSDP): Efficacy Trials.* Report of a meeting at the Center for International Child Health, Institute of Child Health; March 2002; London.

12. Micronutrient Initiative and UNICEF. *Vitamin and Mineral Deficiency: A Global Progress Report.* Ottawa, Canada: Micronutrient Initiative, 2004. http://www.micronutrient.org/reports/reports/Full_e.pdf.

13. Sommer A, Tarwotjo I, Djunaedi E, et al. Impact of vitamin A supplementation on childhood mortality: a randomized controlled community trial. *Lancet* 1986;1:1169.

14. West K, Katz J, Khatry S, = et al. Double blind, cluster randomized trial of low dose supplementation of vitamin A or beta-carotene on mortality related to pregnancy in Nepal. *BMJ* 1999;318:570–575.

15. Humphrey J, Illif P, et al. Effects of a single large dose of vitamin A, given during the post-partum period to HIV-positive

women and their infants, on child HIV infection, HIV-free survival, and mortality. *J Infect Dis* 2006;193:860–871.

16. Zinc Investigators' Collaborative Group. Prevention of diarrhea and pneumonia by zinc supplementation in children in developing countries: pooled analysis of randomized controlled trials. *J Pediatrics* 1999;135:689–697.

17. Scholl TO, Hediger ML, Shall JI, Khoo CS, Fischer RL. Dietary and serum folate: their influence on the outcome of pregnancy. *Am J Clin Nutr* 1996;63:520–525.

18. Green NS. Folic acid supplementation and prevention of birth defects. *J Nutr* 2002;132(8 suppl):2356S–2360S.

19. Castilla E, et al. Preliminary data on changes in neural tube defect prevalence rates after folic acid fortification in South America. *Am J Med Genet* 2003;123A(2):123–128.

20. Sphere Project. *The Sphere Humanitarian Charter and Minimum Standards in Disaster Response.* 2004 revised edition. Oxford, UK: Oxfam Publishing, 2004. http://www.sphereproject.org/handbook/index.htm.

21. Salama P, Spiegel P, et al. Lessons learned from complex emergencies over past decade. *Lancet* 2004;364(9447):1801–1813.

22. Spiegel P. Quality of malnutrition assessment surveys conducted during famine in Ethiopia. *JAMA* 2004;292:613–618.

23. SMART 2005. Measuring mortality: nutritional status and food security in crisis situations—the SMART protocol. Version 1. Final draft. January 2005.

24. Salama P, Assefa F, et al. Malnutrition, measles, mortality, and the humanitarian response during a famine in Ethiopia. *JAMA* 2001;286:563–571.

25. Myatt M, Feleke T, et al. A field trial of a survey method for estimating the coverage of selective feeding programmes. *Bull World Health Organ* 2005;83(1):20–26.

26. World Health Organization. The WHO child growth standards. 2006. http://www.who.int/childgrowth/standards/en/.

27. United Nations Standing Committee on Nutrition. SCN endorses the new WHO growth standards for infants and young children. April 27, 2006. http://www.unsystem.org/scn/publications/html/who_growth_standards.htm.

28. Hill Z, Kirkwood B, Edmond K. *Family and Community Practices That Promote Child Survival, Growth and Development: A Review of the Evidence.* Geneva: World Health Organization, 2004:21–26.

29. World Health Organization. *The Optimal Duration of Exclusive Breastfeeding: Report of an Expert Consultation.* Geneva: World Health Organization, 2001. http://www.who.int/child-adolescent-health/New_Publications/NUTRITION/ WHO_ CAH_01_24.pdf.

30. Picciano MF. Nutrient composition of human milk. *Pediatr Clin North Am* 2001;48:53–67.

31. US Department of Health and Human Services. *Healthy People 2010.* 2nd ed. With *Understanding and Improving Health and Objectives for Improving Health.* 2 vols. Washington, DC: US Government Printing Office, 2000.

32. Nduati R. John G, Mbori-Ngacha D, et al. Effect of breastfeeding and formula feeding on transmission of HIV-1: a randomized clinical trial. *JAMA* 2000;283:1167–1174.

33. World Health Organization. *The Management of Nutrition in Major Emergencies.* Geneva: World Health Organization, United Nations High Commissioner for Refugees, International Federation of the Red Cross and Red Crescent Societies, and World Food Programme, 2000.

34. Collins S, Dent N, Binns P, et al. Management of severe acute malnutrition in children. *Lancet* 2006;368(9551):1992–2000.

35. CTC Research and Development Programme. *Community-Based Therapeutic Care (CTC): A Field Manual.* Oxford, UK: Valid International, 2006.

36. Collins S. *Community-Based Therapeutic Care—A New Paradigm for Selective Feeding in Nutritional Crises.* London: Overseas Development Institute, 2004. Humanitarian Policy Network paper 48.

37. Emergency Nutrition Network. *Operational Challenges of Implementing Community Therapeutic Care: ENN Report on an Inter-Agency Workshop, Washington DC, February 28–March 2, 2005.* Oxford, UK: Emergency Nutrition Network, 2005:6.

38. Guerrero S, Mollison S. Engaging communities in emergency response: the CTC experience in Western Darfur. In: Humanitarian Policy Network, eds. *Humanitarian Exchange.* London: Overseas Development Institute, 2005:20–22.

39. Myatt M, Khara T, Collins S. A review of methods to detect cases of severely malnourished children in the community for their admission into community-based therapeutic care programs. *Food Nutr Bull* 2006;27(suppl):S7–S23.

40. Ashworth A. Efficacy and effectiveness of community-based treatment of severe malnutrition. *Food Nutr Bull* 2006;27 (suppl):S24–S48.

41. Heller L. Nutritional support for children with HIV/AIDS. *AIDS Reader* 2000;10109–114.

42. Duggan C, Fawzi W. Micronutrients and child health: studies in international nutrition and HIV infection. *Nutr Rev* 2001;59:358–369.

43. World Health Organization. *Nutrient Requirements for People Living with HIV/AIDS: Report of a Technical Consultation.* Geneva: World Health Organization, 2003. http://www.who.int/nut/documents/hiviads_nut_require.pdf.

44. World Health Organization. *HIV and Infant Feeding: A Guide for Health Care Managers and Supervisors.* Geneva: World Health Organization, 2003.

45. Integrating nutrition therapy into medical management of human immunodeficiency virus. *Clin Infect Dis* 2003;36(suppl 2).

46. Guerrero S, Bahwere P, Sadler K, Collins S. Integrating CTC and HIV/AIDS support in Malawi. *Field Exchange* 2005;25:8–10.

47. Bhagwati, J, Fogel R, Frey B, et al. Ranking the opportunities. In: Lomberg B, ed. *Global Crises, Global Solutions.* Cambridge, UK: Cambridge University Press, 2004.

Primary Care in Global Health 7

Alain J. Montegut, Cynthia Haq, Debra Rothenberg, and Leon Piterman

LEARNING OBJECTIVES

- To understand the definitions of primary care and primary health care
- To understand the development of primary care historically and its global importance today
- To understand the role of primary care in health systems and how countries with inadequate primary health care are adversely affected
- To be able to compare and contrast four countries with different health policies, priorities, and resources

Primary health care is a phrase introduced to our lexicon in the 1970s. However, it is an approach to health care that in fact has been present for centuries. It is important for us to understand the roots of primary health care in general practice as well as its current practice to fully understand its role in society and health. It is also important to distinguish between primary health care as a comprehensive strategy for prevention, health promotion, and treatment at the community level and *primary care*, which is a Western concept of the point of patients' initial contact with the health care system and providers.

Health care has become a major issue for many countries in the 21st century. Health care includes economic, social, political, and technical issues. The questions that surround national debates regarding health care around the globe are similar. How do we best promote health and treat disease? Who should provide this care? How should the system be organized? What is the right balance and mix of health providers, and how should they be distributed? What health services should

be provided for all, and who should pay? How much should health care cost? For individuals and families, these questions can be synthesized as follows: How do I attain the highest possible level of health, and how do I access health services in times of need?

This chapter focuses on primary health care and how it is organized and practiced around the globe. It offers a definition of primary health care and looks at how it is delivered in different health care systems. It explains how primary health care can have an impact on disease and on health indicators. It looks at what some goals could be for improving health systems through advocacy for primary health care education and delivery and discusses health workforce issues as they relate to models for training of primary health care physicians and other members of primary health care teams. The chapter focuses on primary care physicians because of the limitation of space; however, we recognize that there are many other health professionals who often compose the primary health care team.

Additionally, the chapter explores how four countries with vastly different political and socioeconomic conditions have tried to improve health in their countries—some through the advent of strong primary health care delivery systems, others through systems based on specialist care, and others who have selected primary health care as the central theme for health care reform and are in their infancy of implementation. It is hoped that the reader will gain an appreciation for the complex challenges involved in improving opportunities for health for all.

THE HISTORY OF PRIMARY CARE

Healing has been practiced for centuries around the globe. In fact, in the premodern era it was practiced in broadly similar ways. The healer was often an elder of the community who over time had gained respect and knowledge. Disease was felt to come from both natural and supernatural causes. Often the causes were felt to be spiritual, involving the entry or exit of spirits to or from the body. Primary care has its roots in the premodern era, when healers had strong ties within communities and used this status to improve the health of the members of the community. Over time some of these healers became known as *physicians,* the person who "heals or exerts a healing influence";[1] others became nurses, midwives, pharmacists, and allied health professionals, among others. Traditional healers continue to provide health advice and treatment worldwide as well.

Over time, the art of healing was joined with the science of prevention. The Yellow Emperor, the first sovereign of civilized China, wrote the *Neijing* roughly 2000 years ago, which has come to be known as *The Yellow Emperor's Classic of Medicine.*

> *"In the good old days the sages treated disease by preventing illness before it began, just as the good government of emperor was able to take the necessary steps to avert war. Treating illness after it has begun is like suppressing revolt after it has broken out.*
>
> *A superior doctor arrests disease at the skin level and dispels it before it penetrates deeper. An inferior doctor treats illness after it passess the skin.*
>
> *A good healer cannot depend on skill alone. He must also have the correct attitude, sincerity, compassion, and a sense of responsibility"[2]*

Hippocrates later articulated the importance of a holistic approach to health. In Plato's *Phaedrus* we learn that "Hippocrates the Asclepiad says that the nature even of the body can only be understood as a whole," and "it is more important to know what sort of person has a disease than to know what sort of disease a person has."[3]

The Renaissance brought the beginning of modern medicine in 1543 with the publication of the first complete textbook of human anatomy, *De Humanis Corporis Fabrica* by Andreas Vesalius. Vesalius was a classicist by education. He knew Greek and Latin and had studied the ancient writings and extolled them. He was considered a true humanist; in his teachings, he was able to blend the approach to the whole person with his science. The evolution of the physician as scientist and humanist continued.[4]

The ensuing three centuries brought many changes in the science of medicine. Alongside progress in medical science most of the world continued to use traditional healers. However, in countries that were becoming industrialized through the 19th and early 20th century, physicians and nurses assumed the primary responsibility for patient care. Before the political changes of 1917 in the Soviet Union, there was a rich tradition of general practice. The Zemstvo physicians combined traditional medical care with the humanitarianism and reformism of the contemporary populist movement. These physicians believed that if medical

care was to be effective, it had to be given in tandem with improvements in the sanitation, nutrition, and living standards of the time.[5]

In the United States, the generalist was also the primary physician. This was advocated by William Osler in an article entitled "Internal Medicine as a Vocation" published in the *Medical News* in 1897: "By all means, if possible, let [the young physician] be a pluralist, and—as he values his future life—let him not get early entangled in the meshes of specialism."[6]

The end of the 19th and early part of the 20th centuries brought with them desires for reform in medical education. The Medical Act of 1858 in Great Britain[7] and the 1910 report entitled *Medical Education in the United States and Canada: A Report to the Carnegie Foundation for the Advancement of Teaching,*[8] authored by Abraham Flexner, offered recommendations that would change the face of medical education in these countries and then the world. The activities generated by these reports developed standards for the accreditation of medical schools and policies related to the qualifications of physicians. Although these reforms raised the quality of medical education, they concurrently caused a disproportionate reduction in the number of physicians serving disadvantaged communities

The role of the generalist physician continued to evolve during this period. There was a progressive separation of the role of community-based general practitioners from physicians and surgeons who specialized and held hospital appointments. In this division the general practitioner became the doctor of first contact working in the community, whereas consultant physicians and surgeons controlled the hospitals with their scientific and technical facilities. Patients who needed these additional services were referred by their general practitioners.

As medical education reforms evolved through the early part of the 20th century, so did the need for good generalist physicians. In his book *A Time to Heal,* Flexner wrote that

> The small town needs the best and not the worst doctor procurable. For the country doctor has only himself to rely on: he cannot in every pinch hail specialist, expert, and nurse. On his own skill, knowledge, resourcefulness, the welfare of his patient altogether depends. The rural district is therefore entitled to the best trained physician that can be induced to go there.[9]

In nonindustrialized parts of the world, the value of the generalist health care provider of first contact was also recognized. *Barefoot doctors* were farmers who obtained basic medical training and worked in rural villages in China to bring health care to areas where urban-trained doctors would not settle. There had been scattered experiments with this concept before 1965, but with Mao's famous 1965 speech about health care[10] it became institutionalized as part of the Cultural Revolution, which radically diminished the influence of the Weishengbu, China's health ministry, which was dominated by Western-trained doctors. In Vietnam, a national Commune Health Center system was created in the 1950s; it was staffed by health care workers initially, but then began to receive staffing by generalist physicians in the late 1960 and 1970s.

Health care professionals of first contact have evolved and become more stratified in response to advances in medical sciences and therapies. Health care services are often organized into four overlapping levels of care: primary health care, which is the focus of this chapter; secondary medical care, which includes consultations by specialists for patients with more unusual problems; tertiary care, which is care for patients with disorders that are so uncommon in a population that the primary care physician would not be expected to maintain skills in caring for them; and emergency care, which is initial care for urgent problems or trauma.[11]

DEFINITION OF PRIMARY CARE

In 1978, the World Health Organization (WHO) convened a conference in Alma Ata, the capital of the Soviet Republic of Kazakhstan. It was attended by 3,000 participants from 134 governments and 67 international organizations. The purpose of the conference was to look for ways to improve health. Ideas about primary health care had been discussed in many countries and across many organizations. The outcome of this conference was a declaration entitled "Health for All by the Year 2000." The declaration provided a framework for the definition of primary health care as being essential, practical, affordable, scientifically sound, and the main focus of overall social and economic development. The needs fulfilled by primary health care will vary depending on the location, burden of illness, demographics, and socioeconomic circumstances of the community.[12]

As distinct from secondary or tertiary care that is provided in hospitals, primary health care is principally provided in the community. Care may be provided by public or private practitioners and includes efforts to coordinate services across sectors.

In economically developed countries, primary health care professionals include family doctors, nurses, pharmacists, and a variety of allied health professionals. In less economically developed countries, primary health care may be delivered by health workers who have received shorter courses of training, such as barefoot doctors in China or Aboriginal health workers in Australia. These health workers are often community members and therefore knowledgeable of the communities they serve; they provide a vital link to other health care providers.

Primary Care and Its Relationship to Disease

As countries struggle to provide the highest possible level of health care services at the lowest cost, researchers have analyzed how the organization and composition of health services affect health outcomes. There are many determinants of health for individuals and for populations. The basic determinant, of course, is the gene pool, but this is "heavily modified by the social and physical environment, by behaviors that are culturally or socially determined, and by the nature of the health care provided."[13] Across all countries, evidence shows us that health outcomes are often adversely affected by poverty both within and between countries.

Although health services are one of the determinants of health, greater spending on health care is not necessarily associated with improved health outcomes. Very strong evidence exists that access to comprehensive primary health care improves health outcomes. Increasing the ratio of primary health care physicians to specialists improves health outcomes even more.[14]

The benefits of primary health care become apparent by reviewing the relationship between primary care orientation and the health indicators of the population. An important indicator of health outcomes is the mortality rate of children younger than 5 years (Figure 7-1). These data reveal clusters of countries with similar rankings on a logarithmic scale.[15] It is unfortunate that even though these data are from 1995, the rankings today have changed very little. The issue is easily put into perspective when one looks at the actual under-five mortality rates for some of these countries: Uganda, 195/1,000; Cambodia, 135/1,000; Vietnam, 30/1,000; and China, 40/1,000. These rates are quite high when compared with Russia at 21/1,000, the United States at 9/1,000, and Australia at 6/1,000. Although economic factors play a significant role in determining health outcomes, there is mounting evidence that development and access to primary health care services play an important role as well.

Data have been analyzed from Western industrialized countries, looking at the strength of primary care as evaluated based on nine characteristics of health systems' infrastructure (Table 7-1) and six practice characteristics of the patients' experiences in receiving care (Table 7-2). A scoring system was developed to assign a relative value to the countries studied based on their level of primary care. The countries with higher rankings in primary care were found to have had better health indicators. Additionally, those countries that had weak primary care infrastructures had higher costs and poorer outcomes.[11,16]

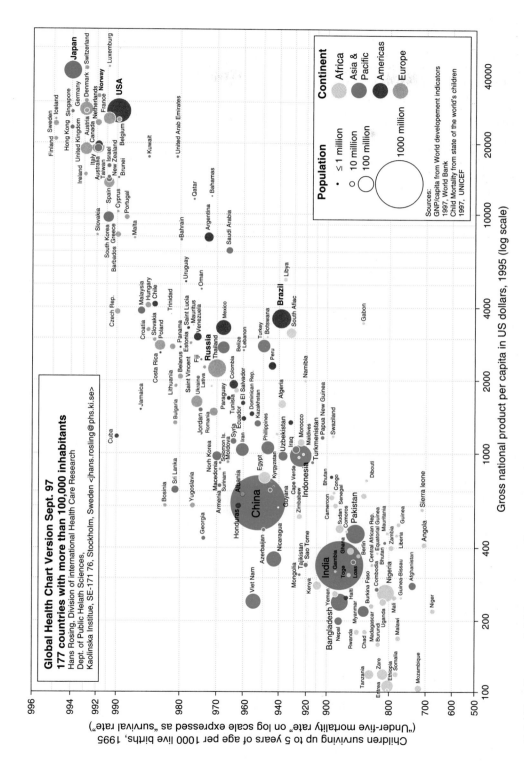

Figure 7-1. Mortality rate of children younger than 5 years.

Table 7-1. Health system characteristics.

Extent to which the system regulates the distribution of resources throughout the country
Mode of financing of primary care services
Modal type of primary care practitioner
Percentage of active physicians involved in primary care versus those in conventional specialty care
Ratio of average professional earnings of primary care physicians compared with other specialists
Requirement for cost sharing by patients
Requirement for patient lists to identify the community served by practices
Twenty-four-hour access arrangements
Strength of academic departments of primary care or general practice

From Starfield B, Shi L. Policy relevant determinants of health: an international perspective. *Health Policy* 2002;60:201–218. (Reproduced with permission.)

A correlation also exists between primary care and age-standardized mortality. With a 20% increase in the number of primary care physicians, there is an associated 5% decrease in mortality (40 fewer deaths per 100,000). Most important, the effect is greatest if the increase is in family physicians. One more family physician per 10,000 people (an estimated 33% increase) is associated with 70 fewer deaths per 100,000 (an estimated 9% decrease). In contrast, an estimated 8% increase in the number of specialist physicians is associated with a 2% increase in mortality.[17] An association also exists between primary care and infant outcomes. The greater the supply of primary care physicians, the lower the infant mortality and percentage of low-birth-weight infants. An increase of one primary care physician per 10,000 is associated with a 2.5% reduction in infant mortality and a 3.2% reduction in low birth weight.[18]

Numerous studies have demonstrated that earlier detection of diseases such as breast cancer,[19] melanoma,[20] colon cancer,[21] and cervical cancer[22] improves with greater access to primary care. A decrease in total mortality and the mortality for heart disease and stroke is also correlated with increased access to primary care.[23] Increased access to primary care results in better health outcomes and lower costs.[24]

Almost all of the evidence concerning the benefits of primary health care systems comes from industrialized countries. There are few data from developing countries. A study in Indonesia that looked at primary health care and infant mortality rates showed that as the government shifted spending away from primary care and toward the hospital and technological sector, there was a worsening of infant mortality.[25]

Table 7-2. Practice characteristics.

First-contact care
Longitudinality
Comprehensiveness
Coordination
Family-centeredness
Community orientation

From Starfield B, Shi L. Policy relevant determinants of health: an international perspective. *Health Policy* 2002;60:201–218. (Reproduced with permission.)

HUMAN RESOURCES FOR HEALTH

People are at the heart of all effective health systems. Health professionals and their support staff, or human resources for health, organize and provide services and health education and assess outcomes. A wide array of skills is required for the effective delivery of comprehensive primary health care services; these services may be delivered by a variety of personnel.

Ample evidence exists that the number, quality, and distribution of health personnel strongly affect health outcomes. For example, birth outcomes are strongly associated with the presence of a skilled birth attendant at deliveries. A minimal density of health workers is needed to ensure that all women will have access to a skilled attendant.

The WHO estimates that there is a total of 59.2 million full-time health workers worldwide. Approximately two-thirds of these workers are health services providers; the other one-third are health management and support workers.[26]

Individual health professionals are usually integrated into teams to deliver primary health care services. Primary care physicians, nurses, and outreach workers are of particular importance to well-functioning primary health care teams. They are called upon to assess and treat a wide range of patients at the community level, including those with urgent or complex disorders. They function to bridge the gaps between patients and health resources, between individual and public health, and between communities and secondary and tertiary care services.[27]

A primary health care team is composed of people who contribute to delivering health services. Each team is unique: local conditions determine the members, relationships, and responsibilities of the team; regional and national conditions influence the resources and contexts in which the teams operate. Enormous diversity exists in the composition of primary health care teams. They often consist of physicians, nurses, medical assistants, midwives, social workers, community health workers, and others who provide direct patient care. Supportive members of the team may include receptionists; administrative professionals and administrators; health educators; and laboratory, pharmacy, and radiology personnel. Consultative members of the team may include those who provide specialized health services or those with expertise in community health.[28,29]

Flexibility in the makeup of primary health care teams is necessary for dealing with the unique circumstances and resources of a particular community. For instance, not all of the above-mentioned personnel may be available, in which case others may assume essential roles. Achieving a sustainable and balanced health workforce requires the coordination of many sectors of society: educational institutions, policy-making bodies, communities, and financiers (Figure 7-2).

Access to care is increased when primary care services are provided at the community level, usually through primary care team members. Access is determined by availability, convenience, proximity, affordability, and acceptability.[13] Under ideal circumstances, continuous access to health care services is provided to patients through coverage arrangements at the point of first contact, along with referrals for patients who require services that are not available at the local level. When patients can readily access primary health care services in the community, they are less likely to seek hospital services, which are often less convenient and more expensive.

Continuity of care involves an ongoing personal relationship with an individual; alternatively, it may be shared among team members. Continuity is enhanced when patients can identify and readily access their own primary health care providers. Similarly, continuity is expedited when providers identify a specific group of patients for whom they are responsible. In some practice arrangements, doctors may supervise the care provided by nurse practitioners, medical assistants, and other health team members to ensure continuity of care for a greater number of patients. In these situations, doctors will focus their efforts on the care of patients with more complex conditions, while nurses and other health professionals provide preventive services and manage less complex patient problems.

Achieving the right distribution of health workers is challenging within and between countries. Health professionals tend to congregate in urban areas, resulting in rural shortages in most nations. Additionally, there are absolute shortages of health workers in many areas of the world, most notably in the sub-Saharan African region, where it is estimated that there is a shortage of a million health workers to meet even the minimal standards for delivery of essential health care services (Figure 7-3).

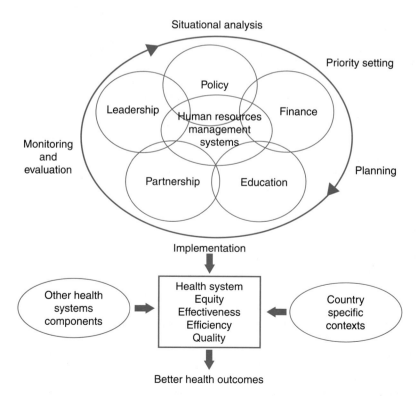

Figure 7-2. Human resources for health technical framework: achieving a sustainable health workforce.

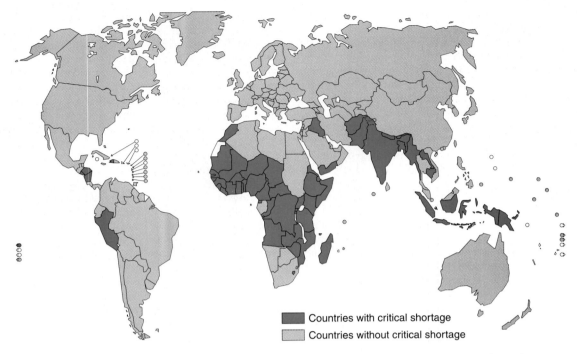

Figure 7-3. Countries with a critical shortage of health service providers (doctors, nurses, and midwives).

Health professional education requires eligible students, intact educational institutions, sufficient faculty, and years of investment. Health professionals are likely to practice in environments to which they have been exposed in training. If students do not see primary care as attractive, they are unlikely to pursue primary care careers. Therefore, much of the education of the primary health care workforce should be in well-supported primary health care and community settings.

Train, sustain, and retain refers to the steps necessary to prepare, deploy, and support health professionals where they are needed. Health professionals do not work in a vacuum. They require a system that encourages and supports their efforts and provides adequate facilities with good working conditions. If salaries are too low or facilities are inadequate, it is difficult to recruit or retain workers where they are needed (Figure 7-4). There is an ongoing relationship between education, labor and health services markets, and the human resources considered necessary in each sector.

International comparisons of primary health care outcomes in economically developed countries suggest that the greatest differences in health between countries are associated with the degree to which the following principles have been implemented in their health services delivery system[13]:

- Equitable distribution and financing of health care services
- Similar level of professional earnings for primary care physicians and specialists

- Comprehensiveness of primary health care services
- Absent, or very low, requirements for co-payments for primary health care services
- Primary care physicians providing first-contact care and entry into the health delivery system
- Person-focused longitudinal care

Globalization has resulted in the flow of ideas, goods, and people around the world. Powerful economic forces lure many health professionals to greener pastures and better facilities. Strong global, national, and local alliances are needed to ensure that health professionals are not only trained to meet the needs of communities but also that they are retained to practice in areas where they are needed (Figure 7-5).

CASE STUDIES FROM AROUND THE WORLD

The cost of health care has been rising across the globe, and countries have been trying to reorganize the delivery of health care in many ways. The evidence that provision of primary care and the existence of a sound primary health care infrastructure lead to improved health has led many countries to choose this model on which to base reform. Other countries have continued to base their systems on a disproportionate share of secondary and tertiary care.

This section of the chapter discusses four countries to illustrate disparities in health care delivery systems

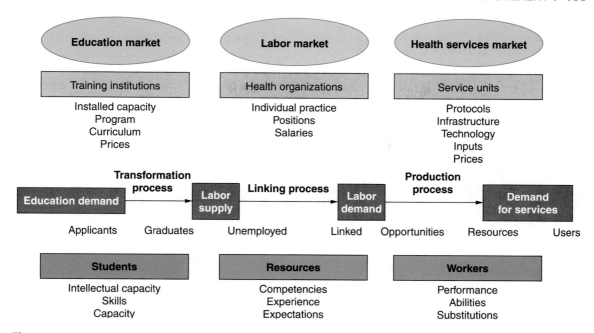

Figure 7-4. Relationship of education, labor, and health services markets with human resources.

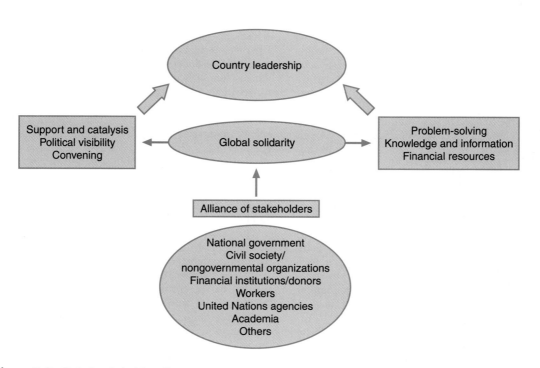

Figure 7-5. Global stakeholder alliance.

around the globe. These examples were chosen specifically to demonstrate inequalities and disparities in health. They demonstrate that wealth is not an indicator for improved health for all and that creative solutions to provide primary care are important for all countries.

Australia

Australia has a population of approximately 20 million people who come from 200 countries, with almost a quarter of the population having been born outside Australia. The country consists of a federation of seven states and territories, with the commonwealth or federal government providing national leadership, and state governments providing leadership at state or territory levels. A third level of government determines municipal policies. These three layers of government are all involved in determining health policy and delivering health services at different levels. The commonwealth government, through the Health Insurance Commission, assumes primary responsibility for the dispersion of funds and for underwriting the national universal health insurance scheme, known as Medicare, and the Pharmaceutical Benefits Scheme, which provides subsidized medication. All citizens who are employed pay around 2% of their income as a levy to support the universal health insurance system. Total health expenditure in 2001–2002 was $66.5 billion, or 9.3% of the gross domestic product (GDP).

In addition to the public health insurance scheme, citizens may avail themselves of private insurance that entitles them to private hospital care under the doctor of their choice and partly covers a range of ancillary health services such as dentistry, psychology, physiotherapy, podiatry, and pharmacy that are not routinely covered by Medicare. This mix of private and public health care has been a feature of the Australian health system for many years and was enshrined in legislation in 1972.

In 1986, Australia joined with other countries through the Ottawa Charter[30] to identify action to achieve the objectives of the WHO's Health for All by the Year 2000 initiative, launched in 1981 at the first International Conference on Health Promotion held in Ottawa, Canada. The conference was primarily a response to growing expectations for a new public health movement around the world. Discussions focused on needs within industrialized countries, but took into account similar concerns in all other regions. In keeping with the Ottawa Charter, Australia has identified a number of national health priorities that receive attention both directly through funding of health care as well as indirectly through research funding (Table 7-3).

Primary care in Australia is delivered by a range of health practitioners and suffers from a lack of integration of medical services in the private sector, where most doctors practice, and other sectors, where services are delivered

Table 7-3. National health priorities as defined by the Ottawa Charter—Australia.

Cardiovascular disease
Cancer
Mental health
Injury
Diabetes
Asthma
Musculoskeletal disease

by allied health professionals, particularly through government agencies. Practitioners participating in the primary health care system include physicians (largely general practitioners or family physicians—these terms are used interchangeably in Australia) and allied health professionals. In addition, several hundred community health centers, funded by state governments, provide access to both medical and allied health services largely for those who cannot afford private health care.

In Australia, general practitioners (GPs) are the major providers of primary health care and the first point of contact with the health system. Around 40% of Australian doctors work as GPs, their numbers totaling almost 21,000.[31] Their training is discussed later in this chapter. General practitioners are the gatekeepers of the health system; patients are unable to gain direct access to specialists without referral from a GP. Although most patients (around 85%) have an identifiable GP, there is no government restriction on the number of GPs that a patient may attend. Fees charged by GPs and specialists are underwritten by Medicare, with patients able to claim 85% of the government-recommended fee as a rebate from Medicare.

The most frequent problems managed by GPs and the percentage they represent of total problems are as follows: respiratory (13.7%), musculoskeletal (11.7%), skin (11.5%), circulatory (11.5%), endocrine and metabolic (7.7%), and psychological (7.4%).[32]

To overcome the lack of integration between general practice and other segments of the health sector, the government has over the past 15 years introduced a number of strategies designed both to improve and monitor quality of care within general practice as well as facilitate linkages between GPs and other components of the health system, particularly those in the public sector.

The first of these strategies was introduced in 1990 and led to the creation of the Divisions of General Practice as well as the introduction of mandatory continuing professional development linked to vocational registration for general practice. Patients attending vocationally registered doctors receive a 15% to 20% higher rebate on their consultations, which means that these doctors charge higher fees without risk of penalizing their patients. The other major development resulting from the strategy review was the establishment of the Fellowship of the Royal Australian College of General Practitioners (FRACGP) as the only recognized end-point of vocational training. Since 1995, the only pathway to vocational registration has been through the Fellowship exam.

The second major review took place in 1998[33] and led to the formation of the Primary Care Research Evaluation and Development (PCRED) program, established to support primary care research. The 1998 strategy also introduced the Enhanced Primary Care Package, which included a number of reforms for funding general practice consultations, immunization in general practice, computerization of practices, and teaching medical students in practices. Another important reform included the Better Outcomes in Mental Health Program, introduced in 2001, that enables GPs who have undertaken appropriate training to charge extra for consultations that involve assessment and/or management of patients with mental illness or psychological problems.

Although attempts have been made to improve integration between general practice and other providers of primary health care, Australia has not moved as far or as rapidly as the United Kingdom and New Zealand in reforming the integration of general practice with public-sector providers of primary care. Primary Care Partnerships have been established in some states, in particular, Victoria. Also, a number of projects are under way to improve the hospital—general practice interface, for example, preadmission planning and discharge planning.

Medical schools in Australia provide courses to prepare physicians for internship, further training, and practice. Medical school programs range from 4 years for students who have completed college to 6 years for students who enter medical training directly from secondary school. On completion of medical school, all doctors must then complete a compulsory internship year before commencing vocational training in their chosen specialty. Training for general practice consists of an additional 3 years; 2 of these are spent in hospital residency rotations, and 1 year is spent in accredited general practices where they undergo supervised training. Doctors choosing to become rural GPs are required to undertake an additional year in order to acquire special skills in emergency medicine, surgery, and anaesthetics.

The training curriculum is set by the Royal Australian College of General Practitioners; however, the training itself is coordinated through a government authority known as General Practice Education and Training, Australia. Around 650 new trainees enter the program each year. One of the notable changes that has occurred over the past 5 years is an increase in the number of overseas-trained doctors undertaking training in general practice. Over one-third of the new entrants into the training program are now doctors whose basic degree is from overseas. On completion of training, doctors present for the Fellowship of the Royal Australian College of General Practitioners. All Australian universities now have general practice as a major part of their undergraduate curriculum.

Australia has a chronic shortage of GPs (and other health professionals), particularly in rural areas.[34] This has been attributed to factors such as feminization of the workforce, with approximately 70% of GP trainees being women who work part-time when their training has been completed or even undertake part-time training. There is currently active debate about whether nurse practitioners and other allied health workers should undertake some of the roles traditionally carried out by GPs to overcome some of these workforce shortages. Five new medical schools have been created in the past 5 years to provide long-term solutions to the workforce problem.

Uganda

Uganda is an East African nation of 27 million situated on the equator. The country faces challenges typical in many sub-Saharan African nations. Following independence in 1962, Uganda experienced widespread civil war that ended for most of the country in 1986 but continues in the north today. HIV/AIDS was identified in Uganda in the early 1980s and spread rapidly, reaching a peak of 30% prevalence in the early 1990s and now infecting 6% of the population. Health outcomes are strongly linked to poverty: 82% of Ugandans live on less than $1 per day. The target of health for all remains distant in the context of extensive poverty, low educational levels, a high burden of infectious diseases, and insufficient health resources.

Uganda's health outcomes stagnated and even worsened for some conditions from 1990 to 2005. The WHO and the Ugandan Ministry of Health (MoH) document a mean life expectancy of 49 years, an infant mortality rate of 81/1,000, an under-five mortality rate of 140/1,000, a maternal morality rate of 880/100,000, and a population growth rate of 3.1%, with more than 38% of children suffering from chronic malnutrition.[35] More than 75% of years of life lost due to premature deaths are attributable to ten preventable diseases. Perinatal and maternal conditions (20.4%), malaria (15.4%), acute lower respiratory tract conditions (10.5%), HIV/AIDS (9.1%), and diarrhea (8.4%) account for more than 60% of the total disease burden.[36]

Uganda's health care services are provided through parallel traditional, public, and private systems of care. Many Ugandans first seek health services from traditional and complementary medical practitioners (TCMPs). These practitioners are often more accessible at the community level than Western-trained health professionals, and are aware of cultural and contextual factors. TCMPs include birth attendants, herbalists, spiritualists, bone-setters and many others. Most have learned their skills through apprenticeship. Some provide beneficial services such as psychosocial support and counseling; others engage in harmful practices such as cutting and burning. Efforts are under way to license and train TCMPs to work in partnership with Western-trained health professionals.

Private medical practitioners provide health services throughout Uganda. Private health services include mission hospitals and health centers; such centers provide care to patients for minimal or sliding fee scales. Many health professionals employed by the public sector also offer private services after public working hours.

The Ugandan MoH supervises public health services "to ensure that all the people of Uganda attain a good standard of health." The Ugandan health system is organized through a hierarchy of public health centers and hospitals (Table 7-4). Although public health services are officially provided free of charge, patients are often required to purchase drugs, tests, and other medical supplies that are not available through the public sector.

The Health Sector Strategic Plan (HSSP) developed by the MoH provides a strong framework from which to improve health care services. The HSSP seeks to provide primary health care services to all through the Uganda National Minimum Health Care Package (UNMHCP). The package is designed to provide services to address common causes of death and disability; it includes maternal and child health services, control of communicable and noncommunicable diseases, health promotion, disease prevention, and community health initiatives.[37]

The public health system was decentralized in 1997 to strengthen primary health services and to promote increased autonomy and accountability at the local level. The MoH provides guidance, funding, and supplies to the districts; district health directors oversee services and distribute supplies and resources to health centers.

Table 7-4. Health care delivery system in Uganda.

- Health Center I: Village health team—1,000 population; census, health education and preventive services
- Health Center II: Parish level—5,000 population; primary ambulatory services
- Health Center III: Subcounty level—20,000 population; preventive, promotive, curative, basic laboratory
- Health Center IV: County level—100,000 population; preventive, curative, rehabilitative, emergency surgical
- District Health Services: District level—500,000 population
- Regional Referral Hospitals: 2,000,000 population; above plus select specialty care and outreach services
- National Referral Hospital: 27,000,000 population; above plus comprehensive specialty care, research, and teaching

The Ugandan health system is based upon the principles of primary health care:

- Accessibility: Services are available at the local level.
- Equitability: Services are distributed according to the population.
- Preventive, promotive, and curative services are targeted at common conditions.
- Community participation is emphasized, through decentralization to districts and local leadership.

Although the Ugandan health system is strategically designed to provide primary health care services to the population, financial and human resources are inadequate to deliver these services consistently. The cost of providing the package was estimated at $28 per person per year in 2004, yet the government of Uganda could afford only $12 per person. Consequently, shortages of basic supplies, drugs, and equipment are the norm in most public health facilities.

Ugandan health professionals include a broad spectrum of community health workers, social workers, pharmacists, laboratory technicians, radiologists, nurses, medical officers, physicians, and dentists. Uganda has a very low density of skilled health professionals; the majority of these are employed in the public sector. In 2003, the MoH employed 2,074 doctors and 9,510 nurses and midwives for a population of more than 25 million.[38] The doctor-to-population ratio is 1:12,500 at best and as low as 1:50,000 in some parts of the country. Most health professionals are concentrated in urban areas, whereas 88% of Uganda's population is rural.

The education and training of health professionals in Uganda occurs in two major universities (Makerere and Mbarara), a number of smaller private colleges, vocational training centers, and mission health centers. The training, competencies, certification and licensing, and responsibilities of health professionals are subject to great local variation. Shortages of almost every category of health professional are common, especially in rural areas and in the war-torn regions of the north. Consequently, health professionals often find themselves assuming responsibilities for which they have not been adequately prepared.

The education of Ugandan physicians follows the British model. Medical students are selected based on their performance in secondary school and entrance examinations. Medical school consists of 5 years of training; the first 2 years focus on the basic sciences, and the last 3 years include clinical rotations. All graduates must complete a 1-year internship with at least two 6-month rotations in internal medicine, pediatrics, surgery, or obstetrics and gynecology. The majority of physicians then enter general practice. A small percentage of physicians pursue additional specialty training. At this time, surgery is the only specialty that offers a board examination and certification. Roughly one-third of Ugandan-trained physicians leave the country for greener pastures within 5 years of graduation. Many senior health professionals and faculty members have succumbed to war or HIV/AIDS.

Ugandan nurses, medical officers, and community volunteers play a major role in the delivery of primary care. Nurses are trained to provide general and surgical nursing care, midwifery skills, mental health counseling, and health education and management. Medical officers, who have completed 2 or more years of vocational training, provide primary care; some receive further training to perform special procedures such as cesarean sections or cataract surgeries. Community volunteers with appropriate training and supervision frequently provide valuable outreach and health education services.

The shortage of primary care physicians and other health professionals is of great concern to the MoH. University and MoH officials, practicing physicians, nurses, and representatives of nongovernmental organizations (NGOs) met in Kampala in June 2005 to assess the problem and develop recommendations.[39] It was agreed that in-country training is urgently needed and is the most cost-effective way to achieve a critical mass of health professionals in Uganda. Recruitment, training, and deployment of family physicians (also known as community practice physicians) were identified as key priorities for improving health services. It was resolved that there should be training and posting of family physicians at general hospitals and at each Health Center Level IV. The MoH set a goal of preparing at least 400 new Ugandan family physicians.

Makerere and Mbarara University faculties and staff are collaborating in efforts to develop a common core curriculum and to develop and expand a network of decentralized training programs through distance education. Senior house officers (postgraduate residents) will be able to learn as they deliver clinical services at selected community-based training sites; their learning will be enhanced through case discussions, self-directed study, and short visits to well-established training centers.

Ugandan faculties are actively collaborating with international colleagues to enhance their capacity, build linkages, and recruit resources to strengthen their departments. Family physicians and faculty from East and South Africa, Europe, the United States, and Canada are already involved in and assisting these efforts. The evolving East African Community, with its emphasis on regional cooperation, may provide additional incentives for Ugandan, Kenyan, and Tanzanian faculty and governments to harmonize efforts and share resources to educate, monitor, and support family physicians and other health professionals. Coordinated efforts among key stakeholders such as the MoH, NGOs, the private sector, and international donors are critical for strengthening the health system, training, recruitment, posting, and long-term maintenance.[27]

Vietnam

The Socialist Republic of Vietnam, a country with more than 80 million people and a distribution of 80% of the population in its rural areas, does better than many other developing countries in its region on some health indicators, but not all. The infant mortality rate of 18/1000, life expectancy at birth of 71 years, and under-five mortality rate of 24/1,000 are comparable with those in some of the more developed countries in the region, but the prevalence of malnutrition and preventable communicable disease is still quite high.[40] The leading causes of death have changed little over the last decade, with head injury and other injuries leading this category. Even though the total expenditure on health has been 5.3% of the GDP,[40] with public health expenditures being only 20% of this,[41] there has been a strong political commitment to provide health care to all in Vietnam.

In the 1950s this commitment to health care for all led to the development of a medical network of 10,000 commune health centers across the country. The MoH trained a cadre of health care workers for each of these health centers over the next two decades. Although there have been attempts since that time to introduce generalist physicians into these health centers, this has met with limited success. Many of the barriers experienced by other countries around the world to bringing physicians to rural areas exist in Vietnam as well. As a result, midwives, nurses, and assistant physicians have primarily staffed the commune health centers. One decade ago, only 15% of the commune health centers were staffed with physicians. Currently, 40% of the commune health centers, both urban and rural, have general doctors; however, these doctors do not have postgraduate medical education and are perceived as being poorly trained.[41]

There are eight institutions training physicians in Vietnam: two medical universities under the direction of the MoH, and six medical colleges under the direction of the Ministry of Education. Vietnam's current system of training physicians is based on the French system of medical education.[42] Candidates are eligible to enter 6 years of medical school directly after completion of high school. Medical training consists of classroom academics, with the basic sciences taught in the first 2 years, the medical sciences in the next 2 years, and then clinical rotations within the hospitals during the final 2 years. Very little time is spent in outpatient centers outside the hospital system. At the end of the undergraduate medical education, the physicians are called "general doctors." They all are immediately faced with compulsory service in outpatient services in urban areas or in village community care centers according to the needs outlined for the distribution of manpower by the provincial health directors.[43] Many graduates elect to decline the service and so become unemployed.

Following a minimum of 3 years of work in the community, physicians may then take a competitive examination specific to a desired specialty. Two to 6 years of postgraduate training is required for specialties such as internal medicine, pediatrics, obstetrics, and surgery. Until recently, there were no postgraduate or continuing medical education requirements for general practice physicians (Figure 7-6). Postgraduate specialty training begins with a 2-year program, at the end of which the graduate is classified as a first-degree specialist in that discipline. That physician may then practice in that discipline or continue with additional training to obtain the second-degree certification. Physicians may also pursue research and academic tracks within the disciplines by pursuing master's- and PhD-level training.

The health care delivery system in Vietnam is hierarchical (Figure 7-7). The expectation is that medical care will be entered at the commune health center level and that referrals will then be made to the next level of care. With the advent of the private sector, the expectations of patients regarding the quality of their medical care have increased and they are less likely to follow the traditional avenues of health care delivery. In a 1991 survey in Cu Chi Province, only 10% of the population sought services from the commune health centers, 15% to 20% sought services directly from the hospitals, 40% sought services in the private sector, and the rest sought services at the district health level. In the urban areas, a more affluent family can go to a private physician or to a hospital clinic, where there is a 90% chance of being seen by a physician.[44]

In 1996, a report entitled *Strategic Orientation for People's Health Care and Protection from Now to the Years 2000 and 2020* was published from the proceedings of the VIIIth Congress of the Communist Party of Vietnam. It noted the accomplishments in health workforce training, while recognizing that "the ratio of physician per population remain[ed] low."[45] It also recognized that there were "only a few physicians working in the communes." The report set out new goals for the health care delivery system. These included goals for the continued improvement of the health care indicators and policies by which these goals should be reached. In particular, these new policies included streamlining the organizational structure, developing a national health care network to provide quality health care to all, and improving training programs with criteria for new and annual retraining. Provisions were made for the development of training networks. The report spelled out that in the "training of community health doctors, [the] commune doctor should be [trained] different[ly] from . . . doctors who . . . work in hospitals. To do this a training environment should be created so that trainees will acquaint themselves with the environment that they will work in the future."[45]

This document also promotes increased investment in health-related activities. Since 1985, with the inception of the government policy of "Doi Moi" (change and newness), Vietnam has been moving toward a market-oriented socialized economy. This has allowed for the development of health care delivery on a private fee-for-service basis and the early advent of purchased health insurance products. The MoH believes that a planned public-private health care mix can maximize

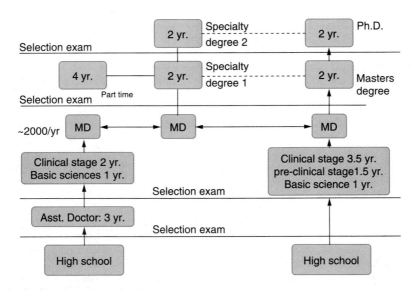

Figure 7-6. Medical education system in Vietnam.

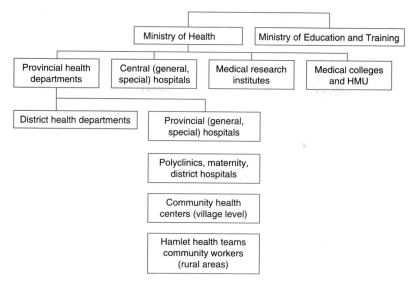

Figure 7-7. Health care delivery system, Vietnam.

access and efficiency to promote the rational growth of health care.[46]

The MoH of Vietnam, acknowledging the difficulties it was having meeting the people's needs for primary health care services, began to investigate alternative approaches to meet this need in 1995. As a result it commissioned a needs assessment to investigate the current status of the primary health care system and to make recommendations for change in the Vietnamese health care system.[47] The request highlighted the special interest by the ministry on focusing on primary health care delivery at the rural, community level.

The consultation spanned 4 years and included site visits to multiple areas of the country and discussions with many stakeholders. By the end of the needs assessment, it became clear that the MoH was seeking to develop a primary care physician with a patient-centered, family-focused, community-oriented model of training. The criteria for a primary care physician as described by the MoH included comprehensiveness and continuity of care. The stakeholders in the needs assessment from the medical faculties of Hanoi, Ho Chi Minh City, and Thai Nguyen, along with the consultants, recommended to the MoH that its objective should be "to create educational programs that will lead to a specialty that will be the cornerstone for the delivery of primary health care to the people of Vietnam." This report was accepted by the MoH in March 2001 and created the specialty of family medicine in Vietnam.

Since 2001, with support from international colleagues, four medical schools have initiated training of family physicians. Two models have evolved. The first is

the usual postgraduate training model, in which a physician, after having served in the community in a general practice, may take an entrance examination and then enter a 2-year program that, when completed, results in the awarding of a First Degree Specialist in Family Medicine. The second model is a part-time model of education. This was developed to engage the current rural general practice workforce in enhancing their knowledge and skills. In this model, the commune health center or district health center physician enters the program after successful completion of the entrance examination. Learning is divided into 3-month blocks, between which the physician returns to his or her practice for 1 to 2 months. In 3 years' time, the successful graduate of this training model is also awarded the First Degree Specialist in Family Medicine. Since the inception of training, there have been 69 graduates from four programs.

To date, the training is being done by specialty physicians who have been trained from 1 month to 1 year in faculty development fellowships in US family medicine residencies and who have received ongoing support through Training of Trainer workshops by US consultants. Through outside support, a Family Medicine Faculty Development Center at the Hanoi Medical University has been created to produce master's-and PhD-level family medicine faculty.

Finally, the MoH has recently adopted new policies that include the mandatory creation of Departments of Family Medicine in all medical schools and the requirement that by 2020 commune health center physicians must be specialty trained.

United States

The United States, a country of 294 million people, spends a greater share of its GDP on health than any other nation. In 2003 this figure rose to $1.7 trillion, a 7.7% increase from the previous year and 15% of the GDP.[48] Despite the amount of money spent, the United States ranks far from number one for health outcomes as compared with countries that spend from 7% to 8% of their GDP on health, such as Sweden, Spain, Portugal, and the United Kingdom.[35] In fact, with the exception of the average length of life left for those who have already attained 80 years of age, the United States ranks last or near last on most rankings of the major health indicators for industrialized nations.[49]

In spite of this significant health care expenditure, increasing numbers of Americans are without health insurance or adequate access to care. The United States is the only industrialized nation lacking a government program to ensure financial access to health care services for all. The patchwork of both public- and private-sector safety nets still leaves 45.5 million adults between 18 and 65 years old (or 18.5%) without health insurance and many more with only sporadic coverage.[50]

As noted in the introduction to this chapter, it is important to distinguish between a primary health care system and "primary care"—or the place of first contact for health. The United States ranks poorly in the strength of its primary care orientation; there is currently no overarching system of physicians, nurse practitioners, and physician assistants who serve as the point of first contact for all patients in the United States.[16]

The medical system in the United States is rooted in specialization. In fact, the term *primary care* was not a part of the medical lexicon in this country until the mid-1960s. The American Board of Medical Specialties (ABMS) currently recognizes more than 70 specialties and subspecialties. The first of these, ophthalmology, was established in 1908, while the boards of pediatrics and general internal medicine were established in 1935 and 1936, respectively. The American Board of Family Practice, not established until 1969, preceded only five other currently recognized specialty boards: thoracic surgery (1970), nuclear medicine (1971), allergy and immunology (1971), emergency medicine (1979), and medical genetics (1991).

The medical specialties presumed to provide first-contact care in the United States are known as generalists. The type of physicians who fall into this category is somewhat controversial—some statistical sources include "general obstetric/gynecology" under this rubric. For the purposes of this chapter, this specialty is not included as primary care and has been excluded from the following statistical citations. According to the Bureau of Health Professions, approximately 32% of all practicing physicians in the United States in 2003 were "generalists." Of these, 12% were in family or general practice, 14% in general internal medicine, and 5% were pediatric providers.[48] Although there were more "generalists" (i.e., physicians without residency training) practicing in this country prior to 1950, the current percentages have remained stable for the past 30 years.

By contrast, specialist providers represent more than 60% of the physician workforce, and their numbers continue to increase in spite of government efforts to encourage medical graduates to enter primary care. According to the *Dartmouth Atlas of Health Care*, there were 65 primary care providers and 121.7 specialists per 100,000 residents in 1996. The distribution of primary care physicians varies regionally, however, with a range from 33.8 per 100,000 residents in McAllen, Texas, to 105.1 per 100,000 in White Plains, New York (Figure 7-8).[51]

As is evident from the distribution of both primary care and specialist physicians, access to primary care depends, in part, on its geographic availability. In an effort to address the needs of medically underserved areas, the federal government created the Community Health Center (CHC) program in 1965. These not-for-profit health centers provide care in federally designated medically underserved areas and/or underserved population groups. Federally qualified health centers (FQHCs) can be CHCs, health care for the homeless, school-based health programs, migrant health centers, and health care for public housing. There are currently over 3,000 FQHC clinics in the United States. Although they form a partial safety net, these centers serve only 25% of people living below the poverty line and only an eighth of all uninsured Americans.[52]

In addition to geography, another factor determining access to health services is insurance status. Note that the United States has a "peculiar welfare system that is neither wholly private nor public."[53] The majority of Americans (61%) under age 65 get their health insurance through employer-provided programs. Joint federal and state programs for the poor (Medicaid, State Children's Health Insurance Plans, Medicare, and military programs) provide insurance for another 16%, and 5% pay for private insurance, leaving 18% of the population without any insurance coverage.[50]

Although tax incentives encourage employer participation, providing employee health insurance is not mandated by law. As many as 41% of smaller businesses did not offer health insurance as a benefit in 2004. Of all the people who receive health insurance through employer-linked programs, about half are themselves employed, while the other half benefit as an employee's dependent.

Medicare and Medicaid are federal-and state-sponsored programs created during President Lyndon Johnson's tenure. He signed Title XIX of the Social Security Act of 1965, the law creating both of these programs, in July 1965. Medicaid is a federal-state matching program, in which both the federal and state governments must contribute a specified percentage of total expenditures. Today, Medicaid provides insurance to 13% of the non-elderly population—a larger proportion than any other single insurer.

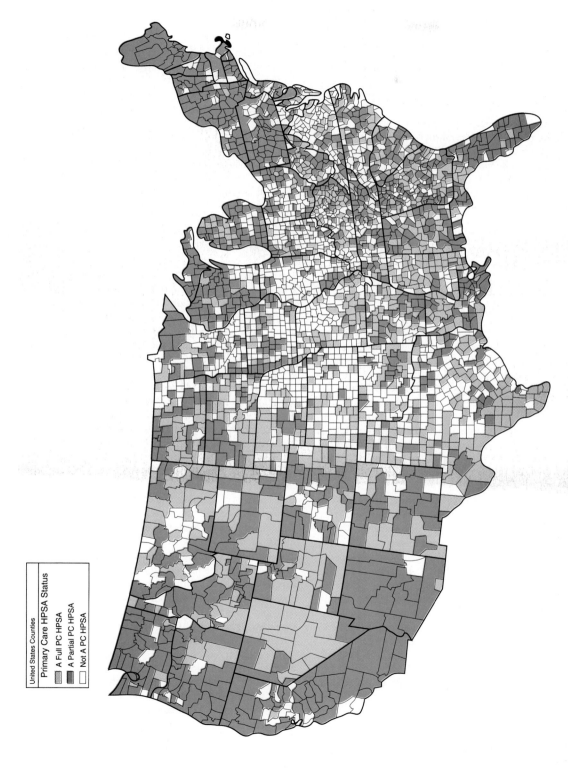

United States Counties

Primary Care HPSA Status

- A Full PC HPSA
- A Partial PC HPSA
- Not A PC HPSA

Figure 7-8. Primary care physician distribution in the United States; PC HPSA designates a primary care health personnel shortage area.[51]

As reflected in the ratios of specialist to generalist physicians noted previously, the distribution of health providers in the United States is out of balance. Taken together, the data in several recent population-based investigations of health outcomes and quality indicators in US counties suggest that optimal health outcomes occur when 40% to 50% of the physician workforce is made up of family physicians, general internists, and general pediatricians.[54] Since, as previously noted, only 32% of the physician workforce are currently primary care physicians, there is a need for more generalists. The remedy for this imbalance, however, will not soon be fulfilled. The number of medical students choosing to enter general pediatrics, general internal medicine, or family medicine has been declining since its peak in 1998. Currently, fewer than 40% of graduates from US medical schools expect to enter generalist practice. In the Match, or residency program selection process, of 2007, the proportions of positions filled by US graduates were 73% for pediatrics, 56% for internal medicine, and 42% for family medicine.[55]

COMPARING CASES: POLITICAL WILL AND PRIMARY CARE

We have defined primary health care as an integrated system based in the community that provides first-contact, continuous, comprehensive, and coordinated care. The four country cases illustrate a variety of primary care systems in practice and provide examples of the spectrum of governmental commitment to ensuring adequate primary health care for their populations. The four countries represent two each from the developed (Australia and the United States) and developing (Uganda and Vietnam) worlds. They represent some extremes—for example, the US per capita spending on health care or Uganda's HIV/AIDS disease burden. Though they do so on widely different scales and with huge variation in available resources, all four countries confront challenges of developing adequate workforce to support the primary care needs of their populations.

There is a striking difference in each country's commitment to providing health for all. In some cases, the desire to provide such care is explicit. Recall Vietnam's government report declaring its commitment to "developing a national health care network to provide quality health care to all" or Uganda's explicit commitment to supervise public health services "to ensure that all the people of Uganda attain a good standard of health." More indirectly, we can discern a commitment to primary health care for all in Australia by the existence of a national universal health insurance scheme, and a contrasting lack of governmental commitment to such access in the United States, where 18.5% of adults under 65 are without any health insurance.[56]

This lack of health insurance has consequences for access to primary care. In an article comparing primary care in five developed countries, Schoen and her colleagues noted the outlying characteristics of the United States, where about one in ten adults had no usual person or place where they sought first contact care and nearly one in five could not report a usual doctor.[57] This contrasts with Australia, another of the countries included in the study, where 88% of adults identified a particular doctor as their usual source of care. Of note, adults with lower incomes in all five countries were particularly affected by cost of care; this was especially striking in the United States, where 57% of respondents who were below the median income reported either not seeing a doctor when sick, not getting recommended tests or follow-up care, or not getting prescription medications because of costs in the past year. By comparison, 35% of Australians with below-median incomes did not seek such care. The best-scoring country for this was the United Kingdom, where only 12% of adult respondents with below-median income did not seek needed care.

As noted previously, Dr. Barbara Starfield has developed a method of ranking countries on primary health care.[13] Based on average scores on 11 essential features of primary care, she has ranked countries in the developed world on a scale from 0 to 12 (Figure 7-9). Using this ranking, we can see that the United States is worst in primary care rank and also worst in the average of health care outcomes. Australia fares somewhat better in both categories.

Starfield also ranks these countries for their primary health care score as compared with their per capita health expenditures. This comparison illustrates the high-expenditure yet inferior-primary-care score of the United States compared with Australia (Figure 7-10).

Such primary health care rankings are not available for Uganda and Vietnam. However, by comparing health outcomes and expenditures for the four countries (Tables 7-5 and 7-6), we can compare and contrast several salient issues. Each of the four countries makes a disparate financial commitment to health. Note that although the United States spends about 15% of its GDP on health, more than half of that expenditure is from private sources. Compare this with Australia, where the national universal health insurance system funds 70% of health care costs. Vietnam and Uganda have much more limited resources, each spending about $6 per capita on health, with comparable expenditures as represented by percentage of GDP. In spite of the low expenditure, Vietnam does relatively well on health outcomes, with a life expectancy at birth of 71 years and a low under-five mortality rate compared with Uganda.

It is perhaps most striking to see the difference in political will of countries such as Uganda and Vietnam, where systems are deliberately designed to provide primary health care to the entire population, in comparison with the United States, where the need for a delivery system that ensures a source of good primary care and minimizes inappropriate services remains controversial.[58]

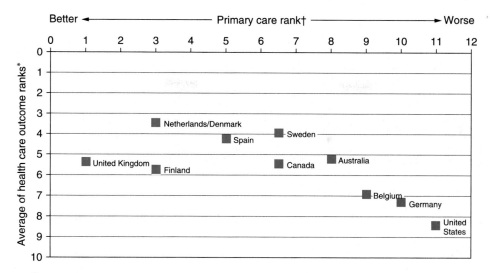

*The average health care outcome rank is an average of ranks for the following outcome measures: patient satisfaction, expenditures per person, 14 health indicators, and medications per person.

†Primary care rank is a rank of primary scores. The primary score is derived form the average of scores on 11 features of primary care. (See Starfield B. Primary care: concept, evaluation, and policy. New York: Oxford University Press, 1992)

Figure 7-9. Primary care rank versus average of health care outcome ranks. From Starfield B. Is primary care essential? *Lancet* 1994;344:1129–1133. (Adapted with permission.)

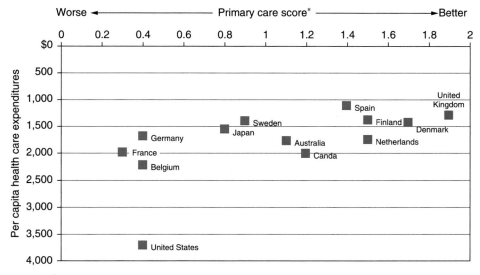

*The primary score is derived form the average scores on 11 features of primary care. (See Starfield B. Primary car: concept, evaluation, and policy. New York: Oxford University Press, 1992).

Figure 7-10. Per capita health care expenditures versus primary care score. From Starfield B. Policy relevant determinants of health: an international perspective. *Health Policy* 2002;60:201–221. (Adapted with permission.)

Table 7-5. Health outcomes.

	Life expectancy at birth (y)	Under-five mortality ratio (per 1,000)	Children receiving measles vaccine by age 2 (%)	Births attended by skilled personnel (%)
Australia	81	5	93	100
Uganda	49	138	82	39
United States	78	8	93	99
Vietnam	71	23	83	85

Adapted from World Health Organization, *The World Health Report 2005: Make Every Mother and Child Count* and *The World Health Report 2006: Working Together For Health*. Geneva: World Health Organization, 2005, 2006.

CONCLUSIONS

This chapter tries to answer the questions posed at the outset, which health care policy makers are asking. It looked at four countries and how their health care policies are evolving and how they affect the health of their people. The goal is common: improved health. The approaches found around the globe to achieve this goal through the structuring of health care delivery systems are dissimilar.

The evidence from the industrialized countries is clear: where primary care is the fundamental basis for access to health care systems, the costs are less and the outcomes better. The evidence is yet to be determined in the developing world. To date, however, there is no correlation between government spending on health care and the health of the population. Will the outcomes from the developing world be any different?

In the Declaration of Alma-Ata, primary health care is defined by seven principles. These can be summarized by stating that a solid system of primary health care "reflects and evolves from the economic conditions and sociocultural and political characteristics of the country and its communities"; "addresses the main health problems in the community, providing promotive, preventive, curative and rehabilitative services"; and "relies, at local and referral levels, on health workers, including physicians, nurses, midwives, auxiliaries, . . . community health workers, [and] traditional practitioners."[59] The four countries used in this chapter's case studies have followed these principles, with different outcomes.

Perhaps the soundest principle is that we know that "health for all" can be achieved by providing health care access that is first-contact, continuous, comprehensive, and coordinated and provided to populations undifferentiated by gender, disease, or organ system—that is, through primary care.

STUDY QUESTIONS

1. Define primary heath care and describe the various components and health personnel requirements.

2. Compare the primary care systems of Australia and the United States and relate their systems to health outcomes.

3. How can countries use limited resources to most efficiently improve the health of their populations?

Table 7-6. Health expenditure.

Year 2003	Total expenditure on health as % of GDP	Gov't expenditure on health as % of total health expenditure	Private expenditure on health as % of total health expenditure	Gov't expenditure on health as % of total gov't spending	Per capita gov't expenditure on health at average exchange rate (US$)	Out-of-pocket expenditure as % of private expenditure on health
Australia	9.5	67.5	32.5	17.7	1,699	67.8
Uganda	7.3	30.4	69.6	10.7	5	52.8
United States	15.2	44.6	55.5	18.5	2,548	24.3
Vietnam	5.4	27.8	72.2	5.6	7	74.2

GDP, gross domestic product; gov't, government.
Adapted from World Health Organization, *The World Health Report 2005: Make Every Mother and Child Count* and *The World Health Report 2006: Working Together For Health*. Geneva: World Health Organization, 2005, 2006.

REFERENCES

1. Answers.com. Physician. http://www.answers.com/topic/physician.

2. NI, M. *The Yellow Emperor's Classic of Medicine*, Boston: Shambala Publications, Inc., 1995.

3. U.S. National Library of Medicine, History of Medicine Division. Greek medicine: Hippocrates and the rise of rational medicine. September 2002. http://www.nlm.nih.gov/hmd/greek/ greek_rationality.html.

4. University of Virginia Health System. Vesalius the humanist. June 2004. http://www.healthsystem.virginia.edu/internet/library/historical/artifacts/antiqua/vesalius.cfm.

5. Weber S. Soviet health delivery. *Health Social Work* 1977;2(1):8–25.

6. University of Nebraska Medical Center, World of Rural Medical Education. Osler and rural practice. http://www.unmc.edu/Community/ruralmeded/osler.htm.

7. Crowther MA. The invisible general practitioner: the careers of Scottish medical students in the late nineteenth century. *Bull History Med* 1996;70(3):387–413.

8. Flexner A. *Medical Education in the United States and Canada.* New York: Carnegie Foundation for the Advancement of Teaching, 1910.

9. University of Nebraska Medical Center, World of Rural Medical Education. Flexner's impact on American medicine. http://www.unmc.edu/Community/ruralmeded/flexner.htm.

10. Wang S. Chinas health system: from crisis to opportunity. *Yale-China Health J* 2004;3:5–50. http://www.yalechina.org/publications/healthjournal/davis.pdf.

11. Starfield B. Is primary care essential? *Lancet* 1994;344:1129–1133.

12. World Health Organization. *Primary Health Care.* Geneva: World Health Organization, 1978:25.

13. Starfield B. *Primary Care: Balancing Health Needs, Services, and Technology.* New York: Oxford University Press, 1998.

14. Starfield B, Shi L, Grover A, Machinko J. The effects of specialist supply on populations' health: assessing the evidence. *Health Affairs* Web Exclusive, March 15, 2005.

15. United Nations Statistics Division. Millennium Development Goals indicators. http://millenniumindicators.un.org/unsd/mi/mi_series_results.asp?rowId=561.

16. Starfield B, Shi L. Policy relevant determinants of health: an international perspective. *Health Policy* 2002;60:201–218.

17. Shi L, Macinko J, Starfield B, et al. The relationship between primary care, income inequality, and mortality in US states, 1980–1995. *J Am Board Fam Pract* 2003;16(5):412–422.

18. Shi L, Macinko J, Starfield B, et al. Primary care, infant mortality, and low birth weight in the states of the USA. *J Epidemiol Community Health* 2004;58(5):374–380.

19. Ferrante JM, Gonzalez EC, Pal N, Roetzheim RG. Effects of physician supply on early detection of breast cancer. *J Am Board Fam Pract* 2000;13(6):408–414.

20. Roetzheim RG, Pal N, Van Durme DJ, et al. Increasing supplies of dermatologists and family physicians are associated with earlier stage of melanoma detection. *J Am Acad Dermatol* 2000;43(2 pt 1):211–218.

21. Roetzheim RG, Pal N, Gonzalez EC, et al. The effects of physician supply on the early detection of colorectal cancer. *J Fam Pract* 1999;48(11):850–858.

22. Campbell RJ, Ramirez AM, Perez K, Roetzheim RG. Cervical cancer rates and the supply of primary care physicians in Florida. *Fam Med* 2003;35(1):60–64.

23. Shi L, Macinko J, Starfield B, Xu J, Politzer R. Primary care, income inequality, and stroke mortality in the United States. A longitudinal analysis, 1985–1995. *Stroke* 2003;34(8):1958–1964.

24. Franks P, Fiscella K. Primary care physicians and specialists as personal physicians. Health care expenditures and mortality experience. *J Fam Pract* 1998;47(2):105–109.

25. Simms C, Rowson M. Reassessment of health effects of the Indonesian economic crisis: donors versus the data. *Lancet* 2003;361(9366):1382–1385.

26. World Health Organization. *The World Health Report 2006: Working Together for Health.* Geneva: World Health Organization, 2006.

27. Boelen C, Haq C, Hunt V, Rivo M, Shahady E. *Improving Health Systems: The Contribution of Family Medicine—A Guidebook.* Singapore: Wonca (World Academy of Family Doctors), Bestprint Publications, 2002.

28. Kark SL. *The Practice of Community-Oriented Primary Care.* New York: Appleton-Century-Crofts, 1981.

29. Pritchard P. *Manual of Primary Health Care: Its Nature and Organization.* 2nd ed. Oxford, UK: Oxford Medical Publications, 1981.

30. International Conference on Health Promotion. Ottawa charter for health promotion. November 1986. http://www.who.int/hpr/NPH/docs/ottawa_charter_hp.pdf.

31. *General Practice in Australia: 2004.* Canberra: Commonwealth of Australia, Department of Health and Ageing, 2005.

32. Britt H, Miller G, Knox S, et al. *General Practice Activity in Australia 2003–2004.* Canberra: AIHW, 2004. AIHW Cat. No. GEP16.

33. General Practice Strategy Review Group. *Report of the General Practice Strategy Review Group.* Canberra: Commonwealth of Australia, Department of Health and Ageing, 1998. http://www.health.gov.au/hsdd/gp/gpsrgrpt.htm.

34. Humphreys JS, Jones MP, Jones JA, Mara P. Workforce retention in rural and remote Australia: determining the factors that influence length of practice. *MJA* 2002;176:472–476.

35. World Health Organization. *The World Health Report 2005: Make Every Mother and Child Count.* Geneva: World Health Organization, 2005.

36. Ministry of Health, Republic of Uganda. *Annual Health Sector Performance Report.* October 2003.

37. Ministry of Health, Republic of Uganda. *Health Sector Strategic Plan II.* March 2005.

38. Ministry of Health, Republic of Uganda. *Human Resource Inventory, Government of Uganda Payroll.* November 2003.

39. Proceedings of the National Dialogue on the Future of Family Medicine in Uganda, June 8, 2005. Unpublished manuscript, Makerere University. Available from Ms. Evelyn Bakengesa, Dean's office (ebakengesa@med.mak.ac.ug)

40. World Health Organization. *World Health Report 2005 Statistical Annex: Annexes by Country (P–Z).* Geneva: World Health Organization, 2005. http://www.who.int/whr/2005/annex/indicators_country_p-z.pdf.

41. Trong Le Ngoc, Professor, Vice Minister of Health, Socialist Republic of Vietnam. Personal interview, March 2000.

42. Singer I. The medical education project in Vietnam. *JAMA* 1975;234(13):1405–1406.

43. Project of Vietnam–Netherland. Strengthening in teaching epidemiology and primary healthcare in 8 medical faculties in Vietnam: survey to evaluate the knowledge, attitude and skills of medical curriculum in 8 medical faculties, 2000–2001. Draft version.

44. Gellert GA. The influence of market economics on primary health care in Vietnam. *JAMA* 1995;273(19):1498–1502.

45. Socialist Republic of Vietnam Ministry of Health. *Strategic Orientation for People's Health Care and Protection in the Period of 1996–2000 and Vietnam's National Drug Policy.* Hanoi: Socialist Republic of Vietnam Ministry of Health, 1996.

46. Dung PH. The political process and the private health sector's role in Vietnam. *Int J Health Plann Manage* 1996;11:217–230.

47. Montegut A, Cartwright C, Schirmer J, Cummings S. An international consultation: the development of family medicine in Vietnam. *Fam Med* 2004;35(5):352–356.

48. National Center for Health Statistics. *Health, United States, 2005: With Chartbook on Trends in the Health of Americans.* Hyattsville, MD: National Center for Health Statistics,2005.

49. Starfield B. The importance of primary care to health. *Medical Reporter* June 1999. http://medicalreporter.health.org/tmr0699/importance_of_primary_care_to_he.htm.

50. Kaiser Commission on Medicaid and the Uninsured. *The Uninsured: A Primer. Key Facts About Americans Without Health Insurance.* Washington, DC: Kaiser Family Foundation, 2006. http://www.kff.org/uninsured/7451.cfm.

51. *The Dartmouth Atlas of Health Care* [online]. 1998. http://www.dartmouthatlas.org.

52. Starfield B, Shi L, Macinko J. Contributions of primary care to health systems and health. *Milbank Q* 2005;83(3):457–502.

53. Gottschalk M. *The Shadow Welfare State: Labor, Business, and the Politics of Health Care in the United States.* Ithaca, NY: Cornell University Press, 2000.

54. Association of Departments of Family Medicine. News. *Ann Family Med* 2005;3:468–469.

55. Results and Data 2007 Main Residency Match. NRMP, AAMC, Washington, DC, 2007. nrmp@aamc.org.

56. Phillips RL Jr, Starfield B. Why does a U.S. primary care physician workforce crisis matter? *Am Family Physician* 2004;70(3):440, 442, 443–446.

57. Schoen C, et al. Primary care and health system performance: adults' experience in five countries. *Health Affairs* 2004;October 28. http://content.healthaffairs.org/cgi/content/full/htlhaff.w4.487/DC1.

58. Starfield B. Insurance and the U.S. health care system. *N Engl J Med* 2005;353(4):418–419.

59. World Health Organization. *Primary Health Care. Report of the International Conference of Primary Health Care, Alma-Ata, USSR, 6-12 September 1978.* Geneva: World Health Organization, 1978. Health for All Series, no. 1.

Tuberculosis and HIV/AIDS

8

Lisa V. Adams and Godfrey Woelk

LEARNING OBJECTIVES

- *Describe the global epidemiology of tuberculosis*
- *Understand how tuberculosis is transmitted, diagnosed, and treated*
- *List the components of the DOTS strategy and describe some of the current controversies*
- *Discuss the current challenges to controlling tuberculosis in resource-limited settings, and developments expected in the future*
- *List criteria to guide selection of a successful tuberculosis control project*
- *Describe the history, pathogenesis, diagnosis, and transmission of HIV/AIDS*
- *Describe the treatment of HIV/AIDS, including the prevention and management of opportunistic infections*
- *Outline the policy and operational issues on treatment rollout, with particular reference to low- and middle-income countries*
- *Discuss HIV/AIDS prevention strategies and their potential effectiveness and limitations at different stages of the epidemic*
- *Know where to find additional resources for both tuberculosis and HIV/AIDS*

INTRODUCTION

Tuberculosis (TB) and human immunodeficiency virus/ acquired immunodeficiency syndrome (HIV/AIDS)—one a scourge nearly as old as humankind itself and the other a disease that emerged only two decades ago—are responsible for a significant burden of today's global morbidity and mortality. When occurring separately, each is a challenge to cure or treat, but when occurring together they constitute a deadly pair. In many parts of the world, especially in many resource-poor settings, they are inextricably linked. In sub-Saharan Africa, for example, where the co-epidemics have converged to require a joint programmatic response, most patients consider a diagnosis of one to indicate a simultaneous or eventual diagnosis of the other. Because of the large overlap that exists between both epidemics in the poorest parts of the globe, these diseases have been grouped in a single chapter. Tuberculosis and HIV/AIDS will be considered first separately and then together in this chapter.

Global Epidemiology of Tuberculosis

Tuberculosis is ubiquitous. Approximately one-third of the world's population—2 billion people—is infected with *Mycobacterium tuberculosis* (MTB). Under ordinary circumstances, about 10% of people infected with MTB will develop active TB disease during their lifetime. The World Health Organization (WHO) estimates there were 8.8 million new cases of TB in 2005 (7.4 million in Asia and sub-Saharan Africa), with roughly 60% of these cases being reported to public health programs and the WHO.[1] In the same year there were an estimated 1.6 million deaths due to TB; making it the leading cause of death from a curable infectious disease.[2]

The vast majority of TB patients—nearly 80%—live in just 22 countries in the world. The list of 22 high-TB-burden countries is dominated by the resource-poor countries of sub-Saharan Africa and Asia (Table 8-1). The global incidence rate of TB peaked in 2005; the total number of new TB cases has continued to grow due to increasing case-loads in the African, Eastern Mediterranean and South-East Asia regions. (Figure 8-1).[1] With approximately 75% of TB cases in resource-poor countries occurring among those in their most economically productive years (between the ages of 15 and 54), the human and economic toll on these countries has been devastating.

The persistence of TB through the years is multifactorial, with key factors being neglect by governments, poorly managed TB control programs in the past,

Table 8-1. Countries with a high burden of tuberculosis.

1. India
2. China
3. Indonesia
4. Nigeria
5. Bangladesh
6. Pakistan
7. South Africa
8. Ethiopia
9. Philippines
10. Kenya
11. Democratic Republic of Congo
12. Russian Federation
13. Vietnam
14. United Republic of Tanzania
15. Brazil
16. Uganda
17. Thailand
18. Mozambique
19. Myanmar
20. Zimbabwe
21. Cambodia
22. Afghanistan

From World Health Organization. *Global Tuberculosis Control: Surveillance, Planning, Financing.* Geneva, World Health Organization, 2007. WHO/HTM/TB/2007.376. (Reproduced with permission.)

poverty, population growth, and migration. More recently, the HIV epidemic has contributed to the rising number of TB cases in sub-Saharan Africa. HIV is a significant risk factor that increases the likelihood of progression from TB infection to disease from 10% over a lifetime to 10% each year. Tuberculosis has become the leading cause of death among HIV-infected individuals, accounting for about one-third of AIDS deaths worldwide. In some of the worst-affected countries in sub-Saharan Africa, up to 70% of patients with acid-fast bacilli (AFB) smear-positive pulmonary TB are also infected with HIV.[1]

The emergence of significant levels of multidrug-resistant TB in some parts of the world has also hampered global efforts to control TB. Strains of TB that are resistant to standard (first-line) anti-TB medications have been documented in every country; however, certain countries of eastern Europe harbor the greatest burden of drug-resistant TB. Confirming our worst fears, the emergence of TB strains resistant to virtually all anti-TB drugs (now termed *extensively drug-resistant TB or XDR-TB*) has been reported in several countries.[3]

Global Epidemiology of HIV/AIDS

The global epidemiology of HIV infection is not so different from that of tuberculosis. Recurring themes include the heavy case burden borne by sub-Saharan Africa

and the relationships between HIV infection and poverty, prior lack of access to effective prevention strategies and treatments, and the fact that HIV is also killing those in their most productive years, in many cases wiping out generations in the hardest-hit countries.

It was estimated that just over 40 million people were living with HIV infection in 2005, the highest number ever estimated. AIDS resulted in the deaths of just over 3 million people worldwide in 2005, and an additional 5 million people were newly infected in the same year.[4] Sub-Saharan Africa remains the worst-affected area, with approximately 26 million HIV-infected inhabitants, roughly two-thirds of the total global burden.[4] However, the numbers of people infected with HIV in eastern Europe and Central and East Asia have also grown in the past few years. The proportion of HIV-infected adults who are women continues to increase, reaching 46% globally and 57% in sub-Saharan Africa; the latter is home to 77% of all women with HIV infection.[4]

Heterosexual sex has become the primary means of HIV transmission worldwide, although in some regions injection drug use (often combined with an exchange of sex for drugs) is still a major route of transmission. Efforts to control HIV/AIDS were originally focused on preventing new infections, but in the past decade have included the scale-up of care and treatment programs to provide life-prolonging antiretroviral therapy.

TUBERCULOSIS

Pathogenesis of Tuberculosis

Tuberculosis is caused by the bacterium *Mycobacterium tuberculosis. M. bovis, M. microti, M. africanum,* and *M. canettii* are very similar genetically to MTB, and together they comprise the MTB complex.[5] Although any of the MTB complex organisms may cause tuberculosis, MTB is the most common, especially in the tropics. MTB is an obligate aerobic, non-spore-forming, nonmotile bacillus with a large lipid content in its cell wall. MTB grows slowly, with a generation time of approximately 15 to 20 hours as compared with less than 1 hour for most common bacteria. MTB bacilli are referred to as *acid-fast bacilli* (AFB) because of the ability of their lipid-rich cell walls to retain red carbol-fuchsin stain even after de-colorization with acid and alcohol during the Ziehl-Neelsen staining procedure.

MTB is transmitted when a person with active tuberculosis coughs, sneezes, or talks and expels MTB bacilli into the air. These respiratory secretions contain droplet nuclei that become aerosolized and can linger in a contained airspace for up to 8 hours. Droplet nuclei are tiny, generally only 5 to 10 μm in diameter, which allows them to be transported to the terminal air spaces when inhaled. Once in the terminal air sacs, the MTB bacilli are taken up by alveolar macrophages. Through

Estimated TB incidence rate, 2005

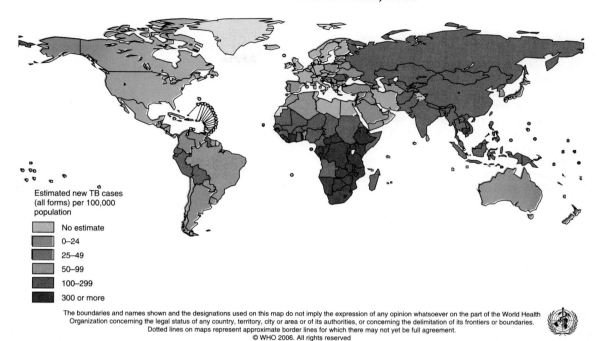

Estimated new TB cases
(all forms) per 100,000
population

- No estimate
- 0–24
- 25–49
- 50–99
- 100–299
- 300 or more

Figure 8-1. Distribution of tuberculosis in the world in 2005. From World Health Organization. Global Tuberculosis Control: Surveillance, Planning, Financing. Geneva, World Health Organization, 2007. WHO/HTM/TB/2007.376. (Reproduced with permission.)

hematogenous or lymphatic spread or by direct extension, MTB bacteria may spread to virtually any organ in the body. In most cases, the bacteria are "walled off" by macrophages and other cells that contain the infection through granuloma formation. In some cases, particularly in children, initial infection with MTB can result in primary disease that has the hallmarks of hilar or mediastinal lymphadenopathy with or without a visible opacity, the "primary lesion," in the lung. If successfully contained, the MTB will continue to grow very slowly over the person's lifetime. This scenario is latent TB infection. Left untreated, MTB will stay dormant and never cause active disease in 90% of people who are otherwise healthy. If a person is HIV infected, this risk of developing active TB increases from a 10% *lifetime* risk to a 10% *annual* risk.

If the person's immune system is not able to contain the MTB infection, the bacteria will begin to multiply more rapidly and the person will develop active tuberculosis. In addition to HIV infection, poor nutrition, diabetes mellitus, chronic renal failure, and certain medications (e.g., steroids) can result in varying degrees of immunosuppression that will increase the likelihood of progression from latent TB infection to active TB disease. Pulmonary tuberculosis is the most common form of the disease, accounting for over 80% of cases (in populations without large

numbers of HIV-infected individuals). Extrapulmonary tuberculosis can affect any organ other than the lungs, but most commonly affected are the pleura, lymph nodes, spine, genitourinary tract, nervous system, or abdomen. Extrapulmonary tuberculosis is more common in HIV-infected individuals and young children.

The classic symptoms of active pulmonary tuberculosis are a cough that persists for more than 2 weeks with sputum production and occasional hemoptysis, weight loss, and fevers with night sweats. Chest pain and fatigue are also commonly seen. Fever and weight loss are more common in tuberculosis patients who are also HIV-infected. On physical exam, weight loss and tachycardia (due to the fever) may be noted. Respiratory signs are variable and may include crackles, wheezes, or bronchial breathing; alternatively, breath sounds may be completely normal.

Diagnosis of Tuberculosis

Any person presenting to a health care facility with a cough for 2 or more weeks in a TB-endemic country should be considered a "TB suspect" and appropriately evaluated. The patient should submit three sputum samples for smear microscopy (and mycobacterial culture where available). Under ideal conditions (and in areas without a high HIV prevalence), sputum smear microscopy using Ziehl-Neelsen staining will identify approximately 65% of adult pulmonary tuberculosis cases.[6] Identification of these cases is a high priority because these are the cases that are infectious and therefore responsible for the majority of instances of transmission of tuberculosis. Immunofluorescence using fluorochrome stain is a newer microscopy technique that is becoming available in the major cities of some resource-poor countries. MTB can be identified more quickly using this method because smears can be scanned under a lower magnification. Results of smear microscopy, regardless of the stain used, are recorded based on the number of TB bacilli observed on the slide, which reflects the severity of the disease and the infectiousness of the patient.

Laboratory culture of MTB, considered the gold standard or definitive test for MTB disease, can require up to 8 to 12 weeks using standard culture technique (e.g., Lowenstein-Jensen media) for MTB growth to be detected. Liquid media using automated equipment such as the BACTEC system (Beckton Dickinson, Sparks, MD) can detect MTB growth as early as 2 to 3 weeks, but its expense has limited its availability in resource-poor settings. Because of the lag time to obtain results, mycobacterial culture is not helpful in making rapid individual diagnoses but can be useful in detecting paucibacillary disease in HIV-infected individuals. Although access to mycobacterial culture is increasing in TB-endemic countries, it is rarely available at laboratories other than those of academic centers or the country's national reference center(s).

Chest radiography is often used to aid in the diagnosis of pulmonary tuberculosis when none or only one of the sputum smears examined is positive for AFB or to evaluate concomitant lung pathology in a patient with extrapulmonary TB. Chest x-rays are more helpful in diagnosing tuberculosis in children, who, due to their paucibacillary disease and insufficient tussive force, usually have AFB-negative sputum smears. In adults, a chest x-ray may show one or more infiltrates, particularly in the upper lung lobes, with or without cavitation, fibrosis, or retraction. However, no radiographic findings are absolutely diagnostic of pulmonary TB, and even a normal chest x-ray cannot rule out the diagnosis. This is especially true in HIV-infected individuals, where the chest x-ray appearance is often atypical (e.g., normal) in those with severe immunocompromise. The tuberculin skin test (TST, also referred to as the *PPD test* because it is composed of purified protein derivative) is rarely used to diagnose TB in adults in resource-limited settings. The TST has both poor sensitivity and specificity for active TB disease (the TST has been shown to be negative in up to 25% of patients with culture-confirmed TB), and its interpretation is complicated in areas where HIV infection is prevalent (increasing the potential for false negative results) and where Bacille Calmette-Guérin (BCG) vaccine is used (increasing the potential for false positive results).

In the absence of typical laboratory and radiographic findings, a small portion of patients will be diagnosed on the basis of the treating physician's clinical judgment.

Extrapulmonary tuberculosis, representing approximately 20% of all TB cases, presents a greater diagnostic challenge. Without the benefit of the standard sputum smear test for AFB and because of the limited availability of mycobacterial culture, the initial diagnosis is often presumptive, based on clinical findings, and confirmed retrospectively by a positive response to antituberculosis treatment. Where available, diagnosis may also rely on the results of specialized diagnostic tools such as ultrasound, biopsy, or aspiration. If extrapulmonary tuberculosis is suspected or confirmed, the patient should also be evaluated for pulmonary tuberculosis. Children younger than 2 years are at risk for developing serious disseminated forms of tuberculosis, specifically miliary tuberculosis or tuberculous meningitis.

Treatment of Tuberculosis

Treatment of tuberculosis requires a multidrug regimen for at least 6 months. When taken without interruption, the standard regimen using first-line drugs will cure over 90% of patients with drug-susceptible tuberculosis. Tuberculosis treatment is divided into two phases: the 2-month initial phase, when rapid bacterial killing occurs, and the 4-month continuation phase, when further sterilizing activity occurs. The two most effective drugs against tuberculosis in our arsenal are isoniazid and rifampin. Both bactericidal agents, they are used throughout tuberculosis treatment. Pyrazinamide, also bactericidal, is only active in an acid environment and therefore only effective during the 2-month initial phase of therapy. A fourth agent, ethambutol, is added to the regimen to prevent the emergence of drug resistance should the primary strain have underlying resistance to any of the other three drugs used.

Treatment regimens based on patient characteristics have been standardized by the WHO (Table 8-2). Different regimens are used for patients suspected of having drug-resistant tuberculosis (see "The Problem of Drug Resistance," later in this chapter). In general, adults and children, regardless of their HIV status, are treated similarly. Whenever possible, fixed-dose combination tablets should be administered because their use will facilitate correct prescribing and patient adherence and simplify drug ordering and stock control. Anti-TB drugs can be obtained by countries at low or no cost from the Global Drug Facility, a program administered by the Stop TB Partnership in Geneva. A 6-month course of anti-TB therapy costs as little as US $11.

Monitoring patients on therapy to ensure a therapeutic response is achieved is crucial. Patients with sputum smears positive for AFB should have follow-up sputum smears examined after the initial phase of therapy and again toward and at the end of therapy.

Table 8-2. Tuberculosis treatment regimens.

TB diagnostic category	TB patients	TB Treatment regimens[i]	
		Initial phase	Continuation phase
I	New smear-positive patients; new smear-negative PTB with extensive parenchymal involvement; concomitant HIV disease or severe forms of extra-pulmonary TB[ii]	**Preferred** 2 HRZE[iii] **Optional** 2 (HRZE)[iv]$_3$ or 2 HRZE[iv]	**Preferred** 4 HR 4 (HR)$_3$ **Optional** 4 (HR)$_3$ or 6 HE[v]
II	Previously treated sputum smear-positive PTB: - Relapse; - treatment after default	**Preferred** 2 HRZES/1 HRZE[vi] **Optional** 2 (HRZES)$_3$/1 HRZE$_3$	**Preferred** 5 HRE[vi] **Optional** 5 (HRE)$_3$
	- treatment failure of Category I[vii] in settings with: - adequate program performance; - representative DRS data showing high rates of MDR TB and or capacity for DST of cases, and - availability of Category IV regimens	Specially designed standardized or individualized regimens are often needed for these patients.	
	in settings where - representative DRS data show low rates of MDR TB or individualized DST shows drug-susceptible disease or in settings of - poor program performance, - absence of representative DRS data, - insufficient resources to implement Category IV treatment	**Preferred** 2 HRZES/1 HRZE **Optional** 2 (HRZES),/1 HRZE$_3$	**Preferred** 5 HRE[vii] **Optional** 5 (HRE)$_3$
III	New smear-negative PTB (other than in category 1) and less severe forms of extra-pulmonary TB	**Preferred** 2 HRZE[viii] **Optional** 2 (HRZE)$_3$ or 2 HRZE	**Preferred** 4 HR 4 ((HR)$_3$ **Optional** 4 (HR)$_3$ or 6 HE
IV	Chronic (still sputum-positive after supervised re-treatment); proven or suspected MDR. TB cases[ix]	Specially designed standardized or individualized regimens	

[i] Numbers preceding regimens indicate length of treatment (months). Subscripts following regimens indicate frequency of administration (days per week). When no subscripts are given, the regimen is daily. Direct observation of drug intake is always required during the initial phase of treatment and strongly recommended when rifampicin is used in the continuation phase and required when treatment is given intermittently. FDCs are highly recommended for use in both the initial and continuation phases of treatment.

[ii] Severe forms of extrapulmonary TB are listed elsewhere.

[iii] Streptomycin may be used instead of ethambutol. In tuberculous meningitis ethambutol should be replaced by streptomycin.

[iv] Intermittent initial phase therapy is not recommended when the continuation phase of isoniazid and ethambutol is used.

[v] This regimen may be considered in situations where the preferred regimen cannot be applied as recommended. However, it is associated with a higher rate of treatment failure and relapse compared with the 4 HR continuation phase regimen. Intermittent initial phase treatment is not recommended when followed by the 6HE continuation phase regimen.

[vi] Daily treatment is preferred. However, thrice weekly treatment during the continuation phase or during both phases is an acceptable option.

[vii] Treatment failures may be at increased risk of MDR TB, particularly if rifampicin was used in the continuation phase (See Section 4.9). Drug susceptibility testing is recommended for these cases if available. Treatment failures with known or suspected MDR TB should be treated with a Category IV regimen.

[viii] Ethambutol in the initial phase may be omitted for patients with limited, non-cavitary, smear-negative pulmonary TB who are known to be HIV-negative, patients with less severe forms of extrapulmonary TB, and young children with primary TB.

[ix] Drug susceptibility testing is recommended for patients who are contacts of MDR TB patients.

H, isoniazid; R, rifampin; Z, pyrazinamide; E, ethambutol; S, streptomycin.

WHO CDS TB 2003.313 Treatment of tuberculosis: guidelines for national programmes, third edition Revision approved by STAG, June 2004.

Treatment decisions are made based on these results. Treatment of TB is complicated by its long duration and multidrug regimen. Therefore, monitoring of adherence is essential (see "The DOTS Strategy to Control Tuberculosis," later in this chapter). In addition, monitoring of adverse reactions should be performed at each medical visit; when toxicity is severe, adjustments to the regimen may need to be made. HIV-infected patients respond well to TB treatment, although regimens may need adjustments when patients are also receiving antiretroviral medications because of potential drug-drug interactions between rifampin and protease inhibitors and non-nucleoside reverse transcriptase inhibitors.

The Role of Bacille Calmette-Guérin Vaccine

The BCG vaccine, a live bacterial vaccine first used in 1921, is currently given to about 100 million children each year.[7] Determination of its efficacy in preventing various forms of TB has yielded variable and inconsistent results. In a meta-analysis of efficacy studies, BCG vaccine was found to have an overall 51% protective effect against all forms of TB, a 64% protective effect against TB meningitis, and a 78% protective effect against disseminated TB.[8] However, this analysis did not exclude studies with "mycobacteria-experienced" patients (i.e., patients who have or may have had prior mycobacterial infection). In mycobacteria-naïve patients (i.e., those without prior mycobacterial infection, such as newborns), BCG efficacy is much higher, at 80%.[9]

Currently, the WHO recommends BCG vaccination at birth in high-TB-burden countries. Furthermore, the WHO recommends BCG vaccination of neonates in high-HIV-prevalence areas given the high risk of developing TB and the low risk of serious adverse reactions in HIV-exposed neonates. There are no data to support BCG revaccination or booster inoculations.[7] Despite its effectiveness in protecting infants and young children from life-threatening forms of TB, high rates of BCG vaccination have not led to a decreased incidence of TB cases worldwide because of the vaccine's limited role in preventing infectious pulmonary TB among adults.[6]

Controlling Tuberculosis

The goals of tuberculosis control are to reduce morbidity and mortality from the disease until tuberculosis no longer poses a threat to the public's health. To achieve this, it is necessary to ensure the accurate and timely diagnosis and successful treatment of each patient with active tuberculosis disease, particularly those capable of transmitting the disease. This will prevent both further transmission to uninfected individuals and the emergence of drug-resistant tuberculosis strains.

THE DOTS STRATEGY TO CONTROL TUBERCULOSIS

Historically, attempts to treat TB were highly ineffective and could take several years. Some improvements in lessening the TB burden in industrialized countries were achieved through better nutrition, less crowded living conditions (which decreased the likelihood of close contact to and shared airspace with others with infectious TB), and the sanatoria movement (which removed infectious TB patients from the community); however, TB was still associated with a 50% mortality rate. In the 1950s, tuberculosis treatment was revolutionized by the development of new drugs that, given in combination, cured tuberculosis and eliminated the need for lengthy hospitalizations. However, despite the availability of effective treatment, tuberculosis remained a public health problem.

Years after the development of anti-TB drugs, it became apparent how difficult it is for patients to complete their full course of therapy. The practice of *directly observed therapy* (DOT), in which a trained individual watches patients take each dose of their medicines, was developed to address this problem. By ensuring regularity and completion of treatment, patients whose treatment is observed have been shown in some settings to have decreased mortality from tuberculosis compared with those whose treatment is not observed.[10] In addition, the discovery of the highly effective drug rifampin made it possible to cure the majority of TB cases in 6 to 9 months. The new rifampin-containing regimen became known as *short-course therapy*. These two dramatic breakthroughs in TB treatment formed the basis of the DOTS approach: directly observed therapy, short course.

However, short-course therapy administered under direct observation was still not enough to control tuberculosis; an even more comprehensive approach was needed. Developed by Dr. Karel Styblo of the International Union Against Tuberculosis and Lung Diseases (IUATLD) based on his work in Africa in the 1980s, the DOTS strategy was launched in 1994 and today is the internationally accepted approach to tuberculosis control. Endorsed by the WHO, the DOTS strategy is a five-pronged comprehensive approach that builds on the administration of therapy under direct observation (Table 8-3). By 2005, the National TB Programs (NTPs) in 183 countries worldwide

Table 8-3. The DOTS strategy.

The five components of the DOTS strategy are as follows:

1. Sustained political commitment
2. Case detection by quality-assured sputum smear microscopy
3. Treatment of TB cases with standard short-course chemotherapy regimens under proper case-management conditions, including direct observation of treatment
4. Uninterrupted supply of quality-assured anti-TB drugs
5. Recording and reporting system enabling outcome assessment and management of program effectiveness

Note: The DOTS strategy is an all-or-none approach; all elements must be implemented.

were implementing the DOTS strategy, with 83% of the world's population living in areas covered by DOTS.[1]

The DOTS strategy has been studied in a number of different settings and found to be successful under a variety of conditions. For example, a DOTS demonstration project was implemented in China in 1990, with support from the World Bank, among 2 million people in five pilot counties near Beijing. By the end of 1991, this project was achieving phenomenal results: cure rates more than doubled, reaching 94%. This provided the basis for a larger World Bank–funded project covering half of the country, which has since cured over a half-million TB patients. In addition, the DOTS strategy is one of the most cost-effective public health interventions.[11]

EVALUATING TUBERCULOSIS CONTROL ACTIVITIES: GLOBAL TARGETS

At the heart of the DOTS strategy is the evaluation of patient outcomes to assess the effectiveness of TB control activities. This process—referred to as *cohort analysis*—allows the determination of, among other outcomes, the treatment success rate of a cohort of patients who started treatment in the same quarter or year. In 1991, global targets were set for TB control by the World Health Assembly based on data from mathematical modeling that showed that achievement of two key targets—detection of 70% of sputum smear-positive TB cases and cure of 85% of those cases—would cut TB incidence in half within 10 years. More recently, the Millennium Development Goals added the following targets for TB control: to reverse the rise in TB incidence globally by 2015 and to halve the 1990 prevalence and death rates in most regions by 2015. Both sets of targets are the benchmarks by which NTPs measure their overall success.

CRITIQUES AND CHALLENGES OF DOTS

Although the DOTS strategy has achieved dramatic success in many settings in comparison with earlier, disorganized tuberculosis control efforts, its shortfalls must also be considered. Perhaps most notable is that DOTS does not address the two most pressing issues affecting tuberculosis control today: namely, tuberculosis control in an HIV-endemic setting and treatment of multidrug-resistant tuberculosis (MDR-TB). Recognizing these important omissions, additional policy framework and clinical guideline documents have been developed to provide guidance to tuberculosis control programs that build on the DOTS strategy. Emphasizing the DOTS-first approach, the management of MDR-TB is referred to as *DOTS-Plus*.

Other aspects of the DOTS strategy have also received some important criticism of late.[12] Concern has been expressed that the emphasis on treating smear-positive patients left a sizable proportion of patients (i.e., AFB-smear-negative patients, children, and patients with extrapulmonary disease) as a low priority, with little support for the development of new diagnostic tools to detect smear-negative cases.[12] Similarly, reliance on the 100-year-old technique of smear microscopy provided little impetus for investment in newer and more sensitive and specific diagnostic measures. As long as the DOTS strategy was hailed as "the answer," the research community could stop pursuing the questions.

Directly observed therapy has been the subject of much heated debate in the international tuberculosis control community. Considered a heavy burden on health care systems and impractical in rural or remote areas, DOT, once a cornerstone of TB treatment, is being challenged. Some studies have shown that similar cure rates can be achieved when treatment is self-administered, challenging the dogma about the essential nature of DOT.[13,14] Lessons from programs rolling out antiretrovirals in resource-poor settings are demonstrating that patients can take long courses of therapy (life-long in the case of antiretrovirals) with appropriate support and education but without the need for direct observation. Whereas DOT in some settings is arranged to support patients, it has been criticized as punitive and burdensome in other settings. It is becoming clear that no one-size-fits-all approach can be accepted in every situation.

THE PROBLEM OF DRUG RESISTANCE

Drug-resistant tuberculosis is wholly a human-made phenomenon. With tuberculosis, the public health consequences of inadequate or incomplete treatment are worse than no treatment. Drug-resistant strains emerge through spontaneous mutation of the bacilli and will be selected as the dominant strain whenever inappropriate therapy (e.g., therapy with a single agent) is used. Single-drug exposure can occur due to improper prescribing, irregular drug supply, incorrect administration, or poor drug quality. Today, we are paying the price for poor tuberculosis control efforts in the past. The rapidly rising rates of drug-resistant TB in many countries (e.g., the former republics of the Soviet Union) are due in large part to previous poor treatment adherence—specifically, a failure of patients to take drugs consistently and/or to complete the prescribed course of treatment. Treatment of drug-resistant TB is more complicated than treatment of drug-susceptible TB; specifically, it is longer, less effective, and vastly more expensive. Consequently, the very ability of public health systems to control TB is threatened by the rising rates of drug-resistant cases.

Multidrug-resistant TB is defined as MTB resistant to *at least* isoniazid and rifampin—our two most powerful anti-TB drugs. Treatment of MDR-TB requires treatment with second-line drugs, which are generally from the following classes: aminoglycosides, polypeptides, fluoroquinolones, and carbothionamides; the category also includes cycloserine and para-aminosalicylic acid. Regimens to treat MDR-TB strains should contain at least four drugs to which the organism is known (or highly likely) to be susceptible. A typical initial phase for MDR-TB treatment may contain five or more drugs, including an injectable agent that is given for a minimum of 6 months. Under ideal program conditions, MDR-TB cure rates can approach 70%. In general, second-line drugs are less effective and more toxic than first-line drugs. When rifampicin can no longer be used because of resistance, treatment must be extended to 18 to 24 months to achieve cure. In addition, treatment of MDR-TB can be 100 times more costly than treatment of drug-susceptible TB.

The WHO estimates there are between 300,000 and 600,000 new cases of MDR-TB each year.[3] The most recent report of the WHO/IUATLD Global Project on Anti-tuberculosis Drug Resistance Surveillance found drug-resistant TB in 74 of the 77 settings evaluated between 1999 and 2002, and, as had been shown in the two previous surveys, MDR-TB was found in all regions of the world. In addition, patients who had received some treatment for tuberculosis in the past were more likely to have drug-resistant TB, and have resistance to more drugs, than previously untreated patients.[15]

In response to the growing problem of drug-resistant TB, interventions building on the DOTS strategy using second-line drugs were needed; thus, the DOTS-Plus strategy was created. Because the first priority in controlling MDR-TB is preventing its further emergence, a solid DOTS-based program must be in place before instituting DOTS-Plus. However, in MDR-TB hot spots such as Estonia, Latvia, and certain areas of Russia and China, where rates of MDR-TB have already reached high levels, additional measures, including the treatment and cure of resistant cases using second-line drugs, are needed to control MDR-TB. DOTS-Plus includes the designation of specialized treatment centers for MDR-TB, special clinical guidelines for management of MDR-TB patients with second-line drugs, and actions to make second-line drugs available for such treatment. Similar to the Global Drug Facility provision of first-line drugs, the Green Light Committee was established to provide quality-assured second-line drugs at reduced costs to carefully monitored programs.

DOTS-Plus has been shown to be cost-effective in a variety of settings, and reasonably high cure rates (approximately 70%) have been achieved.[16] By September 2005, over 10,000 patients with MDR-TB had received treatment through 35 programs in roughly 29 countries. In recognition of the success of DOTS-Plus projects worldwide, the WHO published new guidelines in 2006 on the management of MDR-TB.[16] Compiled by a team of international experts, these guidelines build on the extensive data collected over the years and represent the best available knowledge on the management of MDR-TB. In compliance with the new Global Plan to Stop Tuberculosis to treat all patients with tuberculosis, this document represents a significant shift in policy toward MDR-TB management: rather than a luxury reserved for programs with appropriate resources or for those suffering the highest levels of drug resistance, management of MDR-TB is now an integral activity of an NTP.

The newest threat to global tuberculosis control is the emergence of MTB resistant to isoniazid, rifampin, and to two additional drug classes (Fluoroquinolones) and either aminoglycosides or capreomycin termed *extensively drug-resistant tuberculosis*, or XDR-TB. Results from a survey of international reference laboratories conducted from 2000 to 2004 revealed that 20% of isolates were MDR-TB and 2% were XDR-TB. Population data from the United States, Latvia, and South Korea showed that 4%, 19%, and 15% of their reported MDR-TB cases, respectively, were XDR-TB.[3] XDR-TB may pose a true insurmountable obstacle to global tuberculosis control; if allowed to propagate, it could result in an epidemic of essentially untreatable tuberculosis. The report of these data is a call to action for the expansion of activities to detect drug-resistant TB accurately and rapidly and treat it effectively to prevent further spread of XDR-TB.[3]

CURRENT CHALLENGES TO TUBERCULOSIS CONTROL IN RESOURCE-POOR COUNTRIES

Tuberculosis control activities must be considered in the context of the country's health system. If ignored, these factors may thwart efforts to control the disease; however, if leveraged appropriately, they can contribute to the goals of the NTP.

Role of the Private Sector In many countries, particularly in Asia, a substantial private health care sector exists and is the source of care for a sizable proportion of TB patients. If the role played by the private sector is not recognized by the NTP and the opportunity for collaborating with private practitioners is not seized, many patients will be treated outside of the auspices of the NTP without any assurances of quality or adherence to international guidelines for diagnosing and treating tuberculosis. As a result, diagnosis may be delayed, which can have an adverse outcome for the patient and will allow continued transmission of tuberculosis in the community.

Where a significant private-sector role exists, a wise NTP leadership will acknowledge the potential for private-sector involvement and seek to build collaborative relationships with private practitioners to support their involvement in the NTP's activities. A few countries, notably the Philippines and India, have established sophisticated public-private partnership schemes, which outline different levels of engagement and collaboration—from simple referral mechanisms to full participation in the diagnostic and treatment activities supervised by the NTP. In most of sub-Saharan Africa, public-private collaborations are newer ventures, and in some settings have not met with the same level of success as demonstrated in Asia. This area of involvement is constantly evolving as both the public and private sectors explore potential collaborations based on their specific country and health system context.

Issues of Access and Community-Based Care Health care access is an issue not only in rural areas, where health outposts may be understaffed or nonexistent, but also in urban areas, where overcrowded health facilities are unable to handle the large patient volume. In response, programs that train and utilize community health workers to extend the health care system's reach have been created. Beginning with the WHO-coordinated Community TB Care in Africa project in 1996, the experience and results of numerous models of community-based care have been shared among policy makers, NTPs, community-based organizations, and nongovernmental organizations (NGOs). In rural villages as well as urban slums, together these agencies have contributed to the development of innovative methods of providing patient-centered care and patient- and community-level education as well as contributing to the identification of tuberculosis patients—all of which allow the NTP to expand the availability of services that are reflective of the community's needs. It is essential that all community-based efforts be designed and executed in close collaboration with the NTP.

Health Care Worker Shortage   Most resource-poor countries are experiencing some degree of health care worker shortage. The shortage is most severe in the countries of sub-Saharan Africa, where both limited resources and the AIDS epidemic significantly contribute to the shortage. For example, one government hospital in Malawi with 1,000 patients is staffed by only one doctor and one nurse because the rest of the staff has died.[17] Because of poor working conditions, unlivable wages, and concerns about health worker safety, many local physicians and nurses emigrate and seek employment in Europe and the United States, resulting in the well-known "brain drain" phenomenon. With only 3 to 6 physicians per 100,000 population in high-TB-burden countries such as Ethiopia, Tanzania, and Uganda, these countries fall short of the WHO-recommended minimum of 20 physicians per 100,000 population.[17] A response to the shortage of health care workers is outside the scope of NTP activities and requires a systematic and sustained directive led by the Ministry of Health involving all health care partners, to which the NTP can contribute through appropriate capacity building and the provision of incentives for retaining tuberculosis control staff.

A Dangerous Duo: Poverty and Stigma   Both poverty and stigma challenge the success of tuberculosis control. Tuberculosis is both caused by and a cause of poverty: on average, a person with TB loses one-third of his or her annual income. Additionally, the poor are overrepresented among TB sufferers. The stigma associated with TB can be powerful, and is only worsened in countries where TB is closely linked to HIV/AIDS. Patients with tuberculosis have been ostracized from their families and communities, and being witness to this behavior can lead people with a protracted cough to delay seeking care.

Efforts to address both the stigma of TB and its relationship to poverty have been undertaken by governments, NTPs, the WHO, and NGOs. Addressing poverty in tuberculosis control requires a multifaceted approach across several sectors to address economic impoverishment and the accompanying vulnerabilities and marginalization. The health system must be willing to undertake a pro-poor and equity-based approach to address the special needs of the most disadvantaged groups.[18] This approach, coupled with public education activities to address stigma (such as media campaigns and the use of celebrity TB survivors, which have been successful in some countries), is needed to address these significant challenges to tuberculosis control efforts.

ON THE HORIZON

Future Plans for Tuberculosis Control   Launched on World TB Day in 2006, the Second Global Plan to Stop TB 2006–2015 provides a road map for accelerated progress toward controlling tuberculosis over the next decade. Specifically, the plan sets out activities and the financial requirements necessary to achieve the following objectives: to expand equitable access to quality tuberculosis care; to treat 50 million patients with tuberculosis, including 800,000 with MDR-TB, and enroll 3 million on antiretroviral medications; to introduce the first new anti-TB drug in 40 years by 2010, with a shortened regimen by 2016; and to have safe, rapid, and inexpensive diagnostic tests and a safe, effective, and affordable vaccine by 2010 and 2015, respectively. The cost of implementing this plan—US $56 billion—is the largest sum requested for tuberculosis control to date.

Potential New Diagnostic Tests   Both sputum smear microscopy and the tuberculin skin test, the two 100-year-old TB diagnostic tests most commonly used in resource-poor settings, lack the sensitivity and specificity desirable in a diagnostic test. As discussed, mycobacterial culture, albeit a more sensitive diagnostic tool, is still an imperfect tool because of the delay in availability of results.

Published data on two new commercial ex vivo interferon-gamma assays using two MTB-specific antigens (ESAT-6 and CFP-10) suggest that these rapid tests have a higher specificity than TST for detecting tuberculosis.[19,20] Evaluation of these tests, which require only a single blood sample, has focused on their use in detecting latent infection rather than active disease. Their use is currently limited in the field setting by the need for relatively rapid specimen transport to a laboratory with the appropriate equipment and a trained technician. In addition, their current market-value costs are prohibitive for resource-limited countries. A nonprofit entity, the Foundation for Innovative New Diagnostics (FIND), was launched in 2003 to speed the development of new diagnostic tools for tuberculosis. In addition, new techniques are needed for the rapid detection of drug-resistant strains of tuberculosis.

New Drugs and Treatment Regimens   A faster and simpler therapy for tuberculosis is essential to achieve successful tuberculosis control globally. Several important breakthroughs have occurred in recent years that reveal new possibilities for anti-TB drug discovery. Specifically, the MTB genome was sequenced in 1998, which has advanced efforts to find novel ways to combat this pathogen. Recent public-private collaborations, led by the Global Alliance for TB Drug Development, have ensured swift movement of potential compounds through the development pipeline. New compounds, such as the diarylquinoline R207910, hold promise for effective, shorter tuberculosis treatment with no evidence of cross-resistance.[21] In addition, the use of fluoroquinolones (e.g., moxifloxacin) in a multidrug regimen may shorten the duration of tuberculosis treatment from 6 to 4 months. Phase III clinical trials of moxifloxacin are under way.

Typically, because of regulatory requirements and competition between companies, new drugs are developed consecutively. In 2006, the Global Alliance supported a new approach to testing medications for TB by combining two drugs produced by competing pharmaceutical companies, moxifloxacin and the new compound PA824 (a nitroimidazopyran) in a single clinical trial.

New Vaccine Candidates Given the lack of adult protection afforded by the current BCG vaccine, a new vaccine against tuberculosis is greatly needed. Research on live mycobacterial vaccines (using highly attenuated strains of MTB), inactivated vaccines (using nontuberculous mycobacteria) and subunit vaccines (using individual components of MTB) is currently under way. Most of these candidates will likely be tested as booster vaccines in persons who received BCG at birth. An inactivated vaccine has been shown to boost immune responses to mycobacteria in HIV-infected patients,[22] and a large efficacy trial is under way in Africa. In addition, a subunit vaccine candidate, MVA85A, which works by boosting a person's immune response years after they have received BCG vaccine, has been shown to be safe and effective at producing a high number of T-helper cells in recipients who have previously received BCG.[23] This vaccine is currently being studied at sites in Africa. Despite the momentum in vaccine development, most experts predict that a usable vaccine is unlikely to be available before 2015.

GUIDANCE TO STUDENTS: CRITERIA FOR SELECTING A TUBERCULOSIS CONTROL PROJECT

Students working on global health projects may encounter tuberculosis in two different circumstances: when working on a specific TB project or as one of the many diseases endemic in their overseas setting. The following guidance is intended to help students in both scenarios select well-designed projects and activities.

Most students working overseas on tuberculosis control will do so under the auspices of an NGO. Some hallmarks of well-designed and well-planned NGO tuberculosis control projects are as follows:

1. **A strong and close collaboration with the NTP or its local authority.** In every setting, the NTP retains ultimate responsibility for all tuberculosis control activities, and to work independent of the NTP jeopardizes tuberculosis control efforts in that setting.

2. **Project activities are designed and executed in accordance with national and international guidelines.** Despite the critiques demonstrating the limitations of DOTS, it is still the strategy that provides the foundation for good tuberculosis control (Box 8-1). If the project is not in compliance with the basic tenets of the DOTS strategy, it is unlikely to receive support from the national and/or international tuberculosis community and, of greater concern, it may pose the risk for doing more harm than good (e.g., dispensing medications before a full course of therapy for that patient is assured can lead to the emergence of drug resistance).

3. **In addition to collaboration with the NTP, ideally the organization will have local partners and respected national and international technical advisors.** The use of local partners increases the acceptability and sustainability of the activities, and even the most TB-experienced NGO will seek input from regional WHO officers or other key technical agencies to ensure high quality is achieved.

4. **Community education activities are instituted only if adequate diagnostic and treatment facilities exist.** Many NGOs focus their projects on community health education campaigns, and many have particular expertise in this area. Nonetheless, education campaigns intended to increase detection of tuberculosis cases when appropriate diagnostic and treatment services *are not yet available* will result in increased numbers of incompletely treated cases and increased drug resistance. The best way to avoid this practice is to ensure that all educational campaigns are closely coordinated with the NTP, which ought to have the best assessment of the availability of diagnostic and treatment services.

5. **The organization has a proven track record in tuberculosis control in the region.** Researching the organization (e.g., via its website or available reports) is critical. Seeking comments from previous volunteers or staff and from colleagues working at partner agencies is another means of assessing the organization's performance and quality of work.

6. **Close collaboration with the HIV/AIDS control program in HIV-endemic areas.** Activities to control HIV and TB must be coordinated between the two programs. There are varied examples of how joint TB/HIV activities can be implemented, but most important is that services are organized to ensure proper screening and provision of appropriate

---

BOX 8-1. A MODEL TUBERCULOSIS CONTROL PROGRAM

The national TB control program (NTP) in Vietnam is often cited by the World Health Organization as a model program in terms of organizational structure and program results. The NTP is fully integrated in the general health system at the district and commune levels. In remote areas where access to primary care services is limited, the program works through village health workers and links with commune health posts. Since 2003, Vietnam has achieved 100% DOTS coverage (i.e., DOTS has been implemented countrywide). Furthermore, Vietnam has exceeded the two global TB targets of 70% case detection rate and 85% treatment success by achieving 82% and 92%, respectively. Vietnam has a 5-year NTP action plan in place for 2006 to 2010 and has successfully trained NTP staff at all levels through domestic and overseas training courses. Vietnam's NTP has involved most public hospitals, medical college hospitals, prisons, military services, and a number of private practitioners in TB control. In addition, Vietnam's NTP strives to empower communities and people with TB by organizing TB health education workshops for TB patients, social and local government leaders, and the general public at the commune level and studying the knowledge, attitudes, and practices of populations in the central and northern provinces. Vietnam has also made significant progress in monitoring TB/HIV, established pilot sites for the management of multidrug-resistant TB, developed TB networks in mountainous and remote areas, and conducted other outreach to populations at risk for TB.

Vietnam is one of the best examples of the successful combination of DOTS implementation, political commitment, adequate resources, and good strategic planning.

Adapted from World Health Organization. *Global Tuberculosis Control: Surveillance, Planning, Financing.* Geneva: World Health Organization, 2004, 2006. WHO Global Reports 2004 and 2006.

---

care to individuals with one or both diseases (see "HIV and Tuberculosis: Two Diseases, One Patient," later in this chapter, for further details).

Students who encounter TB care and control as part of a related but not TB-specific project (e.g., work in a primary care clinic where patients with suspected TB are evaluated) can still apply (or adapt as necessary) these criteria to the TB control activities that intersect with their work. Students are also reminded of the importance of evaluating and documenting the outcomes of their project. Various forums exist for sharing student work in TB control, and the value of student contributions should not be underestimated.

HIV/AIDS

AIDS first came to the attention of the public health community in the United States in 1981.[24–26] The clustering of cases of rare skin (Kaposi sarcoma) and lung (*Pneumocystis carinii* pneumonia) diseases in young, apparently healthy, homosexual men sounded warning bells of an unusual condition. Prior to that, Kaposi sarcoma, a skin cancer, had largely been confined to older men and women from the Mediterranean and African regions. *Pneumocystis carinii* pneumonia had usually been observed among those whose immune systems had been severely suppressed due to treatment or illness, such as cancer patients or destitute and sickly elderly men. Because AIDS appeared first among homosexual men, the initial epidemiologic investigations focused on lifestyle practices.

Soon after, AIDS cases were reported in entirely different populations in the United States and Europe, such as injection drug users (IDUs),[27] hemophiliacs,[28–30] recipients of blood transfusions,[31,32] newborn infants,[33,34] and a few travelers from central Africa who went to Europe for medical treatment.[35] Initially, drugs were implicated as a potential cause, because homosexuals often used sexual performance-enhancing drugs such as amyl or butyl nitrate ("poppers"). At the same time, it was hypothesized that AIDS might be caused by immune reactions resulting from frequent immunostimulation by foreign proteins and tissue antigens from sperm and blood products. Similar to healthy homosexuals, hemophiliacs and IDUs were often found to have inverted ratios of infection-fighting cells. This was thought to result from frequent immunostimulation.

However, the observation of AIDS in the other disparate populations and the emerging epidemiology of the disease suggested an infectious cause.[36] The search for an infectious cause of AIDS eventually focused on viruses, particularly those that were known to cause immunosuppression. It was eventually postulated that a variant human T-cell lymphotrophic retrovirus (HTLV) might be the causative agent of AIDS.[37–41] The reasoning was that the recently discovered (in 1980) HTLV-1 was the only known virus at the time that infected T helper lymphocyte cells.[37] Moreover, HTLV was known to be transmitted through the same routes as the causative agent of AIDS: sexual contact, blood, and from mother to baby.[40] Eventually a variant of HTLV, termed HIV-1 (human immunodeficiency virus type 1), was isolated in 1983.[40,41]

Pathogenesis, Diagnosis, and Transmission

HIV infection causes AIDS through the depletion and eventual exhaustion of immune responses, leading to clinical illness and eventually death in most people. The virus binds on a receptor, penetrates the cell, organizes the infected cell to be able to make the viral genetic material, synthesizes proteins for virus particles, assembles the virus particles, and releases them from the cell. HIV is a retrovirus; this class of virus integrates with the genetic material of the host cell, which is unlike the actions of most other types of viruses. In this way, HIV establishes a permanent infection within the body. The virus attacks lymphocytes, white blood cells that are part of the body's immune defense system. In particular, the T4 helper or inducer lymphocytes that activate B cells to produce antibodies and regulate other cells to fight infections in different ways are invaded. This type of cell contains a significant amount of CD4 surface protein, the cell receptor to which HIV binds. In addition, macrophages, cells that engulf and destroy viruses, and dendritic cells also contain CD4 proteins, making them targets for invasion by HIV.

Thus, HIV seems to damage the immune system by the weakening of the T4 response in the following ways:

- Through invasion of the dendritic cells that stimulate the T4 cells to respond to foreign organisms
- Through invasion of the T4 cells and the suborning of the cell reproductive processes to produce more virus, with the subsequent destruction of the T4 cells
- By facilitating uninfected T4 cells to clump around infected T4 cells, thus immobilizing them

The infected macrophages are not killed: most continue to produce HIV virus particles, and some establish a latent state of HIV infection. Although the body mounts a vigorous immune response to the virus through the production of antibodies, the sheer rapid replication of the virus, its latency, and virus variation will eventually lead to the exhaustion and ultimate collapse of the immune system. The variability of the virus is particularly problematic because it has led to immunologically distinct subtypes that vary by region, making vaccine development difficult.

Two main types of HIV exist: HIV-1 and HIV-2. HIV-1 is more predominant and can be classified into three groups: group M, the "major" group; group N, the "new" group; and group O, the "outlier" group. Group O seems to be restricted to west-central Africa, and group N, which was discovered in 1998 in Cameroon, is extremely rare. Over 90% of HIV-1 infections are in group M, and there are at least nine genetically distinct subtypes (or clades): A, B, C, D, F, G, H, J, and K. In addition, two viruses of different subtypes in the same person can sometimes create a new hybrid virus, *circulating recombinant forms* (CRFs). For example, the CRF A/E is a mixture of subtypes A and E. Many people refer to the CRF A/E as "subtype E." Subtypes B and C are the most widespread viruses, with subtype C predominant in southern and eastern Africa, India, and Nepal, and subtype B most common

in the Americas, Australia, Europe, Japan, and Thailand. Subtype C has caused the world's worst epidemic and accounts for about half of all infections. New subtypes will emerge as virus recombination and mutation continues to occur, and the current subtypes and CRFs will continue to spread to new areas with the global pandemic.

The geographic distribution of some of the current subtypes appears to be associated with specific modes of transmission, particularly subtype B, which is possibly more readily transmitted by anal intercourse and intravenous drug injecting (via blood, essentially). Subtypes C and CRF A/E, on the other hand, appear to be more efficiently transmitted through vaginal intercourse (a mucosal route). The different subtypes appear to affect disease progression as well. Studies in Senegal and Uganda found that patients infected with subtype C, D, or G developed AIDS earlier and died sooner compared with patients infected with subtype A.[42,43]

HIV infection is diagnosed through the detection of antibodies. The most common HIV antibody test is an enzyme-linked immunosorbent assay (EIA or ELISA test). The current ELISA tests are more than 99.9% accurate. ELISA tests are also available for saliva (e.g., OraQuick; OraSure Technologies, Bethlehem, PA), and there are now antibody tests that can give results in less than 30 minutes (the rapid tests). Examples of these are Uni-Gold Recombigen HIV (Trinity Biotech, Dublin, Ireland) and Determine HIV 1/2 (Abbott Diagnostic Division, Hoofddorp, The Netherlands). The tests can detect HIV-1 and HIV-2 and the major subtypes of group M.

Although the antibody test is very accurate, there are times when it can produce false positive or false negative results. A false positive result obviously can be very distressing to the individual concerned. Aside from a transcription or a laboratory error, the most likely reason for this is that the prevalence of HIV in the population concerned may be very low. Despite the accuracy of a test, screening in populations with low prevalence will result in a high proportion of false positives. This is an argument why, aside from the cost, general screening for HIV in, for example, the United States, where the prevalence is less than 1%, is not advisable. From the point of view of program managers, though, a more troublesome concern is the occurrence of false negatives.

Aside again from transcription or testing protocol errors, false negatives for HIV can occur for two reasons. The most common is when the individual has been infected but the body has not yet begun the manufacture of antibodies. After initial infection, production of antibodies can take as long as 6 months (although in most cases it is 2 to 6 weeks), so that during that time, the individual will test negative on the ELISA tests, which test for antibodies, yet will actually be HIV positive. This period, known as the *window phase*, is a dangerous time. As with initial

Table 8-4. The progression of HIV infection to AIDS .

Stage	Description
HIV infection	Initial infection with HIV (i.e., through sex or blood contact)
Window period (2–6 weeks; occasionally several months)	No signs or symptoms of disease; no detectable antibodies to HIV.
Seroconversion (brief period that occurs after 2 to 6 weeks, up to a few months)	The development of antibodies. This may be associated with flu-like illness, glandular fever-like illness, or occasionally encephalitis. Illness at seroconversion is sometimes called acute HIV syndrome. About 50% of people experience this illness.
Asymptomatic HIV (duration from less than 1 year to 10 to 15 years or more)	ELISA tests are positive, but there are no apparent signs or symptoms of illness. The incubation period. It may be associated with persistent generalized lymphadenopathy (PGL), persistent swollen glands.
HIV/AIDS-related illnesses (duration months or years)	Increasing signs and symptoms of disease, because HIV is damaging the immune system. Initially not life threatening, but becomes progressively so with the course of the disease.
AIDS (usually less than 1 to 2 years in the absence of treatment)	The terminal stage of HIV infection. The immune system is severely weakened, allowing life-threatening opportunistic infections, including cancers.

From Jackson H. *AIDS Africa: Continent in Crisis.* Harare, Zimbabwe: Southern Africa HIV/AIDS Information, 2002, p. 43. (Adapted with permission.)

infection, there is a large amount of circulating virus, making the individual particularly infectious. The immune system has not yet begun to effectively suppress viral replication, because it is still in the process of identifying the invader and producing the appropriate antibodies.

The course of HIV infection and ultimately AIDS goes from a largely asymptomatic phase to that of severe disease and death over a period of 10 to 15 years or more. There is, however, significant individual variability in the disease progression. Table 8-4 shows the progression of HIV infection to AIDS.[44] In full-blown AIDS, where the immune system has been severely weakened, the second reason for a false negative finding with an ELISA test is that so few antibodies are being produced that the test can no longer detect them. False negatives can also occur in the rare instances of individuals who never mount an immune response.

As HIV increasingly damages the immune system, signs and symptoms of various infections become visible. In babies this occurs faster than in adults; although the signs and symptoms vary, one of the first signs of HIV disease in babies may be a general failure to thrive and grow. In general, the clinical manifestations of AIDS can be grouped into opportunistic infections, that is, infections by microorganisms that would not normally cause disease in healthy individuals (e.g., *Pneumocystis jiroveci* pneumonia,* funguses, and to some extent tuberculosis); cancers (e.g., Kaposi sarcoma, a skin cancer); weight loss; and mental impairment.

THE WHO STAGING SYSTEM

The WHO has developed a four-phase clinical staging system to describe HIV progression in adults and adolescents (Table 8-5).[45] The WHO staging system is useful in resource-poor countries because it obviates the need for CD4 testing. CD4 testing is expensive, requiring equipment (a capital cost) and reagents (a recurrent expense); for many resource-poor countries, it is unaffordable on a national scale presently.

What is notable is that different regions appear to have different prevalences of opportunistic infections. In developing countries, the most prevalent HIV-related infection is tuberculosis.

HIV TRANSMISSION

HIV transmission occurs when the HIV-contaminated fluid of an infected person comes into contact with the bloodstream or mucosal lining of an uninfected person. There are three modes of transmission: birth, blood, or sex. Perinatal transmission can occur during pregnancy, delivery, or through breastfeeding.

Transmission during pregnancy can occur when the mother has high levels of circulating virus (viremia) due to seroconversion or to her precipitating into AIDS, and particularly during the third trimester, when small tears sometimes occur in the placenta, facilitating the entry of cells from the mother's bloodstream into the baby's. HIV transmission during delivery is also enhanced by viremia; by the occurrence of sexually transmitted diseases at the time, particularly syphilis and herpes simplex (HSV2); the prolonged rupture of membranes; and trauma (cuts and tears) during the process. Delivery is a particularly risky time for HIV transmission to the infant because of the infected maternal secretions.

---

*This is the new and current name for this organism, but the acronym PCP, for *Pneumocystis carinii* pneumonia, remains in use.

Table 8-5. WHO clinical staging system for HIV infection and disease.

Clinical stage 1: Asymptomatic

1. Asymptomatic/acute HIV infection
2. Persistent generalized lymphadenopathy (PGL)
3. History of acute HIV infection

And/or performance scale 1: asymptomatic, normal activity

Clinical stage 2: Early (mild) disease

1. Weight loss, <10% of body weight
2. Minor mucocutaneous (skin) problems (e.g., seborrheic dermatitis, prurigo, fungal nail infections, recurrent oral ulcerations, angular cheilitis)
3. Herpes zoster within the past 5 years
4. Recurrent respiratory tract infections (e.g., bacterial sinusitis)

And/or performance scale 2: symptomatic, normal activity

Clinical stage 3: Intermediate (moderate) disease

1. Weight loss, >10% of body weight
2. Unexplained chronic diarrhea, >1 month
3. Unexplained prolonged fever (intermittent or chronic), >1 month
4. Oral candidiasis (thrush)
5. Oral hairy leukoplakia
6. Pulmonary tuberculosis within the past year
7. Severe bacterial infections, (e.g., pneumonia, pyomyositis)

And/or performance scale 3: bedridden <50% of the daytime during the last month

Clinical stage 4: Late (severe) disease, AIDS

1. HIV wasting syndrome (weight loss >10% body weight, with diarrhea >1 month or chronic weakness and prolonged fever >1 month)
2. *Pneumocystis carinii* pneumonia
3. Toxoplasmosis of the brain
4. Cryptosporidiosis with diarrhea, >1 month
5. Isosporiasis with diarrhea, >1 month
6. Cryptococcosis, extrapulmonary
7. Cytomegalovirus (CMV) disease of an organ other than the liver, spleen, or lymph nodes
8. Herpes simplex virus (HSV) infection; mucocutaneous, >1 month, or visceral
9. Progressive multifocal leukoencephalopathy (PML)
10. Mycoses (e.g., histoplasmosis, coccidioidomycosis)
11. Candidiasis of the esophagus, trachea, bronchi, or lungs
12. Atypical mycobacteriosis, disseminated
13. Nontyphoidal *Salmonella* septicemia
14. Extrapulmonary tuberculosis
15. Lymphoma
16. Kaposi sarcoma (KS)
17. HIV encephalopathy (progressive disabling cognitive and/or motor dysfunction, interfering with activities of daily living)

And/or performance scale 4: bedridden >50% of the daytime during the last month

Breastfeeding mothers can also transmit HIV to their infants. Again, this is facilitated by the mother's viremia and by cuts and sores on the mother's nipples and in the child's mouth. In the absence of treatment, about one-third of babies born to and breastfed by HIV-positive mothers will become HIV positive, with about one-third becoming infected during pregnancy, one-third during delivery, and another third through breastfeeding.

The prevention of maternal-to-child transmission (PMTCT)* of HIV was one of the first antiretroviral prevention interventions implemented in low-resource countries. This was made possible particularly with the efficacy of single-dose nevirapine (NVP), the low cost of the drug, and the practicalities of implementation. Nevirapine given in a single dose to the mother in labor and a single dose to the baby at 2 to 3 days old reduces transmission by about 47%.[44,46] The mother can also be given a tablet to take home when labor begins (many mothers in resource-poor countries have their babies at home), and the baby can be dosed 3 days after the birth, perhaps when having a BCG vaccination. However, certain controversies have remained regarding the PMTCT program.

One of the controversies has been that, until recently, antiretroviral therapy was not offered to the parents when the mother tested positive in the antenatal care clinic, yet she was given NVP to prevent transmission to her baby. Consequently, in many programs, the uptake of the PMTCT program was low because the number of mothers agreeing to counseling and testing was low. With the introduction of opt-out testing, in which mothers first have a group talk on PMTCT and then are tested unless they specifically decline, the number of mothers being tested has increased significantly.[†] Another controversy with the PMTCT program in many countries is the use of NVP. Even single-dose NVP has the potential to cause resistance, and some countries have abandoned its use altogether. Some have moved to longer-course regimens, whereas others have added another antiretroviral drug. These adjustments add to the cost of the program and to the logistics of implementation.

Another controversy is breastfeeding. The use of NVP does not prevent the transmission of HIV through breastfeeding. Ideally, HIV-positive mothers should not breastfeed. However, in many less-resourced countries, this is not feasible because the cost of formula feeding is beyond the reach of most mothers, and clean water may not be

---

*This is also known as the prevention of parent-to-child transmission (PPTCT) to emphasize that *both* parents are responsible for the potential transmission of HIV to the baby.

[†]In a town adjacent to Harare, capital of Zimbabwe, 98% of mothers attending antenatal care in the period from July 2005 to June 2006 were tested. Prior to opt-out testing, only 26% of mothers were tested in 1999 to 2002.

accessible or available. Mothers are also stigmatized if they do not breastfeed, because breastfeeding is very important in many cultures. Consequently, ministries of health, especially in sub-Saharan Africa, recommend that babies born to HIV-positive mothers should be exclusively breastfed for 4 months, and then abruptly weaned. In the absence of formula feeding, exclusive breastfeeding is less risky than mixed feeding (breast and formula).

Transmission of HIV through blood can be through blood transfusion, through contaminated needles, or through other medical procedures and delivery. The highest risk of HIV transmission is through transfusion of HIV-infected blood (90%), and although blood for transfusion is screened for HIV in almost all countries now, there is still a risk because of the window period and because the screening tests are not perfect.

Transmission through contaminated needles can be through the sharing of needles during injection drug use or through accidental needlesticks between HIV-infected persons and health workers. Injection drug use is a very efficient mode of HIV transmission. According to the UNAIDS 2006 report, injection drug use accounts for 80% of HIV cases in eastern Europe and Central Asia.[47] The reason for this efficiency is that during the process of injecting the drug, blood is drawn into the syringe to check that the needle has reached a vein, and then the contents of the syringe are injected repeatedly into the vein to ensure that all the drug goes in. If someone else then uses the same needle and syringe, traces of blood (and virus) are readily passed directly into the next person's bloodstream.

Transmission through needlestick injuries and other medical procedures (e.g., surgery, deliveries, blood splashes) is low. Various studies show a range of HIV infection from 0.13 to 0.39 cases per 100 exposures by cut or needlestick injury among health staff.[48]

Sexual transmission of HIV is the most common mode globally. About 70% of HIV infections worldwide are contracted through vaginal sexual intercourse.[44] Anal intercourse (male-to-male sex, or male-to-female sex) is the most risky form of intercourse because it involves a slight tearing of the anus, thus involving the exchange of both semen and blood. In countries such as the United States, Australia, western Europe, and parts of South America, men who have sex with men, the majority of whom practice anal intercourse,[49] constituted the initial risk profile for HIV.

Medical Care and Treatment of HIV/AIDS

MEDICATIONS

Antiretroviral therapy (ART) is the most effective means of preventing opportunistic infections (OIs), and many programs link the prevention and treatment of OIs with ART. Although rapid progress has been made to make ART more widely available (1.3 million received ART in

2005, up from 240,000 in 2001), still only one in five of those who need it is receiving ART.[47] The prevalence of OIs varies by region; for example, tuberculosis is the most common opportunistic infection globally and particularly in sub-Saharan Africa and Asia, whereas PCP is the most common OI in North America and Europe. Table 8-6 presents OIs that have primary and secondary prophylactic medications. ART is taken for life and generally drugs for OI prophylaxis are taken for life, although they could be stopped if CD_4 counts can be measured regularly and the immune system recovers. These activities need to be integrated into daily living.

The prevention and treatment of OIs should be complementary via a holistic approach. The efficacy of many medications is enhanced when the individual is well nourished, has good hygiene, is not stressed or tired, has a positive approach to life, and has access to an acceptable standard of living. Addressing food security and poverty, as well as access to medical care, is an important principle underlying effective medical care and treatment of HIV/AIDS. The prevention and treatment of OIs should include prevention of reinfection (abstinence and/or condom promotion), psychosocial support (counseling and support groups), and nutrition care and support.

Many people in resource-poor countries suffer from underlying nutrition deficiencies, particularly micronutrients, which are exacerbated with the acquisition of HIV. This situation then increases vulnerability to opportunistic infections and facilitates the progression to AIDS. In addition, the individual needs good nutrition to be able to better tolerate many of the antiretroviral drugs.

COUNSELING

Counseling should also be part of the care and treatment of HIV/AIDS. The counseling should involve consideration of what a positive result might mean in the patient's life, whom the result will affect (e.g., a spouse or regular sexual partner), to whom and how the patient will tell his or her results, and what long-term support services are available. There should also be ongoing counseling; this might include knowledge of HIV and AIDS, adherence to drug regimens, coping with stigma, repeated illness episodes, and death and bereavement. Terminal and bereavement counseling should include finances and signing powers, and, for dependents, wills and funeral arrangements.

Counseling, nutrition, and the treatment and prevention of OIs form an important part of the care of people living with HIV/AIDS, the heart of which should be ART. As stated earlier, with the advent of ART the incidence and prevalence of opportunistic infections have been reduced. The first antiretroviral drug marketed was azidothymidine or zidovudine (AZT/ZDV). It belongs to a class of drugs called nucleoside reverse transcriptase inhibitors (NRTIs). These drugs block HIV reverse transcriptase and prevent the copying of the viral genetic code (RNA) into the

Table 8-6. Major opportunistic infections for which primary or secondary prophylactic drugs are available.

Condition	Treatment drugs	Prophylaxis
Candidiasis (oral, esophageal, vaginal)	Fluconazole	Treatment of individual episodes rather than prophylaxis because resistance is common
Cytomegalovirus (CMV—ocular, gastrointestinal, disseminated)	Ganciclovir or foscarnet	Valganciclovir Foscarnet
Cryptococcus (meningitis, pneumonia, disseminated disease)	Amphotericin B deoxycholate and/or flucytosine	Fluconazole
Histoplasmosis (pneumonia, disseminated disease)	Itraconazole or amphoteric in B deoxycholate	Itraconazole
Herpes virus (skin, genital, oral, esophageal, ocular, disseminated)	Famciclovir Acyclovir	Famciclovir Acyclovir (but risk of resistance development)
Mycobacterium avium complex (MAC— pulmonary, disseminated)	Clarithromycin plus ethambutol	Clarithromycin plus/minus ethambutol Azithromycin plus/minus ethambutol
Mycobacterium tuberculosis (pulmonary, extrapulmonary, disseminated)	Isoniazid, rifampin; pyrazinamide, ethambutol	Isoniazid (9 months) where positive skin test (latent TB infection)
Pneumocystis carinii pneumonia (PCP)	Trimethoprim-sulfamethoxazole (TMP/SMX, co-trimoxazole)	TMP/SMX
Toxoplasmosis (central nervous system)	Pyrimethamine and sulfadiazine plus leucovorin	Sulfadiazine and pyrimethamine plus leucovorin
Penicilliosis[a]	Amphotericin B, then itraconazole	Itraconazole
Leishmaniasis[a]	Pentavalent antimony (or sodium stibogluconate)	Pentavalent antimony (or sodium stibogluconate)
Isospora belli[a]	TMP and SMX	TMP and SMX
Chagas disease[a]	Benznidazole	Benznidazole

[a]Geographic opportunistic infections of special consideration.
From Centers for Disease Control and Prevention. Treating opportunistic infections among HIV-infected adults and adolescents: recommendations from CDC, the National Institutes of Health and the HIV Medicine Association/Infectious Diseases Society of America. *MMWR* 2004;53(RR15). (Adapted with permission.)

genetic code (DNA) of infected host cells by imitating the building blocks of the DNA chain. The resulting DNA is incomplete and cannot create new virus. Table 8-7 lists the currently approved HIV antiretroviral drugs. The non-nucleoside reverse transcriptase inhibitors (NNRTIs) block HIV reverse transcriptase and prevent the copying of infected host cells by binding to the enzyme and making the active site ineffective. The most recently marketed drug class is the protease inhibitors. These drugs block the enzyme protease and prevent the assembly and release of HIV particles from infected cells. To avoid the rapid development of resistance, drugs are given in combination. A combination that is in current use for first-line therapy in southern Africa is stavudine, lamivudine, and nevirapine, marketed under the name Stalanev.

In poor-resourced countries, first-line ART utilizes the older classes of drugs (the NRTIs and NNRTIs) because of the cost of protease inhibitors. Cost is an important consideration in ART. Even though the cost of HIV drugs has decreased considerably, the cost of providing ART to all who need it in many African countries is huge and not easily affordable. The WHO estimates that in the least developed countries, where populations are living on less than a $1 per day, ART costs between $300 to $1,200 per annum. In addition, many health systems in poor-resourced countries are weak and need to be strengthened to be able to roll out ART nationally; this entails a cost even greater than that of the drugs. There are insufficient numbers of doctors, nurses, counselors, and laboratory personnel, and these cadres need to be trained, motivated, and retained. Patient monitoring and adherence to treatment are critical to the success of the ART program; consequently, national health systems need to be able to routinely carry out CD4 and viral load testing to be able to assess the immune system function and the amount of HIV virus that can be detected. Enormous capital and recurrent costs are associated with equipping national health systems to be able to provide these monitoring

Table 8-7. Currently approved HIV antiviral drugs.

Drug class	Chemical/generic name	Trade name
Nucleoside reverse transcriptase inhibitors	AZT/azidothymidine/zidovudine	Retrovir
	DDI/dideoxyinosine/didanosine	Videx
	DDC/dideoxycytidine/zalcitabine	HIVID
	3TC/lamivudine	Epivir
	D4T/stavudine	Zerit
	Abacavir	Ziagen
	Tenofovir	Viread
Non-nucleoside reverse transcriptase inhibitors	Nevirapine	Viramune
	Delavirdine	Rescriptor
	Efavirenz	Sustiva
Protease inhibitors	Saquinavir	Fortovase/Invirase
	Indinavir	Crixivan
	Ritonavir	Norvir
	Nelfinavir	Viracept
	Amprenavir	Agenerase
	Lopinavir/ritonavir	Kaletra
	Atazanavir	Reyataz

functions. Low-cost diagnostic tools are in development for at least CD4 measurement and viral load.*

The WHO has developed guidelines as to when to treat and to assist in monitoring. Patients with clinical stage 3 or 4 and a positive HIV test would be eligible for ART. These stages approximate to a compromised immune system, which has been set in sub-Saharan Africa at a CD4 count of 200 or below. In the United States, patients are eligible for ART when they have a CD4 count below 350. Treatment efficacy or failure is adjudged on clinical grounds; essentially, whether the patient is getting better, gaining (or not losing) weight, and is not experiencing opportunistic illnesses. However, the correlation between the CD4 count and the clinical signs and symptoms is not perfect, and there are reports of patients with very low CD4 counts still being able to function normally.

Prevention of HIV/AIDS

HIV/AIDS prevention remains the key to the control of the epidemic. Various prevention strategies have been effected over the years; these strategies vary according to the stage of the epidemic. When the HIV prevalence is still low (<1%) and the epidemic is confined to high-risk groups, different preventive interventions are used compared with when the epidemic has become generalized in the population. In generalized epidemics, there should be a focus on population- or community-level change, because simply concentrating on high-risk groups will no longer be effective. High-risk groups, from which epidemics can spread to become generalized, include commercial sex workers (CSWs), men who have sex with men (MSM), injection drug users, and mobile men (migrant workers, military personnel, truck drivers, etc.).

In the early stages of the epidemic, targeting of high-risk groups can slow the epidemic and prevent it from becoming generalized. Some countries, by acting early and vigorously, have been able to do this. Examples include Senegal, Thailand, and Australia. Despite being a predominantly Moslem country, Senegal was able to reduce the incidence and prevalence of HIV by encouraging condom use among CSWs through the legalization of commercial sexual activities, education on and provision of condoms, and the regular examination for and treatment of sexually transmitted infections (STIs).[50] Similarly, Thailand has been successful by developing interventions for CSWs and the army. Thailand adopted a 100% condom use policy for CSWs, which was enabled by the commercialized nature of sex work (the existence of brothels), allowing for the enforcement of this policy.[51,52] The implementation of this policy was facilitated through peer education programs for the CSWs.[52] Peer education was also the means through which behavior change among young men in the Thai army was facilitated and HIV prevalence reduced.[53] In Australia, the epidemic

---

*See, for example, Guava Technologies' development of a low-cost CD4 assay system (http://www.guavatechnologies.com) and the publication of an article on a low-cost monitoring system for HIV viral load (Drosten C, Panning M, Drexler JF, et al. Ultra sensitive monitoring of HIV viral load by a low cost real-time reverse transcriptase-PCR assay with internal controls for the 5′ long terminal repeat domain. *Clin Chem* 2006;52:1258–1266).

among IDUs was reduced through a policy of needle exchange.[54] A program in Sidney, Australia, included bleach distribution, community outreach, and expanded drug treatment. The needle exchange policy, which remains controversial in countries such as the United States, is predicated on a harm reduction approach, whereby the prevention of illness and death through HIV, and the possibility of transmission to others, is considered more important than prosecution for illicit drug use. Table 8-8 summarizes the evidence regarding various HIV/AIDS prevention interventions.

ABSTINENCE, FAITHFULNESS, AND CONDOM USE

The abstinence, faithfulness, and condom use (ABC) policy remains the cornerstone of many HIV/AIDS prevention programs. Abstinence is a controversial strategy, because there is widespread consensus that youth should abstain, but less consensus about providing the knowledge and skills (including information on condom use and where they can be obtained) necessary to protect themselves should they not abstain. Moreover, although the message of abstinence until marriage has increased the age of sexual debut,[55] there is a tendency

Table 8-8. Summary of evidence base of interventions for HIV prevention.

Intervention/program area	Impact at population level	Impact at individual level	Comments
Abstinence	Temporary impact on young people through delayed debut, but tendency to have more rapid HIV acquisition in their 20s: "catch up" observed; less relevance for adults	While observed, 100% effective	"ABC" formulation has considerable baggage and has had less relevance for women. However, all three prongs are relevant and need reformulating for greater complementarity; avoid either/or formulation.
Be faithful	Appears to have been key to reduced incidence and prevalence in Uganda, Kenya, and Zimbabwe	100% effective if fully maintained by two HIV-negative people (or in a polygamous union)	Concurrent relationships appear to be a key epidemic driver because of very high infectivity in acute/incident infection.
Condoms, male	Appear not to have had strong impact in generalized epidemics (though central to concentrated, sexually driven epidemics elsewhere)	At least 80% to 90% protective if consistently and correctly used: the most protective device currently available for individual protection	Challenge is to achieve correct and consistent use (over 80%). Easiest in commercial sex, and then casual sex; least in more stable partnerships, concurrent or not
Condoms, female	Contribute to number of protected sex acts where available	Highly protective against HIV STIs, and pregnancy	Advantage of female use.
STI treatment	Limited impact on HIV prevention because only targets bacterial STIs, and misses 50% of those needing treatment (asymptomatic)	Untreated STIs greatly increase HIV transmission risk; more so if ulcerous	Only reaches small proportion of infected individuals; increasingly in southern Africa, viral STIs predominate, not bacterial, and treatment misses these.
STI control and prevention	More impact in concentrated than generalized epidemics, but crucial for young people in generalized epidemics	As above	Greater potential to reach large numbers, especially important for young people.
HSV2	Recent infection with HSV2 doubles the risk of HIV transmission, with recent infection with HSV2 more risky than chronic infection	HSV2 treatment reduces HIV shedding and thus reduces infectivity	Research is under way into HSV2 suppression.

Table 8-8. Summary of evidence base of interventions for HIV prevention. (Continued)

Intervention/program area	Impact at population level	Impact at individual level	Comments
Male circumcision	Strong observational data of protective impact at population level; includes correlation with lower incidence and prevalence of HIV in African and other populations; one randomized, controlled trial complete; two (Kenya and Uganda) under way	50% to 75% protective for men, possibly some direct protection for women; many other health benefits for males (e.g., for penile cancer, some STIs, phimosis) and for females (esp. reduced risk of cervical cancer)	Countries vary in their readiness to consider male circumcision where it is not traditionally practiced. UNAIDS and WHO are developing tools, guides, and manuals for safe male circumcision practice and programming. Major challenges include avoiding behavioral disinhibition and unsafe practices.
Counseling and testing	Little population-level impact shown, although essential as an entry point to care and treatment, and for PMTCT	Some behavior change shown in discordant couples and in HIV-positive clients	Concern that "know your status" campaigns must link with effective and available post-test services for HIV-positive and HIV-negative clients, or they may not be effective.
Behavior change interventions for young people	Talloires' consultation in 2004: strongest evidence for behavioral impacts of radio with other media and TV/radio with other media; certain designs of curriculum-based sex and HIV education shown to be effective for young people in school when adult led, with no evidence of increased sexual activity	Increased individual access to youth- (and gender-) friendly health services also shown to be important for general SRH in various studies. Young men and women recognized as essential to reach with effective multipronged strategies.	Data indicate behavior changes through different strategies that are likely to have an impact on HIV incidence in young people. Community interventions with young people: weak evaluation designs and incomplete information, so not possible yet to assess impact clearly of different approaches. Look out for Talloires' final report.
Female diaphragm	RCT under way in Zimbabwe and South Africa; South African study linking with candidate microbicide Acidform Gel	By covering the cervix, likely to confer a degree of protection, but extent not known	Diaphragm is potentially protective to some degree and is entirely female controlled. Could be used with microbicide when available.
Microbicides	None yet available; many candidate microbicides in phase I to III trials in Malawi, Zimbabwe, South Africa, Zambia, Uganda, and outside the region	Not clear what level of protection; hoped at least 50%	Won't be available till 2010 or later, but great potential as female-controlled method. Some countries need to be involved in trials of candidate products.

STI, sexually transmitted infection; HSV2, herpes simplex virus 2; PMTCT, prevention of maternal-to-child transmission; SRH, RCT, randomized controlled trial. SRH, sexual and reproductive health.
From the Southern African Development Community (SADC) Expert Think Tank Meeting on HIV Prevention in High Prevalence Countries in Southern Africa; May 10–12, 2006; Maseru, Lesotho. (Adapted with permission.)

for "catch-up"—the rapid acquisition of HIV soon after becoming sexually active. Young women may not benefit from the strategy of abstinence because, despite being abstinent until marriage, a number of them become infected by their husband soon after marriage.

Faithfulness is a key prevention strategy, especially in the context of multiple concurrent relationships in a generalized epidemic. The high risk of HIV transmission during the acute stage of infection makes this form of sexual networking extremely dangerous, and concurrency is an important driver of the HIV/AIDS epidemic in southern Africa.[56,57] Because concurrency typically involves stable relationships with one or more partners outside the primary relationship, there is a diminished likelihood of condom use with these partners.

Condoms have been proven to be effective against HIV transmission,[58] but condom use is usually low in marriage and other long-term stable partnerships. Access to condoms is still low, and UNAIDS estimates there is only 19% condom coverage in sub-Saharan Africa.[47]

Female condoms, which have the potential for providing a female-controlled prevention method, have been insufficiently programmed and scaled up for population impact.

Condoms, of course, also protect against STIs. Control and treatment of STIs is an important strategy to prevent HIV; however, treatment is likely to be more effective when the epidemic has not yet become generalized. In a generalized epidemic, STIs are less important as facilitators of HIV. In many countries where genital herpes (herpes simplex type 2, or HSV2) is the dominant STI, it is not yet clear what treatment will reduce the risk of HIV from this infection. HSV2 has emerged as a major risk factor for HIV transmission and acquisition.

MALE CIRCUMCISION

Three recent trials in South Africa, Kenya and Uganda were stopped early, as they demonstrated a protective effect for men ranging from 50% to 65%. There is a further trial in Uganda examining the effect of circumcision on HIV/infected men, and there is also some evidence of the protective effect of circumcision on male to female transmission.[59,60,61]

VOLUNTARY COUNSELING AND TESTING

Voluntary counseling and testing (VCT) has been the mainstay prevention strategy in much of sub-Saharan Africa, even in the absence of ART. However, aside from being effective for couples, and possibly for HIV-positive persons, its efficacy on a population-wide basis is not clear. With more widely available treatment programs, VCT has become important as an entry point for such programs and for the prevention of maternal-to-child transmission of HIV.

BEHAVIOR CHANGE INTERVENTIONS

Mass media approaches and certain curriculum-based HIV and sex education designs for in-school youth are effective in producing behavior change among young people.[62] Behavior change approaches should be theory driven. The theories range from those that are individually focused (i.e., the health belief model and the theory of reasoned action/planned behavior[63]) to those that focus on groups and communities (i.e., the ecological model and the theory of the diffusion of innovations[64]). The theory of reasoned action/planned behavior emphasizes beliefs, attitudes, intentions, and subjective norms as being important in behavior, whereas the diffusion of innovations theory, which seeks to explain how new ideas and practices spread in a community, gives attention to knowledge, persuasion, decision making, implementation, and confirmation. A number of theories are used in combination in developing behavior change approaches.

FEMALE DIAPHRAGM

Because the female diaphragm covers the cervix, the site most vulnerable to HIV infection, the diaphragm is a potentially protective device that is female controlled.

Female-controlled interventions have a high priority because of the gender imbalance and consequent power relations imbalance.

MICROBICIDES

Microbicides have generated a lot of interest, particularly as a female-controlled prevention method that, unlike the female condom and to some extent the diaphragm, is invisible to the partner. Until 2000, there was excitement that microbicides would soon become an important HIV prevention tool, because there was an effective candidate product: nonoxynol-9. However, studies showed that nonoxynol-9 irritated the vagina and hence had the potential to increase HIV transmission.[65] This product was subsequently abandoned. Work is ongoing on other candidate microbicides, but no new product will be available for public use for at least 3 years.

ROLE OF ADVOCACY

Advocacy—lobbying or campaigning for a particular decision or perspective—is extremely important in HIV/AIDS prevention. It involves information, education, and communication strategies; groups and individuals to partner with or lobby; and a position or decision to advocate. Individuals or groups who are highly visible, organized, networked, and influential can be powerful advocates. Uganda was able to reduce its HIV infection rate because of the visible commitment of its president, together with a multisectoral approach and widespread societal involvement.[66] Advocacy is often linked to policy development, articulation, and implementation. Policies are frameworks that guide decision making. For example, policies on HIV and injection drug users may include strategies for needle exchange or the provision of bleach to clean the injection equipment. A policy may also exist whereby all newly diagnosed TB patients are screened for HIV.

HIV/AIDS Programs

In many countries, NGOs were the first to begin to respond to the HIV epidemic. Although many governments have begun to roll out prevention and treatment programs, HIV/AIDS prevention, and to some extent treatment, still remains a major focus for NGOs. However, governments are ultimately responsible for the well-being of their people. HIV/AIDS programs should meet the following criteria:

1. **The program should work within the framework of the national AIDS control program.** The national AIDS prevention and control bodies vary from country to country. Some countries have a national AIDS control program within the MoH, where the functions of AIDS control are largely focused on program logistics and technical aspects. Other countries have tried to promote a multisectoral approach and tried to engage a

---

BOX 8-2. ACCESSING HIV/AIDS CARE IN LOW- AND MIDDLE-INCOME COUNTRIES: SOME OF THE CHALLENGES

Tandi came to the clinic because she was suffering from a chronic cough she had had for some time. She had lost a lot of weight—her bones were beginning to stick out—and she had had a skin disease, the marks of which were still visible over her face and much of her upper body. She had a fever and felt sick. To be able to come to the clinic, she had borrowed money for the fee. After waiting two hours, she was finally seen by the sister-in-charge.

After examination, the sister-in-charge referred her to the hospital, where she would be seen by a doctor. The sister-in-charge wanted to call an ambulance for her, since she was concerned that Tandi was too weak and ill to go on her own. Tandi, however, refused, for she did not have money to pay the ambulance. Instead, she would take the cheaper public transport even though she would have to take two buses. When Tandi eventually got to the hospital, it was nearly evening. She had to queue again, and pay again. Tandi waited in the queue for three hours.

When a doctor examined her, he told her that he needed to order some tests for her to see how well her body's defense

(immune) system was functioning and to find out what was causing her cough. He told her what these tests were likely to cost. However, Tandi had already spent all the money she had borrowed. In fact, she had been hoping that she could save some of it to buy food for herself and her two children, aged 6 and 10. The doctor then gave her a prescription for some medicines, which included an antibiotic called Bactrim. At the hospital pharmacy, they only had the Bactrim. They told Tandi to go and buy the other medicines. Tandi then set off home, walking, because she had no more money.

Two days later, after the neighbors had found her collapsed in bed, she was taken back to the hospital. The neighbors and friends had made a collection for her, which helped to pay for the hospital stay. When Tandi came out she was better: she had gained some weight, and the cough had become a little better. Her relatives and friends felt that she should go to her aunt in the rural areas, because the rent was due for her room and she could not pay for it. Hopefully, in the rural areas, she could go to a mission hospital where the fees were not as expensive.

---

range of stakeholders, including civil society, which are formed into a board of a coordinating agency that is a separate entity. The board directs and oversees the work of the executive director and his staff. In this model, a major function of the coordinating body, in addition to coordination, is advocacy. The actual programs (e.g., condom promotion) remain in the relevant section of the MoH.

Since 2004, UNAIDS has been promoting the *Three Ones* principle:

- One agreed-upon HIV/AIDS action framework that forms the basis for the partners working together
- One national AIDS coordinating authority, which has a broad-based multisectoral mandate
- One agreed-upon country-level monitoring and evaluation system

2. **All programs should have monitoring (assessment of whether and how the program activities are being carried out) and evaluation (assessment of the extent to which the programs are likely to make an impact) components.** This means that there should be a baseline assessment before the program is implemented. Sometimes this has not been the case, and subsequently there were attempts, usually not very satisfactory, to evaluate this retroactively. The monitoring and evaluation system should fit into the national monitoring and evaluating system.

3. **To optimize the impact of any prevention control and treatment program, there should be a number of interventions implemented at the same time.** These should include voluntary counseling and testing (especially as an entry point to ART); ongoing counseling facilities and support groups; and information, education, and communication (IEC). Depending on the target groups, the IEC should involve abstinence, being faithful to one mutually faithful partner, and/or correct and consistent condom use. There should also be a sexually transmitted disease treatment and control intervention. If the target population includes women of childbearing age, there will be a need for a PMTCT program. Stigma continues to blight HIV/AIDS activities, and in some instances TB control, and efforts should be made to reduce stigma through advocacy activities, the support of opinion leaders and decision makers, and efforts to encourage greater openness.

4. **Especially in high-prevalence areas, there is a need for strong links with the TB control program.** Screening for TB as a standard procedure among individuals who test positive for HIV is being actively considered, as is screening for HIV among people who are found to have TB. In both instances, treatment should be available.

5. **In areas where there are high levels of AIDS-related illness and death, prevention, control and treatment programs should be linked to**

mitigation activities. These activities include home-based care for persons living with HIV/AIDS (PLWH), including discharge planning and links to hospital care services; orphan care; nutrition support and income generation activities; and poverty alleviation.

HIV/AIDS AND TUBERCULOSIS: TWO DISEASES, ONE PATIENT

The links between TB and HIV are well established. HIV is driving the TB epidemic in much of the world, especially in sub-Saharan Africa, and increasingly in Asia and South America. TB is the leading cause of morbidity and mortality among those with HIV infection. The overlap has resulted in the phrase "two diseases, one patient" to remind health care workers that although health systems may be designed by separate disease control programs, they may be treating the same patient.

Tuberculosis and HIV appear to enjoy a dangerous biological synergy. Untreated HIV results in progressive immunodeficiency that predominantly affects cell-mediated immunity, which increases the risk for developing OIs such as TB. As immunosuppression from HIV progresses, so does the frequency and severity of OIs, which are associated with overall increased mortality rates. In recent years, it has also been shown that HIV-infected individuals with TB disease had higher adjusted mortality rates and incidence of non-TB OIs than HIV-infected individuals who did not have active TB.[67] It has been postulated that the immune activation induced by TB leads to a burst of HIV replication and, subsequently, irreversible, accelerated HIV disease progression. Thus, TB and HIV participate in a negative feedback loop, each negatively affecting the other.

Recognizing this undeniable overlap and the need for a coordinated response to both epidemics, in 2002 the Strategic Framework to Decrease the Burden of TB/HIV was developed. In the document reporting this framework, it was acknowledged that "tackling tuberculosis should include tackling HIV as the most potent force driving the tuberculosis epidemic; [similarly,] tackling HIV should include tackling tuberculosis as a leading killer of PLWH."[68] This seminal manual was followed by several others over the next few years that provided policy guidance and implementation guidelines for collaborative TB/HIV activities.

The key concepts of a coordinated TB/HIV strategy include the following: (1) establishing mechanisms for collaboration, such as joint coordinating and planning bodies, and conducting surveillance to capture the overlap of patients with both diseases; (2) decreasing the TB burden among PLWH by intensified screening for TB among those diagnosed as HIV infected, using isoniazid preventive therapy among PLWH, and reducing TB transmission through appropriate infection control

measures in congregate settings; and (3) decreasing the burden of HIV among TB patients by providing VCT to those diagnosed with TB, counseling about HIV prevention, using co-trimoxazole preventive therapy and (when eligible) ART, and ensuring HIV care and support.[69] Guidelines that describe what joint TB/HIV activities to implement, how to implement them, and by whom were created by the WHO to support national TB control and HIV/AIDS control program managers in operationalizing this strategy.

Establishing Mechanisms for Collaboration on Controlling Tuberculosis and HIV

Collaboration between the national programs for TB control and HIV/AIDS control should occur at every level—from the central offices at the national level down to the district or facility level. At the national level, joint coordinating and planning bodies or committees should exist. Surveillance to capture the HIV prevalence among TB patients should be conducted. Evidence of joint activities at the facility level, where a student is most likely to encounter the product(s) of joint planning and coordination, may be through coordinated and, ideally, seamless services for patients with TB and HIV. Care that is fragmented suggests a lack of adequate planning and coordination from control program managers.

Decreasing the Burden of Tuberculosis in People Living with HIV/AIDS

Intensifying case-finding for TB in practical terms is usually done through routine screening of HIV-infected persons for active tuberculosis at the time of their HIV diagnosis. Screening procedures are not defined by the WHO but generally include asking patients about TB symptoms and obtaining a chest radiograph. The value of routine collection of sputum samples for smears and cultures is also being studied. Screening for TB may be done at the HIV testing center or by referring the patient to a TB diagnostic site.

HIV-infected patients in whom active TB has been excluded are generally tested for latent TB infection (LTBI) by TST. If diagnosed with LTBI, patients may be offered isoniazid preventive therapy for 6 months to decrease the risk of recent TB infection progressing to active disease and the risk of reactivation of LTBI. The duration of benefit from isoniazid preventive therapy is limited to approximately 2.5 years,[70] most likely due to recurrent reinfection in TB-endemic settings.

Infection control measures to reduce the risk of TB transmission in health care and congregate settings (e.g., prisons, military barracks) are recommended. Mechanisms to recognize suspected cases of TB and promptly diagnose and initiate treatment among those confirmed are essential to reducing TB transmission. Separation of people suspected of having TB from others (particularly HIV-infected persons) until a diagnosis can be confirmed is an effective, and generally feasible, option. Whenever possible, natural ventilation should be maximized. Every health care and congregate setting should develop and implement its own infection control plan.

Decreasing the Burden of HIV Among Tuberculosis Patients

Many patients do not know their HIV status at the time they are diagnosed with tuberculosis. In settings where the HIV prevalence among TB patients is greater than 5%, patients diagnosed with active TB disease should be provided HIV VCT on an opt-out basis (i.e., it is provided as the standard of care, and patients must decline testing). Health care workers for TB control programs should include HIV prevention methods and education to reduce sexual, parenteral, and vertical transmission of HIV as part of their routine care or make appropriate referrals. Co-trimoxazole preventive therapy to prevent secondary bacterial and parasitic infections is also recommended by the WHO for HIV-infected adults and children. Specifically, co-trimoxazole preventive therapy has been shown to reduce mortality rates in HIV-infected tuberculosis patients.[71] HIV-infected tuberculosis patients should have access to general HIV/AIDS care and support, which includes clinical management (prophylaxis, diagnosis, treatment, and follow-up for OIs), nursing care (promoting hygiene and nutrition), palliative care, home care (including education for household members), counseling, and social support.

HIV-infected TB patients should be offered antiretroviral therapy based on the eligibility criteria of the respective national HIV/AIDS control program guidelines. Co-treatment of active TB and HIV is complicated by drug-drug interactions between rifampin and some NNRTIs and protease inhibitors (PIs). Rifampin stimulates the cytochrome P450 liver enzyme system that metabolizes NNRTIs and PIs and therefore can lead to decreased blood levels of NNRTIs and PIs. Similarly, NNRTIs and PIs can activate or inhibit this enzyme system, leading to altered levels of rifampin. The results can be higher or lower blood levels of these medications, causing ineffective, suboptimal therapeutic levels or increased risk for drug toxicity.

Treating Tuberculosis and HIV/AIDS Together

In patients diagnosed with TB and HIV infection simultaneously, generally the priority is to initiate treatment for TB. Depending on clinical indications, treatment options include starting ART after the initial phase of TB treatment is completed or after the entire course of TB treatment is completed. If indicated, treatment for both HIV and TB can be started concomitantly, but careful management is needed. In this situation, TB can be treated with a rifampin-containing regimen and ART consisting of efavirenz and two NRTIs.

When a patient with HIV-associated TB who has been started on ART and TB treatment simultaneously experiences a paradoxical worsening with exacerbation of symptoms, signs, or radiographic manifestations of TB, immune reconstitution inflammatory syndrome (IRIS) should be suspected. This paradoxical reaction occurs from a reconstitution of the immune system and may be accompanied by a high fever, lymphadenopathy, expanding central nervous system lesions, and worsening of chest x-ray findings.[72] Other possible causes (including TB treatment failure) must be excluded in the evaluation. Prednisone may be helpful in severe paradoxical reactions, although evidence to support its use is lacking.

STUDY QUESTIONS

1. What are the pros and cons of currently available diagnostic tests for TB?
2. Why is TB treatment difficult to complete?
3. What are the main challenges today to controlling TB globally?
4. Why is the prevention of HIV/AIDS of such significant public health importance in transitional and low- and middle-income countries?
5. What are the policy and operational issues in PMTCT and ART rollout in low- and middle-income countries?
6. What HIV/AIDS prevention strategies are likely to be effective in countries without a generalized epidemic?

RESOURCES

International Tuberculosis Organizations

- WHO, Stop TB Department: www.who.int/gtb/
- Stop TB Partnership: www.stoptb.org/
- International Union Against Tuberculosis and Lung Disease: www.iuatld.org
- KNCV Tuberculosis Foundation: www.kncvtbc.nl/Site/Professional.aspx
- The Global Fund to Fight AIDS, Tuberculosis and Malaria: www.theglobalfund.org

Selected Tuberculosis Literature

- *Bulletin of the World Health Organization* 2002;80(6) http://www.who.int/docstore/bulletin/pdf/2002/bul-6-E-2002/80(6)471–476.pdf
- *An Expanded DOTS Framework for Effective Tuberculosis Control* (WHO/CDS/TB/2002.297) http://www. who.int/gtb/publications/dots/index.htm

- *Global Tuberculosis Control: Surveillance, Planning, Financing. WHO Report 2006* (WHO/CDS/TB/2003.316)
  http://www.who.int/gtb/publications/globrep/index.html
- *Guidelines for Implementing Collaborative TB and HIV Programme Activities* (WHO/CDS/TB/2003.319, WHO/HIV/2003.01)
  http://www.who.int/gtb/ publications/tb_hiv/2003_319/tbhiv_guidelines.pdf
- *Management of Tuberculosis: A Guide for Low Income Countries,* 5th ed. (IUATLD, 2000)
  http://www.iuatld.org/full_picture/en/frameset/frameset.phtml
- *TB/HIV: A Clinical Manual* (WHO/HTM/TB/ 2004.329) http://whqlibdoc.who.int/publications/2004/9241546344. pdf
- *Treatment of Tuberculosis: Guidelines for National Programmes* (WHO/CDS/TB/2003.313)
  http://www. who.int/gtb/publications/ttgnp/index.html
- *Tuberculosis Handbook* (WHO/TB/98.253)
  http://www. who.int/gtb/publications/tbhandbook/index.htm

Selected HIV/AIDS Websites

- AIDS Action (USA): www.aidsaction.org
  A network of 3,200 AIDS service organizations sharing information and experiences.
- AIDS and Africa: www.aidsafrica.com
  Provides wide-ranging information on HIV/AIDS in Africa.
- AIDSETI (AIDS Empowerment and Treatment Initiative): www.aidseti.org
  An international activist organization, with two-thirds of its membership living with HIV. It advocates and lobbies for increased treatment access.
- ANNEA: www.annea.org.tz
  An AIDS NGO network incorporating organizations in Kenya, Tanzania, and Uganda.
- Centers for Disease Control and Prevention (US Department of Health and Human Services): www.cdc.gov
  Focuses on health and treatment-related issues and surveillance.
- Education International: www.ei-ie.org/aids.htm
  Dedicated to school health and HIV/AIDS prevention, documenting the widespread ideas and experiences of Education International and its partners.
- Family Health International: www.fhi.org
  Works to improve reproductive and family health around the world.
- Global AIDS Alliance (GAA): www.globalaidsalliance.org
  A transnational alliance of partner organizations.
- Global AIDS Interfaith Alliance: www.thegaia.org
  Facilitates HIV prevention strategies in developing countries through religious and interfaith organizations.
- Global Fund to Fight HIV/AIDS, Tuberculosis and Malaria: www.globalfundatm.org
  International funding mechanism to expand the response to these diseases.
- Global Health Council: www.globalhealthcouncil.org
  The world's largest membership alliance dedicated to improving health worldwide.
- Health Economics and HIV/AIDS Research Division, Natal University: www.und.ac.za/und/heard
  Undertakes research, publication, policy analysis, planning, and information services on socioeconomic development and HIV/AIDS. In particular, produced *AIDS Briefs* and *AIDS Toolkits* on HIV/AIDS and sectoral impacts and responses that can be downloaded from the Web.
- Healthlink Worldwide (formerly AHRTAG): www.healthlink.org.uk
  Works to improve the health of poor and vulnerable communities by strengthening the provision, use, and impact of information.
- International AIDS Economic Network (IAEN): www.iaen.org
  Provides analysis on the economics of HIV/AIDS prevention and treatment in developing countries.
- International AIDS Vaccine Initiative: www.iavi.org
  AIDS vaccine advocacy coalition.
- International Association of Physicians in AIDS Care: www.iapac.org
  Provides information on clinical management and public health policy.
- International Centre for Research on Women: www.icrw.org
  Works to improve the lives of women in poverty, advance women's equality and human rights, and contribute to economic and social well-being.
- International Labour Organisation: www.ilo.org
  Labor organization of the United Nations (UN), with a focus on HIV/AIDS and the world of work.
- Programme for Appropriate Technology in Health: www.path.org
  International nonprofit organization to improve health, especially the health of women and children.
- SAfAIDS (Southern Africa HIV and AIDS Information Dissemination Service): www.safaids.org.zw
  Information service on HIV/AIDS in southern Africa.
- Save the Children UK: www.savethechildren.org.uk
  Supports children in need and is prioritizing HIV/AIDS. The website introduces the organization's work. Among other publications, it has produced *Learning to Live: Monitoring and Evaluating HIV/AIDS Programmes for Your People,* a wide-ranging, practical handbook for policy makers and practitioners.

- Stop Global AIDS: www.stopglobalaids.org
  Civic society pressure group to pressure the US government to provide more resources to fight AIDS in developing countries.
- Teaching-aids at Low Cost: www.talcuk.org
  Provides low-cost materials on HIV/AIDS regarding wide-ranging development issues, with a catalogue of books, slides, videos, and participatory teaching aids.
- UNAIDS: www.unaids.org
  UN coordination agency on HIV/AIDS to lead, strengthen, and support an expanded response to the epidemic; extensive links to UNAIDS, co-sponsors, and many other websites on wide-ranging areas of focus; UNAIDS publications include the *Best Practice Collection* series with Technical Updates, Case Studies, and Key Materials.
- UNDP (UN Development Programme): www.undp.org
  Development agency of the UN, with an HIV/AIDS program concerning human rights, poverty, and development.
- UNODC (UN Office on Drugs and Crime): www.unodc.org
  The drug control arm of the UN, including a focus on intravenous drug use and HIV/AIDS.
- UNESCO: www.unesco.org
  UN focal agency for education, science, and culture, with wide-ranging publications and information on these areas, including a focus on HIV/AIDS.
- UNFPA (UN Population Fund): www.unfpa.org
  Focus on sexual and reproductive health and population and development; publications include the annual *State of the World's Population* and a series of *HIV Prevention Briefs*.
- UNICEF: www.unicef.org
  UN's children's fund, with a strong focus on HIV/AIDS and children, including parent-to-child transmission; publications include the annual update *State of the Children*.
- UNIFEM: www.unifem.org
  Works to promote gender equity and equality and women's rights; focuses on gender issues and HIV/AIDS.
- World Health Organization: www.who.org
  Health agency of the UN, with wide-ranging information related to health care, surveillance, transmission and prevention, voluntary counseling and testing, and other areas.
- World Bank: www.worldbank.org
  Apart from a wide focus on economic development and HIV/AIDS, the World Bank has a multicountry HIV/AIDS Program for Africa (MAP). MAP aims to significantly increase access to HIV/AIDS prevention care and treatment programs.
- Youth Against AIDS: www.yaids.org
  Global network of support for young AIDS activists.

REFERENCES

1. World Health Organization. *Global Tuberculosis Control: Surveillance, Planning, Financing.* Geneva, World Health Organization, 2007. WHO/HTM/TB/2007.376.
2. Dye C. Global epidemiology of tuberculosis. *Lancet* 2006; 367:938–940.
3. Centers for Disease Control and Prevention. Emergence of *Mycobacterium tuberculosis* with extensive resistance to second-line drugs—worldwide, 2000–2004. *MMWR* 2006;55(11): 301–305.
4. Joint United Nations Programme on HIV/AIDS (UNAIDS) and World Health Organization (WHO). *AIDS Epidemic Update: December 2005.* Geneva: UNAIDS/WHO, 2005. UNAIDS/05.19E.
5. Raviglione MC, O'Brien RJ. Tuberculosis. In: Kasper DL, Braunwald E, Fauci A, et al., eds. *Harrison's Principles of Internal Medicine.* 16th ed. New York: McGraw-Hill, 2005: 953.
6. World Health Organization. *Treatment of Tuberculosis: Guidelines for National Programmes.* Geneva, World Health Organization, 2003. WHO/CDS/TB/2003.313.
7. World Health Organization. BCG vaccine: WHO position paper. *Wkly Epidemiol Rec* 2004;79(4):27–38.
8. Colditz GA, Brewer TF, Berkey CS. Efficacy of BCG vaccine in the prevention of tuberculosis: meta-analysis of the published literature. *JAMA* 1994;271(9):698–702.
9. Larkin JM, von Reyn CF. BCG and new vaccines against tuberculosis. In: Schlossberg D, ed. *Tuberculosis and Nontuberculosis Mycobacterial Infections.* 5th ed. New York: McGraw-Hill, 2006:117–122.
10. Jasmer RM, Seaman CB, Gonzalez LC, et al. Tuberculosis treatment outcomes: directly observed therapy compared with self-administered therapy. *Am J Respir Crit Care Med* 20041; 170(5):561–566.
11. World Bank. *World Development Report 1993: Investing in Health.* New York: Oxford University Press, 1993.
12. Médecins Sans Frontières. *Running Out of Breath? TB Care in the 21st Century.* Geneva: Médecins Sans Frontières, March 2004.
13. Pope DS, Chaisson RE. TB treatment: as simple as DOT? *Int J Tuberc Lung Dis* 2003;7(7):611–615.
14. Zwarenstein M, Schoeman JH, Vundule C, et al. Randomised controlled trial of self supervised and directly observed treatment of tuberculosis. *Lancet* 1998;352(9137):1340–1343.
15. World Health Organization/International Union Against Tuberculosis and Lung Disease Global Project on Anti-Tuberculosis Drug Resistance Surveillance. *Anti-Tuberculosis Drug Resistance in the World: Report No. 3.* Geneva: World Health Organization, 2004.
16. World Health Organization. *Guidelines for the Programmatic Management of Drug-Resistant Tuberculosis.* Geneva: World Health Organization, 2006. WHO/HTM/TB/2006.361.
17. Physicians for Human Rights. *An Action Plan to Prevent Brain Drain: Building Equitable Health Systems in Africa.* Boston: Physicians for Human Rights, June 2004.
18. World Health Organization. *Addressing Poverty in TB Control—Options for National TB Control Programmes.* Geneva: World Health Organization, 2005. WHO/HTM/TB/2005.352.
19. Lalvani A, Pathan AA, McShane H, et al. Rapid detection of *Mycobacterium tuberculosis* infection by enumeration of antigen-specific T cells. *Am J Respir Crit Care Med* 2001; 163(4): 824–828.

20. Mazurek GH, LoBue PA, Daley CL, et al. Comparison of a whole-blood interferon gamma assay with tuberculin skin testing for detecting latent *Mycobacterium tuberculosis* infection. *JAMA* 2001;286(14):1740–1747.

21. Andries K, Verhasselt P, Guillemont J, et al. A diarylquinoline drug active on the ATP synthase of *Mycobacterium tuberculosis*. *Science* 2005;307:223–227.

22. Vuola JM, Ristola MA, Cole B, et al. Immunogenicity of an inactivated mycobacterial vaccine for the prevention of HIV-associated tuberculosis: a randomized, controlled trial. *AIDS* 2003;17(16):2351–2355.

23. McShane H, Pathan AA, Sander CR, et al. Boosting BCG with MVA85A: the first candidate subunit vaccine for tuberculosis in clinical trials. *Tuberculosis (Edinb)* 2005;85(1–2):47–52.

24. Gottlieb MS, Schorff R, Schanker HM, et al. *Pneumocystis carinii* pneumonia and mucosal candidiasis in previously healthy homosexual men: evidence of a new acquired cellular immunodeficiency. *N Engl J Med* 1981;305:1425–1431.

25. Masur H, Michelis MA, Greene JB, et al. An outbreak of community-acquired *Pneumocystis carinii* pneumonia: initial manifestation of cellular immune dysfunction. *N Engl J Med* 1981;305:1431–1438.

26. Siegal FP, Lopez, C, Hammer GS, et al. Severe acquired immunodeficiency in male homosexuals, manifested by chronic perianal ulcerative herpes simplex lesions. *N Engl J Med* 1981; 305:1439–1444.

27. CDC Task Force on Kaposi's Sarcoma and Opportunistic Infections. Epidemiologic aspects of the current outbreak of Kaposi's sarcoma and opportunistic infections. *N Engl J Med* 1982;306:248–252.

28. Davis KC, Horsburgh CR Jr, Hasiba U, et al. Acquired immunodeficiency syndrome in a patient with hemophilia. *Ann Intern Med* 1983;98:284–286.

29. Poon MC, Landay A, Prasthofer EF, et al. Acquired immunodeficiency syndrome with *Pneumocystis carinii* pneumonia and *Mycobacterium avium-intracellulare* infection in a previously healthy patient with classic hemophilia. Clinical, immunologic, and virologic findings. *Ann Intern Med* 1983;98: 287–290.

30. Elliott JL, Hoppes WL, Platt MS, et al. The acquired immunodeficiency syndrome and *Mycobacterium avium-intracellulare* bacteremia in a patient with hemophilia. *Ann Intern Med* 1983; 98:290–293.

31. Curran JW, Lawrence DN, Jaffe H, et al. Acquired immunodeficiency syndrome (AIDS) associated with transfusions. *N Engl J Med* 1984;310:69–75.

32. Jaffe HW, Francis DP, McLane MF, et al. Transfusion-associated AIDS: serological evidence of human T-cell leukemia virus infection of donors. *Science* 1984;223:1309–1312.

33. Oleske J, Minnefor A, Cooper R Jr, et al. Immune deficiency syndrome in children. *JAMA* 1983;249:2345–2349.

34. Rubinstein A, Sicklick M, Gupta A, et al. Acquired immunodeficiency with reversed T4/T8 ratios in infants born to promiscuous and drug-addicted mothers. *JAMA* 1983;249:2350–2356.

35. Clumeck N, Mascart-Lemone F, de Maubeuge J, et al. Acquired immune deficiency syndrome in black Africans. *Lancet* 1983;1:642.

36. Francis DP, Curran JW, Essex M. Epidemic acquired immune deficiency syndrome: epidemiologic evidence for a transmissible agent. *J Natl Cancer Inst* 1983;71:1–4.

37. Essex M, McLane MF, Lee TH, et al. Antibodies to cell membrane antigens associated with human T-cell leukemia virus in patients with AIDS. *Science* 1983;220:859–862.

38. Gelmann EP, Popovic M, Blayney D, et al. Proviral DNA of a retrovirus, human T-cell leukemia virus, in two patients with AIDS. *Science* 1983;220:862–865.

39. Essex M, McLane MF, Lee TH, et al. Antibodies to human T-cell leukemia virus membrane antigens (HTLV-MA) in hemophiliacs. *Science* 1983;221:1061–1064.

40. Gallo RC, Sarin PS, Gelmann EP, et al. Isolation of human T-cell leukemia virus in acquired immune deficiency syndrome (AIDS). *Science* 1983;220:865–867.

41. Barre-Sinoussi F, Chermann JC, Rey F, et al. Isolation of a T-lymphotropic retrovirus from a patient at risk for acquired immune deficiency syndrome (AIDS). *Science* 1983;220:868–871.

42. Kanki PJ, Hamel DJ, Sankale JL, et al. Human immunodeficiency virus type 1 subtypes differ in disease progression. *J Infect Dis* 1999;179:68–73.

43. Laeyendecker O, Li X, Arroyo M, et al. The effect of HIV subtype on rapid disease progression in Rakai, Uganda. Abstract no. 44LB. Presented at: 13th Conference on Retroviruses and Opportunistic Infections; February 2006.

44. Jackson H. *AIDS Africa: Continent in Crisis*. Harare, Zimbabwe: Southern Africa HIV/AIDS Information, 2002.

45. World Health Organization. *Clinical Guidelines for HIV/AIDS*. Geneva: World Health Organization, 2002.

46. Guay LA, Musoke P, Fleming T, et al. Intrapartum and neonatal nevirapine compared with zidovudine for prevention of maternal to child transmission of HIV-1 in Kampala, Uganda: HIVNET 012 randomised trial. *Lancet* 1999;354:795–802.

47. Joint United Nations Programme on HIV/AIDS (UNAIDS). *2006 Report on the Global AIDS Epidemic*. Geneva: UNAIDS, 2006:114.

48. Ward DE. *The AMFAR AIDS Handbook: The Complete Guide to Understanding HIV and AIDS*. New York: W.W. Norton, 1999.

49. Joint United Nations Programme on HIV/AIDS (UNAIDS). *2002 Report on the Global AIDS Epidemic*. Geneva: UNAIDS, 2002.

50. Meda B, Ndoye I, M'Boup S, et al. Low and stable HIV infection rates in Senegal: natural course of the epidemic or evidence for the success of prevention? *AIDS* 1999;13:1397–1405. Also see http://www.who.int/inf-new/aids3.htm and http://www.africarecovery.org.

51. Henenberg RS, Rojanapithayakorn W, Kunasol P, et al. Impact of Thailand's HIV control programme as indicated by the decline of sexually transmitted diseases. *Lancet* 1994;344: 243–245.

52. World Health Organization. Thailand achieves sustained reduction in HIV infection rates. In: *Health: A Key to Prosperity. Success Stories in Developing Countries*. Geneva: World Health Organization, 2000. http://www.who.int/int-new/aids1.htm.

53. Celentano DD, Nelson KE, Lyles CM, et al. Decreasing incidence of HIV and sexually transmitted diseases in young Thai men: evidence for success of the HIV/AIDS control and prevention program. *AIDS* 1998;12:F29–F36.

54. Des Jarlais DC, Friedman S, Choopanya K, et al. International epidemiology of HIV/AIDs among injecting drug users. *AIDS* 1992;6:1053–1068, 1992.

55. Asiimwe-Okiror G, Opio AA, Musinguzi J, et al. Change in sexual behaviour and decline in HIV infection among young pregnant women in rural Uganda. *AIDS* 1997;11:1757–1763.

56. Hankins C. Changes in patterns of risk. *AIDS Care* 1998; 10:S147–S153.

57. Morris M, Kretzschmar M. Concurrent partnerships and the spread of HIV. *AIDS* 1997;11:641–648.

58. Weller S, Davis K. *Condom Effectiveness in Reducing Heterosexual HIV Transmission*. Chichester, United Kingdom: John Wiley and Sons, 2004. The Cochrane Library, issue 2.

59. Auvert B, Taljaard D, Lagarde E, et al. Randomized, controlled intervention trial of male circumcision for reduction of HIV infection risk: the ANRS 1265 trial. *PLoS Med* 2005;2(11):-e298.

60. Gray R, Kigozi G, Scrwada D, Makumbi F, et al. Male Circumcision for HIV Prevention in men in Rakai Uganda: a randomized trial. *Lanet* 2007;369:657–713.

61. Gray RH, Kiwanuka N, Quinn TC, Sewan Kambo NK, et al. Male Circumcision and HIV Acquistion and Transmission: cohort studies in Rakai, Uganda, Rakai Project Team. AIDS 2000;14(15):2371–81.

62. Kaisernetwork.org HealthCast. *HIV Prevention Among Young People: Measuring the Impact* [Webcast]. Washington, DC: World Bank, September 8, 2004. http://www.kaisernetwork.org/health_cast/hcast_index.cfm?display=detail&hc=1263.

63. Ajzen I, Fishbein M. *Understanding Attitudes and Predicting Social Behavior*. Englewood Cliffs, NJ: Prentice-Hall, 1980.

64. Rogers E. *The Diffusion of Innovations*. 4th ed. New York: The Free Press, 1995.

65. US Government Accountability Office. *HHS: Efforts to Research and Inform the Public About Nonoxynol-9 and HIV.* Washington, DC: US Government Accountability Office, March 2005. GAO-05-399.

66. Kebaabetswe P, Norr KF. Behavior change: goals and means. In: Essex M, Mboup S, Kanki PJ, et al., eds. *AIDS in Africa*. 2nd ed. New York: Kluwer Academic/Plenum Publishers, 2002:514–526.

67. Badri M, Ehrlich R, Wood R. Association between tuberculosis and HIV disease progression in a high tuberculosis prevalence area. *Int J Tuberc Lung Dis* 2001;5(3):225–232.

68. World Health Organization. *Strategic Framework to Decrease the Burden of TB/HIV*. Geneva: World Health Organization, 2002. WHO/CDS/TB/2002.2, WHO/HIV_AIDS/2002.2.

69. World Health Organization. *Interim Policy on Collaborative TB/HIV Activities*. Geneva: World Health Organization, 2004. WHO/HTM/TB/2004.330, WHO/HTM/HIV/2004.1.

70. Quigley MA, Mwinga A, Hosp M, et al. Long-term effect of preventive therapy for tuberculosis in a cohort of HIV-infected Zambian adults. *AIDS* 2001;15(2):215–222.

71. Zachariah R, Spielmann MP, Chinji C, et al. Voluntary counseling, HIV testing, and adjunctive co-trimoxazole reduces mortality in tuberculosis patients in Thyolo, Malawi. *AIDS* 2003; 17:1053–1061.

72. World Health Organization. *TB/HIV: A Clinical Manual*. 2nd ed. Geneva: World Health Organization, 2004. WHO/HTM/TB/2004.329.

War, Catastrophes, Displaced Persons, Refugees, and Terrorism

9

Sheri Fink and Mark Stinson[†]

LEARNING OBJECTIVES

- *Understand the history of international humanitarian assistance, including the key organizations involved and the principles and laws governing their work.*
- *Know the most common causes of morbidity and mortality in populations affected by conflict, disaster, and terrorism, and the key assessment strategies and public health intervention to consider.*
- *Be familiar with prevention and preparedness approaches to disasters and acts of terrorism, and the roles and limitations of health interventions in conflict mitigation and humanitarian protection.*
- *Be able to apply lessons learned to actual cases involving conflict, disaster, displacement, and terrorism.*
- *Know where to go for updated information on the field of humanitarian assistance and its practice.*

INTRODUCTION

A health professional who wishes to make a positive impact in a disastrous situation faces many challenges. To begin with, goals must be defined. Is the aim of humanitarian medical work to reduce death, sickness, and suffering during a period of acute vulnerability? Or does the work extend to promoting the sustainable development of health systems, and advancing peace, justice, and the respect of human rights? Should the choice to engage in relief work be motivated by religious, political, or military objectives?

Whether or not the aims of the work are narrowly or broadly defined, practitioners need excellent technical skills in evidence-based medicine and public health to avoid doing more harm than good. They must become rapidly familiar with the particular health problems threatening the population in question, and the available resources (structural, human, and organizational) and strategies that exist to cope with them. The most effective aid workers elicit and prioritize the health concerns of those being served; respect, support, learn from, and, when appropriate, guide colleagues; coordinate efforts; maintain flexibility; and strive for equity and efficiency while ensuring that assistance also reaches the most vulnerable populations. These aid workers also dedicate themselves to serving others while taking care to maintain personal health and equanimity in the midst of unfamiliar and stressful situations.

Experienced aid workers realize that their work may put them in danger, and they contribute to individual and group security by respecting sound security protocols, maintaining positive interpersonal relationships (with officials, community members, and colleagues), and collecting and sharing relevant information. In sum, the consummate humanitarian health worker combines compassion, commitment, and integrity with technical proficiency in promoting the delivery of the most appropriate, evidence-based, and up-to-date preventive and curative health services—a tall order in what are often very challenging environments!

The potential dangers, stresses, frustrations, and, at times, monotony of humanitarian work should not be underestimated. Still, far from being a selfless exercise, the rewards of this work are many.

A HISTORY OF HUMANITARIAN WORK

The word "humanitarian" evokes a mysterious figure wearing a stained white coat and operating by candlelight to the percussion of bombs and artillery rounds.

[†]Deceased. Teacher, mentor and healer.

The epithet that graces the frontispiece of the NATO war surgery handbook only reinforces this romantic view of wartime medicine: " . . . How large and various is the experience of the battlefield and how fertile the blood of warriors in the rearing of good surgeons."

In fact, the reality of most aid work differs radically from these images of adrenaline-charged, hands-on crisis medicine. More often effective relief work involves long-running efforts to prevent disease and facilitate access to care. Sometimes, far from being an ideal culture medium for medicine's greatest achievements, the stresses and strains of aid work try the good will and challenge the ethical compasses of those involved in it.

What Is a Humanitarian?

Many groups with different philosophies participate in relief work. Most believe that humanitarian assistance is about relieving suffering and upholding the sanctity of human life in times of conflict and in other situations where the entities that are typically responsible for providing the basic services fundamental to life are not doing so.

The Red Cross movement is the quintessential humanitarian body. Its founder was Henri Dunant, a Swiss businessman who encountered thousands of soldiers of multiple nationalities lying wounded near Solferino, Italy, during the War of Italian Unification in 1859. Dunant assisted the wounded and wrote a book about the experience, highlighting the need for a cadre of pre-trained volunteers ready to assist in emergencies and calling for the establishment of an international relief society.[1] His idea was that aid workers should be allowed to enter the battlefield unharmed as long as they agreed to remain neutral in a conflict.

The Red Cross movement was born out of this idea, and *neutrality, impartiality, independence, volunteerism,* and *humanity* are among the agency's central principles. The Geneva Conventions, discussed later in this chapter, provide the International Committee of the Red Cross (ICRC) with the mandate to protect and assist victims of armed conflict and internal violence. Its activities include, among many others, aiding civilians and prisoners (for example visiting prisoners of war to assess their conditions, transporting messages between family members divided by conflict, and providing medical and surgical assistance), helping to reunite families and trace missing persons, and spreading knowledge about humanitarian law. The ICRC is based in Geneva, Switzerland, and its delegates are Swiss. In addition, nearly 200 countries maintain a Red Cross or Red Crescent society. These societies are members of the International Federation of Red Cross and Red Crescent Societies (IFRC). All of these organizations together form the International Red Cross and Red Crescent Movement.

When Red Cross delegates document violations of the laws of war, they typically make recommendations in confidence to the responsible authorities. This policy of confidentiality helps the organization maintain its unparalleled access, however, does it have its limits? During World War II, ICRC delegates visited concentration camps and did not publicly reveal what they saw. Keeping silent about extreme, persistent human rights violations can be akin to complicity, and now the ICRC occasionally goes public with its findings when governments fail to heed its concerns. For example, the Red Cross challenged the legal basis of detentions at the United States facility in Guantanamo Bay, Cuba. Other relief organizations, such as the non-governmental organization Doctors Without Borders (in French, *Médecins sans Frontières* or MSF) make "bearing witness" to human rights violations and advocating for populations at risk a central part of their humanitarian work. Often aid workers are the only independent outsiders to witness war crimes against civilians.

Who Else Provides Aid?

First and foremost, the majority of assistance provided in conflict and disaster situations, particularly in the critical early days, is performed by local and national— rather than international—agencies and authorities. These include local health providers and health facilities, Red Cross and Red Crescent chapters, civil society organizations, militaries, police, and regular citizens. Too often their work is overlooked or sidelined by international actors coming in to "save the day."

United Nations agencies also play a major role in humanitarian assistance. The UN High Commissioner for Refugees (UNHCR) has a mandate to protect refugees under the 1951 Convention on the Status of Refugees and its 1967 Protocol. In recent years, the agency has also assisted the larger population of internally displaced persons (IDPs), who, unlike refugees, are displaced within their countries of origin. Table 9-1 (Definition of Terms) describes the differences between refugees and IDPs. United Nations agencies and other groups involved in humanitarian work are listed in Table 9-2 (Entities Typically Involved in Relief Work).

The hundreds of non-governmental organizations (NGOs) that exist have diverse histories and philosophies. Some of these non-profit groups were born out of the Red Cross mould. Others offer assistance based on their members' religious convictions to serve the less fortunate. Government agencies, such as the U.S. Agency for International Development (USAID) and the Humanitarian Aid Department of the European Union (ECHO), fund humanitarian assistance at least in part out of the recognition that aid promotes good foreign relations.

Governments sometimes contract out assistance work to private, for-profit companies. In addition, countries have offered the extensive logistical capacities of their militaries to assist in the aftermath of foreign disasters.

Table 9-1. Definition of terms.

Refugee: Defined under international law as a person who "owing to a well-founded fear of being persecuted for reasons of race, religion, nationality, membership of a particular social group, or political opinion, is outside the country of his nationality, and is unable to or, owing to such fear, is unwilling to avail himself of the protection of that country; or who, not having a nationality and being outside the country of his former habitual residence as a result of such events, is unable or owing to such fear, is unwilling to return to it." Article 1, The 1951 Convention Relating to the Status of Refugees.

In 2004 there were an estimated 9.1 million refugees, according to the UNHCR's "The State of the World's Refugees: Human Displacement in the New Millenium." April, 2006.

Internally Displaced Person (IDP): An IDP often flees his or her home for identical reasons as a refugee and faces similar difficulties. IDPs, however, are defined by not having crossed an internationally recognized border. IDPs do not enjoy the legal protections conferred by the 1951 Refugee Convention, but increasingly they are, in practice, being provided with similar assistance according to the UN's 1998 Guiding Principles on Internal Displacement. According to UNHCR, in 2004 there were an estimated 25 million IDPs—there were many more IDPs than refugees because of an increase in internal versus interstate conflicts.

Disaster: A situation or event involving the destruction of property, injuries, and deaths of multiple people, which typically overwhelms local capacity and necessitates outside assistance. Types of disasters include natural (e.g., hydro-meteorological, geological, biological), technological (e.g., mine explosion, chemical spill, other industrial accidents) and human-made (e.g., complex humanitarian emergency).

Complex Humanitarian Emergency (CHE): A disaster that comes about at least in part due to human design. CHE is usually used to describe a disaster that involves multiple components such as large-scale displacement of people in the context of conflict, war, persecution, economic crisis, terrorism, political instability, or social unrest.

Terrorism: There is no internationally agreed-upon definition of terrorism. Terrorism often refers to attacks on non-military targets, such as the deliberate bombing of civilians and the taking and killing of hostages. These kinds of attacks would, if conducted during wartime, violate the laws of war and thus constitute war crimes. Terrorism is sometimes defined as violent, threatening, or criminal acts perpetrated against human victims but aimed against larger targets, usually states, and intended to create fear or terror in the minds of a population.

Civil affairs units of armies involved in military actions in foreign countries may also provide aid to civilians, as Coalition forces did in Iraq. Complexities in the military-humanitarian relationship are explored in Case Study 1.

Local groups listed by the US and other countries as terrorist organizations may also operate wings responsible for providing emergency assistance. For example, Kashmir-based militant groups ran many of the displaced persons camps following the 2005 Pakistan earthquake, and Hezbollah provided aid to victims of the 2006 war in Lebanon. Foreign aid workers should be prepared to encounter these groups in the field.

Coordinating Diverse Agencies

In emergency after emergency, the greatest criticism of the international relief response has been its poor coordination. In recent years, more and more agencies have become involved in humanitarian work. While they operate independently, many have agreed to adhere to a common code of conduct[2] and minimum standards.[3] On-the-ground coordination is typically facilitated by the U.N.'s Office for the Coordination of Humanitarian Affairs (UN-OCHA) or by agencies set up by the governments of affected countries. When arriving in an emergency, it is important to find out about interagency coordination meetings and look for Humanitarian Information Centers (HICs), which are often set up to provide a clearinghouse of information and maps and to keep tabs on "who's doing what where." With advances in satellite and communications technologies, there is an increasing role for technological experts to rapidly establish communications and information networks in emergencies.

The same agencies that respond to conflict-affected populations also tend to respond to major natural disasters. These often occur in parts of the world that are simultaneously affected by conflict, civil strife, and poverty.

CASE STUDY/DILEMMA 1: IRAQ

In late 2002 and early 2003, humanitarian aid agencies prepared to provide assistance to Iraqis in the event of a United States-led military offensive. Non-governmental organizations (NGOs) disagreed about whether to accept US. Government funds to support their work. Some NGO leaders felt that taking the money would allow them to respond to a potential catastrophe, such as massive population displacement or a disease outbreak in a population that had already endured years of sanctions, isolation, and repression. Taking the funds might also give these NGOs a conduit to provide feedback to the United States about the needs of the civilian population. Other NGOs took sharply different positions. Their leaders argued that taking funding from a party to a conflict (belligerent) would compromise the independence of the aid agencies and produce the appearance of taking sides in the conflict.

After the war began, the dilemma deepened. Aid workers disagreed amongst themselves about how they should relate to the US-led coalition and its civil-military operations centers, which were involved in assisting Iraqi civilians.

Table 9-2. Entities typically involved in relief work.

The International Red Cross and Red Crescent Movement:
International Committee of the Red Cross (ICRC) (www.icrc.org), International Federation of the Red Cross and Red Crescent Societies (IFRC) (www.ifrc.org), national Red Cross societies

United Nations Agencies:
Many, including the World Health Organization (WHO) (www.who.int), United Nations Children's Fund (UNICEF) (www.unicef.org), Office for the Coordination of Humanitarian Affairs (OCHA) (ochaonline.un.org), United Nations High Commissioner for Refugees (UNHCR) (www.unhcr.org), World Food Programme (WFP) (www.wfp.org), United Nations Development Program (UNDP) (www.undp.org), Development Fund for Women (UNIFEM) (www.unifem.org), United Nations Population Fund for Activities (UNFPA) (www.unfpa.org)

International non-governmental organizations (NGOs):
Many, including American Jewish World Service (AJWS) (www.ajws.org), American Refugee Committee (ARC) (www.archq.org), CARE (www.care.org), Catholic Relief Services (CRS) (www.crs.org), Doctors of the World (also Médecins du Monde—MDM) (www.doctorsoftheworld.org), Doctors without Borders (also Médecins sans Frontières—MSF) (www.doctorswithoutborders.org), International Medical Corps (IMC) (www.imcworldwide.org), International Rescue Committee (IRC) (www.theirc.org), Islamic Relief (IR) (www.islamic-relief.com), Mercy Corps International (MCI) (www.mercycorps.org), Oxfam International (www.oxfam.org), Save the Children (STC) (www.savethechildren.org), World Vision International (www.worldvision.org)

Local and national non-governmental and civil society organizations:
Many, different in each country

United States government agencies:
US Aid for International Development (USAID) (www.usaid.gov/)
Office for Foreign Disaster Assistance (OFDA) (www.globalcorps.com/ofda.html)
Office of Populations, Refugees and Migration (PRM) (www.state.gov/g/prm/)

Other governmental agencies:
Humanitarian Aid Department of the European Union (ECHO) (ec.europe.eu/echo/index_en.htm)
United Kingdom Department for International Development (DFID) (www.dfid.gov.uk/)
Japan International Cooperation Agency (JICA) (www.jica.go.jp/english/)

Intergovernmental organizations:
International Organization for Migration (IOM) (www.iom.int/)

Military operations:
Peacekeeping Forces
Monitoring Forces
Belligerent Forces (parties to a conflict)
Non-State Militant/Political Organizations
Civilian Military Operations Center (CMOC)
Civil-Military Information Center (CMIC)

Local and national government organizations:
Ministries of Health
Ministries of the Interior

Aid workers cringed when the US-led coalition publicized their work as part of the coalition's effort to win Iraqi "hearts and minds." As insurgent attacks on aid workers grew, many worried about the blurring of the lines between the military, the political, and the humanitarian not only in Iraq, but also in Afghanistan and other countries. Figure 9-1 depicts the medical services one American relief agency provided during the US-led bombing campaign in Afghanistan, ironically treating the wounds a small child sustained from the lingering munitions of a previous war.

Humanitarians in an Age of Terrorism

Terrorism is a major concern for international aid workers, not only because it leads to morbidity and mortality among civilians, but also because aid workers themselves are increasingly the targets of terrorists. In Baghdad, Iraq, in 2003, both the United Nations compound, which housed the UN's political and humanitarian wings, as well as the ICRC headquarters were targeted by suicide bombers.

For their protection in conflict zones, humanitarians had previously relied primarily on an invisible shield

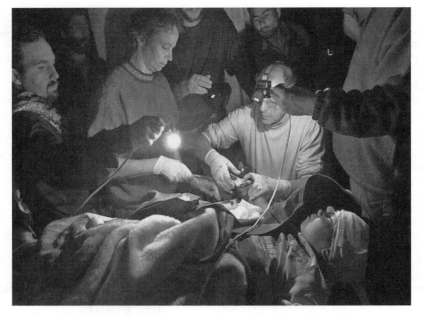

Figure 9-1. December 2001, Afghanistan: NGO personnel work under extremely austere conditions to stabilize a young Afghan boy. The boy was playing with an unexploded Russian heavy machine gun shell, which discharged, amputating his right hand. Apparently the boy's friend struck the firing pin of the shell with a rock causing the explosion. (Photo by Andrew Cutraro/Post-Dispatch/Aurora)

forged from tradition and from the "laws of war", which state that noncombatants, and particularly relief workers, are never legitimate military targets. In fact, isolated attacks on aid workers had become an all-too-common occurrence in the decade running up to the Iraq bombings. Most humanitarians continued to shun security measures that involved armed protection. Aid workers took pains to distinguish themselves from the military, often refusing military escorts, and trusting instead that their widely recognized neutral and impartial status would protect them.

Because the bombers played on the vulnerability of relief workers—the fact that they were soft targets without much in the way of armed protection—the magnitude of the attacks forced a realization among some workers that the promise of protection given by the Geneva Conventions had become inadequate. Some aid workers felt compelled to use armed guards for protection, pragmatic options to avoid having to withdraw and leave the embattled civilians they had traveled across the world to assist. Sadly, many aid agencies have withdrawn from Iraq and other countries because of security concerns and a sense that the "humanitarian space" needed to do their jobs according to their principles has been lost.

Legal Conventions Governing Humanitarian Practice

The major bodies of law that apply to humanitarian work, particularly in times of war and conflict, include International Humanitarian Law (IHL), Refugee Law, and Human Rights Law.

International humanitarian law (IHL) includes, most importantly, the Geneva Conventions of 1949 and Additional Protocols I and II (1977). In 2006 the Geneva conventions achieved universal acceptance; all 194 states in the world have formally agreed to abide by them. IHL requires that belligerents respect the four principles of *discrimination* between military and non-military objects, *proportionality* (the degree of force used should be proportional to anticipated military advantage and should be weighed against the risk of "collateral" damage to civilians), *precaution* to minimize non-combatant risk, and *protection of noncombatants*.

Noncombatants include not only civilians having nothing to do with the fighting, but also injured and captured fighters, refugees, and humanitarian, medical, religious, and journalistic personnel carrying out their duties in the conflict area. IHL gives Red Cross workers and other humanitarians the right to assist war-affected populations without interference or harm, and also certain responsibilities: mainly to practice in accordance with medical ethics and not get involved with fighting (apart from self-defense or protection of patients).

DILEMMA: IDENTIFYING EMBLEMS

IHL requires aid workers to identify themselves with certain emblems for their protection. However, in recent years, aid workers have been specifically targeted by militaries, other armed groups, and terrorists. Some agencies have removed all identifying marks from their clothing and their workplaces. What do you think?

To foster trust in beneficiaries, humanitarian workers long eschewed guns and guards, relying instead on the respect of international law and strong relationships with the community for protection. However attacks on aid workers have occurred frequently in recent years. Humanitarians must consider whether and when hiring private security forces or accepting military escorts will make them more secure and effective in their work, or conversely risk compromising their independence and their access to the most vulnerable populations. How would you decide the best way to ensure your team's security—both for international and national staff?

Refugee law (Convention on the Status of Refugees, 1951, and the Protocol Relating to the Status of Refugees, 1967) gives nations the duty to grant asylum, thus protecting refugees when their home countries have failed to do so. Finally, *human rights law* (based upon the Universal Declaration of Human Rights, 1948; and many other instruments, including those related to genocide (1948), racial discrimination (1965), civil and political rights (1966), economic, social, and cultural rights (1966), women's rights (1979), children's rights (1989), torture (1984), and internal displacement (1998)) protects certain "nonderogable" rights that are not to be limited during time of war or national emergency. These include the rights to life; juridical personality and legal due process; and freedoms of religion, thought, and conscience. Human rights law also prohibits torture, slavery, and degrading or inhuman treatment or punishment in wartime as well as peacetime.

The protection to be afforded noncombatants during wartime is, at base, protection against suffering and death, whether from physical violence, wartime deprivations, or the violation of inalienable human rights. The responsibility for providing this protection rests primarily upon states and members of armed forces. They in turn must allow humanitarian organizations to operate whenever noncombatant needs outstrip the ability of states or militaries to provide for them.

Medical aid workers operating in conflict-affected environments should observe *medical neutrality*. The concept derives from international human rights, humanitarian law, and medical ethics. It refers to the idea that medical professionals must uphold medical ethics (e.g., beneficence, nonmalfeasance, confidentiality) and treat patients according to need, without discriminating based on religion, ethnicity, political views, or even their status as members of a particular military force. Medical professionals must not cause harm to their patients or participate in torture. Medical clinics or hospitals that are used by the military to store weapons or conduct attacks can lose their protected status.

Current Trends

In recent years, the number of refugees falling under the mandate of UNHCR has dropped—from nearly 18 million in 1992 to just over 9 million in 2004. However, the number of IDPs worldwide has increased dramatically—from little over a million in 1982 to an estimated 25 million in 2004. Various factors may have contributed to this trend, for example more international recognition of IDPs as a group; the tendency of potential asylum countries to close their borders to refugees; and an increase in internal conflicts and civil wars where civilians are specifically targeted. It is important to note that situations of displacement have often stretched on for many years or even decades, highlighting the need for international medical assistance and—more importantly—efforts to attain just and durable solutions far beyond the period in which worldwide media attention focuses on the plight of the displaced.

Another worrying trend is the increase in proportion of civilian over military casualties of wars and conflicts. Although statistics are difficult to pin down, there is general agreement that there has been an enormous heightening in the proportion of civilian as opposed to military casualties of conflicts. Most worrisome, civilians are often the intended targets of hostilities, in absolute violation of the fundamental principles of international humanitarian law. Despite the promises made by governments and the United Nations following the failure to protect civilians in the 1990s in genocides that occurred in such places as Rwanda and Bosnia-Herzegovina, the failure of the international community to act decisively to protect civilians in armed conflict was made clear again in the first decade of the twenty-first century in places such as Darfur, Sudan, and the Democratic Republic of Congo (DRC). What did develop, however, was "soft law." Both the United Nations General Assembly (in 2005) and the United Nations Security Council (in 2006) adopted the following statement: "We are prepared to take collective action, in a timely and decisive manner . . . should peaceful means be inadequate and national authorities are manifestly failing to protect their populations from genocide, war crimes, ethnic cleansing, and crimes against humanity."

An increasing number of natural disasters, too, have been reported in the past several decades, affecting an increasing number of people, according to the Center for Research in the Epidemiology of Disasters (CRED) in Belgium. However, the organization's leaders caution that there has been a lack of systematic and standardized data collection to document this trend. Extreme poverty is among several factors that magnify human suffering in disasters. To better understand these factors, specialists separate out three aspects of disasters: The *hazard,* which is the physical or biophysical event itself (e.g., flood, earthquake, tsunami); *exposure,* which is the degree to which people are in danger of falling in the path of a hazard (e.g., the number of people living in disaster-prone areas, how well-built their houses are); and *vulnerability,* which is how susceptible people are to the event due to physical, social, economic, and environmental factors (Do people have the means to escape? Are warning systems in place? How well do medical systems function?). In addition to natural disasters, technological disasters such as industrial accidents affect a great number of people each year worldwide.

PREPAREDNESS AND PREVENTION

Often preparedness and prevention are the last things international medical workers think about when responding to a crisis. However, lightening often strikes twice, with populations affected by one disaster later experiencing another. In the United States, many of those who fled Hurricane Katrina in September 2005 were, several weeks later, displaced by Hurricane Rita. Here are just a few ways international aid workers may promote preparedness and prevention:

- Build the response capacity of local health agencies, hospitals, clinics, and caregivers
- Prioritize physical improvements for health facilities and other critical structures
- Promote safe housing solutions for displaced populations
- Educate the public about potential disaster threats and how to respond to them
- Build human bridges between conflict-affected areas, for example, by hiring staff from various sides of a conflict, bringing together health workers for training programs, and supporting cease-fires for vaccination campaigns.

MEDICAL AND PUBLIC HEALTH PRIORITIES

Humanitarian assistance is both an ancient moral practice and an increasingly professional, social scientific discipline. The failure of humanitarian agencies to avert widespread death and suffering among refugee populations in the 1990s (in particular among Rwandan refugees in what was then Zaire) led to calls for minimum standards in aid, increased qualifications of aid workers, and better research on what does and does not work to decrease morbidity and mortality in affected populations. A result of this work was the 1997 SPHERE Project, which led to a widely used handbook of minimum standards in relief. It covers water and sanitation, food security, nutrition, food aid, shelter and settlement, non-food items, and health services.

SPHERE is based on the idea that aid workers provide assistance not just out of their own desire to relieve human suffering, but also because disaster-affected populations have a right to human dignity and therefore to receive quality assistance. The stated goal of SPHERE is to enhance the quality of assistance and increase accountability on the part of the groups providing it.

Groups that join SPHERE agree to a common set of principles based on international law, including: the right to life with dignity; the distinction between combatants and non-combatants; and the principle of non-refoulement (that refugees must not be forced to return to the country they fled if a danger still exists for them there). The groups also commit to minimizing the adverse effects that aid delivery has too often had in the past, such as paradoxically leaving civilians more vulnerable to attack, or contributing to hostile activities.

SPHERE is not without its critics, including members of Doctors Without Borders and some other agencies. They argue that technical proficiency is not the only means by which humanitarian action should be judged—humanitarians should be held equally accountable for showing compassion, promoting human solidarity, bearing witness to human suffering and upholding justice.

SPHERE also lacks an emphasis on physical protection and the need for humanitarians to press states and other entities to live up to their commitments to protect human rights. This is a critical duty of humanitarians. Human rights groups have also emphasized the importance of measuring and assessing human rights violations in the context of emergencies.

Chief Causes of Morbidity and Mortality in Conflicts and Disasters

In recent years, epidemiological surveillance and research have deepened understanding of the specific causes of morbidity and mortality in war and disaster-affected populations (Table 9-3). The most robust data come from camp situations, which have proven to be ideal settings for epidemiological research at the same time they are disgraceful living arrangements for displaced populations.

Major infectious threats with epidemic potential include diarrheal infections, measles, respiratory infections, and malaria. Infectious disease outbreaks tend to be less common amongst populations displaced by natural disasters than by war. The pre-existing health profile

Table 9-3. Frequent causes of morbidity and mortality in complex emergencies.

Infectious diseases
Traumatic injuries
Emotional distress
Malnutrition/micronutrient deficiencies
Exacerbations of chronic illnesses (often due to treatment
  interruption).

Table 9-4. Initial Rapid Emergency Assessment.

Location of the area assessed
Accessibility
Security
Population data
Vulnerable groups present
Water supply
Sanitary facilities
Shelter and accommodations
Food stocks
Health problems, including the main causes and rates of
  morbidity and mortality in children and adults
Availability of medicines, health workers and health facilities
Other needs of the affected community
Activity of local and international aid organizations
Obstacles to return of IDPs or refugees
Available infrastructure and storage capacity
Electricity supply

of a population affects its experience during displacement. For example, populations with better pre-disaster health status often have a higher proportion of problems due to chronic diseases as opposed to infectious diseases.

Gathering Data: Assessment, Real-Time Evaluation, Health Information Systems, Research

An aid agency hires you to respond to an earthquake. You arrive on the ground ready to act. First, though, you need a little information. What was the population's baseline health status and health infrastructure? What are the immunization rates and incidences of endemic diseases? How many health facilities and health workers were operating here before the catastrophe? Most importantly, you'll want to visit the sites where people are gathered to rapidly assess their size, current health problems, and the health facilities and personnel now available to them. You'll talk to community leaders and health workers, and you'll examine clinic records to glean the information you're seeking.

The key point here? An assessment is a way of saying to a community that you are there to provide what they need and want, not what you *think* they need, or what you readily have at your disposal to give. Generally, the more that foreign aid workers collaborate with and involve affected communities in priority-setting and relief provision, the more useful and sustainable their aid efforts will be.

Table 9-4 (Initial Rapid Emergency Assessment) lists some key aspects of an initial assessment.

Of course, if everyone responding to an emergency conducted an in-person rapid assessment, that would waste time and put too much of a burden on the first responders and community leaders. So you'll want to share data with other agencies at meetings and through computer databases. You may be asked to fill out a standardized rapid assessment form. Joint, multi-agency assessments are also becoming popular, and they might even get you to unexpected places. After the December 2004 tsunami, UN agencies, NGOs, the CDC, and the US military performed a week-long assessment of the Indonesian coastline from the platform of the USS Abraham Lincoln, a Navy aircraft carrier. Also, don't forget, in this information age, to take advantage of Geographic Information Systems (GIS) and related mapping and satellite technologies to help identify populations in need and select groups for assessment.

Once your agency has established itself and is aiding the survivors, there are some critical indicators you need to track.[4] One is the *crude mortality rate* (CMR), the number of deaths per 10,000 population per day. It reflects the general health of a disaster-struck population. Baseline CMR gives a sense of the pre-existing health of the population. It typically falls well below 0.5/10,000/day. During an emergency, the CMR is used to monitor the health of the population. A CMR greater than one per 10,000 per day (or more than two per 10,000 per day for children under five) is considered an emergency. A CMR greater than two per 10,000 per day in the general population (or more than four per 10,000 per day in the under five population) is considered a severe emergency. The nutritional status of children under age 5 is the second basic indicator used to detect health stress on a population.[5]

Other important statistics that reflect pre-existing health status include *maternal mortality*, typically expressed as number of maternal deaths per 100,000 live births; and *infant mortality*, the probability of dying between birth and exactly one year of age expressed per 1000 live births.

SURVEILLANCE

In an emergency, the WHO, nongovernmental organizations, and governmental agencies frequently join forces to establish or enhance a health information system. Medical practitioners are asked to document and report the occurrence of key outbreak-potential illnesses on a daily or weekly basis. Figure 9-2 shows a sample weekly surveillance form including case definitions of

Sample Outpatient WEEKLY Surveillance Reporting Form
Morbidity (disease) and Mortality (death)

Province   District: Sub district:
Town/Village/Settlement/Camp: ……………………………..

Population size   < 5 years ………………   > = 5 years …………………..
Type of Health Facility: Fixed,
                             Mobile with fixed catchments
                             Mobile with varying catchments
  Supporting agency: ………………………

Name and telephone number of reporting officer: …………………………………..

Week from Monday: _____/_____/200_ **to Sunday**____/_____/200_

	Report the number of CASES	MORBIDITY (cases)		MORTALITY (deaths)	
		<5 years	≥5 years	<5 years	≥5 years
A	TOTAL CONSULTATIONS				
B	TOTAL DEATHS				
C	Pregnancy-related death				
D	Neonatal deaths (<28 days)				
E	Acute watery diarrhea				
F	Bloody diarrhea				
G	Malaria conf by rapid test				
H	Other Fever >38.5°				
J	Suspected Measles				
K	Acute respiratory infection				
L	Acute jaundice syndrome				
M	Meningitis				

- Write 0 (zero) if you had no case or death during the week for one of the syndrome listed in the form.
- Deaths might have occurred in the health facility or might have been reported from the community.
- Be careful to report only the deaths that occurred during the week.
- Deaths should be reported only in the mortality section, NOT in the morbidity section.

Case definitions for surveillance are presented on the back.

OUTBREAK ALERT

At any time **you suspect** any of the following diseases, you should alert the Surveillance Coordination by sending an SMS or phone to _____, with maximum information on time, place and number of cases and deaths.

Acute watery diarrhea/Cholera	Bloody diarrhea	Measles	Increase in malaria
Typhoid Tetanus	Hepatitis	Dengue fever	Meningitis

Figure 9-2.   This Outpatient Weekly Surveillance Reporting Form was developed by the World Health Organization and the Indonesian Ministry of Health and used by health workers after the December 2004 tsunami disaster in Aceh.

> **GENERAL OBSERVATION** (e.g. water, sanitation)

WHO RECOMMENDED CASE DEFINITIONS

ACUTE WATERY DIARRHEA

Three or more abnormally loose or fluid stools in the past 24 hours with or without dehydration.

To suspect a case of cholera:
Person aged over 5 years with severe dehydration or death from acute watery diarrhea with or without vomiting.
Person aged over 2 years with acute watery diarrhea *in an area where there is a cholera outbreak.*

To confirm a case of cholera:
Isolation of *Vibrio cholerae* O1 or O139 from diarrheal stool sample.

ACUTE JAUNDICE SYNDROME

Illness with acute onset of jaundice **and** absence of any known precipitating factors **and/or** fever.

ACUTE LOWER RESPIRATORY TRACT INFECTION/PNEUMONIA IN CHILDREN <5 YEARS

Cough or difficult breathing.
    and
Breathing 50 or more times per minute for infants aged 2 months to 1 year.
Breathing 40 or more times per minute for children aged 1 to 5 years.
    and
No chest indrawing, no stridor, no general danger signs.

Note: **Severe pneumonia** = Cough or difficult breathing + any general danger sign (unable to drink or breastfeed, vomits everything, convulsions, lethargic or unconscious) or chest indrawing or stridor in a calm child.

BLOODY DIARRHEA

Acute diarrhea with visible blood in the stool.

To confirm case of epidemic bacillary dysentery:
Take stool specimen for culture and blood for serology. Isolation of *Shigella dysenteriae.*

MALARIA

Person with fever or history of fever within the last 48 hours (with or without other symptoms such as nausea, vomiting and diarrhea, headache, back pain, chills, myalgia) with positive laboratory test for malaria parasites [blood film (thick or thin smear) or rapid diagnostic test].

MEASLES

Fever **and** maculopapular rash (i.e. nonvesicular) **and** cough, coryza (i.e. runny nose) or conjunctivitis (i.e. red eyes).
    or
Any person in whom a clinical health worker suspects measles infection.

To confirm case:
Presence of measles-specific IgM antibodies.

MENINGITIS

Suspected case:
Sudden onset of fever (>38.5) with stiff neck.
In patients under one year of age, a suspected case of meningitis occurs when fever is accompanied by a bulging fontanelle.

Probable case of bacterial meningitis:
Suspected case of acute meningitis as defined above with turbid cerebrospinal fluid.

Probable case of meningococcal meningitis:
Suspected case of meningitis as defined above
With gram stain showing gram negative diplococcus
Or ongoing epidemic
Or petechial or purpura rash

Confirmed case:
Suspected or probable case as defined above
With either
Positive CSF antigen detection for *Neisseria meningitidis*
Or positive culture of CSF or blood with identification of *Neisseria meningitidis*

Figure 9-2. (Continued)

epidemic-potential infectious diseases. A more extensive surveillance form might include mental health problems, injuries, and chronic diseases.

Overworked local medical professionals sometimes view additional data collection and reporting as burdensome. They will appreciate help with the logistics of collecting and compiling forms and communicating results, and they'll appreciate it if all agencies can agree on a single reporting form that complements existing health reporting systems. Cell phone and handheld computer-based reporting systems may help reduce the work involved.

The only reason to gather information is to use it! The goal of surveillance should be to guide programmatic decision-making and health care. Toward that end, it is critical that results—such as regional surveillance reports—be fed back to the practitioners who collected the data.

RESEARCH

Large-scale, population-based studies of nutrition and disease may be needed to truly understand the health problems and needs of the population. Academic researchers and epidemiologists from the US Centers for Disease Control and Prevention often serve as consultants to humanitarian agencies conducting such studies. Because of the extensive resources required to do quality research, it's best to collaborate with other agencies and to work with and empower local and national research bodies.

EVALUATION

You and your colleagues have been working tirelessly for months following a disaster. How are you doing? Real-time and periodic evaluations will help you assess the effectiveness of your organization's work and guide your future efforts. In fact, the donor agencies that give you the money to do your work may demand that you demonstrate your effectiveness. You'll need to track two types of indicators. So-called *process indicators* reflect your actual activities, such as the number of patients seen in your clinic or the number of children you've immunized against measles. More importantly, *outcome indicators* reflect the impact of those activities in a population, such as the number of children who contract malaria or the number of deaths in a refugee camp. To establish whether a particular program is having an effect, you'll need to assess the *baseline* level of each indicator at the beginning of the program. Not all evaluations are quantitative—qualitative measures are important, too. Often agencies hire external evaluators to study their programs.

However, evaluations can be costly, repetitive, and demanding on field staff who are trying to implement programs. So why not collaborate? Aid workers from 50 agencies set up the Tsunami Evaluation Coalition (TEC) after the 2004 Indian Ocean earthquake and tsunami. It was designed to evaluate effectiveness in each humanitarian sector and to study the impact of humanitarian policies.

Key Public Health Interventions

Often aid workers think of the disaster response in phases, beginning with the immediate aftermath (hours to days), followed by an emergency phase (days to weeks), then the late/recovery phase (weeks to months), and finally the rehabilitation and rebuilding phase (months to years). Rather than distinct phases, however, typically a population's needs in the aftermath of a disaster or population displacement vary along a continuum. For some segments of the affected population, emergency needs may linger far into the rebuilding phase. Furthermore, in the context of certain conflicts, for example those involving siege or repeated population displacement, the emergency phase may last for years.

Conversely, some of the public health interventions that are typically conducted in the later phases of a disaster can and should be implemented much earlier if both the need and the capacity to do so exists. Humanitarian and development work have traditionally been funded and implemented separately. However, given that poverty and poor infrastructure contribute to disaster and conflict vulnerability, there is an increasing recognition that some "development" work may be appropriate even in an emergency context. For example, the huge outpouring of generosity for tsunami survivors in Aceh, Indonesia, allowed some NGOs to rapidly begin training midwives. This was critical because of the alarming maternal mortality rate that existed even before the tsunami. Still, it is useful to consider the priorities that take precedence at various points in the disaster continuum.

What follows is a summary of key preventative public health interventions. Treatment guidelines for common medical conditions fall outside the scope of this chapter, but can be readily accessed in the publications of agencies such as Doctors Without Borders[6] and the World Health Organization.

IMMEDIATE AFTERMATH

The immediate health priorities after an acute event include rescue, first aid, trauma care, and protection of the population from further exposure to harm. Depending on the time it takes to organize an external response and move human and mechanical assets to affected areas, the local community will be in charge of providing the bulk of these services.

EMERGENCY

As the emergency phase continues, and help begins to arrive from outside, top priorities include the provision of safe water, safe shelter, food, and adequate sanitation.

Local and regional medical structures often need support. The biggest emphasis of international medical assistance typically should be on primary health care, emergency health care, and preventive health services focusing on the major causes of morbidity and mortality in displaced populations, particularly communicable disease surveillance and control. In some populations, maintaining the treatment of chronic conditions such as diabetes, and renal and heart disease are urgent priorities in situations of disaster or displacement.

The lack of proper safe water supplies and effective sanitation can result in epidemics of diarrheal illnesses, which tend to be the greatest killer in refugee and displaced persons situations due to profound dehydration. Water needs vary, but in general a minimum of 15 liters per person per day is needed for drinking, cooking, and personal hygiene. Survival needs for drinking and food are 2.5 to 3 liters per day. When a choice needs to be made between quantity and quality, assuring an adequate quantity should take precedence. The SPHERE handbook provides guidance on selecting water sources, recommended maximum queuing times, and the minimum number of water taps needed per population. Water quality should be monitored at the point of use, and piped water and all water at risk of contamination should be disinfected (e.g., with chlorine), as should water used in health centers, hospitals, and in feeding centers.

To prevent diarrheal outbreaks, good hygiene practices such as hand washing with soap (or, when unavailable, ash) and water should be promoted. In addition, latrines should be established downwind, downgrade, and away from water/food sources and dwellings. At least one latrine per 20 persons is recommended, but one per 50 is acceptable during the early emergency stage. Latrines must be well maintained and kept clean.

Early availability and institution of rehydration therapy for diarrhea is critical, as the vast majority of diarrhea-related deaths may be prevented with proper oral rehydration alone. Prevention of malnutrition in children with diarrhea is a key priority.

When large groups of people lack access to food or the means to buy it, aid agencies may introduce supplementary or therapeutic feeding programs to address threats ranging from anemia and micronutrient deficiency to acute global or severe protein-energy malnutrition. (See Chapter 6.) The decision to distribute food must be made carefully, based on assessments and with consideration of other more sustainable ways to promote "food security."

In the emergency phase of a disaster at least 2100 kilocalories per person should be assured, with 10–12 percent of energy from protein, 17 percent of energy from fat, and adequate micronutrients provided by fresh or fortified foods. Special supplementation may be needed for young children (nutritious, high energy complementary foods), pregnant or breastfeeding women (additional nutrients and support), and those with AIDS and other diseases. The food provided to a population should be appropriate and acceptable according to cultural practices, religious beliefs and practicality. Careful attention must be paid to food preparation needs.

To promote health and prevent diarrhea and dehydration in infants under six months, exclusive breastfeeding is recommended. International disasters are a magnet for large donations of baby formula, however, formula feeding of infants is to be discouraged in emergencies for several reasons, including the shortage of clean water with which to mix formula. Breast milk substitute should only be used in exceptional cases (such as when mothers have tested positive for HIV). UNICEF and other agencies have established guidelines and training modules for infant feeding in emergencies, which should be included in community health education activities.

If severe malnutrition reaches a certain threshold and distribution in the population, therapeutic feeding programs may be indicated. These involve both nutritional and medical treatment. Traditionally programs have been based at feeding centers, however new protocols are allowing therapeutic feeding to take place in communities, which reduces the hardship on families.

Measles has been a top killer of children in some displaced populations. Rapid organization of a measles immunization and Vitamin A supplementation campaign for children should be considered if local vaccination coverage falls below 90 percent. Because it takes time for immunity to develop following vaccination, health care workers need to be alert to signs of measles, and be prepared to quarantine sick children, trace their contacts, and "ring vaccinate" those children who have been in close proximity.

Emergency mass vaccination against tetanus is usually unnecessary. However, patients who have sustained open wounds and had their last tetanus shot more than five years ago can benefit from a tetanus toxoid booster. Those who have never received a full course of vaccination may require tetanus immune globulin.

In addition to diarrhea and measles, acute onset respiratory infections are extremely common in displaced populations and can lead to significant levels of mortality and morbidity in very young children, the aged, and people of any age who suffer from other illnesses. Refugee populations are particularly susceptible because of close quarters, malnutrition with vitamin deficiency, exposure to smoke, and extremes of temperature. Pertussis (whooping cough) should be considered in populations with poor vaccination coverage. It is commonly misdiagnosed, very contagious, and can lead to asphyxia in infants and dehydration and malnutrition in children.

Closely packed living conditions also provide ideal conditions for malaria to become a major cause of preventable death. Use of insecticide-treated bednets dramatically reduces the incidence of malaria, so bednet distribution and instruction are key public health measures following disasters in endemic areas. Insecticide-impregnated sleeping sheets, insecticide-treated plastic sheeting, and vector control (killing of mosquitoes) through spraying are also useful. Removal of standing water is essential in order to deprive mosquitoes of their breeding grounds. On a personal level, wear long sleeves and pants in the evening, apply insect repellents, and use slow-burning mosquito coils. Aid workers from non-malaria-endemic regions should consider taking chemoprophylaxis. Malaria is more dangerous in pregnant women.

Plasmodium falciparum malaria can be rapidly fatal, so cases must be detected and treated early. Because laboratories may be unavailable in emergencies, and malaria is often chloroquine resistant, aid workers are increasingly using rapid diagnostic tests (RDTs) and treating with artemisinin-based combination therapy (ACT). The Mentor Initiative (www.mentor-initiative.net/about.htm) has useful resources.

Dengue is another mosquito-transmitted febrile illness common in tropical climates. Patients who develop hemorrhagic complications can die rapidly if not transferred or evacuated to a facility where they can receive intensive hemodynamic and hematological support. The white-spotted *Aedes aegypti* mosquitoes that carry dengue feed during the day, so bednets are not sufficient to prevent infection.

Meningitis is a potentially severe health issue in some displaced populations. Eye infections and skin infections are also common acute health problems. In the past, many of the above infectious diseases have resulted from overcrowded conditions and the inadequate provision of shelter. Facilitating better shelter options for catastrophe-affected populations should be a key priority for the next generation of humanitarians. Even where camps are the only option, better planning can reduce the spread of endemic diseases and improve human security, for example, ensuring that women do not have to walk to remote latrines along dark pathways at night. Gender-based violence and rape often plague displaced and conflict-affected populations, and it is important for international medical workers to be aware that this problem might be affecting their patients.

To promote disease prevention, international health agencies often recruit and train local health outreach workers to help monitor for infectious disease outbreaks and other health threats, and to promote good hygiene awareness within their communities and healthy practices, such as breastfeeding rather than bottle feeding of infants. Ensuring access to health services among the affected population is critical. Many displaced persons are reluctant or unable to leave their families or their enclave to seek care.

Aid workers often provide medical supplies, medicines and technical support to local health professionals providing curative services, particularly in health structures that are overburdened, looted, or cut off from usual pharmaceutical supply chains. Aid agencies often stockpile the *Interagency Emergency Health Kit* (2006), the World Health Organization's latest standardized set of essential medicines, supplies and equipment designed to meet the initial primary healthcare needs of a displaced population without health facilities. Each kit serves approximately 10,000 people for three months. International suppliers such as the International Dispensary Association (IDA), Doctors Without Borders (MSF), and UNICEF maintain readily available stockpiles of standardized health kits made of high-quality medicines from approved pharmaceutical companies labeled and proportioned as appropriate for various emergency situations.

Unfortunately, disasters often attract inappropriate, useless, and expired medical donations that end up as a toxic medical waste problem at the exact time and place that communities are least able to deal with them (sometimes these are well-meaning, other times they may be motivated by significant tax breaks for the donor hospital or drug company). Guidelines for appropriate donations have been developed by the WHO and are summarized in Table 9-5 (Guidelines for Drug Donations).

There may also be a need to support higher-level medical services such as orthopedic surgery and intensive care. However, the importance of these types of services may quickly wane after the occurrence of a natural disaster such as an earthquake. Often, well-meaning nations make the public gesture of donating field hospitals or the use of Navy medical ships. When these arrive weeks or months after a disaster's occurrence, they will

Table 9-5. Guidelines for drug donations.

Select drugs based on actual needs
Notify recipients in advance of donation arrival
Ensure that drugs are similar in presentation, strength, and formulation to those used by recipient health workers
Obtain drugs from sources that meet quality standards set by donor and recipient countries and are manufactured according to GMP (Good Manufacturing Practice)
Clearly label drugs in a language understood by local practitioners. Label with International Nonproprietary Name or generic name
Ensure at least one year of shelf life before expiration, except in extraordinary situations
Include detailed packing lists
Cover costs of transport, warehousing, and customs clearances

be appreciated by patients suffering from long-untreated medical conditions in countries with poor health infrastructure. However, much of their capacity may go unused. It is important to support the rehabilitation, reconstruction, and staffing of existing health facilities, to improve patient care in the long term and mitigate future disasters that may occur in the area. As with all services provided by internationals, the emphasis should be on supporting and developing local capacity whenever possible.

In conflict situations, however, attacks on civilians may create an ongoing need for general surgeons capable of treating physical trauma. For example, in the besieged town of Srebrenica in Bosnia-Herzegovina, Doctors Without Borders supplied an international surgeon and surgical support for two years to the town's tiny local hospital. International surgeons have also worked for long periods of time in recent conflicts in Liberia, Sudan, and The Democratic Republic of Congo, among others.

Psychosocial trauma is recognized as a major cause of suffering in emergencies. However, responding appropriately to it depends greatly on cultural context. For example, Western-style focus on debriefing and individual psychotherapy may not be particularly appropriate or helpful in many societies, especially where health-seeking behavior for psychological distress is limited. The most beneficial ways to promote mental health across a population often involve social interventions that help restore a sense of control, safety, and purposeful activity to a community. For children this is especially important. Useful interventions include providing safe spaces for recreation and rapidly organizing the resumption of education. Adults benefit from playing an active role in assisting their families and communities, maintaining mourning customs and religious observances, being informed of and involved in plans for rehabilitation and rebuilding, and having opportunities for income generation and economic activity. For all, family reunification is a top priority, as is identification of the dead.

On the other hand, those with pre-existing psychiatric illness, particularly those who depend on medication, may often experience an exacerbation of their conditions. Emergency psychiatric care and psychiatric medicines should be made available. Access to basic mental health care should be facilitated in both the health system and in the community. All interventions should be designed in collaboration with mental health professionals from within the affected countries, as they will have an understanding of the cultural context.

Many international relief agencies have also committed to rapidly implement the *Minimum Initial Service Package (MISP)*, a set of actions designed to respond to reproductive health needs (including the risks of maternal and neonatal mortality, HIV, and sexual violence) in the midst of acute emergencies. The MISP involves distributing standardized kits (appropriate for various levels of the health system from community midwives up to referral hospitals) that contain equipment, supplies and drugs related to normal deliveries, basic obstetric emergencies, post-rape management, contraception, universal precautions for infection control, and safe blood transfusions. Many factors associated with the transmission of HIV are heightened in a disaster, such as the displacement of people, social instability, worsening poverty due to income loss (which may lead to bartering of sex for food and other resources), sexual violence and rape, poor access to condoms, and the influx of new populations, including reconstruction and relief workers, soldiers, and transporters. The MISP addresses HIV prevention in two key ways: making condoms freely available and ensuring that medical equipment and blood for transfusion are free from infectious agents. We would add that it is crucial to avoid treatment disruption for those being treated for AIDS.

LATER PHASES OF THE EMERGENCY

The MISP ideally forms the basis of re-establishing and ensuring comprehensive reproductive health services in later phases of the disaster response (see Chapter 4).

Other important priorities in the disaster aftermath often include:

Chronic Conditions   Support for detection and treatment of tuberculosis, AIDS, chronic diseases, and psychological conditions. Tuberculosis is the greatest infectious disease killer in the world today, and it is common among displaced populations. Given the need for long-term, consistent therapy, tuberculosis treatment should be a high priority in the later phases of disaster response. Rehabilitation, physical therapy, and prosthetic and orthotic services should be made available for amputees, those with spinal cord injuries, and other survivors of physical trauma.

Child Health   Priorities include re-establishment of the Expanded Program on Immunizations (EPI), Integrated Management of Childhood Illnesses (IMCI), and ongoing nutritional interventions, such as mass deworming of children in populations with high levels of childhood anemia and parasitic infection.

Health Infrastructure   The presence of foreign aid workers is only a temporary situation, but it is an important opportunity to offer training and specialized education to health workers who have had little chance to receive such knowledge or experience. This may lead to longer-term commitments to support formal health education opportunities in the affected country. In addition to medical training, aid workers can support drug supply management, health systems management (particularly where large numbers of health administrators have been killed or have left the area), and laboratory services.

Preparedness and Prevention Helping societies head off future suffering is one of the most important contributions that can be made. Disaster prevention and preparedness are key as are, in the wake of violent conflict, national reconciliation, the re-integration of former soldiers, and the strengthening of civil institutions. Agencies involved in the public health and medical response may not have the expertise or the mandate to carry out this work directly, however these activities clearly merit greater emphasis and awareness than they have historically received from the humanitarian community.

SPECIAL CONSIDERATIONS IN CERTAIN CATASTROPHES

Some health threats are likely to be encountered in many types of crises. The following issues arise less commonly, but also deserve attention.

Dealing with Human Remains

Survivors have a strong need to know what has happened to their loved ones—both for emotional well-being as well as for legal reasons (for example, survivor benefits can be delayed for years if a survivor lacks a death certificate for a spouse). Therefore, it is important to manage the dead with dignity and in a way that facilitates their identification and allows family members to be kept involved and informed.

Typically, dead bodies in natural disasters pose little risk of causing epidemics, so rapid burial—unless dictated by religious need—should not take precedent over identification. The basic requirements for handling human remains include wearing gloves and boots, washing hands, and disinfecting clothing, equipment, and transport vehicles. It is also wise to avoid contact with body fluids such as blood and feces. Most infectious organisms do not survive beyond two days, however, HIV has been found six days postmortem. Toxic gases can build up in confined, unventilated spaces, so body recovery in these situations should be approached with caution.

In certain cases, human remains may indeed pose major risks to the living. These include epidemics of plague, cholera, typhoid, anthrax, and hemorrhagic viruses (naturally occurring or as a result of biological warfare or terrorism), and following chemical attacks where chemical residue may remain on bodies. In these cases, body handling should be left to specialists whenever possible.

In the case of epidemic diseases, chlorine solution or other medical disinfectants are the best choices for disinfection. Family members need to be made aware that traditional practices such as washing the dead and large funerals risk spreading the epidemic—it is best to bury or cremate the body quickly near the site of death with a limited number of people in attendance. Dealing with disposal of bodies in an Ebola virus outbreak requires high levels of protection. In typhus and plague, protective clothing should be worn to avoid infestation with fleas or lice. Those who have contact with bodies in a cholera epidemic should carefully wash with soap and water. Victims who may have active pulmonary TB should have respiratory protection placed over the face prior to moving the body to protect the living from exposure to exhaled infectious material.

Collecting and identifying the deceased has not historically been the purview of humanitarian workers, but given the massive scale of recent disasters, knowledge of this field has become imperative. Identification errors occur frequently in mass disaster situations. When immediate visual identification by close contacts is not possible, rapid use of photography, forensic examination (including fingerprinting and dental examination), and the recording of basic and unique features and personal effects found on bodies should all be used to aid in identification. Bodies rapidly decompose in hot climates, so facial recognition can be difficult after 12-48 hours. If possible, bodies should be kept in body bags or wrapped in sheets and refrigerated or buried temporarily in well-organized graves. Waterproof labels with unique ID numbers should be securely attached to bodies, rather than writing on bodies or body bags, which is easily erased. DNA matching technology has been used to identify thousands of people (e.g., in New York after the 2001 World Trade Center attack, and in Bosnia-Herzegovina after the 1992–1995 war), but requires significant long-term financial commitments and community cooperation.

In Thailand, where a mass identification effort took place following the December 2004 tsunami, the majority of bodies were identified in person or later through photographs, fingerprints, and dental records and only then confirmed with DNA. Sadly, forensic technology was applied inequitably. Soon after the tsunami disaster, victim identification teams raced to Thailand from more than two dozen countries and at first worked independently from Thai scientists to identify foreign tourists. The folly of this approach was soon revealed—within a few days, it was difficult to tell Asian bodies from Caucasian bodies. Only by working together and treating all bodies with equal respect could victims and their relatives be matched. In 2006, the Pan-American Health Association published a field manual for managing dead bodies after disasters, which is available for download from their website (Management of Dead Bodies after Disasters: A Field Manual for First Responders. http://www.paho.org/english/dd/ped/DeadBodiesFieldManual.htm).

Chemical, Biological, and Radiological Threats

Threats from chemical, biological, and radiological (CBR) sources are an ever-present danger from industrial accidents, war, and terrorism. In the run-up to the Iraq war in 2003, several efforts were made to develop guidelines for international aid workers who might be called upon to respond to such incidents or whose work might put them in danger. ("Chemical, Biological, and Radiation Threats: A Guide for Aid Workers," is a training DVD produced by the International Medical Corps and the Center for International Emergency Medicine at UCLA). The conclusion of many experts was that international aid workers were poorly prepared to respond to these threats, and few aid workers had much experience with them.

Key principles in responding to CBR events include:

- **Predeployment preparation:** Learn what CBR threats exist in the environment in which you will be deployed. Consider smallpox vaccination for yourself and your team. It may be wise to include disposable masks, coveralls, gloves, booties, and tape in the gear being taken to the field.

- **Emergency response plan:** Develop and disseminate the plan in advance, including evacuation procedures.

- **Surveillance:** In an environment where CBR threats exist, appropriate indicators should be added to surveillance forms. Signs of dead animals (e.g., rodents, birds) or livestock with difficulty walking suggest the need for immediate evacuation. A single case of smallpox demands immediate action. Clinicians need to be aware of the threat and potential signs and symptoms so they can diagnose sentinel cases.

- **Exposure avoidance and decontamination:** A safe room, such as an entirely sealed inner room, may be useful to take shelter in during the time of the attack. In the case of radiation, take shelter underground or in the interior of a building with thick concrete walls until the cloud passes, if unable to flee in another direction. Only sealed water and food should be assumed to be safe. There will be a need for ample safe water and increased food security.

- **Treatment:** It's important to keep in mind that many of the medicines needed to treat CBR incidents are not included in the WHO emergency health kit.

- **Coordination and information-sharing:** Military in the area may have contamination sensors and equipment for decontamination and treatment of victims. Evacuation may be necessary and will need to be coordinated.

CHEMICAL THREATS

Chemical releases can cause health effects in minutes to hours, affect a large number of people, and persist in the environment. They also pose a risk of secondary contamination. Key principles are first to get away from the threat and then decontaminate. In the Tokyo subway attack using Sarin nerve gas, first responders were also affected. Nerve agents cause symptoms such as miosis (constriction of the pupils) and stumbling. Exposed patients must be treated immediately with atropine or they may die. Blister agents such as mustard gas cause tearing and swelling of the eyes and can cause burns with longer exposure. Decontamination is critical—aid workers can be put in danger by secondary spread. Other potential chemical threats include choking agents, blood agents, tearing agents, and incapacitating agents. Industrial risks include petroleum products, pesticides, and their precursors (such as methyl isocyanate, responsible for the Bhopal accident). Most of the latter will be extremely irritating, and the instinct to get away from the source should be followed. Oil well fires can cause heavy smoke—placing a wet cloth over the nose and mouth can protect against some heavy particles. Useful protective clothing for chemical attacks includes disposable cloth masks, paper coveralls, gloves, and booties (taped to coveralls).

In chemical attacks, key treatment principles, in order of priority, include:

1. Removal from the site of exposure
2. Thorough decontamination, including removal of clothing, blotting of exposed skin, and washing entire body and hair with soap and water
3. Stabilizing and triaging patients

BIOLOGICAL THREATS

Biological threats tend to come from naturally-occurring infectious particles harnessed to produce widespread illness. The CDC maintains a list of high-priority biological agents. Some of the most potentially threatening include smallpox, anthrax, plague, botulism, tularemia, and Ebola and other hemorrhagic infections. It is important that when these are a threat, international aid workers are trained to recognize and treat these illnesses. Many can be prevented and treated by antibiotics. Surveillance and the use of good infection control measures are critical.

RADIOLOGICAL THREATS

Removal from the source and shielding are key. Care for blast and burn injuries is typically the first priority, followed by decontamination. Most external contamination can be removed by disposing of clothing and washing with water and mild soap. Use universal precautions to minimize secondary exposure. The greatest long-term threat of radiologic exposure comes from inhalation of gamma particles from contaminated fallout. Respiratory protection is imperative as even one millionth of a gram of some radiologic compounds can cause lung cancer.

However, a so-called "dirty bomb"—an explosive packed with radiologic material—may cut a wider swath of panic than physical harm.

PARTICULAR NEEDS OF SPECIFIC POPULATIONS

Balanced with the desire to provide the greatest benefit for the greatest number of people, aid workers must keep in mind the particular needs of specific groups within the populations they serve.

Patients Requiring Medical Services Unavailable in the Immediate Area

Some patients require higher level care than they can receive in the immediate area where they have taken shelter (such as a camp-based primary health clinic). Transfers to higher level care frequently do not go smoothly. For example, in a country of asylum, national and local authorities may consider refugees an additional burden on an already overworked health system. The standard of care in tertiary care hospitals may be low, so it is important to remain involved in the care of the transferred patient and possibly support the receiving hospital with materials to compensate for the extra caseload.

In these situations, the fully-equipped and staffed field hospitals that are donated in some emergencies can certainly be of use. Alternatively, sometimes foreign hospitals and doctors offer to treat patients if they can be evacuated. Medical evacuations, while potentially life-saving, are almost always fraught with difficult logistical and ethical concerns. Medical workers become inundated with evacuation appeals from patients and their families, often for longstanding chronic conditions. Desperation for evacuation may lead to corruption and payoffs within the medical system. It makes sense for an experienced, impartial outside organization, such as the International Organization for Migration, to take charge of screening, prioritization, and logistics (travel and repatriation, liaisons with receiving hospitals). Clear medical guidelines for evacuation need to be set and communicated to the community. In some cases, a medical evacuation program has been paired with efforts to improve local and national capacity to provide specialized medical treatment—for example the Medical Evacuation and Health Rehabilitation Program for Iraq (MEHRPI) coordinated by the International Organization for Migration. From 2003–2004, it facilitated the treatment of 250 patients abroad while supporting advanced training for several Iraqi medical professionals. Tragically, the upsurge in violence against civilians and the deterioration of medical services in subsequent years necessitated the re-launch of a medical evacuation program for Iraq.

CASE STUDY/DILEMMA 2: SREBRENICA MEDICAL EVACUATIONS[7]

In April 1994 the town of Srebrenica in eastern Bosnia-Herzegovina had been under siege by nationalist Serb forces for a year, and the town's population was desperate. As the first aid convoys reached the town, an attempt was made to evacuate seriously wounded women and children on returning trucks. Injured men could not be evacuated by road due to the likelihood that they would be taken away by soldiers at checkpoints.

An international doctor noted which patients were to be evacuated by referring to their hospital bed numbers, but the stronger patients forced the weak patients from their beds. Doctors took to marking patients' evacuation priorities with indelible ink on their foreheads. As the selected patients were being brought from the hospital, non-injured women and children surged onto the evacuation trucks, themselves desperate to leave the town. The trucks became so overcrowded that several people died on the hours-long journey. Local authorities accused the United Nations of aiding in the "ethnic cleansing" of the town.

Several weeks later, a cease-fire was established, and the United Nations Security Council designated Srebrenica a "Safe Area." After long negotiations, Serb forces agreed to a medical evacuation of injured men from Srebrenica by helicopter. Male amputees in the town staged a protest when they learned the criteria for evacuation did not include them (see Figure 9-3).

The first attempt at the evacuation had to be scrapped when the helicopter landing area was shelled, but the evacuation began again after firmer security guarantees were received. A senior International Committee of the Red Cross (ICRC) worker and a UN relief worker were in charge of the mission. The Red Cross worker followed every procedure to the hilt, checking each patient, filling out paperwork, and obtaining all required signatures before allowing patients onto helicopters. The UN relief worker had a different approach—he quickly loaded as many men as possible onto the helicopters, whatever their condition, sensing this would be the only chance for them to escape the besieged town.

Over the three-day course of the evacuation, nearly 500 men were airlifted to safety. The war continued for two more years with few other men ever able to leave the town. In July 1995, the forces surrounding Srebrenica launched an attack. In spite of the town's UN protected status, the presence of a Dutch contingent of UN soldiers in the town, and an air support agreement with NATO—there was no international effort to counter the attacking forces militarily. Dutch military doctors in the town were forbidden by their commanding officer from treating injured civilians. During the attack, Serb forces ultimately captured the town and massacred an estimated 8000 men and several women and boys, burying them in mass

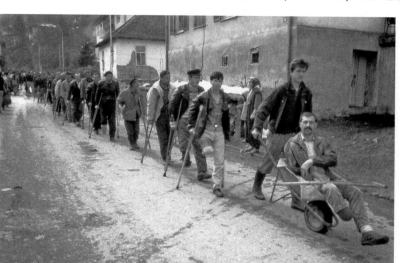

Figure 9-3. April 2003, Srebrenica, Bosnia and Herzegovina: Wounded men, most of them amputees, march through the town of Srebrenica, protesting their exclusion from an aerial medical evacuation out of the besieged enclave overseen by UN and ICRC personnel. (Photo by Philipp von Recklinghausen.)

graves. Two international medical workers from Doctors Without Borders were present in Srebrenica. They managed to save the lives of their national staff by refusing to evacuate without them. The United Nations War Crimes Tribunal for the Former Yugoslavia and the International Court of Justice, both in the Hague, found that the crime of genocide was committed in Srebrenica.

What would you have done if you were in charge of the 1993 medical evacuations? What does this story say about the ability of international medical workers to protect patients in a war zone?

Political, Ethnic, and Religious Minorities and Socially Marginalized Groups

Many recent wars and conflicts have targeted specific groups for displacement and even killing. Providing medical aid to members of these groups is in some sense a political act. As one US government aid official, who requested anonymity, once put it, "You're making a political statement when you say that someone should live when someone else doesn't want them to live." There are two minefields here for aid workers. One is the danger that aid organizations will be steered away from these groups and might not notice their needs. Therefore, minority and marginalized groups need to be identified early and monitoring must be instituted to ensure equal access to aid.

However, another danger is that these groups will receive what appears to those around them as *preferential*

treatment, thus heightening the risk of their further persecution or abuse. This is one reason why good communication and transparency are critical to the work of aid organizations. Explain to authorities and recipients why and how aid is being given, and that it is being given impartially and based on need (and, if true, to "their side," too). To get aid through to vulnerable populations, workers may have to decide when to privately negotiate, when to publicly denounce, and when to consider a proportion of aid stolen by paramilitary soldiers at a checkpoint as a price worth paying.

One of the dangers of committing to providing a high standard of aid to victims of disasters is that it can heighten existing tensions (or create new ones) between populations. For example, the disaster-affected subset of the population may receive more food or higher quality shelter than those around them who are at baseline living in much poorer circumstances. This problem of equity has not yet been resolved satisfactorily by the aid community.

CASE STUDY/DILEMMA 3, ACEH, INDONESIA, 2004

Before the 2004 Indian Ocean earthquake and tsunami, the Indonesian province of Aceh was embroiled in a three-decade conflict between the rebel Free Aceh Movement (GAM) and the Government of Indonesia. Foreigners, including most aid workers, had been banned from working in the province. After the tsunami, the rebel group and the government concluded a peace agreement, and the conflict-affected interior of the province was finally open to aid workers, who were already massed along the coastline responding to the tsunami (see Figure 9-4).

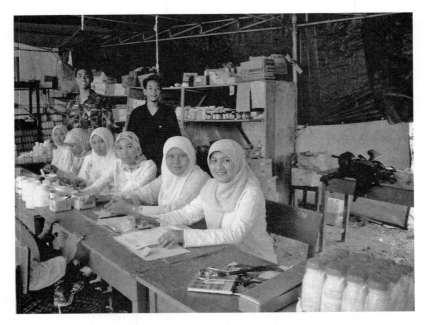

Figure 9-4. February 2005, Aceh Utara District, Nanggroe Aceh Darussalam, Indonesia: Indonesian nurses and doctors who survived the December 2004 tsunami work at an improvised health clinic in a tent camp for displaced persons. Local professionals typically provide the bulk of health care services following a disaster. A Government of Indonesia soldier armed with an automatic weapon is present at the clinic—a common practice discouraged by many international aid organizations. (Photo by Dr. Sheri Fink.)

However, leaders of aid agencies were unsure of whether they could legitimately use tsunami recovery donations to implement programs in areas that were instead primarily devastated by the conflict. Disparities in the provision of aid to coastal vs. inland areas heightened tensions among residents of some of Aceh's conflict-affected districts.

The humanitarian principle of impartiality demands that aid be allotted without any standard other than need. Was it moral, with billions of dollars on the table, to distribute food to children along the coasts while allowing children in the mountains above to die of malnutrition? Is there any justification for rebuilding only tsunami-wrecked health centers but not war-damaged health centers serving sicker children a few miles inland?

Children

UNICEF estimates that half of people displaced by war are children. In a medical sense, children are more vulnerable than adults to the stresses and deprivations of trauma and displacement. They are more prone to dehydration, malnutrition, micronutrient deficiencies, and fatigue compared with adults, and their inexperienced immune systems can leave them more vulnerable to infections. Illnesses and malnutrition experienced early may continue to impact them throughout their lives—for example, studies have shown that malnutrition in childhood can have harmful, long-term effects on the brain and on behavioral development.

Exploitation of children, including child trafficking into labor or prostitution rings, other sexual abuse, and abduction by the military, may take place in camps and other situations of displacement. Child marriage of girls is also common in some cultures, and pressure for girls to marry may increase when many men have lost wives in a disaster. Some aid agencies, such as UNICEF, Save the Children, and IRC, often dispatch a child protection officer with their disaster response team to organize services for children and advocate for them. The 1989 Convention on the Rights of the Child and its Two Additional Protocols (2000) as well as the Geneva Conventions, the Refugee Convention, and human rights law provide a legal basis for child protection work.

Unaccompanied children, children separated from their customary caregivers, orphans, and child-headed households are particularly vulnerable to exploitation. It is crucial to make every effort to preserve family unity. The 2004 Inter-agency Guiding Principles on Unaccompanied and Separated Children provide useful guidance.

Evacuations, including medical evacuations, can cause separation—if at all possible, children should be evacuated with their intact families, or at minimum one caregiver. If this is not possible, a file of personal and family information should travel with the child with copies retained by parents, governmental representatives, and monitoring agencies such as the ICRC's Central Tracing Agency. Evacuation should be to the closest possible location to home and family, and efforts should be made to allow the child to communicate with family members while separated from them.

Any disaster can lead to children being separated from their families. It is important for unaccompanied children to be rapidly identified, registered, photographed, and provided with documentation—all in a way that will not further endanger or stigmatize them or disrupt their community's efforts to care for them. Whenever possible (except, for example, where this could put a family in danger) a concerted search must be made for surviving family members. Typically, the ICRC or UNICEF works with governmental authorities and humanitarian agencies to register and trace separated family members.

Media coverage of suffering children always sparks offers of international adoption. However, experts currently believe that children are better off staying with family members or community members. Many countries have instituted policies barring international adoption following disasters, as it cuts children off from the chance of reuniting with families and maintaining links with their communities.

Likewise, committing these children to orphanages and other institutions should be avoided whenever possible. It is better to place the children with relatives, neighbors, or friends within their communities. Special attention should be paid to the proper health care and nutrition of these children, for example, children under six months should be breast-fed if possible by a lactating woman who tests HIV negative. Ensuring that birth registration takes place during a disaster also helps to protect children.

Psychological trauma is very real for children, and can have long-term impact, but children are also highly resilient. It should not be assumed that children who experience war will be psychologically scarred. In fact, the vast majority are capable of going on to lead productive and happy lives.

To facilitate this, it is important to as quickly as possible establish structures where children can experience normalcy. Resumption of education is particularly important—UNICEF offers "schools in a box," designed for short-term temporary classrooms created in camp settings. Also, child recreation centers are sometimes created where children can enjoy games, safety, and counseling if needed.

Women

Security should always be an utmost priority, as women are frequently victims of physical and sexual assault in unstable circumstances. The Task Force on Gender of the Inter-Agency Standing Committee (IASC) has published *Guidelines for Gender-Based Violence Interventions in Humanitarian Emergencies: Focusing on Prevention and Response to Sexual Violence (http://www.humanitarianinfo.org/ iasc/content/subsidi/tf_gender/gbv.asp)*. Contraceptive and prenatal care programs should be initiated to avoid long-term consequences of unintended pregnancies and premature births. The World Health Organization and MSF have published numerous manuals providing guidelines on such healthcare operations. It is often helpful to involve local women in the provision of health care and health and hygiene education within the disaster or conflict-affected populations. This type of health outreach is important, because many women are reluctant to leave their living quarters to seek medical care out of fear of being separated from children or putting them at risk during travel.

Men

Men are not typically considered a vulnerable group. Indeed, medical aid workers may not think much about the particular problems of men. However, military-aged men are often at risk of being killed by hostile forces or forced into fighting. Men may also be less willing to seek help for physical and especially psychological problems.

The Elderly and Chronically Ill

Elderly people may depend upon others to provide for their food, shelter, and basic needs, and thus they are prone to exploitation and neglect and in need of particular attention. Furthermore, in disasters elderly people are commonly separated from their families and left alone. An effort should be made to identify elderly people who are incapable of caring for themselves, trace and reunite them with family members, and otherwise provide for their care.

In an emergency, providing care only to those who show up for it is not sufficient. No matter how busy medical professionals are, they must also take time to seek out people who may be lying helpless in a corner of a tent with a serious but treatable illness. Such people exist in every disaster—from the camps in Darfur, Sudan, to the Louisiana shelters following Hurricane Katrina.

Elderly people often suffer from chronic diseases that require medicines and ongoing care. Their conditions may be exacerbated by the stress of the disaster or by running out of needed medications. In some recent conflicts, such as Bosnia-Herzegovina and Iraq, exacerbation of chronic diseases accounted for a great deal of morbidity and mortality, in particular from hypertension, diabetes, renal disease, cardiac disease, and stroke. Insulin treatment may be difficult in places where refrigeration is a problem. Cold boxes are often needed.

Renal dialysis-dependent patients require rapid transfer to facilities that have dialysis capabilities, or they will die. While sophisticated cancer treatment is typically unavailable in conflict or disaster situations, cancer patients are often given low evacuation priority due to their poorer prognosis. Shamefully, humanitarian organizations have historically not done a good job of making drugs available to treat their severe pain, such as narcotic analgesics.

People Living with HIV and AIDS

Those who are living with HIV and AIDS when disaster hits may experience problems coping with the physical stresses of displacement. Their survival is at risk from infections and malnutrition, and it is important for them to have access to extra clean water for drinking and hygiene, and to nutritious foods to stay healthy (energy requirements may be increased, and micronutrients are important to maintain immune function). Often chronic diarrhea is a problem. When combined with weakness, this may make it difficult for those with AIDS to reach latrines. Simple inventions, such as a bucket fitted with a toilet seat and toilet lid, can help restore a sense of dignity and improve the quality of life for those with AIDS and those caring for them in difficult circumstances. Aid workers must make efforts to ensure that discrimination does not occur against people living with HIV and AIDS.

HIV prevention activities and information campaigns are important parts of aid programs. In addition, several aid agencies have demonstrated the feasibility of initiating Highly Active Anti-Retroviral Therapy (HAART) in refugee settings. Increasingly, those affected by conflict and disaster may already be taking anti-retroviral treatment, and, due to the likelihood of resistance developing, it is critical that their treatment regimens not be interrupted. In all cases, those living with AIDS should be afforded appropriate medical care to decrease their risk of acquiring opportunistic infections and reduce mother-to-child transmission. Useful resources include *Guidelines for HIV Prevention, Care and Support Among Displaced and War-Affected Populations* (International Rescue Committee, 2003), and *Strategies to Support the HIV-Related Needs of Refugees and Host Populations* (UNAIDS, 2005). Recommendations for AIDS treatment change rapidly, so it is important to consult updated guidelines.

People with Physical Challenges

It is important to ensure that people with limited mobility not be separated from needed equipment, such as wheelchairs or prosthetic limbs, during a disaster. They may also require additional assistance accessing food, shelter, or medical care. Disability should be considered in every aspect of camp and settlement creation, so that drinking water sources, bathing facilities, latrines and other services (e.g. schools and health posts) are made accessible to all. Established settlements should be evaluated and remedied where necessary. Unfortunately, these considerations are typically overlooked, creating hazards for people with disabilities. Handicap International (www.handicap-international.org) is an important agency with expertise in emergency situations.

CASE STUDY/DILEMMA 4: KOSOVO-MACEDONIA BORDER 1999

During the Kosovo war in 1999, many Kosovar Albanians were forced to flee. However, the Macedonian government at first closed its border with Kosovo, trapping roughly 100,000 people in a cold, muddy no-man's land beside the border crossing. Several NGOs and the Macedonian Red Cross created a tented medical treatment area. Two lines of Macedonian police in riot gear stood between the population and the medical area, and the police did not allow family members to accompany sick persons for care. This resulted in several dozen elderly, chronically ill, developmentally disabled, mentally ill, and paraplegic people ending up in the medical area with no family members to care for them. Medical workers were busy with acute medical cases, and they moved these people into a separate "respite" tent and all but forgot about them.

That miserable tent became known as "the tent of the damned." Those who could not walk soiled themselves and were not cleaned. They did not receive enough food or water. Some of them experienced pain and were not given pain killers or treatment. Aid workers made several appeals for help to the Macedonian health ministry, but authorities refused to take these vulnerable patients into care facilities. Several days later, the border area was evacuated. Representatives of the Organization for Security and Cooperation in Europe (OSCE) and UNHCR agreed to transfer the inhabitants of the "tent of the damned" to a local hospital, care facility, or camp. For unknown reasons they were left alone for another cold night in the tent with no nursing care before being transferred. An additional woman died.

People Affected by Mental Illness

Those individuals being treated for pre-existing mental illnesses often run short of their medicines during disasters. In addition, the stressful situations can cause psychological distress or psychological disorders in a portion of the population. In some societies, a great deal of shame surrounds mental illness, and those affected may be hidden away or mistreated. In other cases, depression or a traumatic experience such as rape may decrease the person's motivation to seek medical assistance or even food. All of these problems highlight the need to conduct active "case-finding" in emergency contexts.

Furthermore, medical caregivers must be sensitive to the fact that patients appearing at the clinic with physical complaints may also be experiencing psychological distress. The World Health Organization publishes guidelines on Mental Health in Emergencies (www.who.int).

People with Cognitive Impairments

Displacement can be particularly disorienting for people with cognitive impairments. They too, may require additional assistance to ensure their basic needs are met and to protect them from danger.

A Vulnerable Group: Aid Workers

Providing humanitarian assistance is a risky business. Hundreds of aid workers have been killed on the job in recent years. They have often been intentionally targeted. Many more have been injured or subject to gender-based violence. Every aid worker has the responsibility to ensure that his or her agency provides adequate security training and has a solid security plan. Short courses on security in emergencies are available from organizations including RedR (www.redr.org). In addition, the risks of infectious diseases, traffic accidents and kidnapping may be greater where aid workers do their jobs than in their home countries. Humanitarian work is often stressful, too. The temptation to work until exhaustion should be resisted, as it can reduce effectiveness dramatically and lead to burn-out. Aid workers also run the risk of encountering extremely disturbing situations that may leave a long-lasting psychological impact. Transition to life back home can be difficult. Many have found it helpful to seek professional counseling, which may be provided for free by the hiring agency.

THE ROLES AND LIMITATIONS OF HEALTH PROFESSIONALS IN PHYSICAL PROTECTION AND CONFLICT MITIGATION

Humanitarians are often among the few outsiders present in situations of extreme violence. Their traditional role has been to both assist and protect the vulnerable. While responsibility for ensuring the physical protection of civilians during wartime rests primarily with governments and militaries, humanitarians should also embrace this goal as central to their work. Most important is to regularly examine activities to assess whether they are contributing to or detracting from protection.

Some analysts argue that the mere presence of humanitarian aid workers provides a measure of protection to civilians. However, recent experience has suggested that humanitarian presence may also confer a false sense of protection to a population and may paradoxically represent an obstacle to effective military action aimed at neutralizing aggressive forces. In addition, the presence of desirable aid commodities may make a population more prone to attack. In these cases thought should be paid to making aid less desirable to potential looters, for example by delivering aid in small, family-size packages.

On the other hand, there are several ways that medical aid workers can promote protection by responding to human rights violations, remediating them, and building a positive environment for protection. This is known as the ICRC "egg" model of protection. Aid workers may worry that speaking out directly about human rights violations or war crimes will endanger their access to the people they are assisting. This is a very difficult decision for aid workers. The Active Learning Network for Accountability and Performance in Humanitarian Action (ALNAP, www.alnap.org) has published a Protection Guide that details five options for aid workers responding to protection problems:

1. Public denunciation of those committing atrocities or human rights violations
2. Direct persuasion of those involved to end the pattern of abuse
3. Mobilization or discreet information-sharing with human rights advocates, journalists, peacekeeping monitors, or others who may have the ability to influence military or political leaders to conform to human rights standards and international humanitarian law
4. Substitution or providing aid to assist those at risk of disease, malnutrition, and death
5. Capacity-building or offering support to others providing protection

International medical workers can also promote links between conflicting (or recently conflicting) populations. For example, they can facilitate cooperation between medical workers on different sides of the front lines, or hire staff from different religious or ethnic groups. Medical workers have also been successful in coordinating humanitarian cease-fires to allow vaccinations to take place, a strategy often referred to as "Peace through Health."

Medical workers have used their professional expertise to inform the wider public about the terrible health effects of certain weapons, such as landmines. Indeed, medical professionals played an important part in the Nobel Peace Prize-winning International Campaign to Ban Landmines, which resulted in the 1997 Mine Ban Treaty. The treaty became international law in 1999.

In addition, medical workers have documented the effects of torture and rape on asylum-seekers and furnished evidence in war crimes prosecutions. Physicians, epidemiologists, and others with research expertise have also conducted epidemiologic-style studies of human rights violations that reveal strong evidence about patterns of abuses and can be used in criminal courts. Of course, those committing atrocities are increasingly aware that they may be held to account for their crimes and may try to hide evidence, avoid leaving survivors, or refuse medical workers access to populations that have been targeted.

SUMMARY

The job of an international aid worker is one of great challenge, responsibility, and potentially great rewards. It requires excellent medical skills and a solid understanding of medical ethics and international law. Relief workers often gain a deeper understanding of current events, persistent international health problems, and the human implications of political and military decisions. The work often gives its practitioners a deep sense of purpose. The dedication and humanity of colleagues, particularly those who come from the catastrophe-affected society, is inspiring. At times, however, when dispensing a pill, vaccinating a child, or even documenting an atrocity seems almost purposeless amid the overwhelming violence and destruction, the most important gift an international medical worker can give to those affected is kindness and solidarity.

STUDY QUESTIONS

1. You are an aid worker faced with a disaster involving a large displaced population. List at least ten medical and public health interventions you would consider applying in the short (hours to days), medium (days to weeks) and long-term (weeks to months) situation. List at least three factors you will need to weigh in choosing your priorities, and describe how these factors will influence your choices.

2. Some NGOs rely heavily on government funding to support their lifesaving work. Re-read the Iraq Case Study, above. If an NGO is offered money from a government that is party to a conflict, do you think the NGO should accept the funds in order to serve the population in need, or should it turn them down to avoid undermining the agency's independence? What practical, ethical, or other factors influenced your decision? What other solutions might be possible?

3. In every disaster and war there is a subset of highly vulnerable people who are at risk of suffering more than others suffer. Re-read the Case Study above about the "the tent of the damned" during the Kosovo war. If you were an aid worker on the Kosovo border, what other ways might you have approached the situation? List at least three interventions that might have improved the lives and protected the health of the vulnerable patients.

KEY REFERENCES

Books

Humanitarian Charter and Minimum Standards in Disaster Response. Geneva: Sphere Project, 2004. Also available online: www.sphereproject.org/handbook/index.htm

Mandalakas, Anna, Kristine Torjesen, Karen Olness, et al. *Helping the Children—A Practical Handbook for Complex Humanitarian Emergencies.* Kenyon, MN: Johnson & Johnson Pediatric Institute and Health Frontiers, 1999.

Médecins Sans Frontières. *Clinical Guidelines: Diagnosis and Treatment Manual, Seventh Edition.* Paris: Médecins Sans Frontières, 2006. Also available online: www.msf.org/source/refbooks/ index. htm

Médecins Sans Frontières. *Refugee Health: An Approach to Emergency Situations.* London: Macmillan, 1997. Also available online: www.msf.org/source/ refbooks/index.htm

Noji, E. (ed.). *The Public Health Consequences of Disasters.* New York: Oxford University Press, 1997.

Documents

UNHCR. *Managing the Stress of Humanitarian Emergencies.* Geneva, July 2001. Available online at: http://www.the-ecentre. net/resources/e_library/doc/managingStress.PDF

WHO. *25 Questions and Answers on Health and Human Rights* (via WHO webpage). Health and Human Rights Publication Series, no. 1 July 2002. World Health Organisation. (PDF file 1.03 MB) Available online at: http://www.who.int/hhr/activities/ publications/en/

WHO/UNHCR. *Guidelines for Drug Donations* (via WHO website). Revised 2nd edition, WHO/EDM/PAR/99.4, World Health Organisation and United Nations High Commissioner for Refugees. Geneva, 1999. Available online at: http:// www.who.int/hac/techguidance/pht/essentialmed/en/

WHO. *Mental Health in Emergencies: Psychological and Social Aspects of Health of Populations Exposed to Extreme Stressors.* Geneva: World Health Organization, 2003. Available online at: www.who.int/mental_health/media/en/640.pdf

Websites

Alertnet. Disaster and conflict news. www.alertnet.org.

ALNAP. Active Learning Network for Accountability and Performance in Humanitarian Action. www.alnap.org.

Forced Migration Online. Links to full text versions of many documents related to health in disasters and humanitarian emergencies. http://www.forcedmigration.org/sphere/health.htm

Humanitarian Information Centers. Resources for ongoing emergencies. www.humanitarianinfo.org

Humanitarian Practice Network. www.odihpn.org

Reliefweb. Up to date information on individual disasters and complex emergencies. Job listings for aid workers. www.reliefweb.org

SMART (Standardized Monitoring and Assessment of Relief and Transitions). Assessment tools for humanitarians. www.smartindicators.org

The SPHERE Project. Minimum standards in disaster response. www.sphereproject.org.

UNHCR. Health, Food, and Nutrition Toolkit: Tools and Reference Materials to Manage and Evaluate Health, Food and Nutrition Programmes (via UNHCR website). http://www.

the-ecentre.net/toolkit/home.htm United Nations High Commissioner for Refugees. Geneva, 2001.

WHO. Technical Guidelines for Health Action in Crises. http://www.who.int/hac/techguidance/en/

WHO/PAHO. Health Library for Disasters. World Health Organisation/Pan-American Health Organisation. Geneva, 2003. http://www.helid.desastres.net/

Journals and Newsletters

Disaster Medicine and Public Health Preparedness

Disasters: The Journal of Disaster Studies, Policy and Management

Humanitarian Practice Exchange

Prehospital and Disaster Medicine

REFERENCES

1. Dunant, H. "A Memory of Solferino." International Committee of the Red Cross, 1986.
2. Code of Conduct for the International Red Cross and Red Crescent Movement and NGOs in Disaster Relief. http://www.ifrc.org/publicat/conduct/index.asp.
3. *Humanitarian charter and minimum standards in disaster response.* Geneva: Sphere Project, 2004. Also available online: www.sphereproject.org/handbook/index.htm
4. See Standardized Monitoring and Assessment of Relief and Transition (SMART), an interagency initiative aimed at improving knowledge about the impact of humanitarian assistance. www.smartindicators.org.
5. SMART has developed a methodology (including a survey protocol and software for analysis) that is available to help aid workers conduct rigorous monitoring in emergency situations (www.smartindicators.org).
6. Médecins Sans Frontières. Clinical Guidelines: Diagnosis and Treatment Manual, Seventh Edition. Paris: Médecins Sans Frontières, 2006. Also available online: www.msf.org/source/refbooks/index.htm
7. For a more complete story of war-time Srebrenica, see Fink S. War Hospital: A True Story of Surgery and Survival. Public Affairs, 2003.

Injury and Global Health

10

Jeffry P. McKinzie

LEARNING OBJECTIVES

- *Understand the global impact of injuries, and their relative importance as a cause of morbidity and mortality worldwide.*
- *Know the most common categories of intentional and nonintentional injuries, and their relative importance in the global burden of disease.*
- *Identify recommended focus areas for future research in injury prevention.*

INTRODUCTION

Injury is a leading cause of mortality worldwide, resulting in more than 5 million deaths annually.[1] Global mortality due to injury exceeds that of HIV/AIDS and malaria combined. Deaths due to injury represent only the tip of the "injury iceberg," however. For every person who dies from an injury, there are several thousand injured persons who survive with permanent disability. Additional adverse consequences spill over to affect multiple individuals within the family and community of each injured person.

In 2000, injuries accounted for 9 percent of the world's deaths and 12 percent of the global burden of disease.[1] The relative importance of injuries within the global burden of disease is expected to rise even further, with injury becoming the third leading cause of death and disability by 2020.[2]

Accident vs. Injury

In the past, the term "accident" has been used to describe various categories of unintentional injuries, including those associated with road traffic collisions, falls, burns, and other causes. This traditional view implies that the events leading to injury are random, unavoidable, and unpredictable. Public health officials now recognize that injuries are preventable nonrandom events. After years of historical neglect, injury prevention has become a major area of emphasis within the public health arena. In 2000, the World Health Organization (WHO) established a Department for Injuries and Violence Prevention (VIP) to promote global initiatives in injury prevention and control. The phenomenon of injury has now been taken out of the realm of chance "accident" and placed squarely within the framework of scientific study, where research is being conducted to design effective injury control interventions.

Classification of Injuries

Using the accepted conventions of the WHO,[3] injuries can be divided into two broad categories: intentional injuries and unintentional injuries. Intentional injuries are subdivided into self-inflicted injuries (i.e., suicide attempt or completion), interpersonal violence (i.e., homicide or intentional injury to others), and war-related violence. Unintentional injuries are further subdivided into road traffic injuries, poisoning, falls, fires, and drowning. Most public health experts and organizations, including the WHO, use this classification scheme in discussions of global injury surveillance and prevention.

Mortality vs. DALYs

Mortality due to injuries is a very important indicator of the magnitude of the problem. However, nonfatal outcomes with associated disability and other adverse sequelae must also be considered to fully appreciate the impact of injuries on global health. The disability-adjusted life year (DALY) is an epidemiologic indicator that has been developed to quantify the combined impact of disability and premature death due to illness or injury. One DALY is defined as one lost year of healthy life, either due to disability or premature death. (See Chapter 2.)

Injury Disparities

Although injuries are a leading cause of morbidity and mortality worldwide, the nature and scope of the problem varies considerably by region, age, sex, and socioeconomic status. For example[1]:

- More than 90 percent of the world's deaths due to injuries occur in low-income and middle-income countries.
- Injury mortality among men is twice that among women worldwide.
- Males in Africa have the highest injury mortality rates, and women in the Americas have the lowest injury mortality rates worldwide.
- Young people between the ages of 15–44 years (the most economically productive segment of society) account for almost 50 percent of global injury mortality.

The relative importance of different types of injuries also varies significantly based upon geographic and demographic variables.

- Men have almost three times higher mortality rates from road traffic injuries and interpersonal violence than do women.[1]
- Children ages 0–14 years account for more than 50 percent of DALYs lost due to burn injuries and more than 50 percent of global mortality due to drowning.[1]
- Road traffic injuries are the leading cause of injury-related mortality in most regions except for Europe, where self-inflicted injuries predominate, and in the low- and middle-income countries of the Americas, where interpersonal violence is the most common cause of injury-related death.[3]

More research is needed to clarify the reasons for these disparities and develop strategies to reduce them.

Economic Burden

The global economic burden of injuries is enormous. For example, the annual cost of road traffic injuries alone is estimated at US$518 billion worldwide.[4] In low-income countries, the cost of caring for road traffic injuries is estimated to exceed the amount of development assistance these countries receive. At the individual and family level, medical costs associated with injuries can have a devastating effect on personal finances. This is especially true in low- and middle-income countries, where the majority of injured persons are poor and scarce resources that are needed for other basic necessities must be diverted to pay for medical care. In addition, because injuries disproportionately affect young healthy adults who are in their peak earning years, the loss of earning power due to injury-related death or disability further compounds the economic burden.

UNINTENTIONAL INJURIES

Approximately two-thirds of injuries worldwide are unintentional injuries, with road traffic injuries comprising the largest category.

Road Traffic Injuries

The coroner who attended the inquest of the first road traffic death in 1896 was reported to have said "this must never happen again."[5] More than a century later, road traffic accidents have become the leading cause of injury-related death and disability worldwide. Approximately one-quarter of all injury deaths are due to road traffic injuries. Ninety percent of these deaths occur in low- and middle-income countries. Each year, road traffic crashes kill approximately 1.2 million people and injure or disable between 20 million and 50 million people. Young males between the ages of 15–44 years and vulnerable road users (pedestrians, cyclists, and passengers on public transport) are at the highest risk.[6]

In recent decades, road traffic death rates have decreased significantly in high-income countries, but have increased dramatically in low- and middle-income countries. There is considerable variation among different countries within the same region and economic classification, however. For example, from 1975 to 1998 in North America the road traffic fatality rate decreased by 27 percent in the United States but by 63 percent in Canada. During the same period, road traffic fatality rates in Asia increased by 44 percent in Malaysia but by 243 percent in China. By 2020, road traffic fatalities are projected to increase by 83 percent in low- and middle-income countries, and to decrease by 27 percent in high-income countries. This will result in a predicted 67 percent overall increase in global road traffic deaths. Thus, road traffic injuries are expected to become the sixth leading cause of death worldwide and the third largest contributor to the global burden of disease (DALYs lost) by 2020.[6]

Many factors contribute to the high number of road traffic injuries and deaths in the developing world, including:

- Large numbers of vulnerable road users, such as pedestrians and cyclists, who must share the road with larger vehicles
- Poorly equipped and maintained motor vehicles, which often lack basic safety features such as seatbelts
- Poorly designed and maintained roads with inadequate lighting
- Inadequate establishment and enforcement of traffic safety laws
- Lack of access to quality prehospital and hospital care for injured persons.

The WHO has identified the following five key areas for effective interventions that can reduce the burden of road traffic injuries worldwide: speed, alcohol, seat-belts, helmets, and visibility.[7]

SPEED

Speed is a contributing factor in approximately 30 percent of road traffic fatalities. For every 1 km/hr increase in speed there is a 3 percent increased risk of a crash resulting in injury and a 5 percent increased risk of a fatal crash. Effective interventions include setting and enforcing speed limits, improved road design, and utilization of traffic calming measures such as speed bumps and traffic circles. For example, placement of speed bumps on an accident-prone stretch of highway in Ghana resulted in a 35 percent reduction in the number of crashes, a 76 percent reduction in serious injuries, and a 55 percent reduction in road traffic fatalities at that location.[7]

ALCOHOL

Blood alcohol concentrations greater than 0.04g/dl significantly increase the risk of road traffic crashes. An alcohol-impaired driver has a 17-fold increased risk of being involved in a fatal crash than an unimpaired driver.[8] For any alcohol level, the risk of crash fatality increases with decreasing driver age and experience. Suggested interventions include setting and strictly enforcing blood alcohol concentration limits in drivers, mass media educational campaigns, and utilization of random breath testing. For example, since 1993 in Australia, widespread random breath testing has been credited with an estimated 40 percent reduction in alcohol-related deaths.[7]

SEAT-BELTS

The use of seat-belts has saved more lives than any other road safety intervention. Seat-belts reduce the risk of fatal or serious injury in a crash by an estimated 40–65 percent. In addition, proper use of child restraints can reduce toddler deaths by 54 percent and infant deaths by 71 percent. Suggested interventions include establishment and enforcement of mandatory seat-belt and child restraint use, mass media educational programs, use of audible seat-belt reminders, and child restraint loan programs. For example, a well-publicized police enforcement campaign in the Republic of Korea resulted in an increase in seat-belt use from 23 percent in 2000 to 98 percent in 2001, accompanied by a 5.9 percent decrease in road traffic fatalities.[7]

HELMETS

Head injuries are a major cause of death and disability among users of motorized two-wheel vehicles (mopeds and motorcycles). Nonhelmeted riders have a three-fold increased risk of head injury in a crash when compared to helmeted riders. The proper use of helmets has been shown to reduce the risk of serious or fatal head injury by up to 45 percent. Suggested interventions include establishment and enforcement of mandatory helmet laws, targeted educational campaigns, and development of safe inexpensive helmets that are comfortable in tropical climates. For example, enforcement of the helmet law in Thailand resulted in a five-fold increase in helmet use, accompanied by a 41 percent decrease in head injuries and a 20 percent decrease in deaths.[7]

VISIBILITY

The abilities to see and be seen are fundamental requirements for the safety of all road users. Poor visibility of pedestrians and motor vehicles significantly increases the risk of road traffic injuries. In addition to being relatively unprotected in a crash, pedestrians and cyclists are harder to see than larger vehicles, and are therefore more vulnerable to injury. Inadequate street lighting and insufficient use of reflective equipment and vehicle lights also contribute to poor visibility. Proposed interventions include improved street lighting, increased use of reflective clothing and equipment for pedestrians and cyclists, and requiring use of daytime running lights for motorized vehicles. Crash rates are 10–15 percent lower for vehicles using daytime running lights than for those which do not.[7]

Poisoning

The category of "poisoning" in the injury literature includes unintentional poisoning deaths and nonfatal outcomes. Intentional poisonings and adverse drug reactions are excluded.[9] In 2000, poisoning accounted for 6 percent of all injury deaths and 5 percent of DALYs lost due to injury. More than 94 percent of poisoning deaths occur in low- or middle-income countries.[1]

Europe is the only region where poisoning is a leading cause of death, with one-third of all poisoning deaths worldwide occurring in this region.[1,2] Males in the low- and middle-income countries of Europe have a poisoning mortality rate approximately three times higher than the rate in either sex in any other region of the world, with alcohol poisoning accounting for a significant proportion of these cases. Adolescents and adults between 15–59 years of age account for over 60 percent of the global mortality due to poisoning.[1]

Preventive interventions aimed at reducing the global burden of poisoning injuries include:

- Educational campaigns to inform the public regarding the dangers of accidental poisoning and the importance of proper storage and use of medications and household chemicals
- Establishment and enforcement of laws that mandate the use of child-resistant packaging, adequate labeling, and safer formulations of medications and toxic substances

- Promotion of the use of carbon monoxide detectors in the home, and improving availability of these devices in low-income settings
- Establishment of poison control centers and promotion of their use by the public as a point of first contact following a potential toxic exposure.

In the United States, the introduction of child-resistant packaging, safer product formulation, and interventions by poison control centers and health professionals all contributed to a 45 percent decline in poisoning deaths among children from 1974 to 1992.[10,11] Further investigation is needed to identify ways to adapt these and other interventions for use in limited-resource settings.

Falls

An estimated 391,000 people died worldwide due to falls in 2002, excluding falls due to assault or intentional self-harm. Adults over the age of 70 years, especially women, have the highest fall-related mortality rates in all regions of the world. Children account for the highest fall-related morbidity, however, with almost 50 percent of total DALYs lost due to falls occurring in children under 15 years of age. Approximately one-fourth of all fall-related deaths occur in high-income countries.[1]

Interventions aimed at reducing the risk of injuries due to falls include:

- Public education about fall risk factors and how to modify them in the home
- Establishment and enforcement of laws that promote workplace safety, including fall prevention
- Promotion of exercise programs to improve strength and balance in the elderly
- Education of healthcare providers in how to reduce the risk of falls in the elderly through medication modifications, enhanced vision services, physical therapy, and other therapeutic interventions.

Fires

Fire-related burn injuries were responsible for nearly 322,000 deaths worldwide in 2002.[12] Over 90 percent of burn fatalities occur in low- and middle-income countries. More than half of all fire-related burn deaths occur in Southeast Asia, with two-thirds of these deaths occurring in women. Women in Southeast Asia have the highest rate of burn mortality worldwide. Other groups with statistically higher rates of death due to burn injuries include women in the Eastern Mediterranean region, males in low- and middle-income countries in Europe, and children under 15 years of age in Africa.[1] In addition, for every person who dies due to burn injury, there are many more who experience nonlethal burn injuries, often with permanent disabling sequelae and severe

scarring. Most burn injuries occur at home or in the workplace. Women and children are most often injured at home, especially in communities where open fires are used for cooking, lighting, and heating. Men often sustain burn injuries in the workplace. Alcohol and smoking both contribute to the risk of burn injuries, especially when used in combination. One in four burn deaths in the United States are directly related to careless smoking, and almost half of all burn deaths involve combined alcohol abuse and smoking.[12] Low socioeconomic status is associated with a higher risk of burn injuries in both low-income and high-income countries. Contributing factors may include overcrowded living conditions, inadequate parental supervision of children, and lack of appropriate safety measures.

Scald burns due to contact with hot liquids are also a major source of burn injury. These burns typically occur in the home in association with cooking activities or due to excessively hot tap water. Water heated to 60°C (140°F) can cause a severe burn in 2–5 seconds in an adult and in less than one second in a child. However, it takes up to five minutes for a severe burn injury to occur in water heated to 49°C (120°F), allowing sufficient time for an exposed person to react and remove themselves from the exposure.

Despite advances in burn care in recent decades, primary prevention remains the best approach to reduce morbidity and mortality due to burn injuries. Suggested interventions include:

- Promotion of fire safety education in communities and schools
- Promotion of safer cooking stoves, less hazardous fuels, and enclosure of open fires
- Establishment and enforcement of fire safety standards in the workplace
- Promotion of safer design and construction for single-family and multi-family residential dwellings, incorporating the use of less flammable building materials, smoke detectors, sprinkler systems, and fire escape routes
- Lowering the temperature of hot water taps to 49°C (120°F).

Drowning

Drowning is the second leading cause of unintentional injury death worldwide, exceeded only by road traffic injuries.[13] An estimated 450,000 people drowned in 2000, with 97 percent of these deaths occurring in low- and middle-income countries. Over one-half of all drowning deaths occur in children between the ages of 0–14 years. The incidence of drowning varies significantly by region. For example, the rate of drowning in Africa is more than four times as high as in the Americas, and the rate in the

Western Pacific region is more than twice that of the Americas.[1]

Major risk factors for drowning have been identified.[13] Males have a two-fold increased risk of drowning when compared to females. Factors contributing to the higher risk among males may include increased occupational and recreational exposure to water, and increased high-risk behavior (i.e., swimming alone, drinking alcohol before swimming). Young age is also a factor, with children under five years of age having the highest drowning mortality rates worldwide. Drowning deaths in children are often associated with inadequate adult supervision. Children who live in close proximity to unfenced bodies of water (swimming pools, ponds, irrigation ditches, wells) are at increased risk. Alcohol use increases drowning risk among adolescents and adults, and also contributes to drowning risk in children due to alcohol-related impairment of adult supervision.

Interventions aimed at decreasing the incidence of drowning include:

- Promotion of "learn to swim" and water safety programs within communities
- Mandatory fencing of swimming pools and other water hazards
- Draining unnecessary accumulations of water
- Discouraging by legislation and/or education the use of alcohol while engaged in boating, swimming, or other water-related activities
- Establishing and enforcing boating safety regulations, including essential safety equipment and maximum passenger capacity

INTENTIONAL INJURIES (VIOLENCE)

The WHO defines *violence* as "the intentional use of physical force or power, threatened or actual, against oneself, another person, or against a group or community, that either results in or has a high likelihood of resulting in injury, death, psychological harm, maldevelopment, or deprivation."[14] This definition encompasses three broad categories of intentional injuries: self-inflicted injuries, interpersonal violence, and war. Approximately one-third of injuries worldwide are recognized as intentional; roughly half of these are self-inflicted injuries and the other half are the result of interpersonal violence and war.[15] The incidence of all three categories of intentional injuries is expected to rise, with each category ranking within the 15 leading causes of death and disability worldwide by 2020.[2] More than 1.6 million people die annually due to violence, and many more are injured. Survivors of violence often experience long-term sequelae including physical, sexual, and mental health problems.

Self-Inflicted Injuries

An estimated 815,000 people committed suicide in 2000, making suicide the 13th leading cause of death worldwide.[14] Suicide is sometimes misclassified and unrecognized in official death records due to the social stigma and taboos that are associated with suicide in many cultures. The rate of suicide in the global population varies significantly by age, sex, and geographic region.

- In general, males have a three-fold increased risk of suicide compared to females.
- Suicide rates increase with advancing age. The suicide rate for those age 75 years or older is three times higher than for persons aged 15–29 years.
- The highest suicide rates worldwide are found among males in the low- and middle-income countries of Europe and among both sexes in the Western Pacific region.
- Women in China have a two-fold increased rate of suicide when compared to women in other parts of the world.[1]

In addition, cultural and religious values, socio-economic status, and gender equality issues appear to play some role in the variability of suicide rates in different regions.

On average, the ratio of suicide attempts to suicide completions is 10:1. The likelihood that a suicide attempt will be fatal is directly related to the method chosen. The most lethal methods of suicide include gunshot, hanging, and jumping from a height. The attempt-to-completion ratio tends to be higher among people under 25 years of age who often choose a less lethal method, such as medication overdose.

Suicide attempts are often precipitated by stressful events or circumstances such as the loss of a loved one, divorce, unemployment, financial or legal problems, or problems in interpersonal relationships. These events are common life experiences, however, and the majority of people who experience them do not commit or attempt suicide. Those who are driven to suicide often have pre-existing risk factors that make them more vulnerable. Multiple risk factors have been identified that predispose an individual to suicide and self-injury, including:

- Mental illness, such as depression or schizophrenia
- Alcohol or substance abuse
- Physical illness, especially when painful or disabling
- History of physical or sexual abuse during childhood
- Access to the means to kill oneself (guns, medicines, poisons, etc.)
- History of a prior suicide attempt
- Social isolation[16]

Several approaches have been suggested to decrease the incidence of self-inflicted injuries and suicide, including:

- Early identification and treatment of mental illness and/or substance abuse disorders

- Community-based programs including telephone hotlines, counseling centers, and support groups, especially targeting youth and elderly persons
- School-based interventions designed to identify at-risk youth and refer them to appropriate mental health services
- Media campaigns designed to raise public awareness of the problem and the availability of community resources for those at risk
- Legislative initiatives to restrict access to firearms[16]

Interpersonal Violence

Interpersonal violence is a broad category of intentional injury that includes intimate partner violence, child abuse and neglect, abuse of the elderly, youth violence, sexual assault, and other forms of violence directed by one person or small group of persons towards another. The nature of interpersonal violence can be physical, sexual, psychological, or any combination of these. Deprivation and neglect are also considered forms of interpersonal violence.[14]

Homicide is the ultimate form of interpersonal violence. In 2000, an estimated 520,000 people died as a result of homicide worldwide. For every person who is killed, however, many more survive their injuries, often with permanent physical, sexual, and psychological sequelae. Many survivors also go on to suffer repeated acts of physical and/or sexual violence.

As with other forms of injury, interpersonal violence does not affect all segments of global society equally. Ninety-five percent of homicides occur in the low- to middle-income countries. Three-quarters of all homicide victims are males. The homicide rate among males tends to decline with advancing age, with the highest rate occurring in males aged 15–29 years. The geographic region with the highest homicide rate is the Americas, which includes less than one-sixth of the world's population but accounts for almost one-third of all homicide deaths worldwide. The homicide mortality rate in males in the low- and middle income countries of the Americas is twice that in any other region of the world.[1] Racial, cultural and socioeconomic factors also play a role. For example, in the United States in 1999, the rate of homicide among African-American youths aged 15–24 years was twice that of their Hispanic counterparts, and over 12 times higher than their Caucasian nonHispanic counterparts.

Intimate partner violence occurs in all countries, all cultures, and in all levels of society. Some populations are at higher risk than others, however. Although women can be violent toward their male partners, the vast majority of partner violence is inflicted by men upon women. Surveys conducted among abused women reveal that many victims are subjected to multiple acts of violence over extended periods of time, and many suffer from a combination of physical, sexual, and psychological abuse.

Women are at particularly high risk in societies where marked gender inequality exists, and where sanctions against intimate partner violence are weak and poorly enforced. A significant number of homicides in women are due to partner violence. Studies from various countries reveal that 40–70 percent of female homicide victims were killed by their husband or boyfriend.[17]

Multiple common risk factors are associated with the various forms of interpersonal violence, including:

- Alcohol and substance abuse
- History of childhood exposure to violence in the home
- Family or personal history of divorce or separation
- Low self-esteem and poor behavioral control
- Poverty and income inequality[14]

Violence prevention requires a multifaceted approach. The finding that early childhood experiences play an important role in the subsequent risk of becoming a violent perpetrator suggests an important opportunity to intervene through programs that impact early childhood development and promote family stability. Suggested interventions designed to decrease the incidence of interpersonal violence include:

- Early identification and treatment of alcohol and substance abuse and mental disorders
- Improved surveillance for victims of violence within schools, healthcare facilities, workplaces, and communities, coupled with provision of services to ensure the care and future protection of these victims
- Providing community resources for family therapy and training in parenting skills
- Media campaigns designed to raise public awareness about violence prevention and stimulate community action
- Legislative initiatives to restrict access to firearms
- Establishment and enforcement of strict legal penalties for perpetrators of all forms of interpersonal violence[14]

Collective Violence (War)

Collective violence is defined by the WHO as "the instrumental use of violence by people who identify themselves as members of a group—whether this group is transitory or has a more permanent identity—against another group or set of individuals, in order to achieve political, economic, or social objectives."[18] This category of violence includes armed conflicts between nations and groups, terrorism, gang warfare, genocide, and the use of rape and torture as weapons of war.

During the 20th century, an estimated 191 million people died as a direct or indirect result of armed conflict, making it one of the most violent periods in human history. More than half of these fatalities were among the civilian population. In 2000, armed conflict directly caused more than 300,000 deaths worldwide.[18] As with other forms of violent and nonviolent injury, the number of survivors far exceeds the number of deaths, with many survivors suffering from permanent physical and psychological sequelae. Torture and rape have been used as deliberate weapons of war in some conflicts in order to terrorize and demoralize communities. For example, during the recent conflict in Sierra Leone, many civilians suffered mutilation and severed limbs at the hands of armed forces. During the conflict in Bosnia and Herzegovina, the number of women raped by soldiers is estimated between 10,000 and 60,000.[14] (See Chapter 9.)

In addition to the deaths and injuries that occur as a direct result of armed conflict, there are significant increases in morbidity and mortality that are indirectly related to conflict. Essential infrastructure including healthcare, sanitation, shelter, transportation, and food supply are often disrupted during periods of conflict. This can result in famine and increased vulnerability to disease within the population. Increased mortality is often seen, especially among the most vulnerable populations including infants and refugees. Prevention of collective violence and armed conflicts requires international effort and cooperation across multiple sectors. Goals of the global community should include:

- Reduction of poverty and inequality between groups in society
- Reduction in access to weapons, including biological, chemical, and nuclear weapons
- Promotion and enforcement of international treaties and human rights initiatives[18]

FUTURE DIRECTIONS

Much progress has been made in recent decades in the field of injury prevention. However, there is much left to accomplish and further progress is needed in three important areas:

- **Epidemiology:** Expanded research is needed to more accurately quantify the scope and magnitude of intentional and unintentional injuries, and to delineate risk factors and economic consequences of injury.
- **Prevention:** There is a need to design and evaluate injury prevention interventions, and to identify best practices for implementation among various target populations and geographic settings.
- **Advocacy:** Enhanced efforts are needed to promote education and awareness of injury prevention within the general public, and among policymakers and donor agencies.

SUMMARY

Injuries, both intentional and unintentional, are now recognized as leading causes of morbidity and mortality worldwide. The impact of injuries on the global burden of disease is expected to increase significantly in the coming decades. The causes of injuries are multifactorial, crossing all segments of society. Therefore, injury prevention initiatives must be multidisciplinary in nature, with involvement of public health officials, social scientists, educators, community leaders, politicians, mass media, and others. Significant progress in injury prevention and control has been made in the high-income countries of the developed world. As this progress continues, ways must be identified to adapt successful injury prevention strategies for use within the low- and middle-income countries where the majority of injuries occur.

STUDY QUESTIONS

1. Using the accepted conventions of the WHO, outline the types of injuries discussed in this chapter.
2. List and discuss five key interventions to reduce road traffic injuries worldwide.
3. List and discuss five interventions to reduce morbidity and mortality from burns.
4. List and discuss five interventions to reduce the incidence of drowning.
5. What are some risk factors for suicide? Compare and contrast the importance of these factors in the developing world vs. the industrialized world.
6. List and discuss five interventions to decrease the incidence of interpersonal violence.

REFERENCES

1. Peden, M., K. McGee, G. Sharma. *The Injury Chart Book: A Graphical Overview of the Global Burden of Injuries.* Geneva, Switzerland: World Health Organization, 2002.
2. Murray, C.J.L., and A.D. Lopez. *The Global Burden of Disease.* Cambridge, Mass: Harvard University Press, 1996.
3. Peden, M., K. McGee, E. Krug. *Injury: A Leading Cause of the Global Burden of Disease, 2000.* Geneva, Switzerland: World Health Organization, 2002.
4. Jacobs, G., A. Aeron-Thomas, A. Astrop. *Estimating Global Road Fatalities.* Crowthorne, Transport Research Laboratory, 2000 (TRL Report, No. 445).
5. *World's First Road Death.* London, RoadPeace; www.roadpeace.org. (Accessed 14 January, 2007)
6. Peden, M., et al. *The World Report on Road Traffic Injury Prevention.* Geneva, Switzerland: World Health Organization, 2004.
7. *Safer Roads: Five Key Areas for Effective Interventions.* Geneva, Switzerland: World Health Organization; www.who.int/violence_injury_prevention. (Accessed 14 January 2007)
8. *Road Safety: Alcohol.* Geneva, Switzerland: World Health Organization; www.who.int/violence_injury_prevention. (Accessed 14 January 2007)

9. *International Statistical Classification of Diseases and Related Health Problems, tenth revision. Volume 1: Tabular list.* Geneva, Switzerland: World Health Organization, 1992.

10. Liebelt, E.L., C.D. DeAngelis. "Evolving trends and treatment advances in pediatric poisoning." *JAMA* 1999; 282:1113–5.

11. Rodgers, G.B. "The safety effects of child-resistant packaging for oral prescription drugs: two decades of experience." *JAMA* 1996; 275:1661–5.

12. *Facts about injuries: Burns.* Geneva, Switzerland: World Health Organization; www.who.int/violence_injury_prevention. (Accessed 15 January 2007)

13. *Facts about injuries: Drowning.* Geneva, Switzerland: World Health Organization; www.who.int/violence_injury_prevention. (Accessed 16 January 2007)

14. *World Report on Violence and Health: Summary.* Geneva, Switzerland: World Health Organization, 2002.

15. Murray S. "Global injury and violence." *CMAJ* 2006; 174(5): 620–1.

16. *Facts: Self-directed Violence.* Geneva, Switzerland: World Health Organization; www.who.int/violence_injury_prevention. (Accessed 16 January 2007)

17. *Facts: Intimate Partner Violence.* Geneva, Switzerland: World Health Organization; www.who.int/violence_injury_prevention. (Accessed 16 January 2007)

18. *Facts: Collective Violence.* Geneva, Switzerland: World Health Organization; www.who.int/violence_injury_prevention. (Accessed 16 January 2007)

OTHER USEFUL REFERENCES

1. Krug, E.G., G.K. Sharma, R. Lozano. "The global burden of injuries." *Am J Public Health.* 2000; 90:523-526.

2. National Center for Injury Prevention and Control (CDC) website: http://www.cdc.gov/ncipc/

3. Peden, M., E. Krug, D. Mohan, et al. *Five-year WHO Strategy on Road Traffic Injury Prevention.* Geneva, Switzerland: World Health Organization, 2001.

4. *Preventing Violence: A Guide to Implementing the Recommendations of the 'World Report on Violence and Health.'* Geneva, Switzerland: World Health Organization, 2004.

5. Safe Kids USA website: http://www.usa.safekids.org/

6. *World Report on Violence and Health: Summary.* Geneva, Switzerland: World Health Organization, 2002.

Aging Populations and Chronic Illness

11

Wayne A. Hale, Jané D. Joubert, and Sebastiana Kalula

LEARNING OBJECTIVES

- *Develop an overview of the demography and societal effects of global aging and its relationship to noncommunicable diseases (NCDs).*
- *Understand the increasing contribution of NCDs to the global burden of disease, especially in less developed countries.*
- *Develop a perspective on the rank order of chronic diseases, risk factors, and causes of death when disability effects are included.*
- *Recognize the increasing contributions of development-related risk factors to the expansion of NCDs.*
- *Become aware of institutional and governmental responses to the challenges of managing increasing numbers of older persons and chronically ill patients.*

INTRODUCTION

As countries become more developed, changes occur in their populations that alter the types of problems faced by their health care systems and providers. Successful reduction of deaths at younger ages combined with decreased rates of childbirth eventually shifts the age distributions so that older persons become an increasingly larger portion of populations. Reductions in deaths related to childbirth, undernutrition, infectious diseases, and injuries allow people to live longer and become more vulnerable to chronic diseases. Although these may be secondary to Group I (infectious diseases, perinatal, and nutrition-related) conditions or Group III (injuries), this chapter will focus on the increasingly prevalent Group II [noncommunicable diseases (NCDs)].

Developing as a nation increases access to the products of global markets. As consumers, people often respond to convenience and marketing influences by changing their lifestyle. Generally, as an economy develops its citizens utilize less exertion to meet the demands of life, at the same time that they experience increased access to food calories from nontraditional sources. The resulting increase in obesity and its comorbidities, combined with the adverse effects of increased tobacco and substance abuse, produce the younger onset of many chronic diseases. The more developed countries meet the challenges of these diseases by devoting more resources including manpower. Skilled health care workers are recruited from less developed parts of the world to meet these needs. Initially chronic diseases can be managed medically utilizing these expensive resources, but with time even these resources are unable to prevent functional decline and death.

It is projected that in the near future chronic diseases will become the predominant worldwide causes of death and disability in most countries and that the burden will fall most heavily on the developing areas of the world. Institutions and governments are increasingly focusing on the challenges that this transition in the global burden of disease will present to efforts to improve world health. In the World Bank's April 2006 publication "Global Burden of Disease and Risk Factors," age is noted to have "a particularly strong effect on the pattern and extent of ill health in a population . . . " that is also affected by "the dynamic processes influencing population size and growth, structure, and distribution . . . "[1]

GLOBAL AGING THROUGH DEMOGRAPHIC CHANGE

The worldwide demographics are shifting. People are living longer in most of the world and there is an increasing incidence of chronic illness associated with aging. The following section explains the most important reasons for this change.

Defining Population Aging

Whereas *individual aging* refers to the aging process in an individual, *population aging,* in simplistic terms, refers to the process by which older persons, here defined as persons 60 years and older, become a proportionally larger part of a country's or region's total population.[2] This process, also referred to as *demographic aging,* leads to changes in the age structure of a population, and a higher median age.

Demographic Drivers of Population Aging

Over the last century changes in three principal population factors—fertility, mortality, and migration—contributed to global population aging. It was primarily declining fertility and longer life expectancy that reshaped age structures in most countries of the world by shifting relative weight from younger to older segments of a population, while international migration played a much less important role.[2,3] Although most people intuitively think of changes in longevity when considering why populations age, falling levels of fertility have actually been the most prominent historical determinant in global population aging.[2,4,5]

FERTILITY

While *declining* fertility is the most prominent driver of population aging, fertility-related factors play a multipart role in the aging process. For example, persistently lowered fertility brings about a decline in the proportion of children, which accordingly increases the proportion of older persons. This effect is referred to as *aging from the base of the population structure.*[6] However, past fertility *decline*, such as the lowered fertility experienced in some countries during the Great Depression and World War II, has also led to a *fall* in the growth rate of the older population as the smaller birth cohorts over time reach older ages. On the other hand, past fertility *increase* as experienced in some countries after World War II, has contributed to an *increase* in the growth rate of the older population and from around 2008 until about 2018, these postwar Baby Boom cohorts are projected to augment the numbers of older persons significantly.[4]

While global fertility is estimated to have been persistently high during the 1700s and 1800s at a total fertility rate (TFR) of around 6.0 children per woman, the second half of the 1900s saw a dramatic decline in global fertility levels, declining from 5.0 in 1950 to 2.7 in 2000.[2,7] Resulting from the sustained fertility decline during the 1900s in the more developed regions, the average TFR for 2000–2005 is at the remarkably low level of 1.5, with extremely low levels in countries such as Austria (1.2), Bulgaria (1.1), Greece (1.2), Italy (1.2), Japan (1.3), Slovenia (1.1), and Spain (1.1). Fertility decline in the less developed regions commenced later, generally since 1970, but has proceeded at a faster pace. In these regions the average TFR for 2000–2005 is at 2.9, but large disparities exist among sub-regions. For example, the average TFR ranges from 6.3 in Middle Africa, 4.1 in Melanesia, 3.6 in Western Asia, 2.8 in Central America, to 2.4 in the Caribbean.[2] Although a number of least developed countries still have very high TFRs, such as Afghanistan (6.8), Angola (7.2), Burundi (6.8), Niger (8.0), Somalia (7.3), and Yemen (7.6), rates at and below the conventional replacement level of 2.1 exist in a number of less developed countries such as China (1.8), Hong Kong (1.2), Singapore (1.5), South Korea (1.2), Thailand (2.0), Tunisia (2.1), and a number of Caribbean nations.[2,4]

It is clear that there continue to be numerous nations with high levels of fertility, and that these populations tend to have low proportions of older persons. However, it is important to mention that fertility decline in the less developed regions generally has been much more rapid than experienced in the more developed regions, that the decline is expected to continue,[5] and that a particularly sharp reduction is expected for the least developed countries.[2] This implies that these countries may age sooner and more rapidly than has happened in the developed nations.[5]

MORTALITY AND LIFE EXPECTANCY

It is intuitive to think that once mortality is reduced in a population, that it will automatically lead to aging of that population. However, it is important to realize that mortality reduction influences population dynamics in particular ways according to whether such mortality reduction happens in younger or older ages. Infant and child mortality rates usually are the first to be reduced in a population (and not adult mortality rates). This means that more infants and children survive in that population, and it is therefore common to argue that a mortality decrease in a population usually first leads to a rejuvenation of that population, meaning that there will be proportionally more children in that population, and that its median age is likely to decline.

In general, countries' demographic histories have shown that after such improvements in infant and child mortality, and as fertility rates decline to low levels in such a population, improved chances of survival for adults to older ages becomes a more important factor in population aging.[2] It is therefore usually at a later stage that declines in adult mortality contribute to population aging.

Since the middle of the previous century, life expectancy at birth has increased globally by almost 20 years. Great variations exist between more and less developed regions. Even greater variations exist among nations within the less developed regions, but differences are expected to decrease and more people will survive to older ages. Given current mortality levels, almost 75 percent of newborns in the world will survive to age 60, and about 33 percent to age 80. These proportions, respectively, are projected to increase to about 88 percent and over 50 percent by the middle of this century.[2] Moreover, gains in life expectancy are expected to be higher at older than younger ages. This means that, not only are more persons surviving to old age, but also that once they reach old age, they tend to live longer. UN calculations show that over the next 50 years, global life expectancy at age 60 is expected to increase by 18 percent, whereas global life expectancy at ages 65 and 80, respectively, is expected to increase 19 percent and 22 percent. For the same period in the more developed regions, average life expectancy at age 80 is projected to increase by 27 percent compared to 19 percent at age 60. These figures imply that the older the age group, the more remarkable are the expected relative gains in life expectancy.[2]

In many of the more developed countries, the numbers of persons of extreme old age are of growing importance. Despite the problems with obtaining accurate age data on oldest old persons, researchers in Europe estimated that the number of persons over age 100 in industrialized nations has doubled each decade since 1950, compatible with findings in the United States where a doubling of centenarians has been seen from 1980 to 1990.[4]

According to UN projections, increases in life expectancy at birth began in the mid-1800s, continued during the 1900s, and will continue to increase in all regions of the world to 2050.[2,4]

Despite global gains in life expectancy at birth being the norm, changes in the sociopolitical and epidemiological status quo of some countries have been shown to challenge this historical pattern with particular consequences for the process of population aging. In Eastern Europe and the former Soviet Union, for example, the rate of increase in life expectancy had decelerated sharply by the mid-1960s, and male life expectancy declined during the 1970s and 1980s. In some countries, the decline continued into the 1990s. While causal mechanisms are not clearly understood, the increases in adult male mortality are attributed to a combination of factors including poor diet, increased accident and homicide rates, environmental and workplace degradation, and excessive alcohol consumption.[4,8,9]

In other countries, particularly in sub-Saharan Africa, the HIV/AIDS epidemic has had a devastating effect on life expectancy. As mortality from AIDS usually is concentrated in infant, childhood, and early and middle adult ages, the impact on life expectancy at birth has been shown to be substantial in countries such as Botswana, South Africa, Swaziland, Uganda, and Zimbabwe. Careful analyses of South African mortality data of the 1990s, for example, show marked increases in age-specific death rates in infants and children with a severe increase in young adult mortality. The recent Burden of Disease analysis for South Africa has estimated that HIV/AIDS was the cause of almost 40 percent of premature mortality (measured as years of life lost) in the year 2000, and will account for 75 percent of premature mortality by 2010 if there are no interventions.[10] Further analyses of relevant demographic indicators have shown that these recently increased levels of mortality in infants, children, and young adults have a temporary accelerative effect on population aging.[11] (See Figure 11-1.)

MIGRATION

International migration's role in changing the age distribution of national populations has been far less important compared to fertility and mortality.[2,4] A UN-facilitated assessment of the likely impact of migration as a counterbalance to aging led to the conclusion that, unless the migration flows are of a very large magnitude, inflows of migrants will not be able to rejuvenate national populations.[4] However, there is some evidence that population aging can be influenced in smaller nations, as has been the case in certain Caribbean populations. There the emigration of working-age adults, immigration of foreign retirees, and return-migration of former worker-emigrants, contribute to the aging of these populations.[4]

Urbanization of the Older Population

It is projected that, before 2010, half of the world's people will live in urban areas. Due to the lower fertility and mortality characteristics that commonly occur in cities, this population shift is expected to accelerate the transition to an older world population. However, it should be noted that whereas Latin America has joined North America, Europe, and Oceania in this trend, Africa and Asia remain largely rural populations. Even though the people moving to urban areas tend to be in the young-adult ages, available data show that population aging is occurring in all urban and rural populations, except in rural Africa.[12]

The older population, similar to the pattern in total populations, has become more concentrated in urban areas over the past 50 years. An estimated 73 percent of the population 65 years or older in developed nations lived in urban areas in 1990, compared to 34 percent in developing nations. Regional differences exist, and while older persons in Africa are more likely to live in rural areas than are older persons of other regions, the proportion of urbanized older persons in Latin America and the Caribbean is very similar to the average proportions found in the more developed countries.[12] In spite of the

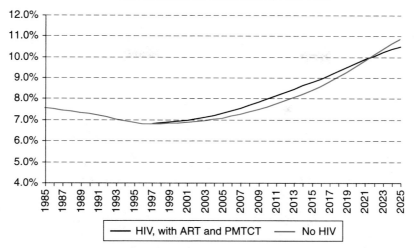

Figure 11-1. Older persons, as a proportion of the total South African population: An HIV scenario with anti-retroviral treatment (ART) and prevention of mother to child transmission (PMTCT), and a no-HIV scenario for the period 1985–2025. From Actuarial Society of South Africa (ASSA): ASSA AIDS and Demographic Models: ASSA2002 Suite. Accessed online at http://www.assa.org.za/ on July 23, 2004. (Reproduced with permission.)

increasing urbanization of today's older populations, rural areas in the majority of nations remain disproportionately inhabited by older persons. This is largely the result of rural-to-urban migration of younger people in search of employment with a small contribution by return migration of older persons from urban to rural areas.[4]

Global Extent of Population Aging

Most, if not all nations, at a time in their history had a youthful age structure, but nearly all nations are now experiencing growth in the numbers of their older populations.[4] In 1950, older persons made up 8 percent of the world population. In 2000, this proportion increased to 10 percent, and in 2050, it is projected to reach 21 percent. These proportions translate to an estimated 205 million older persons in 1950, 606 million in 2000, and nearly 2 billion in 2050, reflecting a tripling of this age group over each of the two consecutive 50-year periods.[2] This implies that the older population over the next five decades will increase by a projected average of 28 million persons every year, or approximately 76,000 per day.

Rectangularization of Population Age Structures

These demographic changes lead to changes in the balance between age groups. The population pyramid is a frequently used manner to graphically represent the age and sex distributions of a population. Historically, the shape has been pyramidal due to the preponderance of people being in younger age groups, with smaller proportions in the older age groups. As the adult age group becomes proportionally larger, the pyramid shape commonly changes to a dome shape, after which it "rectangularizes" as shown in Figure 11-2.[12]

Extent and Rate of Population Aging in the More and Less Developed Regions

In general, the more developed countries are in a more advanced stage of their demographic transitions to lower fertility and mortality, and thus they have the highest percentages of older persons in the world today. Among the world's major regions, Europe has had the highest proportion of older persons for many decades, and it is projected to remain as such for the next five decades. Except for Japan, the world's 25 demographically oldest countries were all in Europe in 2000. Among the oldest by percent of population 60 years and older, were Italy (24.1 percent), Greece (23.4 percent), Japan and Germany (23.2 percent), Sweden (22.4 percent), Belgium (22.1 percent), and Spain (21.8 percent). The North America and Oceania regions have somewhat lower, but still relatively high percentages, with Canada and the United States, respectively at 16.7 percent and 16.1 percent, and Australia and New Zealand, respectively at 16.3 percent and 15.6 percent

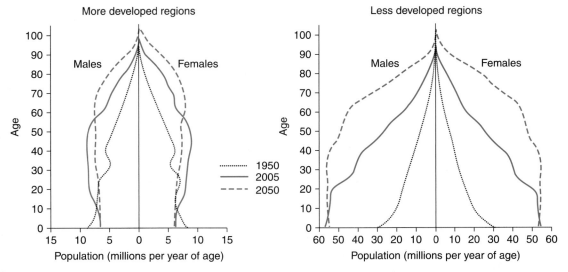

Figure 11-2. Sex and age distributions of world populations, 1950, 2005, and 2050. From The diversity of changing population age structures in the world. Population Division, Department of Economic and Social Affairs, United Nations Secretariat August 2005; p 6. (Reproduced with permission.)

in 2000. All together, almost one in five persons living in the more developed countries were 60 years and older in the year 2000, and this is expected to grow to 28 percent by 2025. Before the middle of the current century, some of these countries may have more grandparents than children under age 18.[2,4,5]

In contrast, 7.7 percent of the population in the less developed regions, and 4.9 percent in the least developed countries was 60 years and older in 2000. Of the UN-classified major areas, Africa (5.1 percent), and of the sub-regions, Eastern Africa and Melanesia (each 4.5 percent), housed the smallest proportions of older persons globally. Some less developed countries were further advanced in demographic change and had higher proportions in 2000, including Tunisia (8.4 percent), Singapore (10.6 percent), Israel (13.2 percent), Argentina (13.3 percent), Cuba (13.7 percent), and Uruguay (17.2 percent). This was still below the average 19.4 percent of the more developed countries.[2]

Proportions by themselves, however, do not give a real sense of the aging momentum in the world's countries. What should be of public health concern is that the total number of older persons and the growth rate of the older population are currently increasing at a much faster rate in the less developed than in the more developed regions. Drastic increases are expected in several developing countries, spanning a wide range of development levels, including Singapore, Malaysia, Columbia, Costa Rica, Mexico, South Korea, Egypt, Guatemala, Morocco, Pakistan, Jamaica, and Malawi.[4]

For the period 2000–2005, the average annual growth rate of the population 60+ in the less developed regions (2.5 percent) was almost three times that of the more developed regions (0.9 percent). Of further concern, is that by 2045–2050, the population 60+ in the least developed countries is projected to be growing at a rate 18 times higher than the corresponding rate in the more developed regions.[2] By the mid-1900s, 54 percent of the world's older population lived in the less developed regions of the world. This proportion increased to 62 percent in 2000, and the trend is projected to intensify over the next few decades to 2050 when almost 80 percent of the world's older persons are projected to be living in the less developed regions. Of the "oldest old," or those 80 years or older, 70 percent are projected to be living in developing areas by 2050. The number of older persons in the less developed regions is expected to more than quadruple from 374 million in 2000 to 1.6 billion in 2050, when four out of the five countries projected to house over 50 million older persons will be in the less developed world (China: 437 million, India: 324 million, United States: 107 million, Indonesia: 70 million, and Brazil: 58 million).[2]

SOCIOECONOMIC EFFECTS OF AGING ON POPULATIONS

As any country ages, it will feel multiple effects throughout society. An aging population not only helps determine the level of health and the types of diseases seen, but all facets of the social, political and economic systems are affected.

Dependency Ratios

Dependency ratios, a commonly used measure of potential social support needs, are a way of describing how the gradual rectangularization of age group distributions will produce socioeconomic effects. These ratios compare the part of the population expected to be in some sense dependent to that part that is likely to be economically productive. This likelihood is estimated using age groupings since aggregate data about individual productivity is not available. Those under age 15 and over age 64 are considered to be unproductive in economic terms, and those aged 15 to 64 are presumed to provide direct or indirect support to those in the dependent ages. It can be argued that these assumptions are not accurate for many populations. For example, in developed countries educational requirements defer productivity until age 20+, and many adults are economically active until 70 or longer. Additionally, in some developing countries with high unemployment levels, productivity in the working age population is not optimal and large proportions do not provide direct or indirect support. Also disability in people aged 15 to 64 may remove them and often a caregiver from the working population. In the future, more accurate measures of the number of worker and dependents will be needed for economic projections, but this measure will be used as an approximation of the burden of dependency for the purposes of this chapter. Dependency ratios for the total world population, and for the more, less, and least developed nations are shown in Figure 11-3.

Due to the large size of their populations, the less developed regions have ratios that are much closer to the world's ratios compared with those of the more developed regions. The total dependency ratio of the world population decreased from around 1975 and is projected to continue declining to around 2015 as those born in years of high birth rates have aged into the productive age groups and as fewer children were produced in succeeding generations. Around 2030 the total dependency ratio is projected to begin to increase due to the rapidly growing older age groups. It is noteworthy that increasing the upper age for the productive age group from 60 to 65 does not have much effect on this trend. In the more developed regions, the increasing total dependency ratio is projected to begin earlier and will be 25 percent higher than that for the world by 2050. About two-thirds of the dependents will come from the older portion of their populations. Less developed nations will continue a low old-age dependency ratio until about 2015 when it will begin to slowly rise. Less than half of their dependents are projected to be older persons by 2050, however, this is a large increase from the approximately 10 percent that older persons contributed in 1950.[13,14]

Delayed Demographic Transition as Productivity Opportunity

Almost all of the increase (from 2.8 to 4.1 billion people) in the world population's working age group will occur in the less developed regions. In contrast, this age group in the developed regions began declining in 2005 and will be 15 percent smaller in 2050. These demographic trends have been said to present an opportunity for the less developed regions to utilize their higher proportion of productive workers to improve economic conditions in their countries. It is, however, important to note that the benefits associated herewith are not automatic, but depend on sound macroeconomic policies that increase employment opportunity, promote productive investment, and ensure a stable socio-economic environment.[12]

Living Arrangements of Older Persons

A recent UN study found that one out of seven older persons live alone, with the majority of these being women. In developing regions, 7 percent of the older persons live alone, whereas 25 percent of those in developed regions do so. The trend in many developed countries for older people to more often live alone has started to decline in some countries, perhaps due to factors such as an increase in the age when children leave home, and possibly also due to greater survival to oldest old ages where a greater need exists for live-in assistance or institutionalization. As people become very old, they have increasing functional disability and eventually need assistance with basic activities of daily living. In some societies, these needs can be managed as three- and even four-generation households become more common. In some developing countries this happens more in families with higher socioeconomic status. In a number of countries, labor migration of adult children has been known as a reason for skipped-generation households, but recent research has found that such households are becoming more common in countries where children live with grandparents due to loss of their parents to HIV infection. Older women are more likely than older men to live in such living arrangements. In more developed economies, the perceived demand for family income is pushing more family members into the work force, leaving fewer caregivers in the home. Ultimately, greater demands are placed on institutions to assist family caregivers. In poor economies, analogous situations of greater labor force participation and less caregivers in the home exist, but little is known about how older persons cope where no institutions, formal home-care, nor assisted-living options exist to help care for dependent older persons.[12]

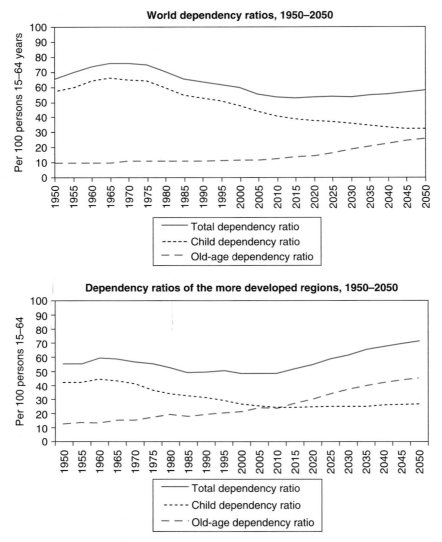

Figure 11-3. Dependency ratios: Total, child, and old-age dependency ratios for the world, more developed regions, less developed regions, and least developed countries, 1950–2050. From Web-based dataset of the Population Division of the Department of Economic and Social Affairs of the United Nations Secretariat, *World Population Prospects: The 2004 Revision*, Medium variant. Accessed online at http://esa.un.org/unpp on 27 June 2006. (Reproduced with permission.)

CHALLENGES OF POPULATION AGING

Any country feeling the effects of a demographic transition to a more elderly population is faced with changes in the socio-economic and political fields. These changes have been very challenging for those countries that have already faced this transition. However, the developing countries must face these issues in a much shorter time frame than in the past. Meeting the challenges in the following section must be a priority of any development plan.

Shifting Age Structures

The shifts in age structures associated with population aging hold important implications for a broad range of economic, political, and social conditions. The older population is growing faster than the total population in both more and less developed nations, and huge increases continue to be experienced in the numbers of older persons. More persons are surviving to older age, and once they reach older age, they tend to live longer.

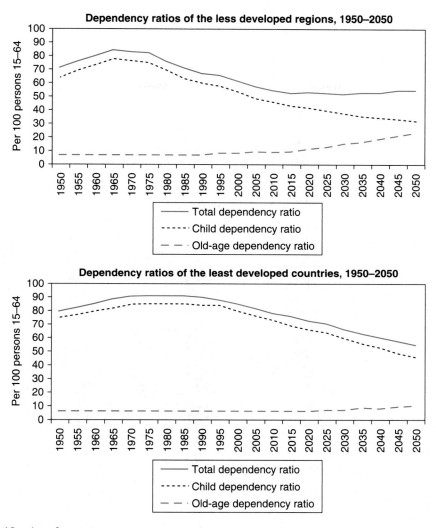

Figure 11-3. (Continued)

As more persons live longer, retirement, retirement funds, social grants, and other social benefits tend to extend over longer periods of time, necessitating changes in social security systems.[2,5] Having more people who live longer is likely to result in rising demands for health services and increasing medical costs. In general, health conditions decline and frailty and disability increase with advancing age, so the growth in the numbers of this oldest old age group is of particular concern. The increase in this group results in an increase in the demand for chronic care, rehabilitative care, palliative care, and other types of long-term care.[15,16] These care needs will promote growing institutional populations and an increased demand for appropriately trained health care staff where institutions are affordable, as well

as an increased demand for informal caregivers where institutions are not an option.

Shifting Fertility, Mortality, and Migration Patterns

An outcome of persistent fertility decline, likely to be of more importance in the less developed nations, relates to the progressive decline in the availability of kin upon whom future cohorts of older persons can rely for support.[2] Fewer family members are available to provide assistance with activities of daily living and disability, life management, financial and subsistence support, and informal long-term care in frailty and severe illness.

As more people live longer through changes in mortality in the majority of the world's nations, various socioeconomic challenges are posed at the societal level. In affected nations, AIDS-specific mortality diminishes a crucial support-base (income-generating and/or caregiving children), producing thereby socioeconomic challenges at societal, community, and individual levels. A number of studies illustrate that older persons are commonly involved with the living and caregiving arrangements of AIDS-sick persons and their dependents in countries as diverse as Cambodia, India, Kenya, Mozambique, South Africa, Sudan, Thailand, Uganda, Zambia, and Zimbabwe.[17–22] Although it is a common phenomenon in some of these countries that many older persons, in particular those in multi-generational households, assist in raising their grandchildren, the AIDS epidemic has brought added responsibilities, concerns, and stressors to many affected older persons. These stressors include caregiving for a relatively unknown disease; a greater burden of housework tasks; dealing with the stigmatization of the disease and those living with the disease; the risk of HIV infection through caregiving activities; extra demands on older caregivers' financial resources to cover health care costs related to AIDS-ill children, costs related to raising and nurturing the dependents of AIDS-ill children, and funeral costs; as well as the loss of current and future financial support from the ill child.[5,17,18]

While international migration usually does not play a major role in population aging, internal migration may pose challenges to the aging of local populations within country boundaries. At the familial or household level, internal migration in some countries, in the form of rural-to-urban movement, may be disadvantageous to older persons who lose their traditional caregiving base (in some communities the only local support base) as children emigrate. At the community and local level a weakened local workforce negatively affects older persons, resulting in a diminished pooling of taxpayers' resources, and, in turn, causing reduced access to health, welfare, or recreation infrastructure and resources in the form of health centers, health personnel, social welfare centers, social workers, and social and cultural events.[23] Lack of amenities, services, and infrastructure, and harsh living conditions in many rural areas pose difficulties for older persons. The provision of health, social welfare, and other support services to ill, disabled, and frail older persons in rural areas continue to present particular challenges to many governments around the world.[4] Also, the provision of services to older persons is likely to present challenges in both urban and rural areas where youthful age structures stimulate an emphasis on infant/child and reproductive health.

These challenges related to fertility, mortality, and migration will be more of a concern in less developed countries with limited resources and less preparedness for an aging population than is the case in more developed countries.

Increasing Female Share

Due to their greater life expectancy, women constitute a large majority of the 60+ population in most countries. The female share increases with age, and women's survival advantages are anticipated to continue so that by 2050 only 38 percent of the 80+ population will be men. This increasing female share is relevant to public policy, because older women are more likely to be widowed, dependent upon social support, and to have less education. They also usually have less work experience and access to income-generating opportunities, assets, and private income sources. The latter socioeconomic characteristics may stem from lifelong gender disadvantages in formal market opportunities, and women's greater burden of providing care for the sick, frail, and disabled. These issues have implications for social support and public planning.[2,5,24,25]

Increasing Prevalence of Chronic Disease and Disability

It is clear that the world is facing unprecedented magnitudes and speed of population aging. The timing and rapidity of population aging are being experienced differently in developed and developing nations, and as the relative size of the youth, working-age, and older-age components of populations change, the shifting weights of these broad age groups are likely to increase social, economic, and political pressures on societies. While population aging has become a well-publicized phenomenon and public concern in most developed nations, there is much less awareness and public concern in developing nations. This is despite the fact that many developing countries are aging at a much faster rate than countries in the developed world, and that the numbers of older persons in developing countries exceed those in developed nations. The rapidity and compressed time frame within which these changes are happening in the developing world, and the fact that it is occurring on relatively larger population bases than in the developed world, pose particular challenges to social and economic institutions in nations with scarce resources.[2]

As individual longevity increases, frailty, chronic disease, and disability rise while physical, mental, and cognitive capacities decline.[15,26] At the societal level, the demographic aging of populations is directly related to fundamental changes in the health and disease patterns within a population as epidemiological change progresses from the predominance of infectious, parasitic, and nutritional disease to the predominance of noncommunicable disease.[23]

THE EPIDEMIOLOGICAL TRANSITION TO NONCOMMUNICABLE DISEASES

Historically, the health status and disease profile of human societies were linked to their level of social and economic development. With industrialization, the major causes of death and disability in more developed societies shifted from a predominance of nutritional deficiency–related and infectious (Group I) diseases to diseases classified as noncommunicable diseases (NCDs, Group II), such as cardiovascular disease, cancer, and diabetes. This epidemiological transition can occur within organ-specific diseases as well as between different disease categories, with childhood infections and malnutrition being substituted by adult chronic diseases and rheumatic heart disease by coronary heart disease.[27,28]

Trends In Communicable and Noncommunicable Diseases

Whereas communicable diseases were previously the main causes of death, improvement in living conditions, the management of infections, and the advent of immunizations caused NCDs to proliferate, especially in Western countries. Noncommunicable diseases (cardiovascular disease, diabetes, cancer, chronic pulmonary disease, and mental illness) have increased the demand for health care in these countries. By the turn of the 21st century, NCDs were present across the globe and showed an increase even in developing countries (see Table 11-1). However, developing countries must still deal with the challenges of the double burden of NCDs and communicable diseases, as the latter have not been eliminated.[29,30]

In the latter part of the 20th century the leading causes of the disease burden were communicable diseases and perinatal conditions resulting from malnutrition, poor sanitation and hygiene, and unsafe water. Though NCDs account currently for less than half of the deaths in developing countries, by 2020 they will account for 80 percent of the global burden of disease.[29,30]

Of the 45 million deaths among adults aged 15 years and over globally in 2002, 8.2 million (18 percent) were caused by communicable diseases and maternal, perinatal, and nutritional conditions combined; 32 million (70 percent) were caused by NCDs; and 4.5 million (10 percent) by injuries. The relative proportion of these causes varies markedly across regions. For example, in Africa, 30 percent of adult deaths are caused by NCDs, compared with 90 percent in developed countries. In Latin America and the developing countries of Asia and the Western Pacific Region, 75 percent of adult deaths are caused by NCDs.[29]

To aid analyses of cause of death and burden of disease, the 192 World Health Organization (WHO) Member States are divided into five mortality strata (A–E) on the basis of their levels of mortality in children aged 0–4 years and in males aged 15–59 years. Three major groupings of countries are used, defined by geography, state of economic and demographic development, and mortality pattern. These groupings are:

1. Developing countries with high mortality (countries in Africa, Latin America, the Caribbean, the Eastern Mediterranean, and South-East Asia)

2. Developing countries with low mortality (countries in Latin America, the Eastern Mediterranean, South-East Asia, and the Western Pacific)

3. Developed countries (North America, Cuba, and countries in Europe and the Western Pacific[29]

Risk factors and disease patterns in these regions differ substantially. In all high mortality developing regions, undernutrition, unsafe water, poor sanitation and hygiene, indoor smoke from solid fuels, and unsafe sex are among leading risk factors. In sub-Saharan Africa, for example, communicable diseases still constitute 7 out of the 10 leading causes of child deaths, and account for 60 percent of all child deaths, with undernutrition causing 1.8 million deaths in Africa and 1.2 million in countries in Asia.[29]

For the industrialized subregions, tobacco, blood pressure, alcohol, cholesterol, and overweight are leading

Table 11-1. Evolution of noncommunicable diseases (NCDs) in developing countries (in millions and percentage distribution 1990–2020).

	Noncommunicable disease	Communicable disease + maternal + perinatal + nutritional	Injuries	Total
1990	18.7 (47%)	16.6 (42%)	4.2 (11%)	39.5 (100%)
2000	25.0 (56%)	14.6 (33%)	5.0 (11%)	45.0 (100%)
2020	36.6 (69%)	09.0 (17%)	7.4 (14%)	53.0 (100%)

From: Boutayeb A, Boutayeb S. The burden of noncommuicable disease in developing countries. Int. J. For Equity in Health 2005; 4(2) June 17, 2006. http://www.equityhealthj.com/content/4/1/2.

Table 11-2. Major burden of disease: leading ten selected risk factors and leading ten diseases and injuries in high mortality developing countries,[a] 2000.[b]

Risk Factors	% DALYs	Disease or Injury	% DALYs
Underweight	14.9	HIV/AIDS	9.0
Unsafe sex	10.2	Lower respiratory infection	8.2
Unsafe water sanitation and hygiene	5.5	Diarrheal disease	6.3
Indoor smoke from solid fuel	3.7	Childhood cluster diseases	5.5
Zinc deficiency	3.2	Low birth weight	5.0
Iron deficiency	3.1	Malaria	4.9
Vitamin A deficiency	3.0	Unipolar depressive disorder	3.1
Blood pressure	2.5	Ischemic heart disease	3.0
Tobacco	2.0	Tuberculosis	2.9
Cholesterol	1.9	Road traffic injury	2.0

[a] Developing countries with high child and high or very high adult mortality (AFR-D, AFR-E, AMR-D, EMR-D SEAR-D).
[b] From WHR 2002. (Reproduced with permission.)

risk factors. Tobacco accounts for about 12 percent of all disease and injury burden. In the low-mortality developing countries, an intermediate picture is seen, with alcohol, tobacco, and high blood pressure accounting for 4–6 percent of disease burden. Indoor smoke from solid fuels, unsafe water, poor sanitation and hygiene are also among the leading risk factors for these areas.[28] (See Tables 11-2, 11-3, and 11-4.)

The tables use Disability Adjusted Life Years (DALYs) for the measure of global burden of disease. DALYs is a metric that combines Years of Life Lost (YLL) due to premature death and Years Lived with Disability (YLD) based on severity and duration of nonfatal outcomes. Thus, one DALY is viewed as one year of "healthy" life lost, and the measured burden of disease is the gap between a population's health and that of a normative global reference population with high life expectancy lived in full health.[29] See Chapter 2 for a more detailed description of these measures.

Global trends show a declining communicable disease burden but HIV/AIDS has become the leading

Table 11-3. Major burden of disease—leading ten selected risk factors and leading ten diseases and injuries, low mortality developing countries,[a] 2000.[b]

Risk Factors	% DALYs	Disease or Injury	% DALYs
Alcohol	6.2	Unipolar depressive disorder	5.9
Blood pressure	5.0	Cerebrovascular disease	4.7
Tobacco	4.0	Lower respiratory infections	4.1
Underweight	3.1	Road traffic injury	4.1
Overweight	2.7	Chronic obstructive pulmonary disease	3.8
Cholesterol	2.1	Ischemic heart disease	3.2
Low fruit and vegetable intake	1.9	Birth asphyxia/trauma	2.6
Indoor smoke from solid fuels	1.9	Tuberculosis	2.4
Iron deficiency	1.8	Alcohol use disorder	2.3
Unsafe water sanitation and hygiene	1.7	Deafness	2.2

[a] Developing countries with low child and low adult mortality (AMR-B, EMR-B, SEAR-B, WPR-B).
[b] From WHR 2002. (Reproduced with permission.)

Table 11-4. Major burden of disease—leading ten selected risk factors and leading ten diseases and injuries, developed countries,[a] 2000.[b]

Risk Factors	% DALYs	Disease or Injury	% DALYs
Tobacco	12.2	Ischemic heart disease	9.4
Blood pressure	10.2	Unipolar depressive disorder	7.2
Alcohol	9.2	Cardiovascular disease	6.0
Cholesterol	7.6	Alcohol use disorder	3.5
Overweight	7.4	Dementia and other central nervous systems disorders	3.0
Low fruit and vegetable intake	3.9	Deafness	2.8
Physical inactivity	3.3	Chronic obstructive pulmonary disease	2.6
Illicit drugs	1.8	Road traffic injury	2.5
Unsafe sex	0.8	Osteoarthritis	2.5
Iron deficiency	0.7	Trachea/bronchus/lung cancer	2.4

[a] Developed countries with very low or low child mortality levels (AMR-A, EUR-B, EUR-C, WPR-A).
[b] From WHR 2002. (Reproduced with permission.)

cause of mortality and morbidity among adults aged 15–59 years (see Table 11-5). Nearly 80 percent of global deaths from HIV/AIDS in 2002 occurred in sub-Saharan Africa. HIV/AIDS has reversed previous gains in life expectancy in these countries.[29]

In contrast to the younger age group, the burden of NCD increases in the older population. (See Table 11-6.) In developed countries, the disease burden of NCDs is over 80 percent in adults aged 15 years and over, while in high-mortality regions the burden is almost 50 percent,

and in middle-income countries it is over 70 percent. Population aging and an increase in the prevalence of risk factors have accelerated the epidemic of NCDs in many developing countries. With a large proportion of the world's population living in developing countries, where morbidity rates and risk factor levels are high and death occurs at a relatively younger age, the absolute number of DALYs attributable to each risk factor is greater in these countries than that in developed countries.[29]

Table 11-5. Leading disease burden (DALYs) among adults (15–59 years) worldwide, 2002.[a]

Rank	Cause	DALYs (000)
1	HIV/AIDS	68,661
2	Unipolar depressive disorders	57,843
3	Tuberculosis	28,380
4	Road traffic injuries	27,264
5	Ischemic heart disease	26,155
6	Alcohol use disorders	19,567
7	Hearing loss (adult onset)	19,486
8	Violence	18,962
9	Cerebrovascular disease	18,749
10	Self-inflicted injuries	18,522

[a] From World Health Report: Today's Challenges, 2003. (Reproduced with permission.)

Table 11-6. Leading disease burden (DALYs) among adults (aged 60+) worldwide, 2002.[a]

Rank	Cause	DALYs (000)
1	Ischemic heart disease	31,481
2	Cerebrovascular disease	29,595
3	Chronic obstructive pulmonary disease	14,380
4	Alzheimer and other dementias	8,569
5	Cataracts	7,384
6	Lower respiratory infections	6,597
7	Hearing loss, adult onset	6,548
8	Trachea, bronchus, lung cancers	5,952
9	Diabetes mellitus	5,882
10	Vision disorders, age-related and other	4,766

[a] From World Health Report: Today's Challenges, 2003. (Reproduced with permission.)

Case Study of Utility of the DALY Measure

At age 56, Mrs. Brown is hospitalized after a stroke paralyzed one side of her body. She is a widow and has been disabled for two years due to depression and complications of diabetes. Her daughter had to quit working two years ago to provide care after Mrs. Brown had a below knee amputation. Their financial resources are exhausted and government assistance is being sought to cover the costs of a nursing home for Mrs. Brown. Her institutionalization is likely to be long-term since her daughter must return to work.

The case study demonstrates how the DALY better represents the total costs to society compared with simply listing patients' diseases and functional limitations. The lost earnings of her daughter and the balance of that loss with the costs of long-term nursing home care are much more difficult to capture. In the United States, the total estimated cost to employers of all full-time employed caregivers was estimated at over $33 billion.[31]. In some nations incentives to keep working-age people in the work force may lead to increased institutionalization of older and disabled people.

Predominant Noncommunicable Diseases

We will now examine in depth the most significant noncommunicable diseases affecting the world today.

CARDIOVASCULAR DISEASE

Cardiovascular diseases (CVD's) are a group of disorders of the heart and blood vessels, and include hypertension, coronary heart disease, peripheral vascular disease and cerebrovascular disease. These diseases predominate among the NCDs.[30] (See Table 11-7.)

In 2002, coronary heart disease and cerebrovascular disease were leading causes of mortality and disease burden globally, accounting for 13 percent of the disease burden among adults aged 15 years and older. Changes

Table 11-7. Deaths caused worldwide by specific diseases (1990–2002).

Deaths (000) and % Disease	1990	2002
Ischemic heart disease	6260 (12.4%)	7000 (12.6%)
Cerebrovascular	4380 (08.7%)	5400 (09.6%)
Lower respiratory diseases	4300 (08.5%)	3700 (06.6%)
COPD	2211 (04.4%)	2700 (04.8%)
Cancer (all types)	6200 (11.2%)	7100 (12.6%)
Diabetes	2400 (05.0%)	3200 (05.6%)

in lifestyle brought about by industrialization and urbanization have led to a rapid increase in CVDs in developing countries. Tobacco use, alcohol, physical inactivity, and an unhealthy diet are all risk factors for CVDs.[29,30] By 2010, CVDs will be the leading cause of death in developing countries.

DIABETES

Diabetes is among the top six causes of disease and deaths worldwide. The number of people with diabetes in the world is expected to increase from 194 million in 2003 to 330 million in 2030, with 75 percent living in developing countries. In contrast to developed countries, diabetes in developing countries often affects a much younger age group. Complications of diabetes such as retinopathy, foot ulceration and amputation, nephropathy, and heart disease exacerbate the burden. Diabetes and its complications are costly to manage and impose great challenges to the health care systems of developing countries.[30,32]

CANCER

Cancer is common in older adults and is a major cause of mortality throughout the world. Over 10 million new cases and an estimated 7.1 million cancer deaths occurred worldwide in 2002. Seventy percent of deaths were attributed to lung cancer alone. It is estimated that between 2000 and 2020, the total number of cases of cancer in the developed world will increase by 29 percent, whereas, in developing countries an increase of 73 percent is expected, largely as a result of an increase in the number of older adults, an increase in tobacco consumption, and changes in lifestyle. These demographic changes may also increase the prevalence of cancers with an infective cause, e.g., cancer of the stomach, liver, and cervix. Lung cancer is currently the most common cancer and its prevalence increases with increasing tobacco consumption. Oral cavity, pharynx, and esophageal cancer types are correlated to alcohol and tobacco use as well as micronutrient deficiency. Colorectal cancer is ten-fold higher in developed countries, while stomach cancer is common in developing countries. The differences in the prevalence of these cancers are mainly due to dietary factors. Liver cancer is common in developing countries. Risk factors for liver cancer are active hepatitis virus infection, alcohol consumption, and ingestion of contaminated food. Breast cancer is five times more prevalent in industrialized countries but the burden of disease is higher in developing countries. If detected early, breast cancer is curable, but 80 percent of cases in developing countries are only detected at an advanced stage. Even if detected early, treatment would be unaffordable in the majority of cases. Cervical cancer constitutes 80 percent of new cancer cases and deaths in developing countries. Effective screening programs and early detection have led to a noticeable decline in cervical cancer incidence and mortality in developed countries. The prevalence is increasing in low- and middle-income countries owing to their limited health care resources and a lack of preventive strategies within their health systems.[29,30]

CHRONIC RESPIRATORY DISEASE

In 1999 respiratory diseases caused 15 percent of the global burden of disease. In 2000 an estimated 600 million people worldwide suffered from chronic obstructive pulmonary diseases (COPD) and 2.5 million deaths were attributed to these diseases. By 2020 COPD is expected to become a leading cause of mortality in the world. In most developing countries, death from respiratory diseases such as COPD and asthma occurs at a younger age because of poverty and its associated increase in respiratory infections and poor access to health services.[30]

NEUROPSYCHIATRIC CONDITIONS

WHO's *World Health Report* for 2003 estimated that neuropsychiatric conditions accounted for 19 percent of the disease burden among adults globally. Mental, neurological, and substance use disorders cause a heavy burden of disease and disability: 13 percent of overall DALYs and 33 percent of overall YLDs globally. Depression, schizophrenia, alcohol problems, and epilepsy are the leading types of neuropsychiatric conditions. The burden of depression is 50 percent higher for women than for men, and women have a higher burden of anxiety disorders, migraine, and late-onset dementias. In addition, a large proportion of people with chronic physical diseases such as diabetes, hypertension, malignancies, and HIV/AIDS suffer from concurrent depression, which significantly interferes with their adherence to health care regimens.[29]

As chronic diseases are better managed and more people live to an advanced age, dementia will become a far greater contributor to disability and death. Traditional risk factors for cardiovascular disease have been associated with an increased risk of both Alzheimer's disease and vascular dementia. A 2005 study showed that the presence of smoking, hypertension, high cholesterol, and diabetes at midlife were associated with a 20 to 40 percent increase in the risk of late-life dementia. This risk increased exponentially with an increase in the number of risk factors.[33]

OTHER CAUSES OF DISABILITY

In high-mortality regions, hearing loss, visual impairment, and HIV/AIDS are major contributors to YLDs. In developed countries and low-mortality developing countries, visual impairment, hearing loss, musculoskeletal disease, chronic obstructive pulmonary disease, and other NCDs (particularly stroke) account for the majority of adult disability. More than 80 percent of global YLDs are in developing countries and nearly half occur in high-mortality developing countries.[29]

Risk Factors

Worldwide, tobacco, alcohol, high blood pressure, diet, and physical inactivity are risk factors for NCDs (diabetes, CVDs, cancer, and respiratory disease). These are preventable diseases. Tobacco is a risk factor for respiratory disease, CVDs, and cancer. Obesity and dietary habits are principal risk factors for Type 2 diabetes. Overall, high cholesterol causes 4 million premature deaths a year, while tobacco causes 5 million, and high blood pressure causes 7 million.[28,30]

In developing countries, urbanization and industrialization lead to a change from a diet rich in fruit, vegetables, and fiber to a diet high in saturated fat, sugar, and salt. The latter diet, combined with tobacco use and low levels of physical activity, is a risk factor for atherosclerosis and CVDs.[29]

TOBACCO USE

While tobacco consumption is on the decrease in most developed countries, it is increasing in developing countries. Eighty percent of smokers worldwide live in developing countries. Tobacco is an avoidable risk factor for NCDs. Tobacco use increases the risk of lung cancer 20–30 fold and the risk of dying from coronary heart disease by two- to threefold. Tobacco is a causative factor of between 80 and 90 percent of esophageal, laryngeal, and oral cavity cancers and exacerbates chronic respiratory diseases such as COPD and asthma.[29,30]

ALCOHOL USE

Alcohol use has increased globally, with major increases occurring in developing countries. In 2000 alcohol use was responsible for nearly 2 million deaths, representing 4 percent of global disease burden. Globally, alcohol is estimated to cause 20–30 percent of esophageal cancer, liver disease, epilepsy, motor vehicle accidents, homicide, and other intentional injuries.[28,30]

LIFESTYLE

Changes in lifestyle have the potential to prevent between 80 and 90 percent of cases of coronary heart disease and Type 2 diabetes, and 30 percent of cancers. Micronutrients block or suppress action of carcinogens, and as antioxidants, prevent oxidative DNA damage. Of the disease burden attributed to a low fruit and vegetable intake, about 85 percent was from CVDs and 15 percent from cancers. Adequate intake of fruit and vegetables can reduce coronary heart disease, stroke, and high blood pressure. High blood pressure and high cholesterol are closely related to excessive consumption of fatty, sugary, and salty foods.[28,30]

Changes in living and working conditions worldwide have led to less physical activity and physical labor. Physical activity improves glucose metabolism, reduces body fat, and lowers blood pressure, thus reducing the risk of cardiovascular disease and diabetes. Participation in physical activity improves musculoskeletal health, controls body weight, and reduces symptoms of depression. Daily physical activity can also help to reduce osteoporosis and falls among older people.[28]

OVERWEIGHT/OBESITY

Overweight (BMI 25–29.9 kg/m²) and obesity (BMI ≥ 30 kg/m²) lead to metabolic changes such as insulin resistance, increasing blood pressure and high cholesterol and triglyceride levels. These metabolic changes promote the risk of CVDs, diabetes mellitus, and many types of cancer. Overweight and obesity are becoming epidemic in both developing and developed countries. In the United States the 2003–2004 National Health and Nutrition Examination Survey (NHANES) survey of adults aged ≥20 years estimated the prevalence of obesity at 32.2 percent with another 34.1 percent of the population being overweight.[34] The prevalence is equally high in many other developed countries and in some developing countries. Of concern is the increase of the disease in children. Overweight/obesity and undernutrition are found side by side in most low- and middle-income countries.

According to the WHO World Health Report (2002), approximately 58 percent of Type 2 diabetes, 21 percent of ischemic heart disease, and 8–42 percent of certain cancers are attributable to obesity. A mechanism by which obesity induces cancer is unclear, but may relate to obesity-induced hormonal changes. Chronic obesity and overweight also contribute significantly to osteoarthritis, a major cause of disability in adults.[28]

The Obesity Epidemic

Obesity and overweight are becoming extremely important risk factors for chronic disease. Obesity has become an epidemic worldwide and it is useful to consider it in detail.

CAUSES OF THE OBESITY EPIDEMIC

The dietary changes and decreased exercise that accompany increasing development appear to be major causes of the obesity epidemic and its associated illnesses. Individual treatments of adult obesity have shown modest efficacy for medications, diets, and lifestyle changes.[35]

As obesity becomes common beginning in childhood, many chronic diseases are occurring at an earlier age. Those countries that have the resources to treat chronic illness and stave off mortal results from one organ failure are finding that these patients then live long enough to develop multiple organ failures. Continued maintenance

of these patients requires dependence on externally powered technological treatments and skilled caregivers. Natural disasters will place these patients at risk of death if the people, power, and supplies for these technologies suddenly become unavailable. Even where these technological supports are available, life expectancies are projected to decline in some developed nations if the obesity epidemic is not controlled.[36] Functional dependency in the young-old (60–70) may become more common and reverse earlier progress toward compression of morbidity into the latter years of life.

OBESITY IN DEVELOPED AND IN DEVELOPING COUNTRIES

Many of the countries leading in economic development have also been the leaders in developing obese populations. In the least developed countries, overweight and obesity remain low. They total about 10 percent in Sub-Saharan Africa and in Haiti, the poorest country in the western hemisphere. Greater obesity generally occurs as a country develops economically.[37] A review of the studies of the relationship between socioeconomic status (SES) and obesity in adults living in developing countries found a pattern for women but not for men. In the majority of studies in low-income countries, the risk of obesity was highest in the highest SES group, but as the country's GNP increased the risk of obesity shifted to the lower SES groups. In the United States in 1974 the lowest and middle SES groups had obesity prevalences respectively thrice and twice that of the highest SES women's level of 7.3 percent, but obesity has increased most rapidly in the latter group. By 2000, the prevalence ranged from 37.8 percent in the lowest SES group to 34.5 percent in the middle and 29.9 percent in the highest. A similar trend has occurred in men, although the middle SES group has been the heaviest, having a prevalence of 29.4 percent in 2000 compared with 23.6 percent in the highest SES and 26.7 percent in the lowest.[38] Being more educated and economically well off appears to have been only transiently protective against the factors producing the obesity epidemic as countries become more developed. Population-wide public health measures to encourage increased physical activity and decreased daily calories should be put in place in concert with research mechanisms able to document their efficacy and lack of perverse incentives. For the effective control of the burden of NCDs, a balance between government, community, and individual action is necessary.

RESPONSES TO THE DEMOGRAPHIC AND EPIDEMIOLOGIC CHALLENGES

Fortunately the leaders in health around the world are paying an increasing amount of attention to the problems of aging. Programs on aging have been developed from the local to the international level. This section will provide some examples of responses to the demographic transition.

International Responses

Various international entities have responded at different levels in various formats to demographic aging, including the International Association of Gerontology (IAG), the International Federation on Aging (IFA), the International Monetary Fund, the Population Council, the Population Reference Bureau, the United Nations, the World Bank, and the World Health Organization. This section and Table 11-8 focus briefly on selected responses from the United Nations (UN) and World Health Organization (WHO). These initiatives often work in conjunction with more general international instruments such as the United Nations Universal Declaration of Human Rights[39] and the United Nations Declaration on the Right to Development[40] that aim to promote fundamental freedoms, care, protection, fair treatment, and the development of all citizens. Various initiatives aiming to guide thinking and the formulation of policies and programs on aging have been started by the Programme on Aging of the United Nations, including some of those listed in Table 11-8. The Second World Assembly on Ageing and the resultant Madrid International Plan of Action on Ageing are remarkable initiatives devoted to a response to the growing global concern about the speed and magnitude of population aging, and continued promotion of the concept of a "society for all ages." Covering the three priority directions of (a) older persons and development, (b) advancing health and well-being into old age, and (c) ensuring enabling and supportive environments, the International Plan provides planners and policy makers with a set of 117 recommendations, tailored to suit both more and less developed country needs.

Within the WHO's Noncommunicable Diseases and Mental Health Cluster, the response of the Ageing and Life Course Programme to aging includes a number of online publications at http://www.who.int/ageing/ publications/active/en/index.html, focusing on topics that are pertinent to population and individual aging. One of these publications, *Active Ageing: A Policy Framework* conceptualizes "active ageing" as a goal for policy and

Table 11-8. Selected international responses to population aging.

Year	Selected International Initiatives
1982	First World Assembly on Aging, and its International Plan of Action on Aging (UN) http://www.un.org/esa/socdev/ageing/ageing/ageipaa.htm
1991	United Nations Principles for Older Persons (UN) http://www.un.org/esa/socdev/iyop/iyoppop.htm
1999	International Year of Older Persons 1999 (UN) http://www.un.org/esa/socdev/iyop/index.html
1999	WHO Minimum Data Set on Ageing and Older Persons (WHO) http://www3.who.int/whosis/menu.cfm?path=whosis,mds&language=english
2002	Madrid International Plan of Action on Ageing (UN) http://www.un.org/esa/socdev/Ageing/waa/a-conf-197-9b.htm
2002	Political Declaration adopted at the Second World Assembly on Ageing (UN) http://www.un.org/esa/socdev/Ageing/waa/a-conf-197-9a.htm
2002	Research Agenda on Aging for the 21st Century (UN and IAG) http://www.un.org/esa/socdev/ageing/ageing/ageraa.htm
2002	Active Ageing: A Policy Framework (WHO) http://www.who.int/hpr/Ageing/ActiveAgeingPolicyFrame.pdf
2002	The Toronto Declaration on the Global Prevention of Elder Abuse (WHO, University of Toronto, Ryerson University, International Network for the Prevention of Elder Abuse (INPEA) http://www.who.int/hpr/ageing/TorontoDeclarationEnglish.pdf
2004	Towards Age-Friendly Primary Health Care (WHO) http://libdoc.who.int/publications/2004/9241592184.pdf
2005	Valetta Declaration (Help the Aged and UN International Institute on Aging) http://policy.helptheaged.org.uk/NR/rdonlyres/ eloqe5kz2upipjiwkmpll5xhil64xkha2bbf3dnrdbnvffevrdqnzkfomwmxsm3tlkdnktlgd7hddkgmkmkex2mhyec/ valetta_declaration_nov05.pdf
2005	The Framework for Monitoring, Review, and Appraisal of the Madrid International Plan of Action on Ageing (UN) http://www.un.org/esa/socdev/ageing/documents/MIPAA_frmwrk.pdf

program formulation, and provides a policy framework for active aging and suggestions for key policy proposals that include the prevention and reduction of the burden of excess disabilities, chronic disease, premature mortality, and risk factors.[41]

Example of a National Response

Table 11-9 includes governmental initiatives undertaken in South Africa where the population is aging at a rapid rate, and where over 7 percent of the total population are 60 years or older. This proportion is the third highest in Africa after the two island populations of Mauritius (9 percent) and Reunion (9.9 percent), and displays levels of population aging similar to that of Brazil (7.8 percent), Mexico (6.9 percent), Samoa (6.8 percent), and Vietnam (7.5 percent).

The commitment toward older persons is shown through these legislative and policy initiatives that contain provisions of either direct or indirect relevance to older persons. For example, the supreme law of the country, the Constitution of 1996, includes a Bill of Rights stating under Section 9, *Equality*, that neither person nor the state may unfairly discriminate directly or indirectly against anyone on the basis of age.[42] The Aged Persons Amendment Act of 1998 provides for every registered dentist, medical practitioner, nurse, or social worker, or any other person who attends to an older person and suspects that he or she has been abused or suffers from an injury, to immediately notify the Director-General of Welfare. The Director-General may issue a warrant for the removal of the older person concerned to a hospital or other such place, and will arrange that the older person receive the necessary treatment. The notifying official shall not be liable as a result of any notification given in good faith, but on failing to comply, shall be guilty of an offense and liable to a fine or imprisonment, or both. It further protects older persons by providing that any person who abuses an older person shall be guilty of an offense, and shall be liable to a fine or imprisonment, or both.[43]

The initiatives in Table 11-9, combined with broader perspectives in local instruments such as the White Paper for the Transformation of the Health System in South Africa,[44] the National Health Act,[45] and the White Paper for Social Welfare,[46] aim at the economic, social, and physical protection of older persons, enhancement of their health and well-being, and promoting access to and affordability of health care.

The government has furthermore observed the 1999 International Year for Older Persons and is signatory to the Political Declaration that commits countries to the 2002 Madrid International Plan of Action on Ageing. It participated in the drafting of the Valetta Declaration at the Commonwealth Heads of Government Meeting

Table 11-9. Selected governmental responses to population aging and a growing number of older persons in South Africa.

Year	Selected Responses
1996	Constitution of the Republic of South Africa http://www.info.gov.za/documents/constitution/index.htm
1998	The Aged Persons Amendment Act http://www.info.gov.za/gazette/acts/1998/a100-98.pdf
1998	The Domestic Violence Act http://www.info.gov.za/gazette/acts/1998/a116-98.pdf
1999	National Guideline on the Prevention of Falls in Older Persons http://www.doh.gov.za/docs/factsheets/guidelines/falls/falls.pdf
2000	National Guideline on the Prevention, Early Detection, and Intervention of Physical Abuse of Older Persons at Primary Level http://www.doh.gov.za/docs/factsheets/guidelines/abuse/abuse.pdf
2000	Guideline for the Promotion of Active Ageing in Older Adults at Primary Level http://www.doh.gov.za/docs/factsheets/guidelines/ageing/ageing.pdf
2001	National Guideline on the Management of Osteoporosis at Hospital Level and Preventative Measures at Primary Level http://www.doh.gov.za/docs/factsheets/guidelines/geriatrics.html
2002	National Guideline on the Prevention of Blindness in South Africa http://www.doh.gov.za/docs/factsheets/guidelines/blindness.pdf
2003	Older Persons Bill http://www.info.gov.za/gazette/bills/2003/b68-03.pdf
2004	The Social Assistance Act http://www.info.gov.za/gazette/acts/2004/a13-04.pdf

in Malta in November 2005 and has shown remarkable support to various international responses by integrating their aims and objectives into the different drafts of the South African policy for older persons, which now has culminated in the Older Persons Bill.[47]

The government provides social services for older persons directly facilitated by the Department of Social Development, and through subsidies to a range of NGOs. Such services include social work services such as organization of community and inter-sectoral programs, and subsidies to community-based care that provides support to community-living older persons. A longstanding governmental commitment is the provision of the noncontributory Older Persons Grant, currently granting R820 (about US$ 116) to age-eligible older persons with an income below a specified amount. South Africa currently faces very high levels of poverty and unemployment, and this grant is often of crucial importance for survival of both the recipients and their families. In a poor continent like Africa, the social security offered to older South Africans through this grant, and the economic impacts thereof, are extraordinary and incomparable.[48,49]

These initiatives show that, at the policy and legislative level, South Africa is responding to population aging and a growing number of older persons, and that it has a commitment toward the well being of its older citizens. These policy and legislative initiatives are good foundations, but need to be followed by a budget allocation and implementation, which will facilitate positive changes in the lives of older persons at the grass roots level.

International Organizations' Strategies Related to Chronic Disease

More information is still needed to understand all the effects of chronic illness and aging. There are programs worldwide that are collecting and disseminating information about aging. The following are some examples of these programs and how they are joining the fight against chronic illness.

GLOBAL BURDEN OF DISEASE STUDIES (GBD) AND THE DISEASE CONTROL PRIORITIES PROJECT

Through World Bank and WHO collaborations, two large projects have served as major international responses toward enhancing global health. These are the Global Burden of Disease Studies, which provide descriptive information about demographic and epidemiological changes and challenges in the world, and the Disease Control Priorities Project, which suggests cost-effective interventions in low- and middle-income countries. These projects include publications with chapters on NCDs, risk factors for disease and injury, as well as demographic change.

WHO STEPS RISK FACTOR SURVEILLANCE PROGRAM

Although the general trend to increasing morbidity from chronic diseases is unquestioned, measurement of risk factor effects is inadequate in many developing countries. WHO STEPS is a tool for surveillance of risk factors that the World Health Organization has developed for use in low and middle-income countries. Step 1 gathers subjective information obtainable by questionnaire, such as habits and socio-demographics. Step 2 collects data from basic physical measurements including height, weight, waist circumference, and blood pressure. These objective measurements are expanded in Step 3 to include blood testing for glucose and cholesterol. Thus information is being gathered on population samples at the level currently feasible for the country with potential expansion of data gathering as financial resources become more available.[50]

INITIATIVES IN COLLABORATION WITH THE FOOD INDUSTRY

In 2003 the WHO began dialogues with the international food and beverage industry regarding positive roles that the private sector could play in promoting good diet and physical activity. The Global Strategy on Diet, Physical Activity, and Health was endorsed by the May 2004 World Health Assembly (WHA) of the World Health Organization. They recognized that supermarkets increasingly dominate retail sales, and that five multinational companies control 50–80 percent of the global markets. Due to the power of food industry advertising, the assembly recommended that governments work with that industry to stimulate the production and marketing of healthier foods. Governments were also encouraged to use mass media to publicize health initiatives such as environmental changes that promote increased levels of physical activity in communities.[51]

RISK FACTOR CONTROL MEASURES

Countries are urged by the World Health Organization and other agencies to develop efficient preventive measures to halt the growing trend of NCDs through control of risk factors. An example of this is the WHO Framework Convention on Tobacco Control (WHO FCTC), which was negotiated under the auspices of the WHO and entered into force in February 2005. The WHO FCTC was developed in response to globalization of the tobacco epidemic. It asserts the importance of demand reduction strategies as well as supply issues and liability. Member states that have signed the convention indicate that they will show political commitment not to undermine its objectives. Further information on the convention can be found at www.who.int/tobacco/framework/ en/. Prohibiting smoking in public areas has been adopted in only a few countries that include South Africa, Brazil, Thailand, Poland, Bangladesh, and Canada. This together with increases in tobacco product prices and government tobacco taxes would produce significant health benefits at very low cost. Promoting physical activity, healthy diet, and controlling alcohol abuse are necessary, but not actively implemented in many countries.

While many developed nations have focused considerable efforts on addressing NCDs, the rising burden of chronic disease in developing countries has received inadequate attention. Improving primary health care for prevention, screening, and early detection of chronic disease may be hampered by inadequate financing, and lack of manpower, but very substantial health gains can be made with relatively modest health expenditure. There are additional factors limiting the control of NCDs, including the emphasis of health care systems on acute care and decision makers' lack of: 1) understanding of economic factors that influence chronic disease risks, 2) information on the burden of chronic disease, and 3) goodwill. In the absence of early detection many people are diagnosed at advanced stages of cancer, cardiovascular disease, and diabetes complications. Without further action it is estimated that in 2020 the disease burden attributed to tobacco will be nearly double its current levels, and there will be a one-third increase in the loss of healthy life as a result of overweight and obesity. For the effective control of the burden of NCDs, a balanced approach to prevention and management is needed at government, community and individual levels.[30,52]

CASE STUDY OF A NATIONAL RESPONSE TO NONCOMMUNICABLE DISEASE

Thirty years ago Finland had the highest death rate from cardiovascular disease. Utilizing interventions including tobacco advertising bans, incentives to lower the fat content of dairy products, and rewards to communities lowering citizens' cholesterol level reduced heart disease death rates by 65 percent and also decreased cancer death rates. During that period of time, life expectancy for men was extended by seven years and for women by six years.[53] Participants in a study in Finland also decreased their incidence of Type 2 diabetes by 60 percent by improving diet and increasing physical activity. They had lower levels of glucose, cholesterol, triglycerides, and blood pressure after a year and continued the improvement through the six years of the study.[54]

SUMMARY OF KEY POINTS FROM A GLOBAL PERSPECTIVE

1. Demographic change has ensured that the number of older people is increasing rapidly throughout the world.

2. Demographic, epidemiological, dietary, and social change have contributed to chronic diseases being reported as the predominant challenge for medical care throughout the world.

3. Developing countries will be most challenged due to insufficient resources and ill-equipped health care systems.

4. As the average age of death increases, the disability effects of disease generally become more significant for a nation's productivity than the death rate. The most recent Global Burden of Disease study has reinforced the importance of including nonfatal outcomes in assessing population health.

5. An economy's success at increasing availability of food, transportation, and discretionary money to buy products such as tobacco often has adverse effects on the health of its population.

6. Medical care can manage the ill effects of risk factors, but must utilize expensive diagnostic and treatment methods to do so. These methods are often not an option to low-income countries, and creative intervention approaches within a prevention paradigm may prove more cost-effective.

7. Companies marketing their products globally and utilizing mass media to promote "desirable" ways of living must consider the health effects on targeted populations.

8. Governments can promote healthier diets and lifestyles by changing incentives.

9. To enhance decision-making and planning for better health, all governments should take responsibility for population health by promoting regular, comprehensive, and consistent descriptions of their country's demography, their burden of disease and injury, and the associated risk factors.

10. Large contributions to global loss of healthy life are associated with a small number of major risk factors. Several risks are relatively prominent in regions at all stages of development. Relatively inexpensive multiple risk factor interventions can make rapid and significant improvements in the ill effects of NCDs.

11. A number of terms exist to describe persons in the later phases of adulthood. We use the term *older person(s)* or *older population* as currently promoted and utilized by the United Nations and the World Health Organization. *Older persons* in this chapter refers to persons 60 years and older. References made to other cutoff points are indicated as such in the text.[2]

STUDY QUESTIONS

1. How would you allocate funds for health care if you were directing your country's budget and $100 million dollars in new money became available annually?

2. What measures might be effective in a developed country whose population is aging to effectively care for a burgeoning retired population while maintaining a work force capable of growing the economy?

3. What methods have been shown effective to help a population growing in affluence make discretionary choices in lifestyle, diet, and habits that promote health?

4. "As the proportion of the world's population in the older ages continues to increase, the need for improved information and analysis of demographic aging increases".[2] Critically argue whether knowledge generation is an important priority in the aging discourse in developed and developing nations.

5. Epidemiological knowledge of the world at the time led to Omran's 1971 Epidemiological Transition Theory, which implies that as countries become more developed their disease profile changes from one of infectious and other pre-transitional conditions to a predominance of NCDs.[55] However, different countries experience different trends in mortality, morbidity, and disability, and more theories of health change have been generated to accommodate such differences. How applicable are these theories to your country's health situation? Demonstrate how demographic and epidemiological changes interact to allow for changing theories.

6. Breslow's classic 1952 paper recognized that weight control is a "major public health problem today" among Americans; 80 years ago, individuals had been charged with higher premiums on insurance because of overweight;[56] and the WHO describes obesity as one of the most blatantly visible public health problems.[57] However, health problems associated with overweight and over-nourishment have gained global recognition only during the past ten years.[58] What factors are responsible for this lag in global recognition of a leading risk factor for chronic disease and disability, and how should health agents, such as health ministries, respond to remedy the situation?

REFERENCES

1. Lopez AD, Begg S, Bos E. Demographic and epidemiological characteristics of major regions, 1990–2001. In: Lopez AD, Mathers CD, Ezzati M, et al., eds. *Global Burden of Disease and Risk Factors*. New York: Oxford University Press, 2006:17.

2. United Nations. *World Population Aging 1950–2050*. New York: United Nations, 2002.

3. Lesthaeghe R. Europe's demographic issues: Fertility, household formation and replacement migration. Working paper of the United Nations Expert Group Meeting on Policy Responses to Population Aging and Population Decline. New York: United Nations, 2000.

4. Kinsella K, Velkoff VA. *An aging world: 2001*. International Population Reports. Series P95/01-1. Washington, D.C.: US Government Printing Office, 2001.

5 Kinsella K, Phillips DR. *Global Aging: The challenge of success*. Population Bulletin 60(1): 1–42, 2005.

6 Pressat R. *Demographic analysis: Methods, results, applications*. London: Edward Arnold, 1972.

7. Batini N, Callen T, McKibbin W. The global impact of demographic change. IMF Working Paper WP/06/9. January 25, 2006. Washington, D.C., IMF, 2006. http://www.imf.org/external/pubs/cat/longres.cfm?sk=18763.0

8. Murray CJL, Bobadilla JL. Epidemiological transitions in the former socialist economies: Divergent patterns of mortality and causes of death. In: Bobadilla JL, Costello CA, Mitchell F, eds. *Premature Death in the New Independent States*. Washington, D.C.: National Academy Press, 1997:184–219.

9. Virganskaya IM, Dmitriev VI. Some problems of medico-demographic development in the former USSR. *World Health Statistics Quarterly* 1992;45:4–14.

10. Bradshaw D, Groenewald P, Laubscher R, et al. Initial Burden of Disease Estimates for South Africa, 2000. *South African Medical Journal* 2003;93:682–688.

11. Joubert JD, Bradshaw D, Dorrington R, et al. Population aging in South Africa in the era of AIDS. Oral presentation at: 18th World Congress of the International Association of Gerontology, June 26–30, 2005; Rio de Janeiro, Brazil.

12. Population Division of the Department of Economic and Social Affairs of the United Nations Secretariat. *The diversity of changing population age structures in the world*. June 5, 2006. New York, United Nations, 2005. http://www.un.org/esa/population/publications/EGMPopAge/1_UNPD_Trends.pdfsearch=%22United%20Nations%20The%20diver

13. Bloom DE, Canning D. Global demographic change: Dimensions and economic significance. July 26, 2006. Harvard Initiative for Global Health, Program on the Global Demography of Aging, Working Paper No. 1. 2005. http://www.globalhealth.harvard.edu/dc_publications.html

14. Web-based dataset from the Population Division of the Department of Economic and Social Affairs of the United Nations Secretariat. World Population Prospects: The 2004 Revision. September 4, 2006. http://esa.un.org/unpp

15. National Academy of Sciences. *Preparing for an Aging World: The Case for Cross-National Research*. Washington, D.C.: National Academies Press, 2001.

16. World Health Organization. *Lessons for long-term care policy*. Geneva: World Health Organization, 2002. September 4, 2006. http://www.who.int/chronic_conditions/en/ltc_policy_lessons.pdf

17. World Health Organization. *Impact of AIDS on older people in Africa: Zimbabwe case study*. Geneva: World Health Organization, 2002.

18. Knodel J, VanLandingham M. Children and older persons: AIDS' unseen victims. *American Journal of Public Health*, 2000;90(7):1024–1025.

19. Knodel J, VanLandingham M, Saengtienchai C, et al. Older people and AIDS: Quantitative evidence of the impact in Thailand. *Social Science and Medicine* 2001;52(9): 1313–1327.

20. HelpAge International and International HIV/AIDS Alliance. *Forgotten families: Older people as carers of orphans and vulnerable children.* London: HelpAge International & International HIV/AIDS Alliance, 2003.

21. Ferreira M, Brodrick K. *Towards supporting older women as carers to children and grandchildren affected by AIDS: A pilot intervention project.* Cape Town: Institute of Aging in Africa, University of Cape Town, 2001.

22. Ntozi J, Nakayiwa S. AIDS in Uganda: How has the household coped with the epidemic? In: Orubuloye IO, Caldwell JC, Ntozi J, eds. *The continuing HIV/AIDS epidemic in Africa: Response and coping strategies.* Canberra: Health Transition Centre, Australian National University, 1999: 155–180.

23. Joubert JD, Bradshaw D. Population aging and its health challenges in South Africa. In: Steyn K, Fourie J, Temple N, eds. *Noncommunicable disease in South Africa, 2005.* Cape Town, South African Medical Research Council, 2006:204–219.

24. HelpAge International. *The aging and development report: Poverty, Independence and the World's Older People.* London: Earthscan, 1999.

25. HelpAge International. *State of the world's older people 2002.* London: HelpAge International, 2002.

26. World Health Organization. Key policy issues in long-term care. Geneva: World Health Organization, 2003. September 4, 2006. http://www.who.int/chronic_conditions/policy_issues_ltc.pdf

27. Yusuf S, Reddy S, Ôunpuu S, et al. Global burden of cardiovascular disease: Part I: General considerations, the epidemiologic transition, risk factors and impact of urbanization. *Circulation* 2001;104:2746–2753.

28. World Health Organization. The World Health Report, 2002: Reducing risks, promoting healthy life. Geneva: World Health Organization, 2002. September 4, 2006. http://www.who.int/whr/2002/en/

29. World Health Organization. *The World Health Report, 2003: Shaping the Future.* Geneva: World Health Organization, 2003. September 4, 2006. http://www.who.int/whr/2003/en/

30. Boutayeb A, Boutayeb S. The burden of noncommunicable disease in developing countries. *International Journal for Equity in Health* 2005;4(2). June 17, 2006. http://www.equityhealthj.com/content/4/1/2

31. Metlife Mature Market Institute. *The MetLife caregiving cost study: productivity losses to US business.* Metlife Mature Market Institute, National Alliance for Caregiving; June 2006:17.

32. Wild S, Gojka R, Anders G, et al. Global prevalence of diabetes. Estimates for the year 2000 and projections for 2030. *Diabetic Care* 2004;27:1047–1053.

33. Whitmer RA, Sidney S, Selby J, et al. Mid life cardiovascular risk factors and the risk of dementia in late life. *Neurology* 2005;64:277–281.

34. Centers for Disease Control and Prevention, National Center for Health Statistics. Prevalence of overweight and obesity among adults in the United States, 2003–2004. August 13, 2006. http://www.cdc.gov/nchs/products/pubs/pubd/hestats/obese03_04/overwght_adult_03.htm

35. Arterburn DE, DeLaet DE, Schauer DP. Obesity: interventions. In: *Clinical Evidence.* BMJ web publication 8/1/06 based on July 2005 search. August 13, 2006. http://www.clinicalevidence.com/ceweb/conditions/end/0604/0604.jsp0

36. Olshansky, SJ. A potential decline in life expectancy in the United States in the 21st century. *New England Journal of Medicine* 2005;352:1138–1145.

37. York DA, Rössner S, Caterson I, et al. *Obesity, a worldwide epidemic related to heart disease and stroke.* Group I: Worldwide demographics of obesity. AHA Conference Proceedings. Prevention Conference VII. *Circulation* 2004;110:e463–e470.

38. Zhang Q, Wang Y. Trends in the association between obesity and socioeconomic status in US adults: 1971 to 2000. *Obesity Research* 2004;12:10.

39. United Nations. *Universal Declaration of Human Rights.* Resolution 217 A (III) of December 10, 1948, adopted and proclaimed by the General Assembly of the United Nations. New York, United Nations, 1948. October 11, 2006. http://www.unhchr.ch/udhr/lang/eng.htm

40. United Nations. *Declaration on the Right to Development.* Resolution 41/128 of December 4, 1986, adopted by the General Assembly of the United Nations. New York: United Nations, 1986. October 11, 2006. http://www.un.org/documents/ga/res/41/a41r128.htm

41. World Health Organization. *Active Ageing: A Policy Framework.* Geneva: World Health Organization, 2002. October 11, 2006. http://whqlibdoc.who.int/hq/2002/WHO_NMH_NPH_02.8.pdf

42. Republic of South Africa. *Constitution of the Republic of South Africa, Act No. 108 of 1996.* Pretoria, Republic of South Africa, 1996. October 11, 2006. http://www.info.gov.za/documents constitution/index.htm

43. Republic of South Africa. *Aged Persons Amendment Act, Act No. 100 of 1998.* Pretoria, Republic of South Africa, 1998. October 11, 2006. http://www.info.gov.za/gazette/acts/1998/a100-98.pdf

44. Ministry of Health. White Paper for the Transformation of the Health System in South Africa. Pretoria, Ministry of Health, 1997. October 11, 2006. http://www.doh.gov.za/docs/policy/white_paper/healthsys97_01.html

45. Republic of South Africa. National Health Act, Act No. 61 of 2003. Pretoria, Republic of South Africa, 2004. October 11, 2006. http://www.info.gov.za/gazette/acts/2003/a61-03.pdf

46. Department of Welfare. White Paper for Social Development. Pretoria: Department of Welfare, 1997. October 11, 2006. http://www.polity.org.za/html/govdocs/white_papers/social971.html?rebookmark=1

47. Republic of South Africa. Older Persons Bill, Bill No. 68 of 2003. Pretoria, Republic of South Africa, 2003. October 11, 2006. http://www.info.gov.za/gazette/bills/2003/b68-03.pdf

48. Institute of Development and Policy Management (IDPM), HelpAge International. *Noncontributory pensions and poverty prevention: A comparative study of Brazil and South Africa.* London: IDPM & HelpAge International, 2003.

49. Case A, Deaton A. Large cash transfers to the elderly in South Africa. *The Economic Journal* 1998;108 (September):1330–1361.

50. STEPS conceptual framework: chronic diseases and health promotion. WHO sites, World Health Organization, 2006. July 26, 2006. www.who.int/chp/steps/framework/en/index.html

51. World Health Organization. Global Strategy on Diet, Physical Activity, and Health. Geneva: World Health Organization,

2004. July 26, 2006. http://www.who.int/dietphysicalactivity/strategy/eb11344/strategy_english_web.pdf

52. Yach D, Hawkers C, Gould CL, et al. The Global Burden of Chronic Diseases. Overcoming Impediments to Prevention and Control. *JAMA* 2004;291:2616–2622.

53. Jamison DT, Breman JG, Measham AR, et al., eds. Cost Effective Strategies for Noncommunicable Diseases, Risk Factors, and Behaviors, In: *Priorities in Health*. Washington, D.C.: The World Bank, 2006:101.

54. Tuomilehto J, Lindstrom J, Eriksson JG, et al. Prevention of Type 2 diabetes with changes in lifestyle among subjects with impaired glucose tolerance. *NEJM* 1994;308:367–372.

55. Omran A. The epidemiological transition: A theory of the epidemiology of population change. *Millbank Memorial Fund Quarterly*, 1971;49:509–538.

56. Breslow L. Public health aspects of weight control. *American Journal of Public Health* 1952;42:116–20. (Reprinted in: *International Journal of Epidemiology* 2006;35:10–12)

57. World Health Organization. *Obesity: Preventing and managing the global epidemic*. WHO Technical Report Series, No. 894. Geneva: World Health Organization, 2000.

58. Haslam DW, James WPT. Obesity. *The Lancet* 366: 2005; 1197–1209.

Emerging Diseases and Antimicrobial Resistance

12

Arif R. Sarwari and Rashida A. Khakoo

LEARNING OBJECTIVES

- *Recognize emerging and re-emerging infectious diseases as threats to global health.*
- *Raise awareness of the national and international response to emerging infectious diseases.*
- *Learn about global issues of antimicrobial resistance of a variety of organisms and their spread.*
- *Understand various concepts of antimicrobial resistance.*
- *Learn about the impact of antimicrobial resistance in patients and communities.*
- *Expand knowledge regarding prevention and control strategies directed against problems of antimicrobial resistance.*

CASE STUDY OF AN EMERGING INFECTION

Severe Acute Respiratory Syndrome (SARS) is a prototypical emerging infectious disease that, largely because of global travel, instead of remaining an obscure respiratory infection in South China, became a global public health crisis. By the time the outbreak ran its course, over 8000 cases were identified from 29 countries with an overall 10 percent fatality rate.

Global attention towards the outbreak was first drawn in March 2003 with the recognition of cases of severe acute respiratory illness among patients in the Guangdong province of China, Hong Kong, Vietnam, Singapore, and Canada. The World Health Organization (WHO) issued a global alert and coined the term Severe Acute Respiratory Syndrome (SARS) for the disease. By April 2003, the WHO had to take the unprecedented step of issuing a travel advisory for the Guangdong Province and for Hong Kong, later broadened to other countries. Eventually, the etiologic agent was identified as a novel coronavirus (SARS CoV), likely a virus that jumped species from the civet (cat-like delicacy in China) to humans. The initial zoonotic transmission was followed by subsequent nosocomial and human-to-human transmission perpetuating a widespread global epidemic. Most patients presented with fever, cough, shortness of breath, and reported either close contact with a person with SARS or a history of travel or residence in an area with recent local SARS transmission. The chest radiograph would reveal findings of pneumonia or acute respiratory distress syndrome (ARDS), with some cases progressing on to require ventilatory support. Supportive treatment remained the mainstay of clinical care.

Initial cases of SARS were reported from Guangdong province of China in November 2002 with almost 800 cases noted by February 2003. A physician with SARS contributed to the subsequent widespread dissemination of the disease by traveling from Guangdong to a hotel in Hong Kong and infecting ten other individuals who then traveled widely, perpetuating outbreaks in their countries of destination.[1] Most severe illness occurred in adults, with children, if infected at all, developing a milder illness. Patients above the age of 60 years had a higher mortality, with a case fatality rate up to 43 percent. Twenty-nine countries in Asia, Europe, and North America were affected with 83 percent of the reported cases hailing from China and Hong Kong. Table 12-1 depicts the timeline of the SARS outbreak.

While most disease transmission occurred by droplet spread (requiring face-to-face contact), airborne transmission with droplet nuclei was strongly suspected as the cause of cases in a large apartment complex in Hong Kong.[2] Transmission to health care workers was a common feature of the outbreak. This was likely precipitated by the high levels of viral shedding in nasopharyngeal

Table 12-1. Timeline of the SARS Outbreak.[a]

November 2002	First cases reported in Southern China.
February 2003	Up to 792 cases reported from Guangdong province, China.
	Index case of symptomatic physician traveling to Hong Kong.
	Transmission to others living in same hotel as index case.
	Widespread dissemination to Singapore, Vietnam, Canada, Thailand.
March 2003	Global alert issued by WHO (March 12th).
	1622 cases reported from 13 countries, with 58 deaths.
April 2003	WHO issues travel advisory to China, Hong Kong, Taiwan, and Toronto.
	5663 cases reported from 26 countries, with 372 deaths.
May 2003	Travel advisories lifted for Toronto.
	8360 cases reported from 29 countries, with 764 deaths.
June 2003	WHO lifts last remaining travel advisory for China.
	100 days into the outbreak (June 19th).
	8447 cases reported from 29 countries, with 811 deaths.
July 2003	Major epidemic in Asia ended.
	WHO declares SARS outbreak contained worldwide.

[a] www.who.int/csr/sars/en/

aspirates early, and in stool later in the disease course, with possible environmental contamination. Infection control guidelines requiring that hospitalized patients be isolated in negative pressure rooms and that all health care workers wear masks, gowns, gloves, and protective eyewear helped finally control the epidemic.

DEFINITION AND BACKGROUND OF EMERGING DISEASES

The global spread of infectious disease can be traced back to the 16th century when Spanish explorers reportedly introduced smallpox, typhus, and measles to the susceptible population of the New World and returned with syphilis. This introduction of new diseases resulted in catastrophic depopulation with approximately 50 million deaths amongst the native South Americans. There has subsequently been a number of major epidemics but by the mid-20th century, primarily with the rapid advances in sanitation and public health, infectious diseases were felt to be a problem of the past. In the United States, infectious disease mortality rates, per 100,000 population, fell from 500 in 1900 to 50 in 1960.[3] This success was reflected in statements such as "… one can think of the middle of the twentieth

century as the end of one of the most important social revolutions in history, the virtual elimination of infectious disease as a significant factor in social life."[4]

This optimism, unfortunately, was short lived as infectious diseases staged a dramatic come back with more than 30 new diseases, including the HIV/AIDS pandemic, emerging in just the past three decades. In addition, old foes like malaria and tuberculosis returned with a vengeance. Among these and other infections, our options for control started shrinking as drug resistance started spreading. In fact, in the United States, between 1980 and 1992, the death rate from infectious diseases increased 50 percent.[3] Attention towards these emerging and re-emerging infections was first drawn by a landmark 1992 report by the Institute of Medicine.[5] This report drew attention to the fact that pathogenic microbes can be resilient and dangerous foes. While it is impossible to predict their individual emergence in time and place, we can be confident that new microbial diseases will continue to emerge. Based on this report, these diseases were defined as:

New, reemerging, or drug-resistant infections whose incidence in humans has increased within the past two decades or whose incidence threatens to increase in the near future.

This concept of emerging infections is flexible, reflecting not only the temporal and geographical interactions between humans and microbes, but also the ability of the medical community to identify them. The relationship between man and microbe is seldom stable. New threats are ever present, confronting public health authorities as well as physicians.

The Institute of Medicine report identified some key factors explaining why infectious diseases emerge or re-emerge. These include:

1. Global travel
2. Globalization of the food supplies and centralized processing of food
3. Population growth and increased urbanization and crowding
4. Population movements due to civil wars, famines, and other man-made or natural disasters
5. Irrigation, deforestation, and reforestation projects that alter the habitats of disease-carrying insects and animals
6. Human behaviors, such as intravenous drug use and risky sexual behavior
7. Increased use of antimicrobial agents and pesticides, hastening the development of resistance
8. Increased human contact with tropical rain forests and other wilderness habitats that are reservoirs for insects and animals that harbor unknown infectious agents

Table 12-2. Major agents of infectious disease identified over the past three decades.

Year	Infectious Agent Identified
1975–1979	Parvovirus B19, *Cryptosporidium parvum,* Ebola, *Legionella pneumophila, Campylobacter* spp.
1980–1984	*Borrelia burgdorferi,* HIV, *E. coli* 0157:H7, *Helicobacter pylori.*
1985–1989	*Ehrlichia* spp., Hepatitis C and E virus
1990–1994	*Vibrio cholera* 0139, *Bartonella henselae,* Sin nombre virus, Human Herpes Virus 8/Kaposi's Sarcoma Herpes Virus
1995–1999	Prions, Influenza A H5N1, Enterovirus 71, West Nile Virus
2000–2004	SARS-corona virus, Human Metapneumovirus

Table 12-2 lists some of the major agents of infectious disease identified over the past three decades.

Examples of Emerging and Re-emerging Infectious Diseases

Although there are many examples of new, emerging, and re-emerging illnesses, several of particular importance worldwide will be discussed. Agents of bioterrorism have assumed great importance and the illnesses associated with terrorism will also be included in this discussion.

DENGUE

Dengue virus infection is an example of an emerging infection with a wide distribution, now found in all continents except Europe and Antarctica (see Figure 12-1). With over 100 million annual infections worldwide among the 2.5 billion individuals at risk, the dengue viruses are arguably the most important arthropod-borne viruses from a medical and public health perspective.[6] A flavivirus, the dengue virus has four antigenically related but distinct serotypes carried by the principal mosquito vector *Aedes aegypti,* which is well adapted to the urban environment.

Both epidemic and endemic transmission is maintained through a human-mosquito-human cycle and no evidence for a significant animal reservoir exists, unlike yellow fever or West Nile virus. Susceptible individuals become infected after the bite of the infected female *Aedes* mosquito and become viremic towards the end of a four- to six-day incubation period. Viremia persists until the resolution of fever, usually in seven days. Mosquitoes become infected if they feed on the viremic individual, and after eight to twelve days are capable of transmission of disease for the duration of their lifespan. They are daytime urban feeders and prefer to bite humans, frequently taking multiple blood meals in a single breeding cycle. Thus transmission among multiple family members is common. *Aedes aegypti* are widely distributed from latitude 45° N to 35° S. While greatly restricted in distribution in the Western hemisphere during the

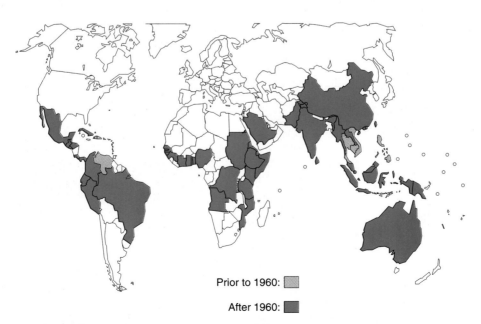

Prior to 1960: ▨

After 1960: ▪

Figure 12-1. Global distribution of cases of dengue, before and after 1960 (http://www.who.int/csr/disease/dengue/impact/en/index.html)

1970s yellow fever control programs, they now have re-infested nearly all their former habitats.

The vast majority of cases of dengue virus infection globally are from areas with hyperendemic transmission—the continuous circulation of multiple dengue virus serotypes, particularly in urban areas. Most clinical cases occur among children as the prevalence of antibody rises with age and most adults are immune. This immunity is, however, serotype-specific and may in fact predispose to more fulminant disease. Instead of a self-limiting, nonspecific, febrile viral illness, individuals with antibodies to one dengue virus serotype but infected with another serotype are more likely to manifest the complications of hemorrhagic fever and dengue shock syndrome secondary to a capillary leak phenomenon. Up to 500,000 such cases occur annually with approximately 25,000 deaths worldwide. There is currently no specific treatment available.

Various factors have been implicated in the increased transmission of dengue virus of late. Warmer temperatures increase the length of time that a mosquito remains infective and crowded conditions increase the potential for transmission. Global climate change with increased global temperatures is expected to further expand the range of *A. aegypti* and dengue virus.

AVIAN INFLUENZA

Avian influenza H5N1 represents an emerging disease with currently focal distribution but with explosive potential, not unlike the 1918 global influenza pandemic that killed 20 million people. The 1918 pandemic caused by H1N1 remains, to date, the greatest infectious disease outbreak in history. This virus was an avian strain that adapted to infect and transmit among humans. Of the three influenza pandemics in the 20th century, two were caused by human-avian reassortant viruses (H2N2 in 1957 and H3N2 in 1968). Genetic reassortment between avian and human viruses leading to a new virus capable of pandemic spread may occur in coinfected persons or intermediate hosts such as pigs that have receptors for both avian and human influenza viruses.

After its initial identification in May 1997 in a young boy who died of influenza in Hong Kong, sporadic transmission of avian influenza H5N1 to about 200 humans in Asia has raised concerns about an imminent pandemic.[7] The virus is now endemic among bird and poultry populations in Eurasia, likely spread by migratory birds, with concerns that the virus will adapt to a strain capable of sustained human-to-human transmission, unlike the current strain where almost all cases are secondary to direct contact with poultry.

Like most new influenza strains, the current H5N1 strain also emerged in Southeast Asia and rapidly spread westward, reaching Turkey by 2006. This spread has continued despite the culling of domestic and agriculture poultry flocks. Human infections have been confirmed in Thailand, Vietnam, Indonesia, Cambodia, China, Turkey, Azerbaijan, and Iraq with a 50 percent case-fatality rate. Human cases from 2006 compared to 1997 show that the virus has undergone some antigenic changes (i.e., antigenic drift).

Clinical presentation may include symptoms related to both the respiratory and gastrointestinal systems. Most patients present with fever, upper respiratory symptoms, diarrhea and pneumonia as documented by chest radiographs. Laboratory abnormalities may include elevated aminotransferases and pancytopenia with complications and death resulting from respiratory failure and multiorgan dysfunction.

The H5N1 avian influenza virus is resistant to amantadine and rimantadine but susceptible to the neuraminidase inhibitors oseltamivir and zanamavir. The latter are most effective early in the course of illness. Unfortunately, strains with a high level of oseltamivir resistance have already been identified from a few Vietnamese patients. In addition to treating the patient, household contacts are recommended to receive post-exposure prophylaxis with oseltamivir (75 mg daily for seven to ten days).

The World Health Organization and governments across the world are currently actively preparing for a pandemic by investing in vaccine development, stockpiling medication, and developing grass root plans to cater to large numbers of patients. As of August 2006, WHO had retained the avian influenza pandemic alert at Phase 3. The following is a description of the six phases of pandemic alert:

Phase 1: Interpandemic phase; low risk of human cases

Phase 2: New virus in animals but no human cases; high risk of human cases

Phase 3: Pandemic alert; no or very limited human-to-human transmission

Phase 4: Clusters of human cases suggesting increased adaptability of the virus; evidence of increased human-to-human transmission

Phase 5: Larger clusters of human cases over longer periods; evidence of significant human-to-human transmission

Phase 6: Pandemic; efficient and sustained human-to-human transmission

WEST NILE

The West Nile virus, another flavivirus, suddenly emerged in North America in August 1999. It was first identified as an outbreak of viral encephalitis in New York with 62 cases and 7 deaths.[8] The virus has since progressively spread westward and 2005 saw activity detected in 48 states and the District of Columbia. An arbovirus extensively distributed throughout Africa, the Middle East, Europe, South Asia, and

Table 12-3. Potential bioterrorism agents by category.

Category A	Category B	Category C
Variola major (Smallpox)	*Coxiella burnetii* (Q fever)	Nipah virus
Bacillus anthracis (Anthrax)	*Brucella* spp. (Brucellosis)	Hanta virus
Yersinia pestis (Plague)	*Burkholderia mallei* (Glanders)	Congo-Crimean hemorrhagic fever (CCHF) virus
Clostridium botulinum (Botulism)	*Burkholderia pseudomallei* (Meliodiosis)	
Francisella tularensis (Tularemia)	*Chlamydia psittaci* (Psittacosis)	Tick-borne encephalitis viruses
Filoviruses (Ebola, Marburg)	*Rickettsia prowazeki* (Typhus)	Yellow fever
Arenaviruses (Lassa, Junin)	Alphaviruses (Encephalitis viruses)	Multidrug resistant tuberculosis (MDRTB)
	Ricin toxin	
	Clostridium perfringens toxin	
	Staphylococcus enterotoxin B	
	Salmonella spp. (Salmonellosis)	
	Shigella dysenteriae (Shigellosis)	
	E. coli O157:H7 (Enterohemorrhagic *E.coli*)	
	Vibrio cholerae (Cholera)	
	Cryptosporidium parvum (Cryptosporidiosis)	

Australia, the North American strain is believed to have been imported from the Middle East, likely through air travel. In the United States, the peak of the outbreak was in 2003 when all but three states in the continental United States reported a total of 9862 cases, 2866 with neuroinvasive disease. Like other arboviral encephalitides, peak incidence was seen in late summer or early fall. Viral transmission has since spread to Canada, Mexico, the Caribbean, and Central America.

Mosquitoes of the Culex species are the primary vectors with birds as the primary amplifying hosts, maintaining a bird-mosquito-bird cycle. Humans are incidental hosts and, unlike dengue, not important for transmission. Most human cases are asymptomatic or present with a nonspecific febrile illness with only 1 in 150 infections resulting in meningitis or encephalitis, especially in the elderly. No specific treatment exists.

West Nile virus transmission in the United States has subsequently also been described with blood transfusions and organ transplantation, the latter often with catastrophic results.

AGENTS OF BIOTERRORISM

In addition to the natural emergence and re-emergence of disease, some biological agents have the potential to be used deliberately to inflict mass casualties. Among weapons of mass destruction, biological weapons are more destructive and cheaper to produce than chemical weapons, and may be as lethal as nuclear weapons. It is estimated that the aerosolized release of 100 kg of anthrax spores upwind of Washington, DC would result in between 130,000 and 3,000,000 deaths, similar to a hydrogen bomb.[9] In 2001, the United States experienced a bioterrorism attack using anthrax powder distributed via the postal system.[10] Three cases of anthrax were confirmed in South Florida in October 2001 with 19 additional confirmed or suspected cases from New York City, New Jersey, Maryland, Pennsylvania, Virginia, Connecticut, and Washington, DC Eleven of these were cases of inhalational anthrax, most occurring in postal employees. The Centers for Disease Control and Prevention (CDC) and FBI continue to investigate this attack.

While the list of potential biologic agents is large, the CDC has identified a number of high-priority organisms as category A agents based on their potential for easy dissemination, person-to-person transmission, and ability to cause panic, social disruption, and high mortality. Category B agents are moderately easy to disseminate and cause moderate morbidity and low mortality while Category C agents include emerging pathogens that could be engineered for mass dissemination in the future because of availability (see Table 12-3). Preparedness and planning for a bioterrorism-related event involves strengthening existing systems for detection and response to naturally occurring epidemics, particularly the emerging and re-emerging infections. Through strong epidemiologic training, development of a communications infrastructure, a network of diagnostic laboratories, and a respect for the threat of biological terrorism, preparedness can be improved and the impact of epidemics, regardless of the origin, can be reduced.

GLOBAL RESPONSE TO THE PROBLEM

In response to the Institute of Medicine report, the CDC developed a strategic plan in 1994 that was subsequently updated in 1998.[11] Four interdependent goals were identified:

1. Surveillance and response
2. Applied research
3. Infrastructure and training
4. Prevention and control

Surveillance systems monitor emerging infectious pathogens and outbreaks of disease. A response is mounted when surveillance data or other information indicates a change in the incidence or distribution of an infectious disease, or when a new or variant strain of a pathogen has become a health threat. Through applied research, scientists answer questions about the etiology, transmission, diagnosis, prevention and control of emerging infectious diseases. Research, surveillance, and response all depend on the public health infrastructure that supports, trains, and equips public health workers, and links them in national and global networks. Training the next generation of public health scientists is a crucial component of the public heath infrastructure. All of the CDC's efforts are ultimately directed at implementing the fourth goal, prevention and control. In many instances, CDC acts as a catalyst, developing and evaluating prevention and control strategies that can be implemented by others.

The Global Emerging Infection Sentinel Network of the International Society of Travel Medicine (GeoSentinel) systematically surveys travelers as sentinels to herald the emergence of new pathogens early enough to develop appropriate public health responses to limit the dissemination of novel microbial threats. Compared to the conventional surveillance based on public health laboratories and local health departments, this is a provider-based consortium of 25 travel medicine clinics located in various countries.

Crucial to the global response has been the incorporation of information technology resources for the rapid dissemination of information. (See Chapter 13.) ProMED-mail (www.promedmail.org), a free e-mail list run by voluntary moderators, was established in 1994 and reports on disease outbreaks in plants, animals, and humans. In February 2003, ProMED-mail reported on the 300 cases of pneumonia in South China identified from November 2002, ultimately recognized as SARS and leading to the WHO-issued global alert by March 2003.

In January 1995 a peer-reviewed, public domain, indexed journal, *Emerging Infectious Diseases* (www.cdc. gov/neidad/EID), was launched with the objective of enhancing the professionals in infectious diseases and related sciences. The monthly journal tracks disease trends, analyzes new and re-emerging infectious diseases, and disseminates information around the world.

The World Health Organization in 1995 created a new division of Emerging and Other Communicable Diseases Surveillance and Control and uses at least two instruments to disseminate information: the Disease Outbreak News (www.who.int/disease.outbreak-news), which immediately alerts to outbreaks detected and verified by WHO, and the Weekly Epidemiological Record (www.who.int/wer), WHO's principal instrument for alerting the world to changes in both the behavior of infectious diseases and recommended measures for control. How all these instruments worked together was well exemplified by the SARS outbreak and its rapid containment.

IMPORTANT CONCEPTS ON ANTIMICROBIAL RESISTANCE

Antimicrobial resistance is widely recognized as a global public health problem. This problem continues to worsen with selective pressure exerted by inappropriate use of antimicrobials and the spread of resistant organisms in health care institutions and the community.

In health care settings, the incidence and prevalence of many resistant strains has been increasing, including but not limited to methicillin-resistant *Staphylococcus aureus* (MRSA), vancomycin-resistant enterococci (VRE), and extended spectrum β-lactamase–producing strains of aerobic gram negative rods. There are increasing reports of multidrug-resistant strains of *Pseudomonas aeruginosa* and *Acinetobacter baumanii,* and additional concern about *Staphylococcus* with intermediate sensitivity to glycopeptides and rare strains showing resistance to vancomycin.

Worldwide there is an increasing population of critically ill and immunosuppressed patients who often require and receive various courses of antimicrobials further increasing problems of resistance. The issue of resistance to antimicrobials is not restricted to hospitals and other health care institutions. Organisms causing community-acquired infections have also demonstrated resistance as noted in the case study that follows. Worldwide there is a problem of antimicrobial resistance of respiratory bacterial pathogens including *Streptococcus pneumoniae, Haemophilus influenzae,* and *Moraxella catarrhalis.* Organisms that cause sexually transmitted disease, such as *Neisseria gonorrhoeae,* and pathogens causing gastrointestinal infections, such as *Shigella* and *Salmonella,* have also demonstrated widespread resistance. The problem of multidrug resistance in *Mycobacterium tuberculosis* (MDR-TB) is well known. In a survey of the international network of tuberculosis laboratories by the CDC and WHO from 2000–2004, of 17,690 *M. tuberculosis* isolates, 20 percent were MDR and 2 percent were resistant to even second-line drugs (XDR).[12] Worldwide MDR-TB has emerged as a threat to public health.

Resistance is not restricted to bacteria but is also present in viruses, fungi, and protozoa. With the ongoing HIV pandemic and the expanding use of antiretroviral therapy, both primary and secondary resistance is being increasingly reported. Difficulty with adherence to antiretroviral therapy poses many challenging issues and frequently results in the development of acquired multidrug resistance. Primary drug resistance is also occurring more commonly, dictating the need for drug susceptibility testing in more patients, where available. Acyclovir resistance of *Herpes simplex* has been reported in HIV-infected patients.[13] Fungal pathogens have also been reported to be resistant, particularly some of the nonalbicans species of *Candida* in which resistance to fluconazole has been well described.[14] Occurrence of multidrug resistant *Plasmodium falciparum* continues to be a significant and serious problem worldwide.

Global spread of antimicrobial resistance can occur with increased travel. Infectious diseases have been known to travel faster and farther than ever before. During the 1990s resistant *S. pneumoniae* was identified in Spain and then rapidly found in Argentina, Brazil, Chile, China, Columbia, Malaysia, Mexico, Philippines, Cambodia, South Africa, Thailand, and United States.

Inappropriate use of antimicrobials also extends to their use in veterinary medicine and agricultural fields. Antimicrobials have been used in food animals in North America and Europe for nearly half a century. There is continued debate about this issue and the impact of this type of antimicrobial use on human health. Commonly used agents include penicillins, tetracyclines, cephalosporins, fluoroquinolones, avoparcin (a glycopeptide that is related to vancomycin), and virginiamycin (a streptogramin that is related to quinupristin-dalfopristin). Antimicrobials are given to these animals for growth promotion, or occasionally for therapy. The percentage of antimicrobials used for animals versus humans is not exactly known. It is estimated that 50 percent of all antimicrobials produced in the United States are administered to animals mostly for subtherapeutic uses.[15] The use of antimicrobials in food animals has been postulated to be associated with antimicrobial resistance among *Salmonella* and *Campylobacter* isolates from humans.[16] Widespread resistance to Streptogramin antimicrobials among *Enterococcus faecium* strains throughout the poultry production region on the eastern seaboard of the United States has been reported.[17] Resistance to various antimicrobial agents has also emerged among pet animals including MRSA, VRE, and multidrug resistant *Salmonella*.[18] White et al. found that 20 percent of samples of ground beef obtained from supermarkets in the United States were contaminated with *Salmonella*.[19] Eighty-four percent of these isolates were resistant to at least one antimicrobial. Another study found that at least 17 percent of chickens obtained in supermarkets in four states had strains of *Enterococcus faecium* that were resistant to quinupristin-dalfopristin.[20] Because of public health concerns about the resistance of glycopeptides among enterococci, avoparcin was banned in Denmark in 1995. In 1996, it was banned from Germany and finally in 1997 it was banned in all European Union member states. After the ban in Denmark, reduction in the occurrence of VRE in the poultry flocks was noted. In Germany there was also a decrease in VRE in poultry meat and fecal samples in the community.

Bacteria possess a large number of mechanisms for the development of resistance.[21] They can undergo mutations in chromosomes and express a latent resistance gene or acquire new genetic material by different mechanisms including direct exchange of DNA via conjugation or by bacterial transduction and extra chromosomal plasmid DNA via transformation. The information encoded in the genetic material makes it possible for the organisms to develop resistance by production of antimicrobial inactivating enzymes, alteration of antimicrobial target sites, or prevention of antimicrobial access to a target site. Transposons and plasmids (extrachromosomal DNA) provide the transfer of genes easily. In addition to exchanging genetic material, transposons and plasmids also may encode genes for active efflux of antimicrobials. An organism may possess more than one mechanism of resistance. A few examples of organisms commonly causing infections and their mechanisms of resistance are detailed to enhance understanding of mechanisms.

Health care–associated MRSA are generally multidrug-resistant. The presence of the Mec gene is a requirement for methicillin resistance. In susceptible *S. aureus*, β-lactams bind to penicillin binding protein PBP 1-3. Mec A encodes for PBP 2a, which has a low affinity for β-lactam antimicrobials. Phenotypic expression of methicillin resistance in the laboratory varies and it is important to follow guidelines for determining the presence of MRSA in the laboratory. The exact mechanism of intermediate resistant strains of *S. aureus* to vancomycin (MIC 8-16 μg/ml) is not known. Thickening of cell walls has been visualized by electron microscopy. It is postulated that vancomycin is trapped in the cell wall because of decreased cross-linking of peptidoglycan strands. Vancomycin resistance of *S. aureus* (MIC ≥ 32 μg/ml) is thought to be due to synthesis of an alternative terminal peptide, D-ala-D-lac, instead of D-ala-D-ala. Vancomycin is unable to bind to this changed peptide.

Inactivation of β-lactam antimicrobials occurs with the production of β-lactamases. Initially described β-lactamases inactivated penicillin and narrow spectrum cephalosporins. Extended spectrum β-lactamases (ESBLs) were initially described in the 1980s. The family of ESBLs is heterogeneous.[22] Their activity against different oxyimino-β-lactams (cefotaxime, ceftazidime, and ceftriaxone) varies but they do not inactivate cephamycins (cefoxitin, cefotetan, and cefmetazole) and carbapenems. ESBLs have been found in aerobic gram negative organisms, predominantly *Escherichia coli* and *Klebsiella*. However, they also occur in other aerobic gram negative rods. Identification of organisms producing ESBLs in the laboratory is important since they are heterogeneous and can be missed.

Enterococci are intrinsically resistant to several antimicrobials. They have become resistant to additional antimicrobials. High-level resistance to ampicillin has been demonstrated in *E. faecium*. Intrinsic resistance of *E. faecium* to ampicillin is thought to be due to the presence of a cell wall with low affinity for PBPs. High-level resistance to ampicillin is postulated to be due to alterations of PBP_5 protein and increased expression of PBP_5. Enterococci show intrinsic resistance to low and moderate levels of aminoglycoside. Unfortunately, strains showing high-level aminoglycoside resistance have also been reported to cause infection. Streptomycin resistance can be caused by mutation or by the presence of streptomycin-modifying enzyme. High-level resistance to gentamicin is due to the production of bifunctional enzymes. High-level resistance to gentamicin and streptomycin results in a lack of synergy with cell wall active antimicrobials.

High-level resistance of enterococci to vancomycin was first reported in Europe. Subsequently, VRE has been reported from many parts of the world. Vancomycin inhibits enterococci by binding to the D-alanyl-D-alanine terminus of cell wall protein. In the peptidoglycan, D-ala-D-ala is replaced with D-alanyl-D-lactate. Binding of vancomycin to this changed terminus is with significantly lower affinity. Different clusters of genes, Van A, B, and D, encode for high-level resistance to vancomycin. Van A is the most common type of vancomycin resistance. It also mediates cross-resistance to teicoplanin. The second most common type of vancomycin resistance is Van B. These organisms are usually sensitive to teicoplanin.

Linezolid and quinupristin-dalfopristin resistant isolates of *E. faecium* have also been reported. Mutations in the V domain of 23S rRNA appear to be related to resistance.[23] Linezolid-resistant strains have even been identified prior to exposure to linezolid. Resistance to quinupristin-dalfopristin occurs via a variety of mechanisms— antimicrobial modifying enzymes, efflux pump, and modification of the target site.[24]

Decreased susceptibility of some organisms to antimicrobials might be difficult to detect during routine laboratory testing. Examples include decreased susceptibility of *S. aureus* to vancomycin, detection of resistance of *S. pneumoniae* to penicillin, and organisms with newer mechanisms of resistance, for example ESBLs. Recently, Tritor has emphasized the importance of quantitative information from MIC testing results in surveillance studies rather than just reporting MIC 50 and MIC 90.

CASE STUDY OF AN ISSUE WITH ANTIMICROBIAL RESISTANCE

Health care–associated MRSA infections were initially reported in the 1960s. They have become prevalent pathogens causing health care–associated infections.

There were sporadic reports of community-acquired methicillin-resistant *Staphylococcus aureus* (CA-MRSA) infections beginning in 1980. Currently CA-MRSA infection has become a common and serious problem. These infections represented between 8 and 20 percent of all MRSA isolates in the United States from 2001–2002,[25] and the current epidemic in the United States has been reported since 1999.[26] Initial reports in the United States occurred with infections among young children. Subsequently, infections were reported in prisoners, men who have sex with men, intravenous drug users, and those competing in contact sports. The most common site of infection has been the skin, which can range from minor to severe, including necrotizing fasciitis. Skin infections caused by these organisms often have necrotic centers and have sometimes been misdiagnosed as "spider bites."[27] CA-MRSA has also been associated with severe pneumonia and sepsis including deaths in healthy persons. Outbreaks of infections have now been reported from many countries in the world including but not limited to the UK, Switzerland, Greece, Taiwan, and Singapore.

CA-MRSA infections are different from those that have previously been health care–associated. However, CA-MRSA types are also now being reported to cause infections in the health care setting. There was a report of an outbreak of seven such cases of skin and soft tissue infections in United States.[28] Genetic fingerprinting showed that the outbreak strain was closely related to the United States 400 strain. An outbreak also occurred among healthy newborns at two hospitals in the United States.[29] Finally, there is one report involving postpartum women. This report documented hospital transmission of CA-MRSA.[30]

The Mec gene is required for *S. aureus* to express resistance. The Mec gene is part of a mobile chromosomal element called staphylococcal chromosomal cassette (SCCmec). Five SCCmec types have been described. Most CA-MRSA have type IV SCCmec. Most CA-MRSA isolates in the United States have been reported as containing genes encoding Panton-Valentine Leukocidin, a cytotoxin that causes leukocyte destruction and has been postulated to cause tissue necrosis. Two clones have been identified in the United States. The US Clone 400 was seen in Native American children initially and subsequently has caused infections throughout the country. The US Clone 300 has now also been reported. Our knowledge of the epidemiology of CA-MRSA is incomplete. It is also possible that there are other sites of colonization in addition to the nose such as the GI tract. Household pets have also been postulated to be potential additional reservoirs for CA-MRSA.

The pathogenesis of infections caused by CA-MRSA is also not clear. Some of the virulence characters are as described above. In addition, we do not have data on host factors that are important for occurrence and transmission of infection. Patients with CA-MRSA pose challenges for clinicians. These patients are usually seen in the outpatient setting with skin and soft tissue infections. Spread of these organisms to health care facilities has occurred. Awareness and recognition of this problem is important. Traditionally used cephalosporins and anti-staphylococcal penicillins are ineffective. Many isolates in the United States have been reported to be sensitive to trimethoprim-sulfamethoxazole and clindamycin in addition to the usual drugs that are used for health care–associated MRSA. There are no clinical trials to demonstrate whether clindamycin or trimethoprim-sulfamethoxazole is actually effective for these infections. Clindamycin presents an additional challenge. Strains that may be sensitive to clindamycin but resistant to erythromycin *in vitro* can contain genes encoding inducible resistance to clindamycin and have potential to develop resistance while the patient is receiving treatment. If the strain demonstrates resistance to erythromycin and sensitivity *in vitro* to clindamycin, it is very important to check for inducible resistance before clindamycin is used. For serious infections, vancomycin is usually recommended. Alternate agents include quinupristin-dalfopristin, linezolid, and daptomycin. However, daptomycin cannot be used if there is an infection involving the lungs. The importance of drainage of infected foci and appropriate debridement cannot be over-emphasized.

IMPACT OF ANTIMICROBIAL RESISTANCE

The issue and problem of antimicrobial resistance has received attention from a wide sector throughout the world including health care professionals, governments, nongovernmental organizations, and the general public. The magnitude of the impact of resistance still remains unknown. An article by Cosgrove and Carmeli outlines some of these issues.[31]

The impact on the patient can be quite serious. Resistance can certainly result in the delay of administration of appropriate antimicrobials to the patient. Multidrug resistance of organisms can certainly limit the choices available for the patient. Alternate agents may be more toxic. Occasionally with multidrug resistant strains, there might not be any options. Some of the alternative agents may not be as effective. The patient is often placed in contact isolation on admission and upon subsequent admissions. The potential barriers to care from contact isolation have been reported.[32] The impact on health care workers has also been reported.[33] With increasing resistance of various organisms, empiric regimens change and patients who may not have infection with resistant organisms on admission are administered empiric therapy to cover the possibility of resistant organisms.

There are many methodologic issues outlined in the literature regarding the measurement of the impact of resistance. Often there are no controls for length of stay before the onset of infection with resistant organisms. The selection of an appropriate control group is essential. It is important to adjust for severity of illness. The patients with infections caused by resistant organisms often have more severe underlying illnesses that may result in adverse outcomes. The appropriate timing for the measurement of severity of illness has been discussed. The assessment of severity of illness more than 48 hours before the first signs of infection is considered important. One must distinguish between all-cause mortality versus attributable mortality. The morbidity has to be determined carefully. Multidrug-resistant tuberculosis is associated with increased morbidity and mortality. One cause is if an appropriate antituberculous regimen is not used early in the course of infection. In developing countries where second-line treatments are not as easily available and where most cases occur, this is likely to have an impact on death rates.

Understanding of the economic impact of antimicrobial resistance on society as a whole is limited. The cost of antimicrobial resistance in the United States was estimated to be $4 billion per year in 1995. The cost is certainly much higher currently. There is an interesting paper by McGowen[34] on the economic impact of antimicrobial resistance. He discusses differing viewpoints of the various stakeholders as far as economic impact is concerned, including physicians, health care businesses, the pharmaceutical industry, and the general public. His paper provides an excellent perspective on assessing the economic impact of resistance. He comments on the follow-up work that is necessary to further define the optimal methods of measurement of this impact including noting the specific perspective from which the assessment is being made.

CONTROL STRATEGIES TO COUNTER ANTIMICROBIAL RESISTANCE

Strategies to prevent, control and improve antimicrobial resistance are critical. A single country cannot adequately address the problem. Collaboration and cooperation among various countries dealing with this issue are very important. In 2001, WHO issued the Global Strategy for Containment of Antimicrobial Resistance.[35] It was difficult to translate this strategy into public health actions. In 2004, the WHO published another paper on the antimicrobial resistance containment and surveillance approach—a public health tool that outlines important areas.[36]

Surveillance

Surveillance systems can be helpful for monitoring the current situation but also for assessment of the impact of any intervention that is made. Surveillance programs are useful for improving recommendations regarding empiric antimicrobial therapy in a variety of settings including the development of appropriate guidelines. Data can be used for giving feedback to users of antimicrobials, helping direct more focused and appropriate infection control efforts, monitoring changes in resistance patterns, providing various comparisons, and carrying out interventions that help prevent the spread of resistant strains.

It is important to track the spread of resistant organisms globally through a variety of surveillance programs.[37] There are numerous types of surveillance programs: local, national, and international. Masterson[38] lists the aims of surveillance programs as specific, measurable, accessible, realistic, and targeted. The World Health Organization has initiated a global program for gathering information on resistant bacteria. WHONET[39] involves a network of microbiologists collecting antimicrobial resistance results in a common database. Quality control and proficiency testing are also included in the program. There are surveillance programs targeting specific organisms and specific antimicrobial agents. There are programs for nosocomial infections such as the National Nosocomial Infection Surveillance System and Surveillance and Control of Pathogens of Epidemiologic Importance (SCOPE), just to give a few examples. There are some surveillance programs that evaluate trends in the antimicrobial susceptibility of pathogens that cause lower respiratory infections. Data have been systematically collected for *S. pneumoniae, Haemophilus influenzae,* and *Moraxella catarrhalis.* The SENTRY program is a multinational antimicrobial surveillance program. It monitors the predominant organisms and antimicrobial resistance patterns of health care–associated and community- acquired infections by using a network of sentinel hospitals. Surveillance programs by themselves are not adequate for preventing the occurrence and spread of antimicrobial-resistant organism infections. Feedback of this information to the users of antimicrobials is important. Sharing of this information with all the stakeholders involved is critical in making a change. Molecular techniques have recently been included in the SENTRY program that should provide further information.[40] The data on the detection of increasing resistance have led to some changes in clinical prescribing practice. A decrease in the incidence of penicillin-resistant pneumococci was observed in Iceland and in the number of cases of multidrug-resistant *M. tuberculosis* in New York. Resistance of *S. pneumoniae* has been controlled by prescription restriction of antimicrobials in Japan, Hungary, Finland, and Iceland. The surveillance program Project Intensive Care Antimicrobial Resistance Epidemiology (ICARE) is a collaborative study between the Hospital Infections Program, a division of health care quality at the Centers for Disease Control and Prevention, and the Rollins School of Public Health. Through this program, it was demonstrated that participation in the monitoring program with comparison to a valid benchmark provided useful data to the participants. The ICUs were associated with a decrease in the use of vancomycin and the prevalence of vancomycin-resistant enterococci.[41]

In European countries antimicrobial resistance has been monitored in selected bacteria from humans since 1998 through the European Antimicrobial Resistance Surveillance System (EARSS). One of the indicator organisms in EARSS is *S. pneumoniae.* The results from eleven European countries demonstrated a linear relationship between the use of β-lactam antimicrobials and macrolides and the proportion of penicillin-resistant *Streptococcus pneumoniae* among all invasive *S. pneumoniae* isolates. Data demonstrated that resistance of *S. pneumoniae* follows a north to south gradient. Southern European countries had higher proportions of these organisms than countries of northern Europe. There was a correlation with antimicrobial use data and antimicrobial resistance.[42]

It is important to include quality improvement programs in the surveillance systems. Surveillance depends on enhancing epidemiologic and laboratory capabilities. Surveillance of the use of antimicrobials in veterinary practice, agriculture, and food animals is also important.

Improving the coordination of the various surveillance programs and distributing the best information for feedback and intervention is critical. It is also very important to use standardized laboratory methods and data elements so that sensitivity results and surveillance data can be compared across widely dispersed geographic areas. Linking of microbiological, clinical, and pharmaceutical data are important also for the prevention and control of resistance. Just reporting the strains as susceptible, intermediate, or resistant can mask any emerging antimicrobial resistance problem. For example, an organism with a decrease in susceptibility may likely still be classified as susceptible. Clinical laboratories that provide data for antimicrobial resistance surveillance purposes should routinely participate in pertinent educational and proficiency testing programs and indicate methods that are used for surveillance. A report from the Interagency Task Force on Antimicrobial Resistance included a number of stakeholders and provided a useful framework for combating antimicrobial resistance.[43]

APPROPRIATE ANTIMICROBIAL USAGE

HEALTH CARE FACILITIES

The CDC in the Action Plan[43] defined appropriate antimicrobial use as "use that maximizes therapy by minimizing toxicity and development of resistance." In the health care institution, an antimicrobial stewardship program is most effectively accomplished through a multidisciplinary group consisting of pharmacists, infectious disease physicians, and representatives from the Microbiology Laboratory. Reviews by Paterson, Weinstein, and MacDougall and Polk outline many strategies.[44,45,46] Guidelines for prescribing antimicrobials for common infectious diseases are also in use in many institutions. There are also national guidelines for the management of common infections. Computerized decision support systems developed by Burke and Pestotnik[47] and Pestotnik[48] at LDS Hospital in Salt Lake City have been used to support physicians in the choice of antimicrobial agents. These programs have been successful. The same group of investigators has demonstrated that computerized support stabilized antimicrobial resistance background in their institution over several years. The approaches used also include streamlining, discontinuing antimicrobials on day two or three if the infection is not documented, or deescalating once susceptibility testing data are available and an appropriate change can be made. A number of approaches have been undertaken in the United States and other parts of the world in terms of the various components of the antimicrobial stewardship programs. These programs have demonstrated several times to have an impact on outbreaks caused by multidrug-resistant pathogens. One example is a decrease in ESBL producing *Klebsiella* infections, VRE, and *C. difficile* infections. The data are more limited on the effect of antimicrobial restriction on endemic resistance of organisms. However, it is still important to continue the programs and monitor these strains worldwide on a more long-term basis. In some parts of the world, particularly in developing areas, some but not all components of the antimicrobial stewardship program may be possible.

PROGRAMS TO PROMOTE APPROPRIATE OUTPATIENT ANTIMICROBIAL DRUG USE

There is widespread use of antimicrobials in outpatient settings particularly for viral respiratory infections. A program was launched in Wisconsin in 1995 to educate physicians and the public about appropriate antimicrobial use. Minnesota served as a control state.[49] Results of pre- and postcampaign questionnaires indicated that the clinicians in Wisconsin perceived a significant decrease in the proportion of patients requesting antimicrobials including requests from parents for their children. The study, however, did not include objective measures of antimicrobial drug prescribing. There were not many differences between physicians in Wisconsin and Minnesota. It was postulated that Minnesota clinicians along the Wisconsin and Minnesota border might have been exposed to the educational materials from this program and advertisement. Also a public education campaign was launched by the Centers for Disease Control and Prevention in September 2003. There are also national guidelines for appropriate use of antimicrobials for common outpatient infections.

ANTIMICROBIAL USE IN FOOD ANIMALS

The Interagency Task Force on Antimicrobial Resistance with Co-Chairs from the CDC the Food and Drug Administration, and the National Institutes of Health and a number of other health care agencies has recommended the following:

- Improvement and understanding of the risks and benefits of antimicrobial use and ways to prevent emergence and spread of resistance
- Development and implementation of principles for appropriate antimicrobial drug use in the production of food animals and plants
- Improved animal husbandry and food production practices to reduce the spread of infection
- A regulatory framework to address the need for antimicrobial drug use in agriculture and veterinary medicine while ensuring that such use does not pose a risk for human health

Infection Control

Infection control principles and practices in the prevention of transmission of resistant organisms in the health care setting are critical. The importance of hand hygiene cannot be overemphasized. Alcohol-based gel is now available widely. However, adherence to hand hygiene continues to be a problem worldwide and it has varied among health care professionals and institutions. Reasons perceived as contributing to poor hand hygiene adherence include:

1. Time required to perform hand hygiene
2. The effect of hand hygiene products on the skin
3. Inadequate knowledge of the guidelines
4. Workload

The influence of role model and group behavior on the reported levels of adherence is important. A campaign sponsored by WHO in 2005 is promoting the use of alcohol-based hand rubs throughout the world. To decrease transmission there is also an emphasis on the importance of the detection of patients who are colonized with resistant organisms so appropriate isolation precautions can be in place before an infection develops.

Increasing availability of molecular techniques for rapid diagnosis and testing for resistance would help to decrease empiric antimicrobial therapy. Infection control in the health care setting will be enhanced also by the development of rapid diagnosis, the understanding of factors that promote the transmission of organisms and future modifications of medical devices that will help reduce the risk of infection.

Vaccines

Vaccines have the potential to prevent infections and avoid dissemination within a population. Currently, these benefits are best exemplified by the new pneumococcal conjugate vaccine.[50] However, we should also have constant surveillance for the emergence of non-vaccine serotypes causing infection. There is potential for different vaccines in the future including those against *Staphylococci*, *Enterococci*, and some of the enteric pathogens.

Education

In addition to education of health care professionals it is very important to educate the public regarding antimicrobial resistance and inappropriate antibiotic use. Education should include the importance of adherence to prescribed antimicrobials including the use of directly observed therapy (DOT). DOT for tuberculosis has resulted in higher cure rates when there is a low level of multidrug resistance.

Health Care Regulations

Antimicrobial use can be affected by reimbursement policies, financial incentives and health care regulations. In developing countries there are issues of ease of availability of antimicrobials over the counter. Self-medication and poor adherence also occur. Since 1999 the Chilean Ministry of Health has enforced existing laws regarding the purchase of antimicrobials without a medical prescription. This regulatory agency has had a very positive impact on antimicrobial use in the outpatient setting. Separation of dispensing and prescribing of antimicrobials is important. An article in a recent issue of *Emerging Infectious Disease*[51] stated the example of the Korean government policy, which prohibited physicians from dispensing drugs and pharmacies from prescribing drugs. This new policy decreased the prescribing of antimicrobial agents and selectively reduced inappropriate prescribing of these antimicrobials for patients with viral infections. The regulatory environment should also extend to prescription of antimicrobials for food animals and for veterinary practice.

SUMMARY

Despite earlier predictions of a world free of infectious diseases, the struggle for survival between humans and microorganisms will continue indefinitely and new etiologic agents and infectious diseases will continue to emerge. The challenge lies in our recognition and response to their emergence. Recent examples, such as SARS, suggest an air of optimism in our global response strategies. However, antimicrobial resistance remains a global problem and a public health threat.

The problem of antimicrobial resistance is not restricted to only health care settings but has also spread in the community. The example of CA-MRSA is of concern and recent data demonstrate its spread back into the health care institutions. There are a variety of mechanisms of resistance and new mechanisms continue to be described. Global strategies for combating antimicrobial resistance issues are available. The implementation of these strategies requires system and behavior changes. Extensive data are available on health care–associated outbreaks and the institution of appropriate antimicrobial restriction and infection control measures to terminate the outbreak. More data on decreasing endemic resistance rates in health care institutions and communities are needed. Global surveillance for resistant pathogens are of epidemiologic importance must be accomplished. Despite many remaining issues regarding the various types of surveillance for antimicrobial resistance, a lot of progress has been made. Sharing of data and feedback on an ongoing basis to appropriate stakeholders and instituting necessary interventions are important. Global travel poses threats for the transmission and spread of emerging infections and resistant organisms rapidly, and interventions require ongoing collaboration and cooperation between agencies and countries, including sharing of data. Some of the processes that are necessary for combating antimicrobial resistance are more difficult in resource limited environments, but are necessary. The use of limited antimicrobials in food animals remains a concern, and a global approach to this issue is critical. With increasing antimicrobial resistance and fewer antimicrobials in the development pipeline, we must strive to avoid the development of a "post-antimicrobial era."

STUDY QUESTIONS

1. Change in land use such as deforestation and reforestation projects have been implicated in the emergence of infectious diseases. What specific examples can be quoted for each?

2. With mass travel assuming such an important role in the global spread of infectious diseases, are there specific technological advances or interventions at airports or other ports of entry that can be implemented to identify the ill traveler?

3. Resistance to antimicrobials is a global problem. What approaches have been most useful in studying this problem? Outline prevention strategies.

4. Resistance to antimicrobials in food animals is also a global issue. Give examples of antimicrobials that are used in food animals and associated with resistance and issues with human health.

REFERENCES

1. Tsang KW, Ho DL, Ooi GC, et al. A cluster of cases of severe acute respiratory syndrome in Hong Kong. *N Engl J Med* 2003;348:1977.

2. Yu IT, Li Y, Wong TW, et al. Evidence of airborne transmission of the severe acute respiratory syndrome virus. *N Engl J Med* 2004;350:1731.

3. Armstrong GL, Conn LA, Pinner RW. Trends in infectious disease mortality in the United States during the 20th Century. *JAMA* 1999;281:61.

4. Burnet FM, White DO. *Natural History of Infectious Diseases.* Cambridge: University Press, 1962.

5. Institute of Medicine. *Emerging infections: Microbial threats to health in the United States.* Washington, D.C.: National Academy Press, 1994.

6. Scheld WM, Armstrong D, Hughes JM. *Emerging Infections.* Washington, D.C.: ASM Press, 1998.

7. Monto AS. The threat of an avian influenza pandemic. *N Engl J Med* 2005;352:323.

8. Nash D, Mostashari F, Fine A, et al. The outbreak of West Nile virus infection in the New York City area in 1999. *N Engl J Med* 2001;344:1807.

9. Office of Technology Assessment, United States Congress. *Proliferation of Weapons of Mass Destruction.* Washington, DC: US Government Printing Office, 1993. 53–55

10. Update: Investigation of bioterrorism—related anthrax and interim guidelines for exposure management and antimicrobial therapy, October 2001. *MMWR* 2001;50:909.

11. CDC. *Preventing Emerging Infectious Diseases: A Strategy for the 21st Century.* Atlanta, GA: US Department of Health and Human Services, 1998. Vol. 47, No. RR-15.

12. Emergence of *Mycobacterium tuberculosis* with extensive resistance to second line drugs worldwide. *MMWR* 2006;55:301.

13. Levin MJ, Bacon TH, Leary JJ. Resistance of *Herpes simplex* virus infections to nucleoside analogues in HIV-infected patients. *Clin Infect Dis* 2004;39:S248.

14. Pfaller MA, Jones RN, Doern GV, et al. Bloodstream Infections Due to *Candida* Species: SENTRY A Surveillance Program in North America and Latin America, 1997–1998. *Antimicrob Agents Chemother.* 2000;44:747.

15. Gorbach SL. Antimicrobial Use in Animal Food—Time to stop. *Editorial N Engl J Med* 2001;345:1202.

16. Angulo FJ, Nargund VN, Chiller TC. Evidence of an Association Between Use of Anti-microbial Agents in Food Animals and Anti-microbial Resistance Among Bacteria Isolated from Humans and the Human Health Consequences of Such Resistance. *J Vet Med* 2004;51:374.

17. Hayes JR, Wagner DD, English LL, et al. Distribution of streptogramin resistance determinants among *Enterococcus faecium* from a poultry production environment of the USA. *J of Antimicrob Chemother* 2005;55:123.

18. Guardabassi L, Schwarz S, Lloyd DH. Pet animals as reservoirs of antimicrobial-resistant bacteria. *J of Antimicrob Chemother* 2004;54:321.

19. White DG, Zhao S, Sudler R, et al. The isolation of antibiotic-resistant salmonella from retail ground meats. *N Engl J Med* 2001;18:345.

20. McDonald LC, Rossiter S, Mackinson C, et al. Quinupristin-dalfopristin-resistant *Enterococcus faecium* on chicken and in human stool specimens. *N Engl J Med* 2001;18:1155.

21. Shlaes DM, Gerding DN, John JF Jr, et al. Society for Healthcare Epidemiology of America and Infectious Diseases Society of America Joint Committee on the Prevention of Antimicrobial Resistance: Guidelines for the Prevention of Antimicrobial Resistance in Hospitals. *Clin Infect Dis* 1997;25:584.

22. Paterson, DL, Bonomo, RA. Extended-spectrum beta-lactamases: a clinical update. *Clin Microbiol Rev* 2005;18:657.

23. Raad II, Hanna HA, Hachem RY. Clinical-Use-Associated Decrease in Susceptibility of Vancomycin-Resistant *Enterococcus faecium* to Linezolid: a Comparison with Quinupristin-Dalfopristin. *Antimicrob Agents Chemother* 2004;48:3583.

24. Hershberger E, Donabedian S, Konstantinou K, et al. Quinupristin-dalfopristin resistance in gram-positive bacteria: mechanism of resistance and epidemiology. *Clin Inf Dis* 2004;38:92.

25. Fridkin SK, Hageman JC, Morrison M, et al. Methicillin-Resistant *Staphylococcus aureus* Disease in Three Communities. *N Engl J of Med* 2005;352:1436.

26. King MD, Humphrey BJ, Wang YF, et al. Emergence of Community-Acquired Methicillin-Resistant *Staphylococcus aureus* USA 300 Clone as the Predominant Cause of Skin and Soft-Tissue Infections. *Ann Intern Med* 2006;144: 309.

27. Moellering, Jr RC. The Growing Menace of Community-Acquired Methicillin-Resistant *Staphylococcus aureus. Editorial, Ann Intern Med* 2006;144:368.

28. Bratu S, Eramo A, Kopec R, et al. Community-associated Methicillin-resistant *Staphylococcus aureus* in Hospital Nursery and Maternity Units. *Emerging Infectious Diseases* 2005;11:808.

29. Centers for Disease Control and Prevention. Community-Associated Methicillin-Resistant *Staphylococcus aureus* Infection Among Healthy Newborns—Chicago and Los Angeles County, 2004. *MMWR* 2006;31:329.

30. Saiman L, O'Keefe M, Graham PL 3rd, et al. Hospital transmission of community-acquired methicillin-resistant *Staphylococcus aureus* among postpartum women. *Clin Infect Dis* 2003;37:1313.

31. Cosgrove SE, Carmeli Y. The Impact of Antimicrobial Resistance on Health and Economic Outcomes. *Clin Infect Dis* 2003;36:1433

32. Evans HL, Shaffer MM, Hughes MG, et al. Contact Isolation in Surgical Patients: a Barrier to Care? *Surgery* 2003;134:180.

33. Khan FA, Khakoo R, Hobbs GR, et al. Impact of Contact Isolation on Health Care Workers at a Tertiary Care Center. *Am J Infect Control* 2006;34:408.

34. McGowen, JE. Economic Impact of Antimicrobial Resistance. *Emerg Infect Dis* 2001;7:286.

35. World Health Organization. WHO Global Strategy for Containment of Antimicrobial Resistance: Executive Summary. 2001.

36. Gunner SS, Tapsall JW, Allegranzi B, et al. The antimicrobial resistance containment and surveillance approach—a public health tool. Bulletin World Health Organization 2004;82:928.

37. Marchese A and Schito GC. Role of Global Surveillance in Combating Bacterial Resistance. *Drugs* 2001;61:167.

38. Masterson RG. Surveillance studies: how can they help the management of infection? *J of Antimicrob Chemother* 2000;72:53.

39. Stelling JM and O'Brien TF. Surveillance of antimicrobial resistance: the WHONET program. *Clin Infect Dis Suppl* 1997;1:S157.

40. Pfaller MA, Acar J, Jones RN, et al. Integration of Molecular Characterization of Microorganisms in a Global Antimicrobial Resistance Surveillance Program. *Clin Infect Dis* 2001;32: S156.

41. Fridkin SK, Lawton R, Edwards JR, et al. Monitoring Antimicrobial Use and Resistance: Comparison with a National Benchmark on Reducing Vancomycin Use and Vancomycin-Resistant Enterococci. *Emerg Infect Dis* 2002;8:702.

42. Bronzwaer SL, Cars O, Buchholz U, et al. A European Study on the Relationship Between Antimicrobial Use and Antimicrobial Resistance. *Emerg Infect Dis* 2002;8:278.

43. Centers for Disease Control and Prevention. A Public Health Action Plan to Combat Antimicrobial Resistance Part 1: Domestic Issues. February 2005.

44. Paterson DL. The Role of Antimicrobial Management Programs in Optimizing Antibiotic Prescribing within Hospitals. *Clin Infect Dis* 2006;42:S90.

45. Weinstein RA. Controlling Antimicrobial Resistance in Hospitals: Infection Control and Use of Antibiotics. *Emerg Infect Dis* 2001;7:188.

46. MacDougall C and Polk RE. Antimicrobial stewardship programs in the health care systems. *Clin Microbiol Rev* 2005; 18:638.

47. Burke JP, Pestotnik SL. Antibiotic use and microbial resistance in intensive care units—impact of computer assisted decision support. *J Chemother* 1999;11:530.

48. Pestotnik, SL. Expert clinical decision support systems to enhance antimicrobial stewardship programs: insights from the society of infectious diseases pharmacists. *Pharmacotherapy* 2005;25:1116.

49. Belongia EA, Knobloch MJ, Kieke BA Jr, et al. Impact of Statewide Program to Promote Appropriate Antimicrobial Drug Use. *Emerg Infect Dis* 2005;11:912.

50. Kyaw MH, Lynfield R, Schaffner W, et al. Effect of Introduction of the Pneumococcal Conjugate Vaccine on Drug-Resistant *Streptococcus pneumoniae*. *Nl Eng J Med* 2006; 354:1455.

51. Harbarth S and Samore MH. Antimicrobial Resistance Determinants and Future Control. *Emerg Infect Dis* 2005;11: 794.

Global Health Communications, Social Marketing, and Emerging Communication Technologies

13

Gary Snyder, Faina Linkov, and Ron Laporte

LEARNING OBJECTIVES

- *Understand how health communications research and campaigns impact the wellness of individuals and communities globally.*

- *Describe the use of mass media, trusted community members, participatory communication, and "edutainment" in health promotion and education.*

- *Define common barriers to health communications research and delivery, particularly in developing countries and with underserved minority populations worldwide.*

- *Explain the principles of social marketing to deliver health information and services and to change behaviors.*

- *Identify ways to engage the media to cover health issues, and to provide content and training to journalists so they can report more accurately about health.*

- *Describe proven and emerging communication technologies worldwide that are accelerating access to knowledge and information and improving health outcome.*

- *Understand the concept of whisking the research into the classrooms of the world through the power of lecture sharing.*

INTRODUCTION

One significant driver of improvements in public health globally over the past 30 years has been the increased understanding and employment of health communication research, campaigns, and technologies, as well as social marketing strategies.

Health communications research provides a picture of the knowledge, attitudes, and behaviors of individuals and communities. Health communications and social marketing campaigns use multiple "channels" to raise awareness and provide culturally appropriate messages about disease, environmental conditions, nutrition, safety, literacy, and a host of other issues. The communicator must understand individual and community needs and wants, as well as the social and political pressures and competitive forces. They will then be able to inform the people of the community in a manner they trust. This process should help the community be more open to receiving the communication and can lead to motivating them to change behavior and, ultimately, to improving their health and productivity.

Interventions to advance global health have centered typically on clinical and research endeavors, but that has been changing over the past three decades. An important missing piece of the prevention-treatment puzzle was the strategic use of health communication and marketing tools that can empower communities with the knowledge and motivation to improve their environment and wellness, and in return, their social and economic potential and sustainability. Many examples of health communications and social marketing success in changing behaviors and improving health now exist. Effective global health practitioners, particularly those working in developing countries, understand the importance of using communications and marketing at all stages of behavior change. In order to impact entrenched beliefs and practices, as well as open up access to new knowledge, health communications and marketing must continue to be an essential piece of global health strategies.

This chapter will explore:

- Health communications research and program development
- Applying a social marketing process to improve and sustain healthier behaviors
- Partnering with media to promote and inform
- Tapping into the latest communication technologies to empower individuals and communities with new health knowledge and increased ways to stay connected, educated, and able to sustain lasting positive behavior changes

HEALTH COMMUNICATIONS AND PROMOTION

Eliminating or diminishing the burden brought on by the overwhelming diseases of our day calls for aggressive clinical prevention, treatment, and research, but also connecting meaningfully with individuals and communities to promote healthy behavior change. Human behavior plays a significant role in the leading causes of disease, disability, and death. By itself or with other strategies, health communications can inform and influence individuals and groups to quit smoking, use contraceptives, sleep under insecticide-treated bednets, fortify with iron the foods they produce, get an annual mammogram, make their own oral rehydration therapies, filter their water, properly fund immunization programs, exercise regularly, refute myths, or begin to change long-held destructive cultural practices.

Health communications has been defined many ways, but essentially it is the use of communications planning, research, strategy, tactics, and evaluation to increase knowledge and motivate action that improves health. Combined with adequate health services, technological advances, necessary infrastructure, and responsive policies, it can bring about sustained changes that transform individual, community, and global health status for the better.

Early use of health communications relied on one-way messages such as "Boil the water!" or "Don't do drugs" that spoke only to the action the researcher or program leader wanted to bring about. By not taking into account what motivated the related action, what kind of need it fulfilled, what social or economic pressures the individual faced, the one-message campaigns had limited impact. But increasingly, health communication professionals have learned that in order to achieve the desired outcome of improved health, solid research and evaluation must be employed. Program development and delivery must reflect the needs, wants, and cultural values of the community (rather than a "top-down," Western mindset approach). Program developers must tap creatively into channels of communication that are easily accessed by the target audience.

Since communication and marketing efforts aim to motivate an individual or group to take some type of action based on their needs and wants, it is useful to understand what may influence an individual within their "social and health ecosystem."

A well-known model involving motivation is Maslow's Hierarchy of Needs shown in Figure 13-1.[1] Maslow constructed this theory based on individual behavior and needs, described in the form of a pyramid. As the basic physiological needs of food, water, shelter, and security are addressed, individuals seek to attain successively "higher needs" such as the social elements of friendship, family, belonging, and love, and then may be motivated by self-esteem, ego, achievement, and respect of others. At the top of the pyramid is the need for self-actualization and fulfillment. Maslow championed this as reaching one's full potential, with motivation not centered on the self, but rather understanding and helping to solve problems of the wider community.

Applied to global health, Maslow's Hierarchy of Needs can be particularly useful in understanding where the greatest needs are of the individual and community, and how to best position messages, materials, and programs to that level or a higher aspired-to level so they have the most meaning and relevance. If a core set of youth aspire to become leaders in their community, communications and marketing can be directed at their "stepping up" and being recognized for taking action that benefits the entire community. They could help develop the message, advertising, and campaign and be featured in it, which could add credibility. Examples include their choosing to be tested for HIV, or the effective "Truth" stop smoking campaign, designed and developed by US teenagers who describe the reality of why they choose not to smoke.

The values realized at self-actualization (acceptance of other views and traditions, lack of prejudice, using creativity and spontaneity, pursuing solutions to broader problems) parallel the qualities needed by global health communications professionals in order to effectively change behavior and improve health conditions. Maslow also exhibited a worldview when, in explaining self-actualization, he defined it as when one transcends cultural conditioning and becomes a world citizen.

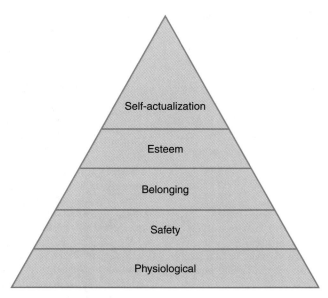

Figure 13-1. Maslow's Hierarchy of Needs.

Connecting Communications to Levels of Influence

There exists many levels of influence that affect a group or individual's behavior, and health communications professionals must take these into account when designing effective strategies. These include: individual, interpersonal, institutional, community, and public policy factors.[2]

Health communications, sometimes referred to as "behavior change communications", can affect *individual* knowledge, attitudes, practices, skills, and dedication related to the desired change. Information and programs aimed at informal *interpersonal* relationships present with family, co-workers, barbers, bus drivers, health professionals, etc., can be effective because they come from known, respected sources. Targeted health messages and calls to action to formal *institutional* groups of like-minded individuals can influence behavior. Organizations can reinforce health information and support programming for their members that promote screenings and expectations of healthier living. Knowing the norms and standards, and gaining the support of trusted *community* leaders, elders, and key peer groups can go a long way toward advancing and sustaining a behavioral change communications process.

Finally, efforts to impact public policy and societal views and laws can be realized through a comprehensive health communications approach that educates, personalizes, and motivates the public, industry, and government to change the norm and take action for the greater good. Examples include work related to transportation and public safety: increasing the wearing of seat belts in the US, reducing the number of passengers allowed by law riding in Kenyan public mini-buses or "matatus," and reducing the number of drunk drivers on American roads.

Behavior Change Communications: Theories, Models, and Frameworks

Effective health communications should start with the use of single or multiple theories and frameworks to build appropriate goals, structure, implementation, impact evaluation, and sustainability with various audiences. Each individual, community, or country presents special challenges and opportunities, and the global health communications professional may combine various theories to understand and influence behavior change related to the problem(s) faced.

Theories and models do not take the place of quality planning and targeted community-based research. However, they can serve as a foundation during the formative stage of planning health communication initiatives and provide insight as to what may motivate and resonate with the audience when the program is rolled out. They can also highlight some of the outcomes that should be considered when designing evaluation and analysis of the impact the communications and marketing are making.

For a summary of some of the most commonly used health communications frameworks, theories and models, see Table 13-1.

Table 13-1. Behavior-Change Theories Used in Health Communications.

Level	Theory/Model/Framework	Description
Individual	Stages of Change Model	Focuses on individuals' readiness to change or attempt to adopt healthy behaviors. Behavior change is a process not an event, and individuals are at different levels of motivation to change.
	Health Belief Model	Centers around: perception of risk of acquiring a health condition; the severity of the consequences; the perceived benefits of adopting the behavior; the barriers and cues to action that may hinder or spur the change. Also factoring into individuals' decisions: are they capable of making the change and sustaining it? Demographic issues and knowledge level play a role.
	Behavioral Intentions Theory	Suggests that the likelihood of intended audiences' adopting a behavior can be predicted by researching their attitudes toward the behavior's benefits, in addition to how their peers will view their behavior.
Interpersonal	Social Learning Theory	Explains behavior as a three-way "triadic reciprocal" relationship in which environmental issues, personal factors, and behavior interact and shape each other.
Community	Community Mobilization Theory	With roots in social networks, it emphasizes active participation and community development where the community helps identify, plan, implement, and solve problems with coordination from outside practitioners. Capacity building and addressing social injustices for the oppressed are hallmarks.
	Organizational Change Theories	Involves processes and strategies for increasing the likelihood of a formal organization adopting healthy policies and programs.
	Diffusions of Innovation Theory	Addresses how new ideas, products, and social practices spread within a society or from one society to another. Examines the innovation, the channels and the social networks involved.
Individual, Interpersonal & Community	Social Marketing Framework	Centers on applying proven marketing technologies and research for developing, executing and evaluating programs that influence voluntary behavior change to improve individual welfare and society they live in. Focuses on research, the customer, and changing behaviors, rather than attitudes/knowledge.

Source: Adapted from United States National Cancer Institute. [6]

Steps for Carrying Out Effective Health Communication Programs

Improving the health of individuals and communities through communications starts with understanding the needs, strengths, and perceptions of the population, and exploring whether the program or desired behavior changes can be successfully adopted. Will the individual, community, organization, or policymaker agree that the benefits to making the change outweigh the costs? What are the barriers to getting a clear picture of the capabilities of those you want to inform and influence? Have programs worked in the past? If not, why? What tools or channels are available to communicate the information in a convincing and credible way? Do you have the resources to impact awareness and motivate sustainable change over time? Who are the trusted individuals that can help carry the messages and bring about the change in behavior?

As seen in Figure 13-2, there are several basic stages involved in developing a successful health communications program. The process is fluid, with steps overlapping, but these represent the basic ingredients:

• Starting with a perceived problem and desired change to bring about

• Finding out more through existing or new research, and setting strategies

• Working with the community closely in development and testing of messages and materials

• Implementing the program

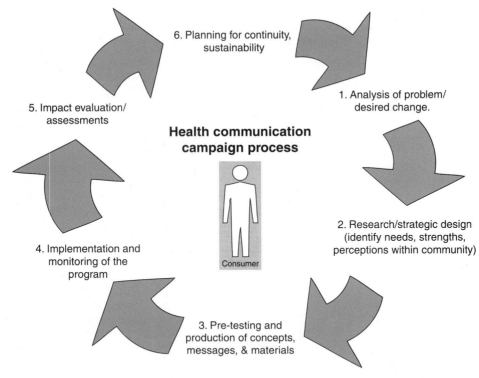

Figure 13-2. Health communication campaign process.

- Assessing its impact on the goals and success
- Planning with the community for sustaining the program and the healthier behavior changes

Successful, strategic behavior change campaigns are also benefit-oriented, can be expanded to scale, and are cost-effective.

Let us take a closer look at what needs to be considered and done at these different stages for behavior change communications to work in the global health setting.

ANALYZING PROBLEMS, CONDUCTING RESEARCH, PLANNING STRATEGIES: A HOPI STORY

You could take several approaches to discerning the initial core problem you want to address through health communications and marketing, implementing and evaluating the program, and sustaining the behavior change. The approach you choose will depend upon your health field, experience, affiliated organization's focus, and familiarity with the region/community you are working in. Since good communication tells a good story, let us put this in terms of a story.

You are part of a clinical team that wants to understand why physicians in the rural clinic keep seeing female patients come in with the same condition of malnourishment and iron deficiency, even though they were provided written instructions on how to prevent it. The three-minute clinic exchange between the Western doctor and the Hopi Indian mother does not provide either party much opportunity for communication or discussion about underlying issues and barriers to her maintaining good nutritional health.

But you, as a health communications researcher, find out who the respected women leaders of the village are and arrange to conduct several interviews with them in their homes, a place where they feel comfortable and more confident. You find in your research that it is culturally inappropriate for a Hopi mother to focus on her own nutritional needs until her children and husband have plenty to eat. Since nutritious food is not abundant, you find she often goes without, skipping meals or not having access to fruits and vegetables after she takes care of the others.

Armed with that knowledge, you design a communications campaign, with the help of the women, that involves the entire family and community, and which supports the message that the mother's health matters much to the health of the family. The strategy will use multiple channels to inform and influence, and you will involve traditional healers giving their blessing that an iron supplement will be safe to add to Hopi meals. You identify women who are leaders to step forth to educate other women and families, and local lay health promoters agree to work with the Western physicians to increase their cultural awareness. A local youth group volunteers to incorporate the "good nutrition for mother" themes into a new play they will perform at the community's Hopi Corn Festival. As part of your strategy, you arrange for radio stations on the reservation to air future public service announcements (PSAs) from women to women about the importance of eating well and staying healthy.

DEVELOPING AND PRETESTING MATERIALS FOR RELEVANCE AND CREDIBILITY

Since you went to medical school at a university in Ohio, you ask the publications office there to help write and print the campaign materials. They produce high-quality publications with content you provide and a script for the PSAs. Slick posters, ads, and brochures in hand, you are understandably excited as you go to the Hopi community center to share the prototypes of the materials. Your presentation is met with uncharacteristic silence and expressions of chagrin.

After some prodding, you hear reasons why these materials will not work. Some Hopis consider the centipede symbol on the cover taboo. The sepia tone photo of the traditional kiva structure inside depicts a ceremonial home where women were only allowed in to serve food and clean. There are only photos of individuals by themselves, which certainly does not express the positive Hopi concept of "Naya," which means people working together for a common good. The music provided for the PSA is Tibetan, not traditional or modern Hopi. Finally, the glossy paper stock is not made from recycled materials—not appropriate given the sacred value Hopis place on the environment and their emphasis on recycling and reusing.

This is why pretesting of materials, health messages, and calls to action with the community for the community are so vital. Sometimes tens of thousands of dollars are spent on campaign materials by well-meaning but Western-mindset communications professionals who bypass pre-testing and then do not understand why the communications campaign failed so miserably to change behavior and improve health.

IMPLEMENTING, EVALUATING, SUSTAINING

You then find right in the Hopi community creative writers, illustrators, designers, student actors, and a printer nearby who understands the Hopi traditions, and re-do the materials so they reflect the Hopi experience and will hopefully resonate with the audience. You meet a fledgling young Hopi filmmaker who agrees to produce a short video aimed at young husbands, an important segment of the market since your research showed the need to include men if the traditional views about food security and mothers were to change. Hearing about the excitement generated by this project, a well-known Hopi actor volunteers to do the vocals for the PSAs and agrees to raise funding for sustaining the effort.

Knowing the importance of evaluation, you included in your earlier research a Knowledge, Attitudes, and Practices (KAP) survey of community members' knowledge of nutrition and family health, attitudes about gender roles in the home, and their current behaviors related to the problem. This sets a benchmark you can measure against in six months to see if the campaign is working.

You kick-off the "Iron Mothers" program by making it one of the featured elements of the Hopi Corn Festival, which includes family health screenings and nutrition counseling from Native American health promoters. The Western clinic physicians assist with the screenings and passing out multivitamins with iron. The creators of the campaign materials are honored for their contributions to strengthening the Hopi community. The PSAs air regularly, a nutrition health column is written weekly for the local newspaper and placed on the new website created for the campaign, and the culturally relevant publications connecting the health of the mother to the well-being of the Hopi community are distributed to homes and businesses. A comic book for kids written in both Hopi and English tells the story of a child who becomes a superhero by keeping his mother healthy and strong. Kids dressed as superheroes help lead a march through a retail section of town, raising social pressure for more affordable access to vitamins and nutrients.

In order to sustain the program's momentum, monthly community events weave in the health message and materials. The high school football team premiers the five-minute video at halftime on the scoreboard. The theater group debuts its nutrition-inspired production, "Food Fight," and the strong, energetic mother character becomes a favorite of the packed house. Pharmacists and discount stores announce an unprecedented cooperative buying strategy to purchase multivitamins and iron supplements in bulk and sell them at a heavy discount to women in the "Iron Mothers" program. Mothers and their spouses and children begin coming to the clinic together each month for screenings and check-ups with the physician and a newly hired Hopi nutritionist.

After six months, the clinical results look good: 80 percent of the women enrolled in the program now show normal iron levels compared to only 35 percent before, and the levels for other women outside the program coming to the clinic have risen as well. You conduct another KAP survey with the families, showing more support from men for helping to keep their wives, sisters, and mothers healthy, and a marked increase in children's understanding of why their mothers need to have fruits, vegetables, and vitamins too.

By all accounts, the "Iron Mothers" health communications and marketing campaign was making a real difference—with individual and community health, but also capacity building. Thanks to the social, community, and business networks built to support it, the tapping of Hopi community talent to help produce it, and the pride of knowing the mothers and the Hopi community were growing stronger because of it, the possibility of sustaining the effort and making it part of everyday life appears high.

This hypothetical campaign worked because it followed the framework for researching, designing, testing, implementing, and evaluating a health communications effort. But it also engaged the community to lend its knowledge, talent, and passion in developing creative ways to keep attention on this problem and to bring about the desired behavior change and health improvement. The program employed research to study the problem and measure success, as well as various communication technologies to deliver the messages. Finally, it always stayed focused on the *consumer* (the mother) and the *benefits* to her, the family, and community.

Cross-Cultural Health and Communications

Health providers, educators, and media wanting to improve their communications and health care outcomes with underserved minority communities such as the Hopi must understand the value and belief systems they bring with them, and link the program's benefits to the deeper values held. An example is the Latino population, which is growing rapidly in the United States, whose core values and beliefs often include:

- *Familismo* (significance of the family to the individual)
- *Collectivismo* (importance of friends, extended family)
- *Simpatia* (need for positive, relaxed relationships)
- *Personalismo* (preference for friendly relations with members of their same ethnic group)
- *Fatalismo* (little belief or experience with prevention—there is little an individual can do to change his or her destiny)
- *Respeto* (deferential treatment to those based on age and position)[3]

Of all of these beliefs, *fatalismo* is perhaps the one that keeps Latinos from taking prevention measures for their health or being motivated to manage a chronic health condition like diabetes. Some feel they cannot do anything about a condition like diabetes, most think insulin is harmful, and many avoid health screenings because of the belief that if you do not know you have the disease, it must not be real.[4]

Many Latinos feel "stress, fear, and anger" bring on diabetes. While "stress, fear, and anger" are not direct causes of diabetes, it is not surprising that Latinos would view them as so, given their cultural values and the need to keep life in *simpatia* or harmony in order to maintain good health. Regarding what motivates them to exercise more may point to the need for health communications researchers, community health providers, and policymakers to consider the Latino belief system centered around *collectivismo*, or the importance of family and friends working together collectively toward a shared goal or interest. This was borne out in a 2006 Columbus, Ohio, survey of new Latino immigrants' knowledge, attitudes, and practice about health and media use. In response to a question about what would help them exercise more, many responded "if friends or family were involved," and "if there were free programs at a park or organization near where the family lives."[5]

Health promotion and communications campaigns can dispel misconceptions about the causes of disease, and build off of strengths in communities, such as *collectivismo* and *simpatia* with Latinos, in designing and implementing health marketing that motivates and changes behavior in a positive way.

Successful outcomes may require a strategy that delivers multiple communications to the audiences that, when combined, influence whether the change can be made. For example, to increase the number of women receiving mammograms, a successful campaign will need to communicate different messages to doctors and women, as well as help push for change in health policy to provide needed resources and technology (see Figure 13-3[6]).

Messages, Methods, and Channels for Health Communications

Health communications professionals possess many outlets and strategies for making sure key messages are relevant, accepted, and acted on. Some of the methods for designing effective campaigns include.[6]

- **Media literacy:** Instructs audiences on how to understand media messages to identify the sponsor's motives, and how to compose messages targeted effectively to the intended audience's point of view
- **Media advocacy:** Seeks to change the social and political environment in which decisions are made by influencing the mass media's selection of stories and by shaping the debate about those subjects
- **Public relations:** Promotes certain messages about a health issue or behavior to the media in order to raise the reporter's knowledge and increase coverage of the topic
- **Advertising:** Places paid or public service messages in the media or public spaces to increase visibility and support for a product, service, or behavior

Communication strategy
a case study: Mammogram

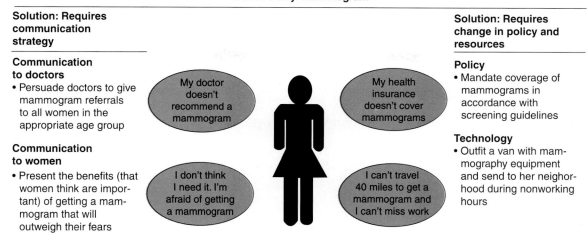

Solution: Requires communication strategy

Communication to doctors
• Persuade doctors to give mammogram referrals to all women in the appropriate age group

Communication to women
• Present the benefits (that women think are important) of getting a mammogram that will outweigh their fears

My doctor doesn't recommend a mammogram

I don't think I need it. I'm afraid of getting a mammogram

My health insurance doesn't cover mammograms

I can't travel 40 miles to get a mammogram and I can't miss work

Solution: Requires change in policy and resources

Policy
• Mandate coverage of mammograms in accordance with screening guidelines

Technology
• Outfit a van with mammography equipment and send to her neighborhood during nonworking hours

Figure 13-3. Communication strategy: increasing mammogram use. From Making Health Communication Programs Work. (Reproduced with permission.)

• **Education entertainment:** Often called "edutainment," seeks to integrate health-promoting messages and storylines into entertainment and news programs; also seeks entertainment industry support for a health issue

• **Individual and group instruction:** Influences, guides, and provides skills to support positive behaviors

• **Partnership development:** Deepens support for a program or issue by attracting the influence, credibility, and resources of profit, nonprofit, or governmental organizations

According to McGuire's "Communications for Persuasion," in order to communicate the message successfully, these five communication elements all must work:

• credibility of the message source
• message design
• delivery channel
• intended audience
• intended behavior[7]

Pitfalls and Possibilities with Health Communications

In all areas but particularly in developing countries, several challenges to effective communication programs exist. These include:

• Developing trust within the community and the culture
• Low literacy rates of the audience you want to address

• Lack of existing quality baseline information and research on the subject
• Environmental disruptions such as floods and earthquakes, and armed conflict can affect roads, telecommunications, and transportation
• Corruption—funds for a program at the local level may never see the local community
• Long-held cultural and spiritual beliefs; traditions that run counter to fact
• Values imposition (by researcher)
• Too much top-down "grasstops" approach to implementation; not enough community or grassroots energy driving the program
• Multiple languages and dialects in region; lack of quality interpreters
• Lack of existing mediums and channels to reach intended community
• Literal translation of images and visuals

The meaning applied by community members to words and pictures can be a barrier to raising awareness of a health condition or attempting to receive feedback about the prevalence of a problem. In its research on HIV/AIDS media reporting, the Kaiser Family Foundation found that the word "prostitute" had a negative connotation but discovered that "sex worker" was more acceptable in some cultures because it more accurately described situations where a woman had no other economic opportunity.[8]

In rural villages of Ecuador, researchers from Ohio University's Tropical Disease Institute carried a placard with them that had an enlarged five-inch photo of the triatomine "kissing bug", the vector for the parasite

Trypanosoma cruzi, which causes Chagas' disease. As they went to each village conducting surveillance, they pointed to the bug on the poster and asked the residents if they had seen it in their homes or community (see Figure 13-4). In each village, the answer was "no," they had never seen a bug like that, which surprised the researchers. Clearly, the kissing bug and Chagas' disease clinical symptoms were present, but the villagers denied ever seeing the bug. Was it because the bug only attacks humans at night while villagers slept? Finally, after further discussion, they realized the community members looked at the size of the bug on the placard literally, and with that cultural prism, understandably responded that they had never seen a five-inch kissing bug in their village.

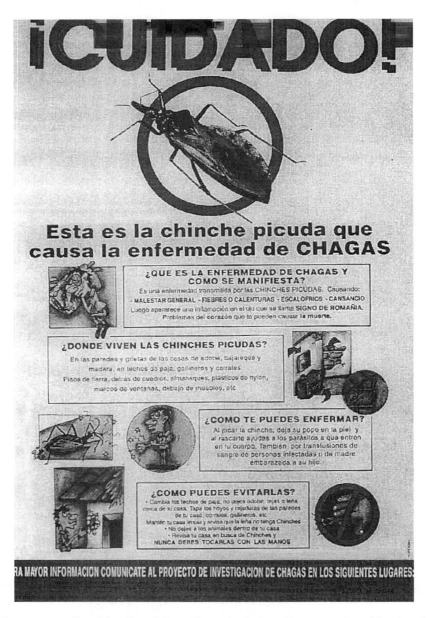

Figure 13-4. Chagas poster, literal size. Ecuadorian villagers had a literal interpretation of the size of this triatomine bug, shown in this poster as being five inches long, and told researchers they had never seen it in their community. From Ohio University Tropical Disease Institute www.oucom.ohiou.edu/tdi. (Reproduced with permission.)

The researchers went back and immediately produced publications with photos depicting the literal sizes of the young and adult triatomines (see Figure 13-5). Re-surveying the same villagers with the new material, they heard "oh yes, of course we've seen *those* bugs . . . they're everywhere!"

SOCIAL MARKETING

A major development in health communications—social marketing—began to take shape as a discipline in the 1970s with the idea that the same marketing principles being used to sell products to consumers could be

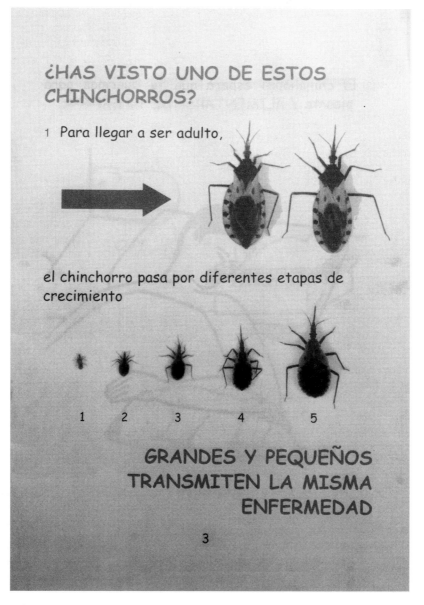

Figure 13-5. Chagas triatomines, book actual sizes. Ohio University Tropical Disease Institute researchers then designed a booklet with the actual sizes of the bugs and showed it to the community. "Oh yes, we've seen *that* bug, that's the chinchero!" From Ohio University Tropical Disease Institute. (Reproduced with permission.)

used to "sell" ideas, attitudes, and behaviors that could benefit the individual, community, and society. As defined by Andreasen, social marketing "seeks to influence social behaviors, not to benefit the marketer, but to benefit the target audience and the general society".[9]

Social marketing aims to change behaviors, first and foremost. Social marketers place a high value on conducting market research to "listen" and determine the needs, wants, and perceptions of the "customer." They recognize that behavioral change will only come about if the researcher focuses the work on where the customer is now. When possible, researchers carefully segment audiences rather than treating them as one mass group, and competing forces that detract from the desired behavior change are addressed by diminishing their appeal and reinforcing the benefits and ease of accessibility of the new "product."

The social marketing process has been used extensively in global health programs for contraceptive use; oral rehydration therapy; literacy; and HIV/AIDS prevention, treatment, and education. In the United States, social marketing can be seen in campaigns to reduce drug abuse, increase the wearing of seat belts, encourage stewardship of the environment, lessen the burdens of heart disease, motivate more people to donate their organs, and stop smoking cigarettes. This framework or mindset centers on determining and delivering the benefits the consumer desires and ensuring the benefits to them outweigh the costs.

Based on marketing principles, but dealing with more complex issues involving behavioral change, social marketing applies the traditionally commercial concepts of the "four P's" of product, price, place, and promotion, and adds a fifth, positioning. When applied to social marketing, these elements become:

- **Product:** The behavior or health idea that the campaign planners would like the consumers to adopt. The product can be an action (e.g., performing breast self-examinations regularly) or material (e.g., fat-free dairy products).
- **Price:** The costs associated with "buying" or adopting the product. Costs can involve sacrifices related to psychological well being (e.g., increased anxiety), sociality (e.g., possibility of ostracism), economics (e.g., financial sacrifice), or time (e.g., inconvenience).
- **Place:** The distribution channels used to make the product available in an easily obtainable way. The consumer must be informed of where, when, and how he or she can obtain the product.
- **Promotion:** The efforts taken to ensure the priority audience is aware of the campaign, the benefits, and how peers are adopting it.
- **Positioning:** The product must be positioned in a way that maximizes benefits and minimizes costs. "Positioning" is a psychological construct that involves the location of the product relative to other products and activities with which it competes. For instance, physical activity could be repositioned as a form of relaxation, not exercise.[10]

Social marketers working to bring about healthier behaviors will conduct an analysis of the individual, community, or organization's environment. This can involve doing a SWOT (Strengths, Weaknesses, Opportunities, and Threats) analysis to examine the audience's strengths and weaknesses, as well as the economic, competitive, regulatory/laws/customs, social, and technological opportunities and threats.

Questions asked during this exploration could be:

- What strengths, skills, and accomplishments does this individual or community have that could be tapped into and built on during a health social marketing campaign?
- What cultural traditions, beliefs, laws, or biases are present that may support or impede the hoped-for behavioral change?
- What's the economic, educational, and social capacity for embracing the change?
- Can the benefits of the proposed change win out over competing desires, habits, and interests?
- Are there sufficient communication channels and resources available to inform and motivate the individual(s) to make the change and sustain it?

Segmenting, Researching, and Sustaining

Effective social marketing health programs tap into other elements of marketing to achieve success. These include: differential advantage, audience segmentation, research, and sustainability.

The differential advantage of a product, service, or behavior change is that feature or benefit that makes it more desirable to adopt than the alternative choices. You may see your differential advantage in a stop smoking campaign to be that it will save the smoker's life. However, focusing on the short-term benefits and advantages, such as better breath, not smelling like smoke, appearing more attractive, or saving money, may be more relevant to the smoker now and have a better chance of success for both the consumer and the social marketer.

Segmenting a population means defining the subgroups based on their common characteristics and traits. Because populations are different, segmentation helps you develop materials, messages, and channels for delivery that are tailored to those you want to inform and motivate, and who may be most at risk yet ready for the change. Segmentation also helps you figure out the individuals or groups who can help you bring about the program and change.

You can segment a population into a priority audience by using the following characteristics to define them:

- **Behavioral:** Health-related activities or choices, degree of readiness to change, information-seeking behavior, media use, and lifestyle characteristics
- **Cultural:** Language proficiency and preferences, religion, ethnicity, generational status, family structure, degree of acculturation, and lifestyle factors (e.g., special foods, activities)
- **Sociodemographic:** Age, gender, occupation, income, educational attainment, family situation, and places of residence and work
- **Physical:** Type and degree of exposure to health risks, medical condition, disorders and illnesses, and family health history
- **Psychographic:** Attitudes, outlook on life and health, self-image, opinions, beliefs, values, self-efficacy, life stage, social class, and personality traits[11]
- **Cohort:** Looks at individuals bound together in history by a series of events. The events may have been the technological upheavals, wars, political crises, and major sociological changes that form and shape an individual's attitudes and beliefs regarding health, prevention, practices. Depending on the timeframe they came of age, these groups can be characterized as worrying about financial security, very accepting of authority, conforming to norms, having great trust in institutions, questioning everything, cynical, conservative, idealistic, team players, always been connected digitally, achieving, and community serving.[12]

Research is at the heart of all successful social marketing programs. In defining the intended audience, their knowledge, attitudes, practices, and sociodemographics, the needed intervention and the outcome goals, market researchers may apply primary and secondary data. Primary data, information collected by observing individuals or asking them questions, address a specific research question. Secondary data were collected previously for another purpose such as the US Census or media access habits, but can be helpful in building a social marketing program.

Observational research is one way to study individual or community behavior. Gender roles within a village could be observed, or how patients of each gender are treated when they first enter a health care facility. This research can show what happens but cannot describe why it happens.

Another common method used is survey research. Surveys can be delivered through telephone interviews, personal in-depth interviews, focus groups, mail, Personal digital assistant (PDA), and web-based applications. Depending on their structure and the skill of the researcher, surveys can yield much about an individual's knowledge, attitudes, and practices related to health. See Figures 13-6

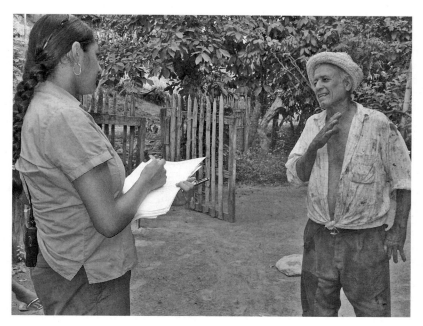

Figure 13-6. KAP survey, Ecuador. Researchers survey the health knowledge, attitudes, and practices of Ecuadorians living in rural villages and mountain towns, as part of Ohio University's Tropical Disease Biology and Communications workshop in 2006. Photo credit: Gary Snyder, University of South Carolina. (Reproduced with permission.)

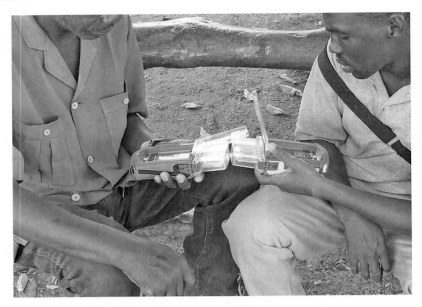

Figure 13-7. Survey technology, CDC. Community researchers in Togo transmit data from PDA to PDA after conducting a survey of villagers' understanding and behaviors related to insecticide-treated bednet use and vaccine access. The PDAs are equipped with a GPS unit to map certain areas of a village or rural area and select a simple random sample of the mapped points, and then guide the interviewers back to the selected households. Community interviewers conduct the survey and enter responses directly into the PDA. All survey data is then combined into a program that analyzes it immediately in the field. Developed by researchers in the Division of Parasitic Diseases at the CDC. Photo credit: Adam Wolkon, CDC Division of Parasitic Diseases. (Reproduced with permission.)

and 13-7 for examples of community-based health surveys being conducted in Ecuador and Togo.

Similar to other health communications, those using a social marketing approach to increase health literacy and produce healthier behaviors employ several channels to send their messages. These channels may be:

- Interpersonal (patient counseling)
- Organizational/community (town hall meetings, workplace campaigns)
- Mass media (newspaper, radio and TV ads, news, letters to editor, opinion pieces, talk shows, and education entertainment)
- Digital communications (Internet and Intranet websites, e-mail, newsgroups, website ads, topic or campaign blogs, podcasts, and various digital social and activist networks on-line)

HEALTH PROMOTERS AND "EDUTAINMENT" TAKE CENTER STAGE

An essential part of any health communications program involves finding out who in the community are the most trusted sources to help deliver information and encourage behavior change. In many cultures, lay health promoters serve this role because of their knowledge and their respected place in the family or community. A broader group called cultural "brokers" can help connect the researcher, educator, or organization to the community as well. These individuals may range from nurses, lay health promoters, and shamans to school counselors, social workers, and youth leaders. By recruiting individuals within the community as leaders, the programs will be more relevant, be communicated by known individuals, and stand a better chance of producing improved health outcomes. An excellent example of a successful program built by the community is the Amupakin midwife initiative in the Napo Province of Ecuador. Native Kichwa lay health promoters and midwives work with the Ecuador Red Cross to provide Kichwa women with a safe childbirth experience that keeps with Kichwa tradition. (See Figure 13-8.)

Latino *promotoras*, trusted professional or lay health workers in the Latino community, have proven to be effective for delivering culturally sensitive health information and increasing knowledge about breast and cervical cancer. Researchers found that having *promotoras* conduct

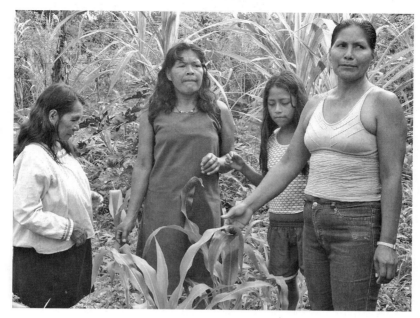

Figure 13-8. Midwives in Ecuador and medicinal plants. Community health promoters and midwives describe the medicinal benefits of nearby plants in the Ecuadorian rain forest in caring for women wanting a traditional childbirthing experience. The innovative program, called Amupakin, has facilities and community-based midwives that provide a safe alternative to hospital deliveries. The program's promotional brochure is simple and colorful, and written in both the native Kichwa language and in Spanish. www.amupakin.org. Photo credit: Gary Snyder, University of South Carolina. (Reproduced with permission.)

the programs improved participants' cancer knowledge and changed their perceptions of the barriers to cancer screening.[13]

Bilingual cultural brokers bridge the gap between the educator or health organization and certain communities, particularly those "hard to reach" because of language, culture, or other differences. They can make the difference whether communications and programming are accepted and believed by the community or not (see Figure 13-9). Examples of their importance can be seen in efforts to provide better health care to the Hmong refugees by overlapping the traditional healer or shaman's approach to treatment with the Western providers' care, or the innovative "Low Rider Bike Project" in California that employed cultural brokers and a community-driven idea to change the lives of at-risk, low-income teenage kids who were joining street gangs.[14] (See Box 13.1)

Research has shown "edutainment", the practice of using mass entertainment to deliver public health messages, raises awareness of issues and motivates action and behavior change. Developing powerful human interest storylines through popular characters that are woven into telenovelas (Spanish language soap opera dramas),

radio dramas, community theater, or other media and shows can have a profound impact on reader, listener, and viewer understanding of health issues and behavior.

One of the earliest examples of how mixing social change content into popular entertainment affects behavior was the Peruvian telenovella, "Simplemente Maria." The central character, Maria Ramos, was a rural-to-urban migrant who moved from the Andes to Lima. She worked as a maid during the day and struggled economically because she was illiterate. She also became a single mother. Her fortunes changed, though, when she decided to start attending adult literacy classes at night and also learned how to become a seamstress. Empowered by her ability to read and her growing seamstress business, she started her own fashion business that became a great success, with Maria becoming known all the way to Paris. Most importantly, during this storyline, enrollment in adult literacy classes in Peru skyrocketed in the 1970s, and rural-to-urban migration accelerated.[15]

Another example of the innovative use of media to reach the audience with human development stories is "Story Story," a successful radio drama broadcast that reaches millions in Nigeria and on the BBC Network. It

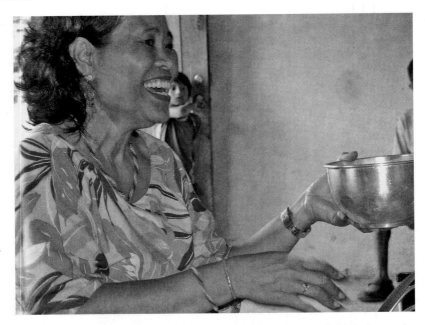

Figure 13-9. Health promoter with community drink. Trusted health educators bridge the gap between researchers and the community's culture. Here a health promoter in a rural Ecuadorian village shares a traditional drink with the community before talking with them about good nutrition and safe water practices. Photo credit: Gary Snyder, University of South Carolina. (Reproduced with permission.)

BOX 13-1. LOW RIDER BIKE CLUB GIVES TEENS HIGH ESTEEM

In the low-income Westside neighborhood of San Bernardino, CA, gangs, substance abuse and violence have been major health concerns. Counseling sessions for at-risk youth were provided but were met with indifference and low participation. Community organizers with the Casa de San Bernardino Westside Prevention Project knew the teens were not coming because participating in antidrug and antiviolence programs was not perceived as "cool." They needed a better way to reach the youth at their level.

Casa leaders found out who the trusted authorities were in the community and recruited them to serve as leaders and cultural brokers to help find an answer. The advisory group identified a symbol of the street culture that would attract high-risk youth: low rider bikes, the ones with glistening handle bars and velvet seats. The Casa group and the community leaders created the Westside Prevention Project Low Rider Bike Club, a program that gives free low rider bike parts to youth for each weekly counseling session they attend. They require regular attendance to maintain club membership.

The result? Over the first two years (2002–2004), more than 200 youth participated in the program, attending individual assessment, and sessions on drug treatment, aggression replacement training, and life and leadership skills. Organizers saw self-esteem and positive behavior rising as the bikes began to take shape. Cultural brokers helped ensure the program was community driven, relevant to the youth, and sustainable. It worked because they centered all efforts on the consumer (the youth) and designed a program that connected with them at their level.

From: Bridging the Cultural Divide in Health Care Settings: The Essential Role of Cultural Broker Programs, National Center for Cultural Competence, Georgetown University Medical Center, Spring/Summer 2004. Bilingual versions available at: http://www.culturalbroker.info/

combines a storyline with discussion of issues raised during the week's shows, centers around everyday people—poor, rich, farmers, teachers, market traders—and covers topics like violence, HIV/AIDS, corruption, environmental sustainability, empowerment of women, education, and citizenship.[16]

Radio, because of its low-cost accessibility and lower literacy demands, has great potential for reaching populations in developing countries with consistent health stories and messages.

In "The Digital World of the US Hispanic II" study, Cheskin found that radio continues to be highly accessed and "culturally relevant" to Latinos. The study showed that Latinos listen to about 15 hours of radio per week, with just more than half of that being to Spanish radio.[17] Radio listening is part of a tradition in Latin America, which has more than 4,000 radio stations (zonelatina.com).[18] Korzenny points out that in the United States, Latinos tend to be concentrated in the service and labor areas of the economy (construction, transportation, agriculture, food service, hospitality), jobs that lend themselves to listening to the radio. Latino radio reminds the listener of home and being "culturally connected . . . in a way English radio cannot." The most effective programming entertains people with humor, music, and storytelling, and brings them information related to their jobs, immigration issues, and education.[19]

A United Nations Acquired Immunodeficiency Syndrome (UNAIDS) effort in India is using television-based programming to address HIV/AIDS-related social stigma. The education-entertainment telecast called "Kalyani," meaning "the one who provides welfare," is an effort to encourage positive health attitudes and behaviors. It addresses HIV-related stigma, discrimination, and treatment through short spots, folk songs, and informative segments with experts. "Kalyani" airs in the capital cities of eight highly populated Indian states, reaching nearly 50 percent of the country's population. The program is reinforced by follow-up action in the form of visits to rural areas in which experts and actors from the show interact with intended audiences. Among the storylines has been a young man who contracted the disease while migrating to a village looking for work. The village initially shuns him but after being educated through a visit by the actors about how HIV is transmitted and how there should be no stigma, the HIV-positive man is accepted and then becomes a champion for HIV prevention in the area.[20]

According to a Porter Novelli Health Styles survey, more than 60 percent of regular prime time and daytime telenovella drama viewers reported that they learned something about a disease or how to prevent it from a TV show. Nearly half of regular viewers said they took some action after hearing about a health issue or disease on a TV show.[21]

In light of the growing potential entertainment channels hold for social change, there have been increased efforts to link public health communication professionals, producers, and scriptwriters together. One initiative, the Hollywood, Health & Society (HH&S) project at the University of Southern California, works with the US Centers for Disease Control and Prevention to provide entertainment industry professionals with accurate and timely information for health storylines.[22]

"Participatory communication" reflects the reality (both strengths and challenges) of communities in delivering health information through entertainment, sports celebrities, radio, TV, periodicals, theater, stories told through photographs (photo-novellas), folk entertainment, music, oral storytelling, emerging digital communications, and trusted community members. The essential elements needed to inform and influence must be a community-grounded approach to the content, real characters that the audience can relate to, vivid storylines that evoke emotion, and information delivered as part of the story but in such a way that motivates the audience members to take action to improve their health. (See Box 13.2)

BOX 13-2. RABIES NO MATCH FOR HMONG PARADE OF STORYTELLERS

Health communication professionals should draw on the strengths of the cultures they work in to communicate messages and motivate behavior change. An example of this occurred in a Hmong refugee camp experiencing an outbreak of rabies. A mass dog vaccination campaign started by the camp's medical staff resulted in zero dogs being brought in for vaccination. Ethnologist Dwight Conquergood, who lived with the Hmong, stepped forward and organized a "Rabies Parade" led by the Hmong. The Hmong played vivid characters from their folktales and culture, explaining through song and dance the story of how rabies is transmitted and why dogs need to be vaccinated. The next day, the health care workers were pleasantly overwhelmed by many dogs brought in by the community to be vaccinated.

From: Fadiman, A. The Spirit Catches You and You Fall Down. New York: Farrar, Straus and Giroux, 1997: 35-37.

MEDIA

Reporters, editors, and publishers can be powerful allies in the push to motivate individuals and communities to adopt healthy practices. This section will briefly explore how to work with the media to get coverage of health issues, what is done to train the media about certain health issues and conditions so they more accurately report on them, and the emerging trend toward more grassroots, community- or citizen-based journalism.

Attracting Media Coverage of Your Issue or Work

Whether you're a public health practitioner in Nebraska, a student volunteer with a women's health nongovernmental organization (NGO) in China, or a trauma counselor in Darfur, understanding the media and partnering with them can help greatly to advance your work and improve health outcomes for the communities you are working in.

Too often, individuals and organizations make the mistake of thinking media are just waiting to tell their story. They do not take the time to understand the editorial interests or focus of the newspaper, radio, or TV station, their capacity (personnel and knowledge level) to adequately cover a story, or the political-social pressures they may need to consider on certain topics. When working with the media, be sure to:

- **Take time to examine what issues or topics are covered most in their newspaper or broadcast program.** Do they cover mainly local or regional news? Is there a health section or segment? If they cover a good deal of business news, can you tie in the economic effects of health problems? What are the trends or issues most important to them and their audience? Do they have the personnel to go out into the field, research, and cover stories, or will they run stories you put together? What is the culture or political situation in their circulation area? Are they independent, government-run, or owned by a corporation? What are the technological capabilities for receiving information and using content? Who are their readers, listeners, or viewers?

- **Develop a relationship with key reporters by showing them you understand their needs, goals, audiences, and constraints.** Appreciate that they have deadlines and return their calls and e-mails promptly. Foster goodwill by being a consistent, reliable, and accurate source of information for them. Contact or send them only press releases that have newsworthiness to their audiences. Never say "no comment" to a reporter because it gives the impression you have something to hide. If you do not know an answer, say "I do not know." Remember, there's no such privilege as "off the record." If you do not want a comment printed or broadcast, do not say it.

- **Position yourself and others in your organization as experts in their fields and valuable sources to the media.** Train others in your organization on how to be responsive to the media, how to conduct an effective interview, and how to get your information out concisely and clearly.

Educating Media About Key Health Issues

Media, particularly in developing countries, play an important part in getting accurate information about serious diseases and problems to the public. Many people and policymakers form their views of diseases and conditions based on how they are presented via the media. Unfortunately, most reporters do not have a health, medical, or science background, may not take cultural or social issues into consideration in their coverage, and may devote minimal time to health issues because of scarce resources. This is sometimes the case with reporting on the complex and sensitive condition of HIV/AIDS. Many in the developing world remain misinformed about AIDS. The role of journalists and communicators is central to containing the crisis in places like Africa and India.

Journalists must continue to be educated about the basics of the disease, how it is prevented and transmitted, what the cultural stigmas are, what treatment is available, and what misconceptions and myths still linger about HIV/AIDS. Training sessions are essential to increase clinical knowledge among journalists about conditions such as HIV/AIDS and malaria, and how to report accurately, ethically, and with clarity.

In order to make it relevant to the media's growing focus on economic issues, global health communicators should connect the impact of disease, and issues like environmental disruption, to the economic effects. How many days of work were lost? What's the cost when a high percentage of a country's most productive age group is dying from HIV/AIDS complications? What's the cost to eco-tourism or agriculture when war or disaster scars the environment? How does environmental degradation impact poverty and foster disease?

Several international groups, such as Internews and UNAIDS "on the ground" programs, as well as the Kaiser Family Foundation's globalhealthreporting.org website, provide in-depth resources and training for media across the world.

Internews, a communications NGO with offices in 23 countries, trains more than 9,000 media professionals each year on how to cover issues like HIV/AIDS and avian flu. It works with local media to produce original programming, build media infrastructure, and advance laws and policies supporting an independent, open media that serves as a "watchdog" to government and industry. Internews' programs are built on the conviction that providing people with access to "vibrant, diverse news

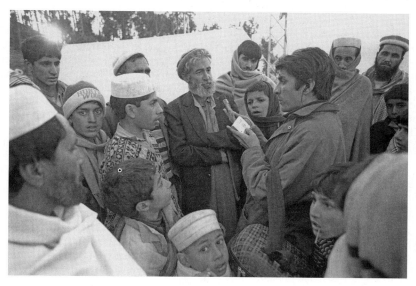

Figure 13-10. Internews at the Pakistan earthquake. Journalist Jamal Swati interviews earthquake survivors in Balakot, northern Pakistan for Internews' radio program of humanitarian information after the October 2005 earthquake. Photo credit: Mark Edwards, Still Pictures/Internews. (Reproduced with permission.)

and information empowers them to participate effectively in their communities, effect positive social change, improve their living standards, and make their voices heard." (See Figure 13-10).

Community Media and Citizen Journalists

Local communities giving voice to their own needs, strengths, and challenges by developing their own content that tells *their* story and that will run in community-owned media can be empowering for education and change. Community radio, for example, makes radio more accessible to all, with content reflecting the local interests, be they economic, health, political, social, environmental, or entertainment.

The World Association of Community Broadcasters, describes community radio as:

> When radio fosters the participation of citizens and defends their interests; when it reflects the tastes of the majority and makes good humor and hope its main purpose; when it truly informs; when it helps resolve the thousand and one problems of daily life; when all ideas are debated in its programs and all opinions are respected; when cultural diversity is stimulated over commercial homogeneity; when women are main players in communication and not simply a pretty voice or a publicity gimmick; when no type of dictatorship is tolerated, not even the musical dictatorship of the big recording studios; when everyone's words fly without discrimination or censorship, that is community radio.

A key strategy in some community-based health communications programs is the use of "behavioral journalism," in which you identify people from the community who have made the desired behavioral change and who can be featured as role models in the media materials and outreach. Having role models within the community helping lead the campaign makes the messages understandable, relevant, and credible. Plus, the community sees proof that change is possible and desirable.

EMERGING COMMUNICATION TECHNOLOGIES

Over the past two decades, we have learned much about how health communications programs can be designed to educate and motivate human behavior toward healthy change globally. One of the most vital tools to generate knowledge and awareness is information communication technologies (ICTs). Advancements in this area are showing great promise at increasing access to information for individuals and communities.

The speed at which the information revolution is occurring is remarkable. Since 1975 the speed and memory of computers has increased a million-fold and prices have plummeted. A $2,000 PC is equivalent to a $10,000,000 supercomputer in 1975. *The Economist* magazine in 1996 pointed out that if automobile technology improved as rapidly as information technology, a car would speed along at 100,000 miles per hour, get 200,000 miles per gallon of gas, and cost $5.00.

This communication technologies explosion over the past few years transformed entire communities and countries, some previously shut off from most communications, and allowed developing countries to leapfrog some costly and time-consuming stages of technology such as the building of telephone land lines. The changes have increased access to and sharing of information that benefits communities in many ways, but also have brought increased costs to individuals and communities as they "keep up" with technology.

Examples of Communication Technology Growth and Use

Access to the Internet has largely been enjoyed by individuals living in North America, Europe, and Australia. But that is changing. As of January 2007, North American residents had the most access to the Internet (70 percent), but the greatest growth in Internet use over the previous six years occurred in Africa (625 percent), the Middle East (490 percent), and Latin America/Caribbean (390 percent).[23] Clearly, the rapid expansion of access to the Internet in developing regions will have a great impact on how health information is shared and what individuals, governments, and societies do with the new knowledge.

Among the many information communication technologies available—Internet, computers, handheld personal digital assistants (PDAs), broadcast media, telecenters, education innovations—one of the most significant developments worldwide has been the advent and adoption of mobile telephones.

MOBILE PHONES: JOURNALISM, COMMERCE, SAFETY OR CONVERSATION

Perhaps no recent technological advancement has been more quickly embraced and life-changing in the world than the mobile phone. For much of the globe, it empowers and connects people. It has become irreplaceable or a "necessary evil" to many as well, particularly in the developing world. Africa, the world's fastest-growing cell phone market, has seen the number of mobile subscribers jump from 7.5 million in 1999 to 79 million in 2004, an annual increase of nearly 60 percent. In India, according to the Cellular Operators Association of India, 50 million Indians now possess a mobile phone, a figure that exceeds the 45 million land line phones in the country. That disparity is even greater in the Congo, which in early 2007 had 4.2 million cell phone subscriber connections compared to just over 20,000 conventional land lines.[24]

Mobile phones are transforming the way news coverage happens—both in its immediacy and in the increased involvement of "citizen journalists." After the terrorist transit bombings in London in 2005, the first short text messages, images, and video to emerge came from people on the trains or at the scene of the disaster using their mobile digital camera phones. Cell-phone videos are transforming TV news, revealing, through the experience of someone at the place where the story is unfolding, the graphic truth. Many media outlets now have technology allowing viewers to quickly upload and transmit their images and video.

Sometimes referred to as "participatory social media," these emerging technologies allow the public to contribute to telling the story and getting the facts out. They also improve communications during natural disasters and give an eyewitness account to the world about atrocities and injustice.

Mobile phones have emerged as a catalyst for development in many countries. They allow access to market information for farmers in India so they know where they can get the best price for their crops and can eliminate long, unnecessary trips to the city if not needed. In China, low-income farmers use text messages to learn about weather forecasts or ways to control pests. For those individuals who cannot afford their own phone, mobile phones in villages are rented out by the minute to callers to make them accessible.

As a key tool of digital commerce, cell-phones are revolutionizing how consumers in African cities conduct financial transactions. With a few presses of the keypad, they can transfer money to merchants or to their bank to pay for supplies or services. Internet access, ATMs, and credit cards may be tough to find in some developing countries, so services have emerged such as Celpay, a company that features Internet banking through mobile phones. Celpay customers can transfer funds through the system and pay bills from their cell phones, and also make deposits into their Celpay accounts at a number of stations in the country.[25] This is particularly significant to the poor who may have never been able to open up traditional bank accounts because they had no credit history and were seen as high-risk.

Several ancillary industries have arisen around the cell phone demand, making it basically a form of currency. Streetside vendors hawk the use of their multiple phones and minutes, and also make money from transferring their minutes to others' phones. Illiterate individuals can pay a fee and have messages typed for them.

A boon for conducting business, the accessibility and relative affordability of the mobile phone have provided families and communities with a sense of security and connectedness to health services that was not available before. In rural areas, disconnected at night from neighbors or health care services, a child suffering from a potentially fatal disease such as cholera or malaria could die before receiving treatment the next day at a clinic several hours away. With the cell phone, they can summon help and transportation, or perhaps get advice from health care workers many miles away. Healthcare workers at remote clinics can call for ambulances using the cell phone, and fishermen on African lakes can call for emergency help if they are threatened by bandits at sea.

Grameen Phone, a pioneering initiative designed to bring mobile phones to villages and rural areas in Bangladesh (which has the lowest number of phones in South Asia), has several million subscribers and more than 120,000 village cellular "pay phones" throughout the country. A large focus is to provide women with the phones in order to build their skills and position them as valuable communication resources for the village. Known as Grameen phone ladies, the women are an essential link for the community to hospitals and to relatives at home and abroad. Their rising status helps balance the distribution of power. The Grameen Foundation (grameenfoundation.org) also has Village Phone programs in the Phillipines, Rwanda, and Uganda that "extend the benefits of affordable telecommunications access in a sustainable, profitable, and empowering way."

Most phones now have a global positioning system (GPS) chip that can be activated to locate wayward hikers, rural accident victims, or injured mountain climbers. GPS-enabled mobile phones can also be used by fishermen to track coming storms or by farmers or disaster relief agencies to detect climate changes that may bring on drought and, subsequently, famine.

Migrant workers or husbands working in cities several hundred miles from home can stay connected regularly via cell phone with family and friends. This helps lessen the sense of isolation, and may make workers away from their social support systems less vulnerable to making unhealthy behavioral decisions.

Like any technology, cell-phones can be abused as well. They have been used for triggering explosive devices remotely, by government officials who force companies to give them free minutes on their cell-phones as bribes, and by rebel armies coordinating their movements. On the flip side, the World Bank started a peaceful disarmament program in the Congo where men and women fighters could turn in their weapons and then be notified through the Celpay cell phone service that they are entitled to job training and a few hundred dollars over the course of a year.

Research conducted by the UK's Department for International Development confirmed that at the village level, "where there has been improvement in access to phone connections, there is a positive impact on livelihoods."[26]

ICTs: Filling the Communication Void of Disasters

Information and communication technologies (ICTs) can save lives through early warning systems and can alleviate hardship and trauma after a disaster strikes by providing accurate information as widely as possible. Media technology plays a large role in the response to disasters and conflicts by communicating with survivors and helping to rebuild communications and communities.

The cyclone preparedness program (CPP), created by the International Federation of Red Cross and Red Crescent Societies in the early 1970s, is credited with saving millions of lives over the past three decades. Its early warning system taps into Asia's largest radio network, and emerging storms tracked by satellite are relayed by radio to 33,000 well-trained volunteers in villages. The volunteers spread the warning to communities that will be affected by using hand-operated sirens or shouting through megaphones from motorbikes. The CPP can alert about eight million people across the coastal region.[27]

One of the greatest challenges following disasters is filling the huge void of communications created when communities and physical spaces are ripped apart. In the race to get supplies to address some of the physical needs, the information response is often neglected. Vulnerable survivors need to know about the status of their loved ones. Logistics about when to expect food and clothing from aid agencies, and when electricity and clean water may be restored, must be shared.

Myths that grow out of ignorance or poor information in refugee camps also must be debunked quickly. Rumors that surfaced after recent disasters, some resulting in fatalities, included:

- Survivors of the Pakistan earthquake coated the inside of their tents with kerosene because they heard it would repel malaria-carrying insects, causing tents to catch fire, resulting in the deaths of a dozen people.

- Rural villagers in Pakistan, seeing bottled water for the first time, refused to drink it, thinking it was unsafe. Instead, they used it for washing and drank polluted river water.

- After the tsunami in Indonesia, survivors heard that dead bodies spread disease, so they immediately tossed the dead bodies into mass graves, causing more distress for families searching for their loved ones.

Internews, the international NGO that specializes in "humanitarian reporting" in post-disaster/conflict environments as part of its mission, helped identify and correct some of these myths by broadcasting interviews with experts and getting the information dispersed. The group also rebuilds media infrastructure and gets accurate, culturally relevant communications out to survivors or loved ones as soon as possible through portable wind-up radios given to survivors and suitcase radio transmitters. Some of the news is created and reported by local individuals such as university students, who are trained in the art of humanitarian reporting.) (See Box 13-3, a case study of Internews' reconstructing of media in Indonesia immediately after the Tsunami of 2005)

BOX 13-3. INTERNEWS: REBUILDING LIVES AND COMMUNICATIONS POST-DISASTER

The December 2004 Asian tsunami destroyed human lives and also wiped out many forms of communication such as radio stations and newspapers, which compounded the suffering of survivors looking for loved ones and trying to rebuild. In stepped Internews, a non-profit NGO that builds media infrastructure before and after disasters, trains local journalists, helps develop local content and capacity and advocates policies to government leaders about the need for open, independent media in democracies.

In the Indonesian province of Aceh, media workplaces were destroyed and stations and newspapers lost many staff members to the tragedy. Displaced survivors yearned for any word of their family and neighbors. Internews, which had been training journalists there for several years, responded by flying in a radio team and equipment to both transmit radio signals and receive them. Here's how Internews and local Acehnese and Javanese journalists rebuilt some of the radio media quickly in a time of extreme crisis.

Internews assembles some of the remaining journalists and engineers from Aceh for training and distributes two portable radio transmitters (sometimes called "suitcase radio stations") so information can be broadcast widely.

Digital receivers and solar panels for energy are given to 36 Aceh radio stations and 147 IDP (internally displaced persons) camps, delivered by boat, raft and motor bike along earthquake-ravaged roads. The receivers allow the stations and camps to pick up the programming.

Internews distributes portable wind-up radios to 785 families. By winding the radio handle, power is generated by a dynamo inside the radio. A few minutes of winding is all that is needed for several hours of listening. Radios have built-in flashlights which are needed by the refugees.

Working with a team of Acehnese and Javanese journalists, Internews goes on the air with "Peuneugah Aceh" (News from Aceh) from a studio built in Banda Aceh. The program airs news about the reconstruction process, relief aid, and missing loved ones, as seen by Acehnese farmers, schoolteachers, market vendors and everyday citizens. Along with the news of housing, assistance, and survival, traditional music, storytelling and even comedy skits make their way into the programming as the survivors begin to rebuild. Stations relayed the program or taped and rebroadcast it. Thousands more wind-up radios were distributed.

The program broadcast news of reconstruction to an estimated audience of one million people through September of 2006.

Adapted from: www.internews.org
See Fig 13-11

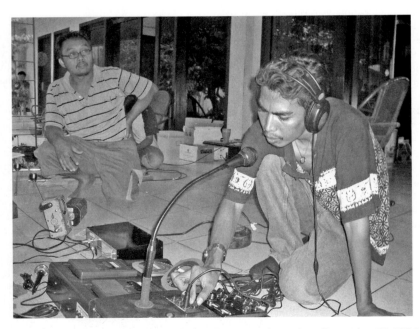

Figure 13-11. Internews at the Indonesia tsunami. After the tsunami struck on December 26, 2004, Internews flew in a radio team and two "suitcase radio stations" to the remote province of Aceh, Indonesia, allowing local stations to get back on the air. Photo credit: Kathleen Reen/Internews. (Reproduced with permission.)

Some other emerging communication technologies that can make significant contributions to improving both access to knowledge and health outcomes in the coming years are:

- **Community-based telecenters in rural areas** provide computer training and access, Internet service, printing, distance education, community radio broadcasts, local content development, online community building; and job training.

- Several hundred cities globally are building, or discussing building, **wi-fi networks** that would make entire metropolitan areas able to provide free wireless access.

- **Solar-powered Green Wi-Fi grid networks** can provide open, wireless access to remote, rural areas in developing countries. Green Wi-Fi (www.green-wifi.org) developed a low-cost, solar-powered system that connects remote areas lacking electricity to a mobile grid. The goal is to provide affordable computing capabilities to everyone in developing areas.

- **The "One Laptop Per Child" project** (http://laptop. org/), designed at the Massachusetts Institute of Technology (MIT), aims to deliver several million $100 laptop computers to children in developing regions normally unable to provide them. The units, targeted toward Arabic, Asian, sub-Saharan, and South American markets, are designed to be durable, and for regions with limited or no electrical access. A crank handle or pedal-powered crank powers the battery and ten minutes of cranking provides an hour's worth of battery life.

- **The Kinkajou Portable Library and Projection System** (http://kinkajou.designthatmatters.org), a creation of MIT's Design That Matters group, projects up to 10,000 pages of information from a microfilm cassette onto a wall. Using a low-cost, renewable battery-powered supply (solar), the innovation provides communities that lack books, teachers, and lighting the opportunity to hold educational programs at night, and delivers a basic curriculum within one cassette. The hope is that this example of "humanitarian engineering" will help tackle global illiteracy. The product costs about $20 total and is being used in villages in Mali, India, and Bangladesh.

- **Laser Virtual Keyboard** (http://www.lumio.com/) is a small rectangular box about the size of a cellular phone that projects an image of a keyboard onto a work surface, and that serves as an actual keyboard. The device could be useful in environments that need to be kept sterile, and where space to carry or use a regular laptop is limited.

- **Health Info Translations** (www.healthinfotranslations. com) is a resource for helping health care professionals teach health education to those patients with limited English skills. Developed by three Columbus, Ohio, medical centers, the goal is to improve doctor-patient communications and health literacy for diverse immigrant communities. Information ranges from what to expect from your surgery, to diet and nutrition, to how to use an insulin pen. The site has patient education content translated into Chinese Simplified, French, Chinese Traditional, Japanese, Korean, Russian, Somali, Spanish, Ukrainian, Hindi, English, Vietnamese, and Arabic.

- **Visual Griots and Photo Blogging** (www.aed.org/ visualgriots) in developing countries is part of empowering individuals and communities to tap into their strengths and tell their own stories. One project, called visual "griots" (the name describing a West African storyteller who furthers the oral tradition of a family or village), includes providing digital cameras to a select number of individuals and having them assert their view of themselves and their world through the photos. Another project featured Ethiopians taking cameras and showing their everyday lives, the work, education, love, struggle, and beauty that typically is not shared by media or known by the rest of the world. This photo blog is housed at www.ethiopialives. net.

- **For survey research, PDAs equipped with a GPS unit** to map selected areas of a village or rural area can then beam and join data in the field without needing a laptop or computer. A GPS program selects a simple random sample of the mapped points and then guides the interviewers back to the selected households. Interviewers from the community (see Figure 13-7 earlier in this chapter) are trained to conduct the survey, enter data directly into the PDA, and then link and combine all the data received into a program that analyzes it immediately in the field. This program was developed by researchers in the Division of Parasitic Diseases at the CDC.[28]

One final example is the **Public Health Supercourse**, which we will examine in detail. The supercourse was developed at the University of Pittsburgh and is an online library of 2,480 PowerPoint lectures on global health research housed in a lecture library on the Internet (www.pitt.edu/~super1/). It is an open source system where scientists across the world share their best lectures for free and every lecture is "copy left," instead of copyright, and thus usable by anyone. The global health research supercourse is used to "whisk research into the classroom" and stimulate research worldwide.[29] The course networks 31,000 faculty members from 151 countries.

Increasingly, health concerns are global. Destruction of the ozone layer might be related to melanomas in Auckland and California, global migrations bring new patterns of disease and risk factors, and the world trade of tobacco impacts risk. Because of the globalization of disease, global sharing of research and education materials has a great potential to improve the translation of knowledge from research to the classroom.

The Internet is the most powerful tool for global research, communication, teaching, and the translation of research into the classroom. It is a transparent, cost-effective medium. It is cheap, and becoming ubiquitous. In addition, the format of the system itself with hypertext links and point and click can lead to powerful new modes of cognitively based training. It is a friendly medium and it breaks down the hierarchy between professor and student, students in Asia and students in Latin America. On the Internet, people are equal. With the power of the Internet, the best scientists of the world can teach the best talents to foster global health research.

The supercourse project has been, as Newton said, " . . . standing on the shoulders of giants" of global health research. Faculty members from across the world are given a web library for free to instruct students. From this library, the faculty members can share their knowledge, education, and training systems with other scientists worldwide. For the future development of this effort, the supercourse team will be employing systems for the information bank that previously have not been used in our discipline, but which have proven to be very valuable in other disciplines. Through a continuous quality assurance/peer review system especially designed for lectures/reviews, the supercourse developers are working to ensure the quality of the educational modules. It is surprising there has been so little research on how to effectively communicate global health research findings to the students of the world. Most faculty are thrown into the classroom with little training, and almost none in lecture development. With the supercourse component, state of the art template web lectures are shared. In addition, continued global monitoring of the lectures provides important feedback as to how to improve them.

With a low estimate of 20,000 students a year seeing a global health research lecture, in ten years, 200,000 will have seen each a lecture. Overall each lecture will take about $4,000 to prepare. In ten years the cost to present each lecture to a student will be $4,000/200,000 or $.02. Contrast this with international talking head lectures where costs can run $100/student/lecture or $4,000 for an hour class of 40. The Internet approach in this case is 200,000 times less expensive, highly cost effective, and accessible to students.

With the supercourse the local teacher is central, and their lectures are improved because of a library of lectures as templates. The goal is to assist the local educators, not replace them. The majority of the lectures are understandable for those educators having a bachelor's degree. The lectures can be modified by the teachers for K-12 grades. They will need to tailor the lectures for their students by simplifying the language and text. However, this is easy to do, so that the educators serve as translators of the top-notch PowerPoint lectures. Oftentimes there are lectures in multiple languages to assist teachers who do not speak English. Although quality control of lecture translations is a very important component of the supercourse, the majority of the translations submitted so far have been of very high quality.

It is not possible to put the lectures up exclusively in PowerPoint format. This was dramatically shown when researchers in Ghana tried to pull down one of the supercourse lectures and it took 18 hours. In addition, the majority of lectures at the CDC could not be seen in Africa. It was like sucking an elephant through a straw. Instead, a system was developed to convert the PowerPoint slides into .gif images. The .gif images can be directly used in PowerPoint, however, they are one-twentieth the size of typical PowerPoint lectures. The slides can readily be put inside of PowerPoint, but are much smaller and easier to distribute than true PowerPoint lectures.

Even with the reduction of size some countries find it difficult to surf US websites. It costs three times more to visit a site in the US than in China for a Chinese investigator. To ease this problem, mirrored servers of the supercourse were built in 42 countries across the world. Every few months these mirrored servers are updated. Most servers are in developing countries; the last five mirrored servers were put into Mongolia, the Sudan, Malaysia, Romania, and Papua, New Guinea. The approximate number of hits on all servers per year is 75 million, making the supercourse one of the highest hit sites in health. Over 10,000 copies of the supercourse CD containing 1,038 lectures and other content were distributed worldwide over a period of five years. The CD is a gift that is meant to be given, and people copy their discs for at least one library and five students. Some of the collaborators have moved well beyond this. For example, every medical school in Brazil, Cuba, and Pakistan has access to the lectures on the CD. The CDs have been distributed to all libraries in the Eastern Mediterranean region of the WHO and are widely distributed across the former Soviet Union.

We must harness the power of the new communication systems to deliver global health research knowledge to scientists around the world. Information sharing through the Internet now is cheap and very effective. The best possible lectures must be delivered to the teachers of the world. With improved information distribution mechanisms like the supercourse, there will be a profoundly beneficial effect on global health.

SUMMARY

1. An important missing piece of the prevention-treatment puzzle had been the strategic use of health communication and marketing tools that can empower communities with the knowledge and motivation to improve their environment and wellness, and in return, their social and economic potential and sustainability.

2. Social marketing seeks to influence social behaviors, not to benefit the marketer, but to benefit the target audience and the general society. Social marketers place a high value on conducting market research to "listen" and determine the needs, wants, and perceptions of the "customer."

3. Other marketing elements used are environment analysis, differential advantage, audience segmentation, and sustainability.

4. Based on marketing principles but dealing with more complex issues involving behavioral change, social marketing applies the traditionally commercial concepts of the "four P's" of product, price, place, and promotion, and adds a fifth, positioning.

5. Surveys can be delivered through telephone interviews; personal in-depth interviews; focus groups; and mail, PDA, and web-based communications. Depending on their structure and the skill of the researcher, surveys can yield much information about an individual's knowledge, attitudes, and practices related to health.

6. Radio, because of its low-cost accessibility and lower literacy demands, has great potential for reaching populations in developing countries with consistent health stories and messages.

7. Research has shown edutainment, the practice of using mass entertainment to deliver public health messages, raises awareness of issues and motivates action and behavior change.

8. Media, particularly in developing countries, plays an important part in getting accurate information about serious diseases and problems to the public. Many people and policymakers form their views of diseases and conditions based on how they are presented via the media.

9. A key strategy in some community-based health communications programs is the use of "behavioral journalism," in which you identify people from the community who have made the desired behavioral change and who can be featured as role models in the media materials and outreach.

10. Mobile camera phones are transforming the way news coverage happens, both in its immediacy and in the increased involvement of "citizen journalists." Camera phones with video allow the public to contribute to telling the story and getting the facts out, improve communications during natural disasters, and give eyewitness accounts to the world about atrocities and injustice.

11. A boon for conducting business, the accessibility and relative affordability of the mobile phone has provided families and communities, particularly in developing regions, with a sense of security and connectedness to health services that was not available before.

12. In order to make it relevant to the media's focus on economic issues, global health communicators should connect the impact of disease, and issues like environmental disruption, to the economic effects.

13. In order to be successful, health communications programs should include community-based cultural brokers and health promoters, and empower the community to help shape, implement, evaluate, and sustain the program.

14. One of the greatest challenges following disasters is filling the huge void of communications created when communities and physical spaces are ripped apart.

15. Emerging communication technologies such as "green" wi-fi networks, solar-powered microfilm projectors containing an entire library of learning, and inexpensive laptops with crank handles for power can help make knowledge and communication more accessible for all.

STUDY QUESTIONS

1. You are a public health researcher and you've agreed to help lead a research and education team from the United States to Darfur to examine how refugees are receiving and understanding their health information. What barriers might you run into while pursuing this work?

2. Social marketing applies marketing principles and methods in order to motivate an individual or group to change behavior. Describe how the five P's would take shape in a campaign centered on motivating seniors to exercise regularly.

3. In the case study involving the Hopi, how would you go about ensuring consistent coverage of the campaign by local and regional media, and what challenges might you confront?

4. You are a journalist with an NGO that specializes in humanitarian reporting. You are the first reporter from your agency to arrive at the scene of an earthquake in Ecuador. The media infrastructure has been destroyed, with minimal personnel and equipment left. Thousands of survivors need information immediately. Describe some of the community-based

health communication approaches and the technologies and media mentioned in this chapter you would use to get accurate information out, and help improve conditions.

5. What is the main strength of the Global Health Network Supercourse project? List two to three problems associated with the translation of information from labs to classrooms.

REFERENCES

1. Maslow, A. *Motivation and Personality*. Psychology Rev 1943; 50(4): 370–396.

2. *Theory at a Glance: A Guide for Health Promotion, Second Edition*. Bethesda, MD: National Cancer Institute, US Department of Health and Human Services, 2005.

3. *Salud Para Su Corazon, Bringing Heart Health to Latinos: A Guide for Building Community Programs*. National Heart, Lung and Blood Institute of the National Institutes of Health, December 1998.

4. Melgar-Quinonez, Hugo, Assistant Professor, Ohio State University Department of Human Nutrition, interview by Gary Snyder, May 24, 2005.

5. Snyder, G. "Knowledge, Attitudes and Practices of Central Ohio Immigrant Latinos Concerning Health and Media Use." MS thesis, Ohio University, 2007.

6. National Cancer Institute. *Making Health Communication Programs Work*. August 2004. NIH Publication No. 04-5145. http://www.nci.nih.gov/pinkbook/

7. McGuire, WJ. Public Communication as a Strategy for Inducing Health-Promoting Behavioral Change. *Pre Med* 1984;13(3): 299–313.

8. *HIV/AIDS Reporting Manual*. Kaiser Family Foundation. http://www.globalhealthreporting.org/reporting.asp?id=18.

9. Andreasen, A. *Marketing Social Change: Changing Behavior to Promote Health, Social Development, and the Environment*. San Francisco: Jossey-Bass, 1995.

10. Alcalay, R, Bell RA. *Promoting Nutrition and Physical Activity Through Social Marketing: Current Practices and Recommendations*. Davis, CA: Center for Advanced Studies in Nutrition and Social Marketing, University of California, 2000.

11. National Cancer Institute. *Making Health Communication Programs Work*. August 2004. NIH Publication No. 04-5145. http://www.nci.nih.gov/pinkbook/.

12. Berkowitz, E. *Essentials of Health Care Marketing*. Sudbury, MA: Jones and Bartlett, 2006.

13. Encarnacion-Garcia, H. "Promotoras de Salud: A Culturally-Sensitive Community Intervention Model for Cancer Prevention Among Hispanic/Latino women." Ph.D. diss., Indiana University, 2004.

14. National Center for Cultural Competence, Georgetown University Medical Center. Bridging the Cultural Divide in Health Care Settings: The Essential Role of Cultural Broker Programs. Spring/Summer 2004. Bi-lingual versions available online at http://www.culturalbroker.info/.

15. Andaló, P. "Love, Tears, Betrayal . . . and Health Messages." *Perspectives in Health Magazine, The Magazine of the Pan American Health Organization* 2003; Vol 8, No 2.

16. UK Department for International Development. "Tell Me a Story." 2005. *Developments*. http://developments.org.uk/data/issue32/tell-story.htm.

17. Cheskin Marketing. *The Digital World of the US Hispanic II*. Redwood Shores, CA: Cheskin, 2001.

18. Zone Latina. http://www.zonalatina.com/Radio.htm.

19. Korzenny, F, Korzenny BA. *Hispanic Marketing*. Burlington, MA: Elsevier, Butterworth-Heinemann, 2005.

20. http://www.unaids.org/en/MediaCentre/PressMaterials/FeatureStory/20060424-india.asp.

21. Beck V, Huang GC, Pollard WE, et al. Telenovela viewers and health information. Paper presented at: American Public Health Association 131st Annual Meeting and Exposition, San Francisco, CA, 2003.

22. Hollywood, Health & Society Project. University of Southern California. http://www.learcenter.org/html/projects/?cm=hhs.

23. Internetworldstats.com, January 2007.

24. Global System for Mobile Communication (GSM) Association. www.gsmworld.com.

25. Sullivan, K. In War-Torn Congo, Going Wireless to Reach Home. *The Washington Post* July 9, 2006. p. A01.

26. UK Department for International Development. *Money Talks*. 2005. *Developments*. http://www.developments.org.uk/data/issue31/money-talks.htm.

27. UK Department for International Development. *What on Earth Is Happening?* 2005. *Developments*.

28. Hightower, A. Using a PDA with GPS to choose a sample and conduct a survey. Presentation at the Multilateral Initiative on Malaria, Yaounde, Cameroon. 2005. US Centers for Disease Control and Prevention, Division of Parasitic Diseases.

29. LaPorte RE, Sekikawa A, Sa ER, et al. Whisking research into the classroom {infopoints}. *BMJ* 2002;324:99.

Economics and Global Health

14

Kevin Chan

LEARNING OBJECTIVES

- *Understand the dual relationship between economics and health: how poverty can affect health and how health problems can result in poverty.*
- *Comprehend the possible linkages between wealth and health and how both absolute and relative wealth have an impact on health.*
- *Describe four key mechanisms by which health can affect wealth.*
- *Show the interrelationships between health and economics looking at three key diseases (Malaria, TB, and HIV/AIDS).*
- *Outline and describe four key factors in choosing the type of health care financing system.*
- *Outline and describe five major financing methods for health care.*
- *Describe and define risk pooling, risk aversion, adverse selection, and moral hazard.*

INTRODUCTION TO ECONOMICS AND HEALTH

Peter Chirwa is a 4 year-old boy in Northern Malawi. His family grows their food on their farm to provide subsistence for the year. When harvests are good, he and his five brothers and sisters eat well throughout the year, but when the harvests are bad, as they have been over the past three years, his brothers and sisters become malnourished and sick. Over the past year, two younger siblings died from malnutrition and pneumonia. Unfortunately, Peter's family is poor and cannot afford to buy food in the market. His family survives on less than 50 cents per person per day, far below the global absolute poverty line of $1.

Peter's uncle lives five houses down. Gaunt and thin and dying from HIV/AIDS, he gazes from his bed to his visitors. He has spent all his money trying to buy the life-saving drugs, but can no longer afford the prices. He will probably die in a few months. His family sits by the bedside caring for him, knowing that their future holds nothing but utter destitution. Just down the road, the devastation from poor health can impoverish families and leave them with no income, opportunity, or hope.

For a long time, it has been recognized that there is a relationship between health and wealth.[1] Three possible different pathways may explain this relationship:

1. Increased wealth leads to health.
2. Improved health leads to wealth.
3. The relationship is caused by a third unknown factor.[2]

Rising incomes increase government and private spending on goods that directly (e.g., purchasing health care and better nutrition) and indirectly (e.g., better housing, water, and sanitation facilities) improve health.[3] (See Figure 14-1.)

In the past decade, there has been increasing recognition that poor health can lead to poverty.[4] These interrelationships are linked with political, demographic, and social pressures.

The first part of this chapter analyzes the growing evidence between "wealthier is healthier"[5] and the counterclaim "healthier is wealthier."[4]

The second part of this chapter focuses on the evidence that the relationship between health systems through their organization, financing, and behavior has an impact on health and economic outcomes. How health systems are financed influences the behaviors of consumers, producers, and intermediaries. It is important to understand how these structures are created, which may in turn, have significant impacts on health and economic outcomes.

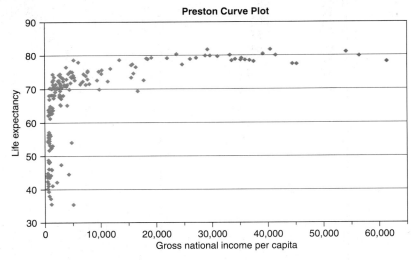

Figure 14-1. Health to wealth correlations. The figures provided are for the year 2004 or the latest year for 179 countries. From World Development Indicators 2006.[67]

THE MECHANISMS FROM WEALTH TO HEALTH

In general, wealthier nations are healthier nations. Higher incomes provide the ability to purchase many of the goods and services that promote better health, including more calories and higher quality food products, access to cleaner water, safe sanitation, and higher quality and more complete health services both at a societal and individual level. Furthermore, more wealth can lead to better education and training.

Preston[1] noted a strong relationship between health and wealth, and suggested that there is a significant gain in health (as measured by life expectancy) with wealth up to $1000 per capita. However, Preston noted that after exceeding $1000 per capita, additional wealth did not lead to significant increases in life expectancy. His classic paper found that between 1940 and 1970, half of the rise in life expectancy was due to improvements in the level of income.

Furthermore, Pritchett and Summers[5] in their paper "Wealthier is Healthier" found that 40 percent of cross-country differences in mortality can be explained by differences in income growth rates. They estimated a 1 percent increase in world income would lead to a reduction of 33,000 infant and 55,000 child deaths.

On a country-wide basis at the microeconomic level, Case[6] examined the impact of a sudden increase in income from South African old age pensions on household wealth. She found that the income protected all household members when the old age pension was put into the overall family income, but when the old age pension was not put into the family income pot, the income only benefited the individual pensioners.

She outlined possible reasons for this advantage to be seen in pooled family incomes, including the ability to purchase more help, better sanitation, improved nutrition, and decreased household psychological stress.

Just as important a finding is that income inequality may lead to poor health. In the Whitehall Study of 10,000 British civil servants, age-adjusted mortality rates were 3.5 times higher for lower grade workers compared to senior administrators.[7–9] This suggests that income differentiation of wealth can make a major impact on country-wide health outcomes. A number of other studies support this finding. Wilkinson[10] in his study of the Organisation for Economic Co-operation and Development (OECD) countries, a group of the wealthiest countries in the world, showed that while greater absolute incomes lead to higher life expectancy, greater inequality had a negative impact on average life expectancy. This relative income inequality holds at the individual level, suggesting that people who make lower levels than their peers have a worse health outcome.[11,12]

Wealth can also increase health via indirect mechanisms like education. The World Development Report in 1993, *Investing in Health*, stated that one of the most effective ways to improve health is to provide primary education to young girls.[13]

THE MECHANISMS FROM HEALTH TO WEALTH

There are four major mechanisms to link health to increased wealth.[14] These four mechanisms are improved productivity, more investment in education (human capital), more investment in physical capital, and utilizing the demographic dividend.

The Role of Health in Impacting Productivity

Healthier individuals are more likely to be productive, since they are more energetic and less likely to miss work due to illness. Furthermore, healthier families need less time off work to care for ill individuals.

A difficulty in looking at health impacts and its role in affecting productivity is the need to separate out the fixed genetic and socially acquired human capital components to health.[15] There is very little to do to change our genetic make-up, leaving us to concentrate on behavioral aspects to improve our health capital.

Strauss[16] believed productivity of labor increased when individuals received more calories. Since increased labor productivity may have had a reverse effect in leading to more food consumption, he used community variation in the price of food as a control variable. A number of subsequent articles have confirmed that nutrition does increase labor productivity.[17–19] Strauss and Thomas[20] in a later work showed that these effects tended to diminish as the daily intake reached approximately 2000 kcal.

Thomas and Strauss[21] highlight two key conceptual links from health to productivity relevant to developing countries. First, the impact of predominantly communicable diseases in developing countries affects individuals throughout their lifetimes, while non-communicable diseases in more developed countries predominantly affect the elderly. Second, since developing countries tend to be labor-intensive, poor health reduces income disproportionately since a higher percentage of the work force is employed in labor-intensive industries.[22] Bhargava, Jamison, Lau and Murray et al.[23] confirmed that higher adult survival rates lead to higher growth rates of income in low-income groups.

Schultz, in a series of papers, looked at the direct impact of health on wages.[15,24,25] He found that "an increase in BMI of one unit was associated with a 9 percent increase in wages for men in Ghana and Cote d'Ivoire, and a percent increase in wages for women in Ghana and a 15 percent increase in Cote d'Ivoire."[15] Similarly, a one centimeter gain in height was associated with a 5 percent increase in wages in Brazil in men, and a 7 percent increase in women.[15] Bloom, Canning, and Sevilla[22] showed that a one-year increase in life expectancy at birth results in a four percent increase in economic output. In summary, better health does lead directly to better wages and overall, macroeconomic output.

When looking at the American South at the beginning of the 20th century, Bleakley[26] found that the eradication of hookworm led to an improvement in wages by 45 percent, and half the wage gap difference between the American North and American South was due to disease factors.

A number of economic studies[27–29] have shown that longer life expectancy and lower rates of mortality led to higher incomes and better economic performance.

Similarly, much work has been done to look at the role of maternal health and nutrition as important determinants of future chronic health problems in children, otherwise known as the "Barker hypothesis."[30,31] Poor health doesn't just have productivity effects in the short term; it may have inter-generational effects that contribute to a country's long-standing poor labor productivity.

Increased Investment in Human Capital

Poor health conditions decrease life expectancy and reduce the amount of human capital investment because individuals have shorter time horizons to regain the costs of the human capital investment. Furthermore, health may directly decrease human capital investments, since children may be sick or have less energy to go to school.

Health plays a fundamental role in developing learning capacity. Damages occur in two specific phases:

1. **In utero:** During the time the child is inside the mother's womb, a number of prenatal insults can occur, including poor genetics, alcohol, smoking, drugs, poor nutrition, infections, and hypertension, which leads to poor brain development.

2. **Postnatal:** There are a number of problems after birth that lead to poor development, including diseases such as meningitis, diarrhea, HIV/AIDS, and pneumonia, and other problems such as head injuries, malnutrition, poor maternal education, inadequate childhood stimulation, and poverty. Any of these insults may lead to poor intellectual development.

Leslie and Jamison[32] state that three general educational issues may occur with poor health:

1. Children may not start school at the typical age.
2. Children may have poor learning capacity once school starts.
3. There may be a gross gender imbalance with a decreased number of female children participating in school.

So what implications does poor schooling have? Mincer[33] showed that an additional year of schooling appeared to increase earnings by 10 percent in the United States and suggested that increasing an average level of schooling should increase economic growth. Bloom, Canning, and Chan[34] showed increasing educational levels may significantly increase sub-Saharan African growth and help Africa escape its poverty trap. In particular, investing in higher education may have a benefit in improving overall economic growth of Africa.

Therefore, poor health may lead to an underinvestment in health capital, and subsequently have a large effect on wages and overall economic development.

Increased Investment in Physical Capital

Like human capital, short life expectancy will reduce the amount of investment in physical capital because of the reduction in time to recuperate investment costs. However, a consequential advantage of longer life is that individuals need to save for retirement, and hence increase the investment in physical capital with the hope of future return.

Disease has a disproportionate effect on poor, rural households. As stated above, there may be a significant reduction in individual productivity. Second, there may be spending to prevent, diagnose, and treat the disease. Third, Nur[35] showed that malaria decreases household savings, as families increasingly spend money to hire labor to compensate for productivity losses from individuals infected with malaria. Therefore, there is less money available to invest in physical capital.

Even the threat of ill health may have an enormous impact. For example, SARS was estimated to cost the city of Toronto $1.5 billion in lost tourism and investment in the city, even though it led to only 44 deaths.[36]

Capturing the Benefits from the Demographic Dividend

The final mechanism for how health improvements could affect economic growth is through the "demographic dividend." The theory is that health improvements trigger a decline in mortality rates, followed by a decline in fertility rates years later. This leads to a large population bulge. This group eventually proceeds through productive working years and produces a large working-age population relative to the young and old-age dependent population. This large working-age to dependent-age population ratio gives a window of opportunity for economic growth, but does not guarantee it. It requires appropriate country-wide conditions (stable politics, good macroeconomic policies, openness to trade, and good health status) to maximize the gains.

Bloom and Williamson[28] suggest one-third to one-half of the East Asian miracle from 1965 to 1990 can be explained by the demographic dividend. Similarly, Bloom and Canning[37] highlight the importance of contraception in reducing fertility and triggering a demographic dividend, leading to the Irish economic boom in the 1980s and 1990s.

ECONOMIC IMPACTS OF THREE KEY DISEASES

Malaria, Tuberculosis and HIV/AIDS are examples of diseases that have the most economic impacts on populations.

Malaria

Each year, 300 to 500 million new cases of malaria occur. This disease kills between 1 to 3 million people a year, mostly children and pregnant women.[38,39] As Gallup and Sachs[40] reveal, countries where a high proportion of the population lived in regions of *Plasmodium falciparum* malaria transmission had annual growth rates 1.3 percent lower than other countries from 1965 to 1990, even after controlling for other standard growth determinants. They conclude that this effect cumulated over time and would reduce the GNP level to half the amount of a nonmalarious country. In subsaharan Africa, malaria does not seem to have a significant class difference.[41]

There are various ways by which malaria could reduce economic productivity. First, there are the private and public medical costs to preventing, diagnosing, and treating malaria. Second, there are the costs due to lost days at work and for taking care of family members who are ill with malaria. Third, malaria has a longer-term consequence, because it can lead to forgone earnings from premature death, decreased labor productivity, and in school-age children, reduced performance in school.[42,43] Sachs and Malaney[38] highlight that, more importantly, malaria can cause significant social costs on school, demography, migration, and savings. Furthermore, the macroeconomic effects may extend to trade, tourism and foreign direct investment.

Historically, there has been a significant reduction in trade between malaria and nonmalaria zones. For example, in the 1950s, when the countries of southern Europe such as Greece, Portugal, and Spain began to eradicate malaria, foreign direct investment from Northern Europe increased rapidly to spur economic growth.[40] Therefore, control of malaria has historically been associated with economic well-being.

Tuberculosis

Tuberculosis infects nine million people and causes two million deaths per year.[44] Over 95 percent of cases occur in developing countries.[45] Tuberculosis predominantly affects working-age populations between the ages of 15 to 54.[46] On average, three to four months of work is lost (resulting in a 20–30 percent loss of annual household income).[47] There is also a significant loss of income if a TB sufferer dies, equivalent to 15 years loss of income over a lifetime.[47]

Without a proper course of treatment, approximately 50–60 percent of those infected will die.[46] Yet, with proper treatment, the life expectancy of an otherwise healthy person would increase by an average of 25–30 years.[48]

Tuberculosis and poverty are inter-linked. Crowded conditions more likely allow the spread of tuberculosis. Yet, tuberculosis can also lead to poverty. The presence of tuberculosis may lead to a significant sale of assets to pay for drugs, reducing food intake in

---

BOX 14-1. TUBERCULOSIS IN RUSSIA

In 1990, when Boris Yeltsin stepped to the top of a tank and declared the fall of the Soviet Union, little did he expect that the opening of the Russian markets would lead to a sudden fall in the ability to control tuberculosis in the country. Why did this occur? What were the steps that led to a sudden rise of tuberculosis and the rise of multidrug resistant tuberculosis?

According to the World Health Organization,[50] the TB incidence in 2002 was 126 new cases per 100,000 population. This rate reflects a significant increase over the 1990 rates of 34 new cases per 100,000 population.[51]

One of the reasons for this sudden increase is that the economic downfall led to significant reductions in spending in social support and health structures (especially public health surveillance and treatment). The result was that infectious diseases could spread rapidly unchecked. One area where this rapid rise occurred most rapidly was within the prison system, which remains overcrowded, and many cases remain untreated.

To attempt to address these shortfalls, Russian officials have increased the training and expertise of health practitioners to implement the widely recognized Directly-Observed Treatment Short course (DOTS). There has been an increasing emphasis on multidrug resistant tuberculosis (MDRTB) treatment and management, including educating and training staff to diagnose and treat MDRTB in prison inmates.

Tuberculosis in Russia shows the importance of economic disintegration and its impact on the social and health networks that can allow disease outbreaks to occur.

---

children due to poverty, and decreasing educational opportunities. Therefore, tuberculosis is a classical example of the poverty and poor health dyad.[49]

HIV/AIDS

HIV/AIDS affects 38.6 million people, with 4.1 million new cases every year and 2.8 million deaths.[52] HIV/AIDS has a large impact on development, since it targets people in prime working ages, accounting for approximately 65 percent of deaths.[53] Studies suggest that HIV/AIDS preferentially affects urban high-income, skilled men and their partners.[54]

Ainsworth and Over[54] list four key reasons why HIV/AIDS is different from other infectious diseases:

1. HIV/AIDS has no cure.
2. HIV/AIDS affects working-age individuals, mostly through heterosexual intercourse.
3. HIV/AIDS decimates social fabrics of care for the young and old and slows down macroeconomic growth.
4. HIV/AIDS has not spared the economic and intellectual elites.

Bloom, Bloom, Steven, and Weston.[55] highlight that HIV/AIDS has reduced the capacity to invest in human capital, which in turn leads to a further inability to identify and treat HIV/AIDS. This reduced capacity leads to a downward "death spiral," resulting in the inability to deal with the consequences of the HIV/AIDS epidemic.

HIV/AIDS has a large impact in sub-Saharan African development. As explained above, HIV/AIDS decreases the working age to dependent age ratios leading to a higher dependency ratio on a smaller work force. Furthermore, with an increasing loss of parents and an increase in HIV/AIDS orphans, there is a disproportionate burden on women and working-age populations to support the orphans. HIV/AIDS and related disease spending is one-third of total health care costs, and over one-half of total public health spending in many countries.[53]

There is evidence that HIV/AIDS is directly affecting companies. Aventin and Huard[56] examined three companies in Côte d'Ivoire and found that a 10 percent increase in the prevalence of HIV/AIDS results in an increase in cost of 6.8 to 10.0 percent. These effects can also be seen at a countrywide level. Arndt and Lewis,[57,58] Bonnel,[59] and ING Barings[60] all report that by 2010, South African gross domestic product (GDP) per capita will decrease by approximately 8 percent due to HIV/AIDS.

HIV/AIDS remains one of the great global health challenges, not just because of the enormous health implications around the world, but also due to its ability to stem economic development. Finding solutions to deliver services, drugs, and prevent disease remain paramount in this struggle.

THE IMPACT OF HEALTH CARE ON THE ECONOMY

One of the largest budgetary items in any government is health care spending. Health care spending accounts for 8 percent of global GDP,[61] but rises to as much as 16 percent of GDP in the United States.[62] In this section, we concentrate on the importance of financing health care and describe the payment systems that help distribute this financing.

FINANCING HEALTH CARE

Every finance and health minister must decide how to finance their country's health care system. Five major methods are used:

- General revenue
- Social insurance
- Community insurance
- Private insurance
- Direct purchaser payment

Most countries use a combination of these different methods. How do we decide which methods to use?

Four key factors determine each country's capacity to successfully finance health:

1. Financial resources
2. Stage of economic development
3. Ability to administer financial services
4. Political will and structure[63]

Financial Resources

The ability to generate revenues may determine a government's ability to use certain methods to finance health care. For example, in many developing countries, *general taxation* may not be feasible when over half the population works in the informal sector and weak enforcement mechanisms are in place. Health care is also just one of many competing departments in the general budget. There may be more emphasis on defense, infrastructure building, and education.

Social insurance requires an administrative structure that allows for the capture of contributions from companies. Often, very small businesses find it difficult to separate out personal profits from wage earnings. In theory, social insurance should be based only on wage earnings, but this is extremely difficult to delineate.

If there is significant social structure and well-being, a social insurance scheme should have a broad reach.

Community insurance refers to the pooling of risks to provide basic health services for a community. This often requires good social co-operation, and tends to be geared toward poorer segments of the population.

Private insurance can occur when people with enough income want to buy more health care services and/or higher quality services. This often leads to two-tiering of the health care system between those that have private insurance that cover more services and those that do not.

Direct purchaser payment systems (user fees and out-of-pocket payment) are used in many developing countries in the world that include payments for drugs, supplies, and services provided when a patient becomes ill or sick. Thus, because the payments tend to be acute in nature, they tend to be higher and may directly cause poverty.

Stage of Economic Development

The stage of economic development is an important factor in determining which financing method to use. Depending on a country's economic well-being, individuals may be able to pay more for health care, and likewise, the country is likely to face increased demand for health care. In general, as income increases per capita, there is an increase in spending per capita on health, especially within the public sector (see Table 14-1).

The implication of a lower level of spending in developing countries is that there is less health capital (beds, hospitals, clinics), service providers (physicians, nurses, and allied professionals), and hospital visits (both inpatient and outpatient). There is also concern that lower income countries have less "fair" access to health care. One of the arguments to improve economic development is that increased wealth can directly lead to better health care systems.

Table 14-1. Health expenditures by income group and region (2002).[a]

Income Group	Total Health Expenditure as % of GNP	Total Expenditures (Across Countries in Group)	Public Sector (% of GDP)	Private Sector (% of GDP)
World	10.2	588	5.9	4.3
Low-income	4.6	30	1.3	3.3
Middle-income	6.0	116	2.5	3.5
High-income	11.2	3449	6.7	4.5
East Asia and Pacific	5.0	64	1.9	3.1
Europe and Central Asia	6.5	194	4.5	2.0
Latin America and Carribean	6.8	222	3.3	3.5
Middle East and North Africa	5.6	92	2.7	2.9
South Asia	4.4	24	1.1	3.3
Sub-Saharan Africa	6.1	36	2.4	3.7

[a] From World Bank. World Development Indicators 2006. Table 2.14.[67]

Ability to Administer Financial Services

One of the challenges governments face is the ability to administer health services. Medical records must be kept, financial tracking and auditing established, and other administrative services developed. These services are dependent on a country or locale's ability to set up and monitor the system, and effectively enforce health care regulation and legislation.

For example, many developing countries may not have the human resources and tracking systems to enforce tax collection. Furthermore, it may be extremely difficult to capture revenues from informal sector employment. These challenges lessen the number of formal workers increased from economic development. However, without these revenues, it may be difficult to develop a strong social insurance or general taxation method to finance health care.

In other countries there may be difficulties in gaining public acceptance of tax collection because of concerns over government corruption and concerns over service delivery. These challenges require a strong trusted monitoring system to ensure transparency of the financial structure and ensure services are provided.

Political Will and Structure

Another consideration is the importance of health care inside the government structure. Competing interests with other sectors such as defense may lead to different priorities. Often, health may be a primary interest (e.g., in Cuba and Canada), but in other countries, health care may take a far less important role (e.g., many developing countries). How government structures health care financing may help determine its priority and importance versus other segments of government.

FINANCING SYSTEMS

We will now examine the major financing systems in use around the world today. However, first we must look at some basic definitions in financing health care.

RISK POOLING

Risk pooling refers to grouping a large number of people together to decrease the variance in health outcomes on an individual basis, and thereby, spreading the financial risk of an adverse event. A health insurance company can help spread an individual's risk by grouping them with people at a similar risk level and spreading the costs between them. For example, if someone has a 1 in 100 chance of getting an illness, and it costs $5000 to treat it, 100 individuals may be willing to put $50 into a joint pool to cope with this illness. Furthermore, this spreading of risk allows for greater precision at the individual level about the possibilities of financial loss.

RISK AVERSION

Another aspect that favors the development of health insurance is that in general, people prefer certainty over uncertainty. Thus, people would rather know that they're paying a small amount every month than one giant lump sum of money when they get ill. *Risk aversion* is an important concept, because it leads to more equivalent payments for health services, rather than lump sum payments when adverse events occur.

ADVERSE SELECTION

Adverse selection refers to the practice of insurers choosing healthier people over sick people for the same insurance since this minimizes the expected costs to be paid. Conversely, sick individuals prefer to purchase insurance over healthier individuals at the same cost.

MORAL HAZARD

Moral hazard is one of the barriers to the implementation of health care insurance. Moral hazard occurs when individuals utilize services more frequently than they would normally, because they have an insurance policy in place.

Direct Purchaser Payment (User Fees, Fee for Service, Out-of Pocket Payments)

The most basic system relied upon to finance health care is to pay directly out of pocket for health care services. These financial systems dominate developing countries. An alternative to this model is the concept of the user fee. This refers to cost sharing, cost-recovery, or co-payment, and has been widely used since the Bamako Initiative in 1987.

The Bamako Initiative was an attempt to decentralize health care to the district level, create an essential drug policy, and provide these drugs to communities.[64] The financing mechanism behind the Bamako Initiative was supposed to be a combination of central government, regional governments, local governments, and individual patients. In theory, user fees were created to aid the development of health services and not to replace government funding. The hope was that there would be a combination of different financing mechanisms, including social insurance, fee for service, and out-of-pocket payment, for drugs, which would lead to a sustainable structure. However, from the Bamako Initiative, governments focused mostly on fee-for-service payment schemes.

In the early 1980s, the World Bank was a major proponent of user fees for health services. They saw it as a major mechanism to finance health care. A significant concern with the implementation of user fees is that they disproportionately affect the poor, who are often reluctant to utilize health care services until they are extremely sick. Yet, there is significant concern that the abolishment of user fees may adversely affect primary health care services, by taking away much needed basic financing for these services.

A recent World Bank publication reverses the position on user fees.[65] In contrast, it focuses on three major ideas: protecting the economic abilities of the poor, building sustainable health care services, and allocating resources more efficiently.

Community Insurance

Finance systems may lead to some collective attempts to pool resources to decrease individual risk. Community insurance is a prepayment scheme that focuses at the community level. Community health insurance may be a village or a group of villages or an employee group that negotiates with suppliers of health care services for discounted health services. In the majority of community health insurance services, primary care is integrated, while secondary and tertiary services are separated.

The advantage of community financing is that in negotiating with health care suppliers, there is a higher incentive for doctors to attend regularly and provide higher quality service. Furthermore, it bypasses the concern of government regulation and corruption in other prepayment schemes. Community financing raises money at the local level, and in turn, the community has clear control of the movement of funds.

Community health care services in many developing countries are comprised of a basic primary health care service provision and contracts with secondary and tertiary institutions for catastrophic health events. There is compulsory membership by all members in the community. A portion of funds are often re-invested in income-generating activities (microfinance) to further encourage investment within the community.

A major disadvantage of community financing is that it requires significant community buy-in, or adverse selection will occur. Furthermore, there are concerns over moral hazard. The financing is also extremely tenuous, especially during financial downturns, when many rural farmers lose their main sources of income. Hence, there needs to be strong community ties and agreements to sustain community health insurance.

Social Insurance

Social insurance is an extension of community health insurance. Social insurance refers to prospectively collecting funds in advance to purchase health care in the future. The first social health insurance program, an amalgamation of many community health insurance schemes, began in 1883 in Germany. Today, the two most common ways to raise funds is either through employers or through the government.

There are three main properties of social insurance. First, insurance must be compulsory. Otherwise adverse selection will play a role and only the sickest will buy insurance. Second, social insurance requires a social compact. There are expectations that individuals will pay and the funds will be used fairly by those within the social insurance scheme. Third, funds are raised and targeted specifically to finance the social health insurance system. In some countries such as France, social insurance is compulsory for all citizens, while in other countries, social insurance is provided only for people in the formal work sector.

Social health insurance funds often have their own health care networks. Often a network of providers negotiates with a social health insurance organization, and draws up a specified list of health care provisions that will be provided.

Countries that have adopted social insurance programs include countries in Europe (France, Netherlands, and Hungary), Latin America (Mexico, Argentina, and Brazil), and East Asia (South Korea, Taiwan, and the Philippines).

Social health insurance schemes increase the pool of resources and funds. This, in turn, because of its negotiation power, leads to a more responsive system. Second, social health insurance systems are easily implemented if formal sector workers can be identified.

There are a number of disadvantages to the social health insurance system. First, it helps finance only those enrolled in the social health insurance system, which are usually formal worker employees. It does not make provisions for the poor and the most vulnerable groups. Second, the cost of social insurance is shifted from employer to employee in the form of lower wages.[66] Third, if there are competing social health insurance systems, they compete to get the healthiest individuals. Fourth, there needs to be an ability to collect the tax revenues and to administrate the financial and health care systems.

General Taxation

In many countries, general taxes may support health care. In general, as countries become wealthier and the government is more able to collect taxes, an increasing amount of health spending is financed through general taxes. Various types of taxes may pay for health care including income taxes, sales and value-added taxes, import taxes, and corporate taxes. In general, revenues for health increase if the economy grows. However, at the same time, health care suffers if there is sudden economic downturn.

The major advantage of general taxation is that there is a strong source of steady revenue. Furthermore, general taxation is politically controllable and it requires a large degree of financial accountability. Depending on the type of taxation used, it may be progressive and improve equity, and it can pool health risks across an entire population. Certain services, such as immunization and public health surveillance, are almost always best covered by general taxation.

Health care faces competition for general tax revenue from other sources of interest including defense, infrastructure development, industry, and education. A major concern with general taxation is that it requires a strong administrative infrastructure and transparency, especially to collect taxes. There is always some concern of favoritism toward certain groups; for example, spending may favor larger urban centers over rural areas.

Private Insurance

Private insurance refers to purchasing insurance on a voluntary basis from individual competitive sellers. A key difference is that the premiums charged are based on a purchaser's risk rather than their ability to pay. One of the clear advantages of private insurance is that it clearly defines the preferences for different levels of services at different income levels. Therefore, private insurance acts as a spur to medical technological advancement. There is also an argument that private insurance empowers individuals to act in their best health interests.

Private insurance is becoming increasingly prevalent in wealthier countries without strong generalized taxation schemes. One of the ways corporations build loyalty in these countries is by providing health insurance as an additional perk for employees. Therefore, companies purchase insurance on behalf of their employees.

Historically, private health insurance is often characterized by the culprit of adverse selection. Insurers prefer to take people who are healthiest, and those that tend to be sickest prefer to get the best insurance possible. A second problem is the poor and the sick tend to find it very difficult to purchase health insurance. The third issue is that there are often high administrative and marketing costs that add to the cost of the health care insurance.

The best example of a private health insurance market is the United States, which has the highest cost of care in the world and almost 45 million uninsured individuals.

SUMMARY

- Health and wealth flow bi-directionally. More wealth can buy better health care services and goods that can improve health. Conversely, better health can lead to more wealth through four key mechanisms: productivity, education, investment in physical capital, and impacts on the demographic dividend.
- Both low income levels and large income disparities can adversely affect overall population health.
- Health care spending is a large part of government spending.

- Four key prioritization methods exist in determining how to finance health care: financial resources, stage of economic development, the ability to administrate financial services, and the political will and structure.
- Key basic concepts in financing health care include risk pooling, risk aversion, adverse selection, and moral hazard.
- Five financing systems include direct purchaser payment, community insurance, social insurance, general taxation, and private insurance.

STUDY QUESTIONS

1. You are a minister of health in a developing country. You would like to improve the health care status of people in your country. What financing system exists now? What type of financing system would you like? Justify why you think this financing system would improve your health care. What criticism could you have from the finance minister and other members of the cabinet?

2. You are the minister of health in China. Explain how avian influenza may affect your economic systems, and what impacts it could have on overall development.

3. "Money, money, money" are the three things needed for better health. Do you agree with this statement? Why or why not?

ACKNOWLEDGEMENTS

The author acknowledges the constructive comments of David Bloom, Rosemary Marotta, and Larry Rosenberg.

REFERENCES

1. Preston SA. Causes and consequences of mortality decline in less developed countries during the Twentieth Century. In: Easterlin RA, ed. *Population and economic change in developing countries.* Chicago: University of Chicago Press, 1980:289–360.

2. Fuchs VR. Time Preference and Health: An Exploratory Study. In: Fuchs VR, ed. *Economic Aspects of Health.* Chicago: University of Chicago Press, 1982:93–120.

3. Fogel RW. Economic growth, population theory and physiology. *American Economic Review.* 1994;84(3):369–395.

4. Wagstaff A. Poverty and Health. Commission on Macroeconomics and Health Working Paper Series. Paper No. WG1: 5. March 2001. www2.cid.harvard.edu/cidcmh/wg1_paper5.pdf. Last accessed: September 21, 2006.

5. Pritchett L, Summers LH. Wealthier is Healthier. *The Journal of Human Resources.* 1996;31(4):841–868.

6. Case A. Does Money Protect Health Status? Evidence from South African Pensions.Princeton University and the NBER, 2001;1–30.

7. Wilkinson RG, ed. *Class and health: Research and Longitudinal data.* New York: Tavistock Publications, 1986.

8. Marmot MG, Theorell T. Social class and cardiovascular disease: The contribution of work. *International Journal of Health Services.* 1988;18(4):659–674.

9. Marmot MG, Smith GD, Stansfeld S, et al. Health inequalities among British civil servants: the Whitehall II study. *Lancet* 1991;337:1387–1393.

10. Wilkinson RG. Income distribution and mortality—a natural experiment. *Health and Illness.* 1990;12:391–412.

11. Deaton A. Inequalities in income and inequalities in health. National Bureau of Economic Research Working Paper Series No. 7141. 1999;1–37.

12. Deaton A, Paxson C. Mortality, education, income and inequality among American Cohorts. National Bureau of Economic Research Working Paper No. 7140. 1–49.

13. World Bank. *World Development Report 1993: Investing in Health.* Oxford: Oxford University Press, 1993.

14. Bloom DE, Canning D. The Health and Wealth of Nations. *Science* February 18, 2000;287(5456):1207–1209.

15. Schultz TP. *Productive Benefits of Improving Health: Evidence from Low-Income Countries.* 2001. (monograph)

16. Strauss J. Does better nutrition raise farm productivity? *Journal of Political Economy.* 1986;94(2):297–320.

17. Deolalikar A. Nutrition and labor productivity in agriculture. *Review of Economics and Statistics* 1988;70(3):406–413.

18. Sahn DE, Alderman H. The effect of human capital on wages, on the determinants of labor supply in a developing country. *Journal of Development Economics* 1988;29(2):157–183.

19. Foster AD, Rosenweig M. A test for moral hazard in the labor market: Effort, health and calorie consumption. *Review of Economics and Statistics* 1994;76(2):213–227.

20. Strauss J, Thomas D. Human resources: Empirical modeling of household and family decisions. In: Behrman JR and Srinivasan TN, eds. *Handbook of Development Economics.* Vol IIIA, Chap. 34. Amsterdam: North-Holland Publishing Company, 1995.

21. Thomas D, Strauss J. The micro-foundations of the links between health, nutrition and development. *Journal of Economic Literature* 1998;36:766–817.

22. Bloom DE, Canning D, Sevilla J. The effect of health on economic growth: a production function approach. *World Development.* 2004;32(1):1–13.

23. Bhargava A, Jamison DR, Lau LJ, Murray CJL. Modelling the effects of health on economic growth. Geneva: World Health Organization, Global Programme on Evidence Discussion Paper, 2000.

24. Schultz TP. Investments in the schooling and health of women and men: quantities and return. *Journal of Human Resources* 1993;28(4):694–734.

25. Schultz TP. Health and Schooling in Africa. *Journal of Economic Perspectives* 1999;13(3):67–88.

26. Bleakley H. Disease and development: evidence from the american south. *Journal of the European Economic Association* 2003;1(2–3):376–386.

27. Barro R and Lee JW. Sources of economic growth. Carnegie-Rochester Conference Series on Public Policy. 1994;40:1–46.

28. Bloom DE, Williamson JG. Demographic transitions and economic miracles in emerging Asia. *World Bank Economic Review* 1998;12(3):419–455.

29. Jamison DT, Lau LJ, Wang J. Health's contribution to economic growth, 1965–1990. In: *Health, Health Policy and Economic Outcomes. Final report of the Health and Development Satellite WHO Director.* Geneva: World Health Organization, 1998.

30. Barker DJ. Fetal and infant origins of adult disease. *British Medical Journal* 1990;301(6761):1111.

31. Fogel RW. Catching up with the Economy. *American Economic Review* 1999;89(1):1–21.

32. Leslie J, Jamison DT. Health and nutrition considerations in education planning: educational consequences of health problems among school-age children. *Food and Nutrition Bulletin* 1990;12:204–214.

33. Mincer J. *Schooling, Earning and Experience.* New York: Columbia University Press, 1974.

34. Bloom DE, Canning D, Chan KJ. *Higher Education and Economic Growth in Africa.* Washington DC: World Bank, 2006.

35. Nur E. The impact of malaria on labour use and efficiency in the Sudan. *Social Science and Medicine* 1993;37:1115–1119.

36. Conference Board of Canada. The Economic Impact of SARS. May 2003. Ottawa: Conference Board of Canada. 1–3.

37. Bloom DE, Canning D. Contraception and the Celtic Tiger. *Economic and Social Review* 2003;34:229–247.

38. Sachs JD, Malaney P. The economic and social burden of malaria. *Nature* 2002;415:680–685.

39. Breman JG, Mills A, Snow RW, et al. Conquering malaria. In: *Disease Control Priorities Project, Second Edition.* www.dcp2.org/pubs/DCP/21.

40. Gallup Jl, Sachs JD. The economic burden of malaria. CID Working Paper No. 52. Cambridge, MA: Centre for International Development, Harvard University, 2000.

41. Filmer D. *Fever and its treatment in the more and less poor in sub-Saharan Africa.* Development Research Group. Washington DC: World Bank, 2000.

42. Chima RI, Mills A. Estimating the economic impact of malaria in sub-Saharan Africa: A review of the empirical evidence. 1998. Unpublished manuscript.

43. Malaney P. *Benefits of malaria control.* Cambridge: Harvard Institute for International Development, 1998.

44. World Health Organization. *2006 Tuberculosis Facts.* Geneva: World Health Organization, 2006. http://www.stoptb.org/resource_center/assets/factsheets/TB_FACTS_SHEET_2006_ENGLISH.pdf

45. Dye C, Floyd K. Tuberculosis. In: Jamison DT, Breman JG, Meashem AR, eds. *Disease Control Priorities, Second Edition.* Washington DC: World Bank, 2006.

46. Murray CJL. Epidemiology and demography of tuberculosis. In: Timaeus IM, Chackiel J, Ruzieka L, eds. *Adult mortality in Latin America.* Oxford: Clarendon Press, 1996.

47. World Health Organization. *The Economic Impacts of Tuberculosis.* Geneva: World Health Organization, 2000.

48. World Health Organization. *Report from a consultation on the socioeconomic impacts of HIV/AIDS on households.* UNAIDS/97.3. Geneva: World Health Organization, 1997.

49. Croft RA, Croft RP. Expenditure and loss of income incurred by tuberculosis patients before reaching effective treatment in Bangladesh. *International Journal of Tuberculosis and Lung Disease.* 1998;2(3):252–254.

50. World Health Organization. *Global Tuberculosis Control: WHO Report 2004.* Geneva: World Health Organization, 2004.

51. Netesov SV, Conrad JL. Emerging infectious diseases in Russia, 1990–1999. *Emerging Infectious Diseases.* 2001;7(1):1–5.

52. UNAIDS. *2006 Report on the Global AIDS Epidemic.* Geneva: UNAIDS, 2006.

53. Haacker M. The Economic Consequences of HIV/AIDS in Southern Africa. IMF Working Paper WP/02/38. 1–41.

54. Ainsworth M, Over M. AIDS and African Development. *The World Bank Research Observer.* July 1994;9(2):203–240.

55. Bloom DE, Bloom LR, Steven D, Weston H. Business and HIV/AIDS: Who me? Geneva: World Economic Forum: 2003;1–9.

56. Aventin L, Huard P. The cost of AIDS to three manufacturing firms in Côte d'Ivoire. *Journal of African Economics.* 2000;9(2): 161–188.

57. Arndt C, Lewis JD. The macro implications of HIV/AIDS in South Africa: A preliminary assessment. *South African Journal of Economics* 2000;68(5):856–887.

58. Arndt C, Lewis JD. The HIV/AIDS pandemic in South Africa: Sectoral impacts and unemployment. *Journal of International Development* 2001;13:427–449.

59. Bonnel R. *HIV/AIDS: Does It Increase or Decrease Growth?* Washington DC: World Bank, 2000.

60. ING Barings. *Economic Impact of AIDS in South Africa: A Dark Cloud on the Horizon.* Johannesburg: ING Barings, 2000.

61. World Health Organization. *World Health Report 2000.* Geneva: World Health Organization, 2000.

62. National Coalition on Health Care. *Health Insurance Cost.* www. nchc.org/facts/cost.shtml.

63. Hsiao W. Financing. In: *Getting Health Reform Right.* Oxford: Oxford University Press, 2004.

64. Camara YB, El Abassi A, Knippenberg R, et al. *State-civil society partnership improves health services delivery for the poorest in West Africa.* Washington DC: World Bank, 2003.

65. World Bank. *World Development Report 2004: Making services work for poor people.* Washington DC: World Bank, 2004.

66. Atkinson A, Stiglitz J. *Lectures in Public Economics.* New York: McGraw-Hill, 1980.

67. World Bank. *World Development Indicators 2006.* Washington DC: World Bank, 2006.

Health Systems, Management, and Organization in Low- and Middle-Income Countries

15

David Zakus and Onil Bhattacharyya

LEARNING OBJECTIVES

- *Explore the application of health services management to low- and middle-income countries.*
- *Understand the structure of health systems.*
- *Understand the concept and dimensions of health system performance.*
- *Explore national, organizational, provider, and patient interventions to improve the performance of health systems.*

INTRODUCTION TO HEALTH SYSTEMS

Have you ever wondered why, in light of great scientific advances, modern communications, and the availability of many cures, treatments, and preventive measures for most diseases commonly found in low- and middle-income countries (LMIC), those diseases still persist and often with great prevalence and incidence? This is the conundrum that we hope to explore further in this chapter, especially as it relates to the organization, management, and delivery of services to reach those in need to either prevent or treat the many diseases, both chronic and infectious, found in LMIC.

In order to start this task, it is important to understand how services that maintain and improve health are provided to individuals and populations in both urban and rural areas.

The perspective that is most often used in understanding the delivery of health and medical services is

that of a "system," which is a set of objects and the relationships between the objects and their attributes or properties. From systems theory we understand a system as a continuum of inputs, processes, and outputs. Therefore, within our understanding of the need for health services, the health system is:

- The totality of the required resources, including human, mechanical, material, and financial
- The formal and informal organization interactions or conversion of these resources in the provision of direct services to individuals and populations to help them maintain good health status or improve their health status when it is perceived in need, either from disease, physical disability, or trauma
- The final product of health, which can vary in definition, but is commonly understood as the state of complete physical, mental, and social (even spiritual) well-being or the ability to live one's life in a manner that is compatible with achieving one's social and individual goals

The last theoretical component of systems is that they are either "closed" or "open." Closed systems are completely self-contained, are not influenced by external events and eventually must die. Open systems, on the other hand, interact with their external environment by exchanging materials, energies, or information, and are influenced by or can influence this environment; they must adjust to the environment to survive over time. The environment can be generally classified as political, economic, social, and technological, as well as physical, the space available and the way system components relate physically to each other.

Health systems are open and must be approached from this perspective. They are open to their local and national environments, and increasingly, to international and global influences. All the world's national health ministries are members of the World Health Organization (WHO), are often accountable to more local government, and usually to the people they serve.

Health systems are one of several determinants of health, and high-performing health systems can improve the health of populations.[1] While there is no perfect health system, an understanding of the system in its current form allows us to gain a comprehensive picture of how it contributes to maintaining health, and thereby also start to understand the various interactions required of its various components.

Theoretically, components within a system can be deterministic, i.e., the components function according to a completely predictable or definable relationship, as in most mechanical systems; or they can be probabilistic, where the relationships cannot be perfectly predicted, as in most human or human-machine systems, like health care. WHO suggests that health system boundaries should encompass all whose primary intent is to improve and protect health, and to make it fair and responsive to all, especially those who are worst off.[1]

What, then, makes a health system good? What makes it equitable? And how does one evaluate a health system or components of it? The World Health Organization published as part of its annual "World Health Report" a complete and noteworthy edition on "Health Systems: Improving Performance."[1] It provided a detailed presentation and analysis of why health systems matter, how well they are performing, choosing interventions and organizational failings, the resources needed, the financing and governance. In summary, it defined four key functions of a health system: "providing services; generating the human and physical resources that make service delivery possible; raising and pooling the resources used to pay for health care; and, most critically, the function of stewardship"[1]

The then Director General, Dr. Gro Bruntland stated: "Whatever standard we apply, it is evident that health systems in some countries perform well, while others perform poorly. This is not due just to differences in income or expenditure: we know that performance can vary markedly, even in countries with very similar levels of health spending. The way health systems are designed, managed, and financed affects people's lives and livelihoods. The difference between a well-performing health system and one that is failing can be measured in death, disability, impoverishment, humiliation, and despair."[1]

The report[1] concluded that:

- Ultimate responsibility for the performance of a country's health system lies with government.
- Dollar for dollar spent on health, many countries are falling short of their performance potential. The result is a large number of preventable deaths and lives stunted by disability. The impact of this failure is born disproportionately by the poor.
- Health systems are not just concerned with improving people's health but with protecting them against the financial costs of illness.
- Within governments, many health ministries focus on the public sector, often disregarding the (frequently much larger) privately financed provision of care.

Health systems have not always existed, nor have they existed for long in their present form. Early attempts to provide organized national and international access to health services have gone through various stages of evolution throughout the last century and will continue to evolve in this century. Early attempts to found national health systems were common throughout Western Europe, starting with the protection of workers, and are now being followed by most countries around the world, in some attempt to provide health care for all their citizens. The first attempt was in Russia following the Bolshevik Revolution in 1917, but it took many more years and a Second World War for most governments to catch on. New Zealand introduced a national health service in 1938; in Britain it was in 1948 with the National Health Service; and in Canada, which is widely known for its health system, national Medicare only came into existence in 1971. The United States remains the only Organisation for Economic Cooperation and Development (OECD) country without a national health delivery system, and Cuba remains a model of what a public system can achieve with limited financial resources.[2]

Today, most countries' health systems have evolved along two lines: the employee/employer payment scheme or the tax-based model, whereby all tax payers contribute all or part of the required financial inputs. Both involve a mix, to widely varying degrees, of public vs. private service provision. Comparing health systems is an often useful exercise, especially for learning new ideas.

The World Health Organization came into being in 1946 and its efforts to promote viable and effective health services culminated with the Declaration of Alma Ata in 1978, which advocated the concept and strategy of primary health care[3] as a means to achieve health for all. While much debate has persisted concerning the value and utility of primary health care, it remains a viable approach for providing an acceptable level of health services in countries at all levels of economic and social development. Debate now centers on how best to deliver services, through public or private providers, and the appropriate mix of financing mechanisms: government expenditure, out of pocket, or various types of insurance.

Health systems matter in the achievement of health, especially for those at the lower end of the socio-economic spectrum, but also for the wealthy. While health systems are complex,[4] proper health system understanding and management offers the potential for coordination of services, and access to these services for those who need them according to their needs. Health service providers may be from the public or private sectors, and how they interact and are coordinated are all issues of great concern within the health system perspective. A systems perspective on health also helps us get out of our "health" box, in thinking that only medical services and technologies are important; rather, through a systems perspective we come to understand that seat belt laws, safe roads, antismoking legislation, firearm registries, dietary recommendations, workplace safety and weather predictions all help to maintain good health.

THE PERFORMANCE OF HEALTH SYSTEMS

We have argued above that health systems are important to people's health, and that some systems seem to achieve more than others, but in order to assess this critically, one must measure it against the objectives of a health system. The World Health Report 2000 defines three objectives for health systems: improving the health of the population they serve; responding to people's expectations; and providing financial protection against the costs of ill-health.[1] Furthermore, it attempts to assess the average level of attainment of a given objective and its distribution across the population. This follows a growing interest in equity, making it an essential element of performance.[5] These objectives and measures will be discussed in a general sense, without specifically referring to those from the WHO report. For the first measure, the health status of a population could be measured by an average, such as life expectancy or infant mortality as well as the range of life expectancy across subgroups within a population. Health systems that systematically neglect certain subgroups while having a good overall average would have a worse performance than one with the same average but more even distribution across subgroups. These subgroups are generally defined by social characteristics such as wealth, education, occupation, ethnicity, sex, rural or urban residency, or religion.[6] These groups are chosen because these characteristics should not affect people's health (though they often do), and health systems should attempt to mitigate these effects where possible by providing access to appropriate services. The difference in health status between these groups—for example, maternal mortality in rural versus urban areas—would be minimized in a high-performing health system. This reflects the degree of distributive justice within a system, which is measured as part of overall effectiveness.

Responsiveness of a health system has also been included as an objective because of interest in governance and a concern for patient preferences, and not only their epidemiologically defined health needs. This is important because patient preference has an impact on health service utilization, as shown by the widespread use of private health services in LMIC, even among the poor and even when free public services are available.[7] Fair financing is an important objective because health care costs are unpredictable and may be catastrophic. For example, in China, family bankruptcies due to medical expenditures account for one-third of rural poverty.[8] Thus, health systems have a responsibility to reduce the financial impact of health care costs and make payments more progressive, such that they are related to ability to pay rather than likelihood of becoming ill.

Functions of the Health System

The formal health care system may not be the only or even the main provider of care to a population, but it nevertheless has several functions that promote the objectives of the system (see Figure 15-1). These are stewardship, the creation of resources, delivery of services, and financing.[1] Stewardship is defined as oversight of the other functions of the health system and it is the one function that is undeniably best done by national governments. However, national governments have tended to neglect this function because of a lack of managerial capacity, data, and the nature of many LMIC health systems, which make this a considerable challenge. The focus of many national health systems has been on service delivery, with the majority of a health system's budget being taken up by recurrent costs, particularly staff salaries. Effective oversight would allow governments to assess the performance of the system with respect to the other functions, and allow it to target certain areas for reform and monitor the impact of health care reforms.

Creating resources refers to investment in health care infrastructure and training of health professionals, which is commonly undertaken by the public sector, though some middle-income countries have large private sectors that include medical schools and high-technology facilities with private financing.[9] Service provision has traditionally been the main role of public health systems, but this is increasingly being questioned because of difficulties with public management in many low- and middle-income countries. These difficulties have included poor incentives for public providers leading to poor quality of care (particularly with regard to responsiveness) and widespread use of private sector providers.[7] As a result, some authors have suggested that the government's role should be to purchase services and monitor the quality, as part of the financing function.

Revenue to fund health systems may come from income tax revenue, like in the United Kingdom; employment insurance schemes, as in most of Latin America; the purchase of private insurance; or out-of-pocket payments

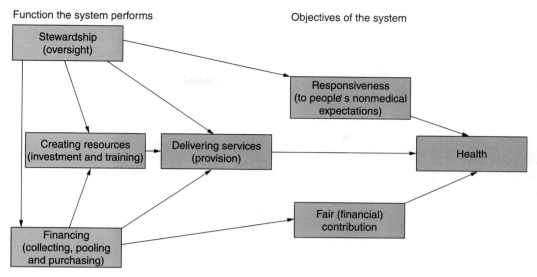

Figure 15-1. Functions of a Health System.[a]
[a] From World Health Report 2000. (Reproduced with permission.)[1]

by patients at the point of care, as in India. Since the health expenditure of individuals is unpredictable, prepayment systems with significant coverage protect patients from impoverishment due to health care expenditures. The financial impact of illness also varies according to how risk of illness (and therefore expense) is pooled. Prepayment systems where insurance premiums are based on ability to pay rather than propensity for illness allow for cross-subsidy from the rich to the poor and from the healthy to sick. In a sufficiently large risk pool, the costs from year to year will be more predictable and with an appropriate mix of young, old, rich, poor, healthy, and sick, the costs will be affordable for all. Health systems that are financed by income tax provide the greatest potential for pooling risk, while those financed primarily by out-of-pocket payments have the worst impact on fair financing. This is because the poor pay a higher proportion of their income than the rich when costs are fixed, and the unpredictable nature of out-of-pocket costs is greater for those with no financial cushion or limited access to credit.

THE STRUCTURE OF HEALTH SYSTEMS

Health systems in industrialized countries are highly structured and were developed in a context of economic stability, with a moderate pace of social change, efficient systems for taxation, strong regulatory frameworks, and sufficient numbers of skilled personnel to run these institutions. These conditions are not found in most low- and middle-income countries.[10] In the second half

of the 20th century, many developing countries established national health systems ostensibly designed to provide comprehensive services for the whole population, much like the UK's National Health Service, which served as an international model. However, countries did not fund or staff these services sufficiently to achieve their stated goals, either due to financial crises or a lack of commitment to universality. Most LMIC governments' incapacity to provide comprehensive health services for the whole population has led to the emergence of other service providers to meet growing patient demand. In these pluralistic health systems, the distinction between public and private are blurred. The more important distinction is between the organized sector, which is subject to some measure of government oversight and the unorganized or informal sector, which operates according to locally negotiated rules and is largely independent of the state.[10]

Table 15-1 shows the types of providers and institutions that support the basic functions of a health system, namely public health, consultation and treatment, provision of drugs, physical support for the infirm, and management of inter-temporal expenditure (i.e., unpredictable and potentially costly health expenses).[11] The providers and institutions are divided into the organized and the unorganized health sectors. The former includes public services run by the government and licensed private providers, while the latter includes marketized services, such as those given by unlicensed private providers, and the non-marketized services provided by household members and neighbors. The importance of the various

Table 15-1. Pluralistic health systems.[a]

Health-related function	Unorganized health sector		Organized health sector
	Nonmarketized	**Marketized**	
Public health	Household/community environmental hygiene		Government public health service and regulations Public or private supply of water and other health-related goods
Skilled consultation and treatment	Use of health-related knowledge by household members	Some specialized services such as traditional midwifery provided outside market Traditional healers Unlicensed and/or unregulated health workers and facilities Covert private practice by public health staff	Public health services Licensed for-profit health workers and facilities Licensed/regulated Nongovernmental organizations (NGOs), faith-based organizations, etc.
Medical-related goods	Household/community production of traditional medicines	Sellers of traditional and western drugs	Government pharmacies Licensed private pharmacies
Physical support of acutely ill, chronically ill, and disabled	Household care of sick and disabled Community support for AIDS patients and people with chronic illnesses and disabilities	Domestic servants Unlicensed nursing homes	Government hospitals Licensed or regulated hospitals and nursing homes
Management of inter-temporal expenditure	Interhousehold/intercommunity reciprocal arrangements to cope with health shocks	Money lending Funeral societies/informal credit systems Local health insurance schemes	Organized systems of health finance: Government budgets Compulsory insurance Private insurance Bank loans Microcredit

[a] From *Beyond public and private? Unorganised markets in health care delivery.*[11]

sectors varies tremendously according to the history and relative capacity of each health system. Health policy recommendations should not be transferred from one context to the next without knowing to what extent they are comparable. In Niger, for instance, 16 percent of deliveries are attended by trained birth attendants, so the vast majority of obstetrical services are provided by family members in the home (in the non-marketized sector) or by a traditional midwife charging fees (in the marketized sector).[9] In Sri Lanka, 97 percent of births are attended by trained personnel, so initiatives to reduce perinatal mortality in these two countries would target very different segments of the health system to achieve similar goals.[9]

For each of the key functions of the health system, it is important to understand in what sector the service is being provided in order to have rational planning of the health system. For example, India expanded the number of primary health centers between 1961 and 1988, in an effort to increase access to care.[12] Government health planners did not take into account the existing capacity of private health providers (which were widely used), nor did they attempt to provide a service that was considered complementary or competitive by patients, who continued to frequent the private sector. As a result, they invested in public service facilities that remained underfunded, understaffed, underutilized, and uncompetitive with pre-existing private and informal providers. For the government to provide adequate stewardship health reforms, policies should take the existing structure and utilization of the health system into account.

APPROACHES TO IMPROVING THE PERFORMANCE OF HEALTH SYSTEMS

Now that we have broadly defined the goals, functions, and the general criteria for assessing the performance of health systems, we will now review a series of approaches to improving performance. We have subdivided these approaches according to the perspective they take, or the

---

BOX 15-1. HEALTH SYSTEM CHALLENGES FOR THE POOR: MEDICAL POVERTY TRAP

One of the goals of a health system is to minimize the financial impact of ill health on the population. In countries with limited insurance coverage, the cost of health services is a common cause of impoverishment.[8] The descent into poverty is the result of a sequence of events that are largely preventable.[13] A breadwinner becomes ill; he or she is no longer able to work, with resultant loss of income. Either the person goes without treatment, or the costs of treatment lead to sale of assets and debt for the family. Food becomes scarce; children become malnourished and may be taken out of school and put to work to support the family. The poor family has been further impoverished, often irrevocably. The adult who has fallen ill may die, increasing the proportion of dependents to providers, and if the adult remains disabled, they are a further burden on the family's resources.

There are many factors which predispose to the sequence of events. The first is untreated morbidity, as poor patients may not consult health providers for financial reasons and may not be hospitalized when it is recommended because they cannot afford it. For example, in China, one-quarter of patients were not hospitalized despite medical recommendations, and of these the majority were for financial reasons.[14] Access to all forms of care may be reduced because user fees are common in many LMIC health systems. Formal and informal user fees are high compared to salaries of the poor, and lack of insurance means that they do not have any financial protection for catastrophic health costs, which often lead to long-term impoverishment. Lastly, the care the poor access is often of low quality, with irrational use of drugs which may be wasteful and potentially harmful. The widespread and unnecessary use of intramuscular and intravenous treatments for conditions such as viral infections is an example of this.[15]

---

level of the health system on which they act. There is the *national or regional perspective*, which refers to policy measures relating to the locus of decision-making within the system, the structure of the health system, and the degree of integration of its component parts. The *local or organizational level* refers to the management of institutions that provide care. Below this is the *provider level*, the management of health service providers. Lastly, the *individual perspective* relates to the engagement or modification of the behavior of health system users.

National Perspectives

The organizational structure and management of national health systems are areas that have profound impact on outcomes. Health system organization can be defined as "the systematic arrangement of various resources, with designated responsibilities and special channels of communication and authority, intended to attain certain objectives. The ultimate objective of organizations in a health care system is to promote or protect people's health, but this ultimate goal is approached through the intermediary role of many agencies with more focused objectives. These agencies may be involved with financing, planning, administration, regulation, provision, or any other health-related function.[16] Loosely, we can include in these agencies:

- Ministries of health and other ministries (e.g., agriculture, finance, labor, transportation, sanitation, education) either nationally or regionally
- Insurance organizations

- Public enterprises
- Private sector players
- Professional groups and unions
- Voluntary organizations
- Health education institutions
- Public participation
- International actors (e.g., WHO)

REGULATION OF HEALTH MATTERS

Governments have often found fertile ground for the implementation of laws to protect citizens from the actions of many parts of the health system, whether they are private or public.

Regulation involves the stipulation and enforcement of various standards and is often regarded as government surveillance. This surveillance can focus on a wide variety of health system components, such as:

- Health professions, including licensing, registration, salary, training, and supply
- Technical specifications and standards, including quantity of high-technology equipment and waiting times for patients to access them
- Pharmaceuticals, including safety and approval for sale, inclusion in supply lists, and pricing
- Hospitals, including governance, accreditation, budgets, physical structures, and even procedures involving wait lists
- Insurance plans and sickness funds

Decentralization

The role of the public sector is in the development, financing, and implementation of policies to guide service delivery. One of the more common recent policies has been decentralization, or the delegating of decision-making power from central to local levels of government. The three key elements of decentralization include: the amount of choice or options that are transferred from central institutions to institutions at the periphery; what choices local officials make with their increased discretion; and what effect these choices have on the performance of the health system.[17] Decentralization can therefore take various forms[16]:

- *Deconcentration* involves passing some administrative authority from central government offices to the local offices of central government ministries.
- *Devolution* involves passing responsibility and a degree of independence to regional or local government, with or without financial responsibility (i.e., the ability to raise and spend revenues).
- *Delegation* involves passing responsibilities to local offices or organizations outside the structure of the central government such as quasi-public (nongovernmental, voluntary) organizations, but with central government retaining indirect control (as in many national Global Fund funded activities).
- *Privatization* involves the transfer of ownership and government functions from public to private bodies, which may consist of voluntary organizations and for-profit and not-for-profit organizations, with varying degrees of government regulation.

Over the past two decades bilateral and multilateral financial and development agencies have been encouraging decentralization as a strategy to achieve greater health outcomes through improved efficiency, effectiveness, equity, participation, and multisectoral collaboration. In theory, it sounds good to decentralize, to get decision-making closer to where the decisions need to be made and where they can have greatest impact. But, as some analysts have concluded, it is important to also understand the political and economic contexts of any decentralization activity. Birn, Zimmerman, and Garfield[18] looked at Nicaragua in the 1990s when decentralization was implemented alongside International Monetary Fund (IMF) structural adjustment policies that favoured budget cuts to social services, including primary health care, promotion of user fees, and privatization. They concluded that decentralization brought few benefits to Nicaragua, particularly in the areas of health policy development, priority setting, and programming; and that it is not sufficient to analyze decentralization as a sector-specific reform that can be ameliorated through technocratic modifications. The political context must also be taken into account, which is consistent with a systems perspective.

Privatization

Most countries of the world have health systems in which both the public and private sectors play a role. The degree to which each is allowed to flourish is usually controlled by the government, though the private sector and multilateral finance and development agencies may also play major roles. The debate regarding whether the public or private sector should be promoted raged through the 1990s and continues today. There is an agreement on a strong government role in regulation, compensating for market failures (particularly in the area of health insurance), and addressing inequalities in access to care. However, whether government should be primarily involved in care provision or should contract it out to the private sector and regulate quality remains an area of contention.

Health markets are fragmented in terms of their structure as noted in Table 15-1, but also in terms of their clientele. The rich tend to use the highest quality private services and the best government referral hospitals, while the poor use low-end government services and informal sector private providers.[10] The rich and powerful push for the development of high-end private facilities and public tertiary care in urban areas, which reduces funds available for the provision of basic care for the poor in rural areas. In this way, health systems often reproduce the inequalities found in society at large.

Private–Public Partnerships

Recognizing that most LMIC governments are not in a position to implement a health system that meets the needs of its more wealthy citizens, they often try to enter into partnerships with the private sector for the delivery of various medical interventions. While historically, most health service delivery was done privately (often by churches), the number of private health system actors, both in the not-for-profit and for-profit sectors, has grown substantially. Many private businesses, especially in the pharmaceutical and health technology sectors, have substantial roles to play, and are now being courted by government to join with them in the delivery of services. However, it is in the voluntary sector or nongovernmental organizations (NGOs) and private voluntary organizations (PVOs) where the greatest growth has been seen in recent years.

Large international NGOs like Oxfam, World Vision, Caritas, CARE, MSF, etc. have been increasingly vocal about their role within the health care system, because they are able to deploy large sums of money and large numbers of personnel quite effectively. Add to these the growing number of private philanthropic organizations, like the Rockefeller Foundation, Ford Foundation, and now the colossal Bill and Melinda

Gates Foundation, and now this part of the private sector is highly competitive with the usual forms of bilateral (national aid agencies) and multilateral (UN agencies and World Bank) aid in the health sector.

With the WHO's emphasis on improving health systems, it became a staunch advocate of partnering with the private sector in dealing with worldwide health problems, including the infectious diseases of public health importance. This led to the creation of the Global Fund for HIV/AIDS, Tuberculosis and Malaria as the lead financial agency. The Global Fund is a partnership between governments, civil society, the private sector, and affected communities, and acts primarily as an agent to review and finance projects. Drug and vaccine development, too, has come more and more under this type of organizational structure. "A large variety of public-private partnerships, combining the skills of a wide range of collaborators, have arisen for product development [and] disease control through product donation and distribution, or the general strengthening or coordination of health services. Administratively, such partnerships may either involve affiliation with international organizations (i.e., they are essentially public-sector programmes with private-sector participation), or they may be legally independent not-for-profit bodies."[19] Widdus concludes that such partnerships show promise but are not a panacea, and should be regarded as social experiments.

Contracting

Health managers easily recognize that they often cannot control all the necessary inputs for ensuring good health and good services to their patients and other clientele. From the open systems perspective they realize that there are many patient-based services that might be more efficiently delivered by organizations outside of their own. This has led to the contracting out of certain services. Services can be described by the degree to which their quality can be measured and the contestability or level of competition for provision of that service. It is best to contract out services whose quality can be easily assessed and for which there is a number of providers competing to provide that service. Examples of these services are laundry, food production, and maintenance. Services whose quality is harder to assess include ambulatory care (for which there is ample competition) and health policy (for which there is much less). The difficulty in contracting out these types of services is that providers may reduce quality while keeping costs constant to increase profit, and the contracting agent may not realize it.

Accreditation

A key component of any health system is the human resources that carry out its daily activities. While the medical profession continues to dominate health services, they have lost some ground to other players such as nurses and allied health professionals in recent years. Hospitals continue to be at the centre of most health systems, though there has been an increasing emphasis on ambulatory and primary care in some countries. But, whether it is a doctor, a nurse, or a community health agent, it is only through the development and implementation of competency-based criteria that patients and communities can be assured that they are getting good health service providers. These criteria are put together into a system of accreditation, which also includes forms of membership, compliance, and enforcement.

Accreditation is common for health professionals and also for major health facilities in the more wealthy countries, but is sorely lacking in the poorer ones. While professional associations provide some control over the training, work, and standards of a particular group of providers (e.g., doctors and nurses), they have varying degrees of credibility in the sense of what they can enforce. A problem, particularly in LMIC, is how to integrate and accommodate traditional healers within the broader health system.[20,21] Large proportions of such populations seek help from traditional practitioners for a wide range of problems. Whether it be an herbalist, a bone setter, or a spiritualist, these practitioners often constitute the first line of health-seeking behavior for many. They present a particular challenge to the coordination of health services, but also to any attempts at accreditation and standardization.

APPLICATION OF THEORIES OF MANAGEMENT AND ORGANIZATIONAL BEHAVIOR

In the management of any organization there is much left to the discretion of the managers. This discretion is informed by knowledge, experience, and intuition. While experience and intuition are personal and acquired over time in a somewhat haphazard way, the knowledge component is one that can be actively worked on in a systematic manner, either through formal education, including continuing education, or informal reading. The validity of such knowledge, then, comes into question, especially that written in the popular press, which is so pervasive in the area of management. However, much can be done to ensure validity of this knowledge through good research.

Research into health systems, policy, and management has now been going on for about 35 years, and the volume continues to increase, though that pertaining to international health and development is scarce, with most of the research looking at private sector companies, and usually those with many employees. However, there is much happening today to promote health system and policy research, especially in the multilateral sector, which has recently seen the birth of the Alliance for Health Systems and Policy Research, and within universities, where more and more young researchers are interested in applying their skills to international health. (A new Centre for Health Systems Studies has just recently opened at the Bangladesh Rural Advanced Committee (BRAC) University and a Canadian group has made an inventory of all the international health systems researchers in their country.[22])

The theoretical perspectives of resource dependency,[23] population ecology, institutionalization, and theories of evaluation are all now utilized to gain more information on how to make health systems and interventions more effective, efficient, and equitable. (Concerning equity, the Global Equity Gauge Alliance[24] is at the forefront (www. gega.org.za).)

Organizational culture is a theory that is particularly relevant to management. By learning from aspects of national cultures, and focusing on issues like values and beliefs, rites and rituals, symbols and heroes, myths and cultural networks, managers who apply them to their workplace can make significant changes to achieve better outcomes in many aspects of organizational life.

Whether a manager is working within a private or public environment, he or she can gain valuable insight by reading the literature on health management,[25] which has now accumulated many years of research experience in understanding the behavior of organizations and the people that work in them. There is also now much literature on leadership, a very important, though often lacking, component of any well functioning health system.

PERFORMANCE OF NGOs, GOVERNMENT INSTITUTIONS, AND PRIVATE COMPANIES

The dominant actors in governance and implementation of health services worldwide continue to change. For much of the period around Alma-Ata- and the 1980s, the WHO held a leading role. Then several of the multilaterals, especially the World Bank, began to occupy a more central role as they created new divisions with a health mandate and increased spending in this area. All the while NGOs were prevalent and gaining in number and importance, especially those with large international profiles and those with strong roots in communities. However, there is some action now on the part of large bilateral donors to take greater control of the development agenda and underfund NGOs who are seen as more independent, but innovative. Private donor agencies are also growing in importance in global health. These trends result in the medium- to small-sized NGOs and community-based organizations having more of a struggle to stay alive and do their work, even though this work is often recognized as being more

effective due to the close proximity to communities, families, and people.

An area that requires further attention is the evaluation of the impact of all levels of organizational involvement in overseas development assistance. It was only after much damage was done that the World Bank and International Monetary Fund began to understand the devastating impact to health and other social services resulting directly from their structural adjustment programs.[26] Governments in high-income countries, with their large bilateral aid agencies, also struggle to understand their effectiveness. NGOs and community-based organizations, while much closer to the people who have the opportunity to directly see the impact of their work, are still in need of good monitoring and evaluation. This evaluation can be done through participatory methodologies that can provide information on outcomes while building capacity.

Provider Perspective

Addressing health system issues from the perspective of providers is important because they are the individuals who do the work of the health care system. Whether they belong to formal professional associations or are unlicensed individuals working in isolation, they collectively make decisions that have a large impact on health resource utilization and, to a lesser extent, population health outcomes. Who are the providers? The broadest definition includes health service providers and health management and support workers.[9] Health service providers are those who directly provide services to patients, while health management and support workers set up and run the infrastructure needed to provide health services. This section will only discuss the former, as there is the most information on this group, though future work may study a broader range of health human resources.

There are numerous challenges facing the health workforce, including the numbers, distribution, skill mix, and working conditions. The WHO estimates that there is a global shortage of approximately 4 million health service providers, though not every region has a shortage.[9] The global distribution of health workers is such that the largest number of health service providers is in the regions with the healthiest populations. For example, the WHO region of the Americas has 10 percent of the global burden of disease, but 37 percent of the world's health workers and 50 percent of the resources for health. On the other hand, Africa bears 24 percent of the global burden of disease with only 3 percent of the world's health workers and less than 1 percent of the global expenditure on health.[9] The distribution within countries is similarly skewed, with most providers in the cities, where health outcomes tend to be better than in rural areas. The skill mix of nurses, doctors, midwives, and public health workers should vary according to the needs of the population, but this is often not the case because these needs are not taken into account in basic training programs. The working conditions of providers are not always conducive to high performance and low pay in the health sector may lead providers to seek informal payments or work in a different field altogether.

The key health human resources issues are:

1. Managing the entry into the workforce
2. Enhancing the performance of existing workers
3. Limiting rates of attrition

Getting the right mix of skills and diversity (racial, gender, and regional) in the health workforce is a key issue for educational institutions. This is being done through reforms in medical and nursing curriculums, the opening of schools of public health (particularly in Asia), and the use of quotas for disadvantaged minorities (this is common in India, where a significant number of university spots are reserved for lower caste and ethnic minority students.[9]

Improving the performance of existing workers is a strategy that may have the greatest short- and medium-term effect, given the time required to train a new generation of health care providers. The key elements to be improved are:

- Availability
- Competence
- Responsiveness
- Productivity

The strategies to achieve this include:

- Matching skills to tasks
- Adequate supervision
- Appropriate financial incentives and remuneration
- Enhancing organization commitment
- Promoting lifelong learning
- Promoting responsibility with accountability[9]

There is extensive literature on improving the appropriateness of care in developed countries and very little from developing countries, but there is no consensus on which methods are most effective for bringing the current practice of health providers in line with "best practice" (based on the best available evidence).[27] Furthermore, approaches that have worked in developed countries may not be as effective in developing countries given the differences in practice environments. Retaining the health workforce is another challenge, as wealthier countries often draw health professionals away from poorer countries (with greater need), or people leave the profession because of low pay or poor working conditions.

Individual/ Patient Perspective

One of the goals of a health system is responsiveness, a term which essentially means that the system provides services that reflect the preferences of its users.[1] This is one of the keys to ensuring that the system is used appropriately, promotes the dignity of patients, and optimizes patient satisfaction. One of the most systematic attempts to understand the perspective and experience of the lower socioeconomic stratum of health system users was conducted by the World Bank and compiled in a report called "Voices of the Poor."[13] It concludes that state services are generally felt to be ineffective, inaccessible, and disempowering by the poor. This is particularly true of health services and education. Preferential treatment is given to those who are well dressed, or have money or influence, while the poor complain of callous, rushed, or ineffective consultations. Many state institutions reproduce the social inequalities that are present elsewhere in society.

Patients generally consult private or informal services for minor acute problems and government facilities for more severe problems. The experience varies in different countries, but generally government health agencies are often not used because they may be difficult to access, may lack medicines, and their staff may be unsympathetic. The barriers to consultation for the poor include:

- Distance
- Transportation
- Time for travel
- Shortage of medicine
- Costs
- Discrimination by staff
- Staff absenteeism
- Ineffective treatment

Health services are very expensive for the poor, when one includes cost of consultation, travel, informal payments, medicine, and lost income. Furthermore, the cost of informal payments in "free" government services is unpredictable and is often regressive, meaning that costs are a much higher proportion of income for the poor than the rich.

USING THE PATIENT PERSPECTIVE TO IMPROVE HEALTH SYSTEM PERFORMANCE: —THE DEMAND SIDE IN HEALTH SERVICE DELIVERY

Though the national, organizational, and provider perspectives mentioned above are key factors in health system performance, ultimately it is the patients who choose which type of health services to seek under which circumstances and which provider instructions to follow and which to ignore. In countries where out-of-pocket expenditure is one of the main sources of health care finance (as in India or China), patients' purchasing power can be harnessed to improve access or quality. Approaches that go through health system users to enhance performance usually refer to the demand side in health services (as opposed to the supply discussed in the previous sections).

The demand side in health care has several meanings.[28] It includes leveraging inputs, such as contribution of land, labor, and time (local representation) from communities to health facilities, as well as the private purchase of health goods like oral rehydration salts or insecticide-treated nets to prevent malaria. It also refers to understanding and changing demand-side behaviors, such as health-promoting behaviors and health-seeking behavior.

The demand side can also be stimulated to provoke changes in provider behavior through consultative processes or involvement in the planning, designing, management, and monitoring of the health service industry. The most direct form of intervention in this area is demand-side financing, which channels resources directly to users who then purchase health services. An example of this is giving vouchers for treatment of sexually transmitted disease to commercial sex workers.[7] These patients then use the voucher to obtain treatment from approved health care providers, who then present the vouchers to a financing agent who reimburses them for their services. Enhancing patient's purchasing power in this way can create a market for services to a group who is either too poor or marginalized to be considered viable customers by existing providers.

Ideally, empowered citizens/consumers use their collective voice to hold providers and policymakers to account for fulfilling their contract to deliver competent, responsive services. The more direct form of accountability is between service providers and users, involving the poor in monitoring and providing services and making provider income dependent on accountability to users. The indirect form of accountability is between government and citizens, where broader political change allows citizens to use democratic means to have input into the reform of health systems.[29]

DETERMINANTS OF THE BEHAVIOR OF HEALTH SERVICE PROVIDERS

In the previous section, we have discussed the various levels at which one can intervene to improve the performance of health systems. Ultimately, health systems should provide the right service to the right patient at the right time in the most cost-effective setting. As one might imagine, this is not often the case in either high-income or low- and middle-income countries. However, the degree to which appropriate management of patients' conditions is practiced in the health system depends on a series of factors relating to the national and organizational context, and the providers and patients themselves. Figure 15-2 is inspired from a model of the determinants of the behavior of private providers by Brugha and Zwi,[30] though it could be applied to all health service providers. The national

context includes the structure of the health system and the degree of interaction between the public and private sector. It also refers to the regulatory environment, the influence of pharmaceutical companies, and the availability of health-related technologies and treatments (which may or may not be effectively regulated by the government). The practice and social environment includes the incentive structure for providers from ownership (e.g., market exposure for private practitioners with recurrent expenses), how providers are paid, their degree of supervision, and the expectations of the community or patients. The next level is the providers, their level of training, opportunities for continuing medical education, the degree to which their knowledge and practice is influenced by the drug industry, and their ability to access timely information on evidence-based practice in the form of guidelines. Lastly, the interaction between providers and patients is affected by a provider's caseload; the number of patients seen in a day; the provider's ability to choose the correct management; and the availability, acceptability, and affordability of treatments. All these factors contribute to the proportion of appropriate and inappropriate management of patients' health conditions.

Case Study: Private Providers in India

The following case study examines the determinants of the behaviour of health care providers in one country (India) in more depth.

NATIONAL CONTEXT

India is a low-income country with a population of 1.065 billion and a GDP per capita of $1,568 at purchasing power parity.[31] Life expectancy is 62 years, though this hides a bimodal mortality profile, with a significant portion of the population still struggling with the infectious diseases associated with extreme poverty and another large group of middle- and upper-class people with predominantly chronic, lifestyle-related diseases.[32] The total expenditure on health care is 6.1 percent of GDP, with government spending about 1.3 percent of GDP on health. This expenditure is lower than many countries with comparable economic development[31,33] and means that 78.7 percent of health expenditure is private expenditure, which compensates for the low level of public investment. Similarly, according to WHO data, 77.5 percent of health expenses are out of pocket at point of service, which indicates a very low level of insurance coverage, less than 10 percent by most accounts.[34]

After independence, the Indian government set up a health care system modeled after the United Kingdom's National Health Service, with comprehensive, free services for all. However, government mostly invested in infrastructure, creating a vast network of facilities that were chronically underfunded.[35] Increasing, unmet demand for

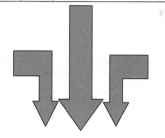

National Contex

- Public/private mix
- Public-private sector relations
- Influence of pharmaceutical companies
- Availability and distribution of diagnostic services and treatments
- Regulatory environment

Practice and Social Environment

- Practice ownership: (public/private/mixed)
- Provider payment system
- Supervision/accountability
- Community/patient/family knowledge and expectations

Provider Knowledge and Attitudes

- Training: type, source and quality
- Opportunities for continuing medical education
- Influence of drug Industry
- Access to practice guidelines

Patient-Provider Interaction

- Ability of provider to choose correct management
- Availability, acceptability & affordability of treatments

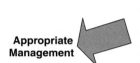

Appropriate Management

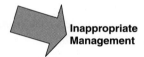

Inappropriate Management

Figure 15-2. Determinants of health service provider behavior. From Brugha R, Zwi A. Improving the quality of private sector delivery of public health services: challenges and strategies. *Health Policy and Planning* 1998;13:107–120. (Adapted with permission.)

services, along with decreasing government investment in health left a gap in which the private sector could flourish. The National Health Policy was to promote the private sector starting from 1982,[36] though the government did little to assess its capacity or monitor its behavior, and did not include it in planning strategies.[12] The result of this has been unrestricted growth of private expenditures on health, with per capita spending increasing by 12.5 percent per year since 1960.[37] The predominance of out-of-pocket spending by patients means that it is very difficult for the government to control costs. In 2001 there were 400,000 registered private providers, of whom 80 percent are in private practice. On top of this, there are an estimated 1.2 million less than fully qualified (LTFQ) physicians, who are unregistered and all practicing in the private sector.

POLICY CONTEXT

The government has made several attempts at regulating the behavior of private providers. The first approach was by establishing the Medical Council of India, which regulates medical education and registers physicians through its branches at the state level. Recent studies have shown that there is no systematic database of its

members[37] and few private providers are aware of, or follow its recommendations.[38] Furthermore, there are allegations that the Council exists more to protect the interests of its members than to protect the public. This claim is supported by the fact that few state councils have ever suspended any members, despite numerous complaints.[37] The perceived failure of self-regulation led to the application of the 1986 Consumer Protection Act to any paid medical service. The argument was that if health care was being run as a business, patients should be able to seek compensation for inadequate services through the consumer courts. This move strengthened the notion of patient's rights, but had the limitation that complainants must prove negligence, and the complexity of most medical malpractice cases requires a level of expertise that the courts or defendants are not equipped to provide. The massive demand for these services has since led to a backlog of 200,000 cases with few funds in the cash-strapped legal system to process them.[37]

PRACTICE ENVIRONMENT

There are no comprehensive studies that describe the practice context of private providers in India, so the results of several smaller studies have been brought together to highlight some of the key elements that affect their behavior. In a study from Ahmedabad, in Gujarat, 92 percent of private providers (PP) surveyed were sole proprietors of their clinics, with unlimited liability.[38] (The high risk associated with this type of business meant that 46 percent of PP used mostly personal equity to establish their practice and 35 percent of PP borrowed more than 50 percent of capital costs at 15 percent interest.) The main risks to the viability of their enterprise in the competitive urban ambulatory care market were fluctuations in patient flow, poor recovery of costs, and increasing operating costs (mostly equipment and location). Three-quarters of physicians in the sample charged fee-for-service based on cost and market price, while others charged a flat fee. Providers stated that kickbacks for specialist referrals, over-prescription of drugs, and inadequate disposal of biohazardous waste were common problems.[38] A study of diagnostic laboratory owners showed that the competition between laboratories in cities has made commissions for physicians based on the cost or number of tests prescribed the norm.[36]

PROVIDER KNOWLEDGE AND ATTITUDES

Many studies have shown that PP tend to be isolated from professional organizations and have few opportunities for continuing medical education (CME) beyond that which comes from pharmaceutical companies.[15,30] In Bombay, there is one medical representative for every four physicians in the city.[39] Companies such as Abbot spend approximately $20 per physician visited per month on marketing, CME, dinners, and gifts. An in-depth qualitative study suggested that physicians who worked in solo practices and had lower levels of training were more likely to "cooperate" with medical representatives to help "move stock" in local pharmacies.[39] Studies on awareness of relevant clinical practice guidelines have shown a moderate level of knowledge.[30]

PATIENT-PROVIDER INTERACTION

There are very few data on this aspect of provider behavior. For common conditions like childhood diarrhea or acute respiratory illness, physicians in several studies had information on the correct approach and access to treatments like oral rehydration salts (ORS) and basic antibiotics.[40] A study in a slum in Karachi, Pakistan, (which is similar to many Indian slums) showed that average consultation time was three minutes plus two minutes for dispensing drugs.[15]

APPROPRIATENESS OF CLINICAL MANAGEMENT

There are a few studies looking at appropriateness of treatments for private providers in India and Pakistan (included because of the similarities between the two countries), but the results are not encouraging. In Bihar, only 15 percent of providers measured respiratory rate in cases of acute respiratory illness in children, despite the

ease and significant diagnostic value of this exam.[40] A study of private providers' management of TB showed 80 different treatments, most of which were not recommended and more expensive.[30] Analysis of prescriptions in the district of Satara, Maharashtra, showed that 19 percent of prescriptions were irrational, 47 percent were unnecessary, and 11 percent were hazardous.[41] Unnecessary injections were given in 24 percent of cases. In the Karachi study mentioned above,[15] a mean of four drugs were prescribed for childhood diarrhea, with 66 percent of patients receiving antibiotics and only 29 percent receiving ORS. Based on the prevalence of bacterial diarrhea in children, it is estimated that less than 10 percent of patients require antibiotics, though all should receive ORS. It is interesting to note that most physicians asked patients about blood in stool or fever (situations where antibiotics would be needed), but went on to give antibiotics anyway, citing that patients would not respect them or go elsewhere if they did not.[15] This underlines the fact that provider knowledge and access to treatments are not the greatest barriers to appropriate care for common conditions. Improving the appropriateness of patient care requires a broad understanding of the determinants of these providers' behavior, and interventions that target various levels (national, organizational, provider, and patient) may be more effective at modifying the root cause.

SUMMARY

The health system perspective is very useful in working towards the improvement of individual and population health by helping to identify management and organizational issues within the health system. Issues of coordination, integration, effectiveness, efficiency, reliability, accessibility, equity, public-private involvement, and community participation are all important to consider in the delivery of health services.[23,42] Added to these various national concerns are now those of globalization.[43] Diseases are crossing borders with high speed and volume, health professionals are migrating to greener fields, technology is becoming more widely available, advocacy is on the increase, and we are all communicating more with each other. How these things can be brought to improve our global health and not denigrate it is the emerging question of the day. Understanding these phenomena and making use of them in the management and organization of health services to meet the growing and changing needs of all is the challenge we leave you with.

STUDY QUESTIONS

1. List the functions of a health system, how they interact, and explain the level of priority given to each function in your country.
2. What are some advantages and disadvantages to nations in decentralization, privatization,

public-private partnerships, and contracting in the health sector?

3. Using the case study of private providers in India as an example, look at the determinants of health service provider behavior in another country. Include the national context, provider knowledge and attitudes, patient-provider interactions, and the practice and social environment.

REFERENCES

1. World Health Organization. *The World Health Report 2000. Health Systems: Improving Performance.* Geneva, WHO, 2000. http://www.who.int/whr2001/2001/archives/2000/en.

2. Spiegel JM and Yassi A. Lessons from the margins of globalization: appreciating the Cuban health paradox. *J Public Health Policy* 2004;25(1):85–110.

3. Zakus D and Cortinois A. Primary health care and community participation: its origins, implementation and future. In: Fried B, Gaydos L, eds. *World Health Systems: Challenges and Perspectives.* Chicago: Health Administration Press, 2002.

4. Glouberman S and Zimmerman B. Complicated and complex systems: what would successful reform of Medicare look like? Discussion Paper No. 8 from the Commission on the Future of Health Care in Canada, July 2002.

5. Gwatkin DR. The need for equity-oriented health sector reforms. *Int J Epidemiol* 2001;30(4):720–723.

6. Braveman P, Starfield B, Geiger HJ. World Health Report 2000: how it removes equity from the agenda for public health monitoring and policy. *BMJ* 2001;323(7314):678–681.

7. Mills A, Brugha R, Hanson K, et al. What can be done about the private health sector in low-income countries? *Bull World Health Organ* 2002;80(4):325–330.

8. Liu Y, Rao K. Providing health insurance in rural China: from research to policy. *J Health Polit Policy Law* 2006;31(1):71–92.

9. World Health Organization. *World Health Report 2006: Working together for health.* Geneva: World Health Organization, 2006.

10. Bloom G. *Private provision in its institutional context: Lessons from health.* London: DFID Health Systems Resource Centre, 2004.

11. Standing H and Bloom G. *Beyond public and private? Unorganised markets in health care delivery.* Background paper for the World Development Report (WDR) 2003/4. Presented at Making Services Work for Poor People workshop; November 2002; Oxford.

12. Berman P. Rethinking health care systems: Private health care provision in India. *World development* 1998;26:1463–1479.

13. Narayan D, Patel R, Schafft K, et al. Voices of the Poor: Can Anyone Hear Us? New York: Oxford University Press, 2000.

14. Zhao ZW. Income Inequality, unequal Health Care Access, and Mortality in China. Population and Development Review 32(3):461–483.

15. Thaver IH, Harpham T. Private practitioners in the slums of Karachi: professional development and innovative approaches for improving practice. In: Bennett S, McPake B, Mills A, eds. *Private health providers in developing countries: serving the public interest?* London: Zed Books, 1997.

16. World Health Organization. *Health care systems in transition: production template and questionnaire.* Copenhagen: WHO Regional Office for Europe, 1996.

17. Bossert T. Analyzing the decentralization of health systems in developing countries: decision space, innovation, and performance. *Soc Sci Med* 1998;47(10):1513–1527.

18. Birn AE, Zimmerman S, Garfield R. To decentralize or not to decentralize, is that the question? Nicaraguan health policy under structural adjustment in the 1990s. *Intl J Health Serv* 2000;30(1):110–128.

19. Widdus R. Public-private partnerships for health: their main targets, their diversity, and their future directions. *Bull WHO* 2001;79(8):159–173.

20. Weeks J. Major trends in the integration of complementary and alternative medicine. In: Fasss N, ed. *Integrating Complementary Medicine into Health Systems.* New York: Aspen Publishers, 2001;12–21.

21. Bannerman RH. The role of traditional medicine in primary health care. In: *Traditional Medicine and Health Care Coverage: A reader for health administrators and practitioners.* Geneva: World Health Organization, 1983;318–327.

22. Haddad S, Zakus D, Mohindra , et al. Promoting Canadian Involvement and Capacity Building in Global Health Policy and Systems Research (GHPSR): Perspectives and Recommendations. Université de Montréal & University of Toronto. Ottawa, Canadian Institutes of Health Research, May 2002.

23. Zakus D. Resource dependency and community participation in primary health care. *Social Science and Medicine* 1998;Vol. 46(4-5):475–494.

24. McCoy D, et al. Global equity gauge alliance: reflections on early experiences. *J Health Popul Nutr* 2003;21(3)0: 273–287.

25. Shortell S, Kaluzny AD. *Health Care Management: Organization Design and Behaviour, Fifth Edition.* Clifton Park, NY: Thomas Delmar Learning, 2005.

26. Abbasi K. The World Bank on world health: under fire. *BMJ* 1999;318:1003–6.

27. Grimshaw JM. Is evidence-based implementation of evidence-based care possible? *Medical Journal of Australia* 2004;180: 50–51.

28. Standing H. Understanding the "demand side" in service delivery: definitions, frameworks and tools from the health sector. DFID Health Systems Resource Centre, 2004.

29. World Bank. World Development Report 2004: Making Services Work for Poor People. Washington, DC: World Bank, 2004.

30. Brugha R, Zwi A. Improving the quality of private sector delivery of public health services: challenges and strategies. *Health Policy and Planning* 1998;13:107–120.

31 World Health Organization. *World Health Report 2005.* Geneva: WHO, 2005.

32. Mahal A, et al. The poor and health service use in India. World Bank Publications, March 2001.

33. Prabhu K, Selvaraju V. Public financing for health security in India: issues and trends. Technical Paper for National Consultation on Health Security, July 2001.

34. Ellis RP, Moneer A, Gupta I. Health insurance in India: prognosis and prospectus. *Economic and Political Weekly* January 22, 2000.

35. World Bank. India: raising the sights: a better health system for India's poor. Health Nutrition and Population Sector Unit, South Asia Region. World Bank, November 3, 2001.

36. Baru R. *Private health care in India: social characteristics and trends.* New Delhi, India: Sage Publications, 1998.

37. Bhat R. Regulation of the private sector in India. *International Journal of Health Planning and Management* 1996;11:253–274.

38. Bhat R. Characteristics of private medical practice in India: a provider perspective. *Health Policy and Planning* 1999;14:26–37.

39. Kamat V, Nichter M. Monitoring of product movement: an ethnographic study of pharmaceutical sales representatives in Bombay, India. In: Bennett S, McPake B, Mills A, eds. *Private health providers in developing countries: serving the public interest?* London: Zed Books, 1997.

40. Chakraborty S, D'Souza SA, Northrup RS. Improving private practitioner care of sick children: testing new approaches in rural Bihar. *Health Policy and Planning* 2000;15:400–407.

41. Whitehead M, Dahlgren G, Evans T. Equity and health sector reforms: can low-income countries escape the medical poverty trap? *Lancet* 2001;358:833–36.

42. Zakus D, Lysack C. Revisiting community participation. *Health Policy and Planning* 1998;13(1):1–12.

43. Waters, WF. Globalization, socioeconomic restructuring, and community health. *J Comm Health* 2001;26(2):79–92.

Global Health Ethics

16

Anvar Velji and John H. Bryant

LEARNING OBJECTIVES

- *Define the emerging discipline of Global Health Ethics and its components.*
- *Expand the dialogue on Global Health Ethics and its relationship to human rights; culture-including race, gender, ethnicity and religion; poverty; and ill health.*
- *Discuss the concept of the "global person" in the milieu of equity, equality, justice, and benchmarks of fairness.*

INTRODUCTION

The world is changing, and one product of this change is the rapid emergence of a new discipline: global health ethics, the theory and practice of ethics in a holistic manner informed by multiple disciplines. These disciplines include public and population health and health systems; biotechnology and other scientific research; philosophy, including ethics; and other fields, such as anthropology, psychology, sociology, economics, religion, and law. Practitioners of global ethics thus include not only health care workers and researchers but also practitioners of international biolaw, philosophers, bioethicists, moral and civic leaders, human rights advocates, environmentalists, experts in religion, social and biological scientists, governmental officials, and nongovernmental organizations. Once considered independent of (and often competing with) one another, this diverse group has converged to achieve a common, overarching goal: the well-being of the *global person*. This collective entity is embodied in each person and transcends differences between groups of people regardless of whether these differences are based on race, ethnicity, political affiliation, economics, culture, education, language, gender, age, or religion.

Whereas the traditional concept of *international* health focuses on bilateral interactions between well-to-do and poor countries, the concept of *global* health reaches beyond the rich-poor dichotomy and geographic borders to the forces that separate the powerful, free, privileged population from the population that is powerless, unfree, and humiliated. In its acceptance of human diversity, global health is an expression of support for human rights. And with human rights as a key value, global health ethics thus provides moral guidance for world health systems and governance.

In recent decades, the development of global health was greatly influenced by the 1978 International Conference on Primary Health Care, convened by the World Health Organization (WHO) and UNICEF in Alma-Ata (Kazakhstan, USSR).[1] At that landmark conference, primary health care was established as a fundamental component of health care, with equity and the right to health care as core features. The conference responded to ongoing global changes, particularly with regard to their ethical dimensions. Because it encompasses clinical/medical ethics, public health ethics, population health ethics, and bioethics, the study and practice of global health ethics are potent tools for alleviating human suffering, poverty, disease, and environmental degradation, both locally and globally. Locally, global health ethics challenges its practitioners not only to identify promising research subjects but also to assure respect for their equity, dignity, and human rights when interacting with them and their communities. Globally, global health ethicists are challenged by the extensive imbalance in research support available to well-to-do countries compared with resources available to poor countries: Ninety percent of all medical research funds are expended by and for the wealthiest countries to address 10 percent—their share—of the worldwide disease burden.

Global health ethicists recognize that individual health security—an essential component of personal well-being—is a human right, which every civil society is obliged (and therefore must be empowered) to protect. This obligation is emphasized in the United Nations Millennium Development Goals, which insist that major obstacles to human social, economic, and health development be addressed. In partnership with global health ethicists, these goals recognize that ethical reform in national and global governance is a necessity in the 21st century amidst the threats and spread of global violence, erosion of health gains accumulated during the past two centuries, and emergence of novel health challenges.

PUBLIC HEALTH ETHICS, CLINICAL ETHICS, AND BIOMEDICAL ETHICS

Public health ethics focuses on the general public good of the population (instead of the individual). The "macro-ethics" of public health transcend both the "micro-ethics" of medicine (with its provider-patient relationship) and "meso-ethics," which operate at institutional levels. Public health concerns envelope health and safety issues at city, state, and country level. The principles and practice of public health may be at odds with the "micro-ethics" of individual rights and autonomy. A case in point is the classical ethical conundrum of mandating quarantine for a patient with a communicable disease such as tuberculosis or severe acute respiratory syndrome (SARS).

Clinical ethics (also called *clinical medical ethics*) is a burgeoning field that focuses on improving the quality of patient care by identifying, analyzing, and attempting to address the ethical problems that arise in clinical practice. Clinical ethics is acknowledged to be an inherently inseparable part of good clinical medicine and includes concerns of the patient's family.[2] Clinical ethics as a discipline consists of research, teaching, committee work, and consultation activities.[2] The primary emphasis of clinical ethicists is the quality of end-of-life care and conflict resolution within the framework of clinical ethics committees. To date, clinical ethics as a distinct discipline has been primarily a phenomenon of developed countries and is based on secular premises: "Clinical ethics is not founded in philosophy, law or theology but instead on the subdiscipline of medicine, centering upon the doctor patient relationships."[2] In many institutions, committees that meet to discuss issues of clinical ethics are called "bioethics committees" or "biomedical ethics committees." As an academic discipline, clinical ethics addresses questions at the clinical level, such as informed consent, autonomy, and death and dying.

Often called "bioethics," biomedical ethics is an academic discipline limited to learned societies and academicians; it is the purview of departments of philosophy. At the national level, bioethical forums discuss institutional and national policies and issues such as health care rationing and access. Bioethics relates to the ethical questions and dilemmas that arise at the interfaces between medicine; biology; cybernetics; politics; law; theology; philosophy; technological research; and the ethics of morality, duty, and obligations. In the global context, newly emerging issues related to human genomic research and other major developments of biotechnology, such as cloning, xenotransplantation, and stem-cell research, have become focuses of bioethics.

The post–World War II emergence of bioethics in the United States evolved around the Protestant values that predominated in US culture. This concept was elegantly encapsulated by Jonsen, who stated, "US Medicine had in the immediate postwar years begun to build a wall around itself and within that wall a complex edifice. Three streams of bioethical concerns highlighted that reality. The therapeutic stream, which brought new treatments, found that it had to exclude persons from them, as the 'God Committees' chose some to live, others to die. The experimental stream, on the other hand, seemed to capture some, entrusting them into treatment they did not want or need, and repelling others from treatment they needed. The scientific stream was perhaps the most ominous, suggesting in the power the remaking of humans in an engineer's image."[3] In the early 1960s, vigorous debate in the "God-Committees" centered on the first genuinely life-supporting, lifesaving technology—chronic hemodialysis.[3]

The second bioethical model is that of "Euro-Ethics." This model also has limited value because it lacks diversity and the notion of plurality. The focus of Euro-Ethics is the philosophy of medicine and epistemology; this focus contrasts with the American model of bioethics, which is more closely aligned with applied and practical ethics.[3]

Nominally and conceptually, the modern discipline of bioethics is seen as an offspring of a Western, predominantly US model characterized by scientific voluntarism or the technological imperative and libertarian or secular morals. This focus demonstrates radical change of the tradition of "*bios* (life) and *ethike* (ethos) through manipulation of life."[4] The discipline of bioethics as viewed by the developing world is "conceptually a synthesis of the advances of science and the mandates of conscience."[4] The Roman Catholic perspective, expressed predominantly in Latin America, is succinctly described as containing bioethical premises based on the principle of holiness of life and on the imperatives of natural law as supported by the moral theology of the Catholic Church.[4]

Can the rules, laws, and principles of secularism be separated from religious rationales and the sanctions of God's reward and punishment? Secularists and religious fundamentalists are at odds on several issues of current relevance in the new millennium. One danger of the Western (and particularly the American) form of biomedical ethics is the "unleashing of absolute individualism and moral atomism of a socially destructive kind."[5] This powerful, incessant drive operates in issues such as euthanasia, assisted suicide, abortion, purchase of organs for transplantation, all forms of reproductive technology and surrogate parenthood, preservation of confidentiality, and use of public health funding for research.[5]

FROM "INTERNATIONAL HEALTH" TO "GLOBAL HEALTH": EXPANDING OUR LANGUAGE AND PERCEPTIONS

Traditionally, medical practitioners have focused on personal health from a limited perspective (prevention, diagnosis, and treatment) and are bound by ethics and covenants traceable to ancient civilizations (India, Persia, Egypt, China, Greece), whereas the new discipline of global health requires a vocabulary that defines health as a state of physical, social, mental, and spiritual well-being that extends beyond absence of physical disease or infirmity. The new dialogue on global health has already outgrown the limitations of current terminology (e.g., "international health"), and no consistent vocabulary yet exists that adequately describes the conceptual framework and operationalization of global health ethics. Language is needed to fully convey the global cultural contexts for such terms as individual and public good, equity, inequality, rights, solidarity, beneficence, autonomy, justice, fairness, dignity, virtue, and responsibility. Indeed, with the onset of globalization—a set of new economic realities amid disappearing political boundaries—the world's thinking must be reoriented to achieve health in this new millennium.

This reorientation is being guided by leaders in the emerging field of global health who contribute their experience and ideas regarding major health-related concerns of social science (e.g., societal discrimination and inequality, health care rights, population displacement, poverty, ethics of environmental practices and technology transfer, access to primary health care services, health care financing, education, global networking) and of natural science (e.g., diagnosis and treatment of diarrheal, respiratory, tropical, and infectious diseases; malnutrition; and global disease burden), summarized in 2 seminal volumes edited by A. Velji.[6]

As an example of steps taken to address ethics, culture, and health care equity globally, a consortium—originally named International Health Medical Education (IHMEC) and subsequently renamed Global Health Education[7]— was founded to address new challenges in global health education.[8] The cofounders of this consortium stated their intent to impart a systemic networking approach to global health education by focusing on marginalized populations around the world. This intent was articulated also in the historic 1997 WHO policy statement, which stated that "Health for All in the 21st century . . . [must be] built on the genuine expressions of moral obligations to protect the vulnerable and to mitigate inequities . . . with . . . science-based and socially sensitive methods."[9]

Accordingly, a Director General of WHO articulated its changing role as the world's health conscience: "the role of WHO . . . must include ethical standard setting to meet today's and tomorrow's needs in such areas as cloning, reproductive health, and access to triple-drug treatment for persons with HIV infection, or the use of interferon for Hepatitis C carriers. Many issues relating to fair access to preventive, therapeutic and rehabilitative technologies should be considered, and ethical guidelines should be prepared."[10]

HEALTH-RELATED ETHICS OF GLOBALIZATION

From the perspective of the developing nations, globalization is manifested as an onslaught of ethico-religious, cultural, technological, economic, and informational changes that disrupt established societies. These globalization-related changes result in the marginalization of vulnerable populations, whose health is further affected negatively by additional phenomena present throughout the world: unethical organ-donor policies, militarization, privatization, unfair trade practices, and economic sanctions.[11–13] All these phenomena cause continuous and sporadic societal paradigm shifts that transcend national boundaries and affect the politics, ecology, economics, education, and health of entire societies. Without a commitment to ethical principles— human rights and freedom, justice, fairness, equity—the weak, disadvantaged global citizen is denied access to education, housing, jobs, and food and is placed in a lopsided struggle against the privileged citizen within a neo-liberal, highly individualistic environment. Lack of ethical intervention will continue to erode health care not only in the developing countries but also in the developed nations.

EQUITY AS A CORE ELEMENT OF GLOBAL HEALTH ETHICS

The enormous size of these challenges calls for ethical policies that benefit the vulnerable and have equity at the core. This essential element was affirmed in the WHO Declaration of Alma Ata[1] and was a centerpiece of renewing the WHO *Health for All* call.[14] Health equity involves more than equality and is not "vague but politically popular desire for social justice"[15]; instead, health equity is "a feasible and tangible process" in which health benefits are received according to measurable need, not on the basis of economic or political status.[15]

Surveillance of equity status is a practical management tool that makes the moral imperatives of social justice feasible.[16] Inequities in health care—and especially in health outcomes—imply presence of a subset of measurable inequalities that are both unfair and avoidable. Equitable distribution of health care is not necessarily sufficient to overcome health inequities; health equity is measured also by the extent to which disadvantaged populations can exercise their human right to justice and fairness in the context of achieving well-being.

EQUALITY AS A CORE ELEMENT OF GLOBAL HEALTH ETHICS

The 19th-century British epidemiologist William Farr is credited with having initiated the scientific study of health inequalities,[17] a central feature of the European tradition, especially in the United Kingdom. Unlike the normative concept of health equity, health inequality is a primarily empirical concept that emphasizes the disparity between rich and poor populations and thereby avoids focusing on the health of the poor.[18] The most daunting challenge of the third millennium is to understand the causes of health inequity and how health care is distributed within and between countries. Central to this concern is the need to create health systems on the basis of fairness, distributive justice, human rights, democracy, and peace-building—a suggestion echoed by a recent Rockefeller Foundation report,[19] which presents diverse dimensions of health equity in 13 countries. The report explores fundamental issues, such as ethics and its measurement as well as causal analysis related to underlying social determinants (e.g., gender, globalization) and argues explicitly that specific fairness-related values are involved in distributing health care and facilitating positive health outcomes. The report discusses remediable health inequalities, including unequal access to resources—financial assistance, education, job security, clean air and water, sanitation, health care—and gender inequality. Within any society, health inequity is both a proxy and a barometer for marginalization, for deficiencies in social justice and human rights, and for lack of democracy.[19]

To be accurate, any ethics-based measurement of inequalities in health care requires a sophisticated technique. Ideally, this measurement technique would consider the distribution of ill health across the full socioeconomic gradient and not only within a selected segment of the population.

The classical health status indicators used for monitoring global health achievement includes rate of infant mortality, overall mortality and morbidity, and combined rates of mortality and morbidity (described by indicators such as quality-adjusted life years (QALYs), disability-adjusted life years (DALYs), and health-life years). However, these indicators fall short of monitoring equity in health care. The Council of International Organizations for Medical Sciences (CIOMS) working group suggested monitoring of other health services indicators, including accessibility, affordability, utilization, and coverage of health care along with its appropriateness and procedural fairness. Moreover, processes of decision making must be visible, and caregivers must be accountable.[20]

The sea-change in the ethical search for cost-effective and equitable care has focused on one vexing philosophical, theological question: How should life be valued? This question subsumes others: Should life be valued in terms of economic and social productivity or in terms of a given duration of life, with its intrinsic value and variation by age, economic productivity, and social status? How do we measure the value of future life versus that of the present? As Morrow and Bryant state,[21] measuring and valuing human life contribute importantly to understanding the disease burdens in populations and to guiding thinking about the most appropriate ways to address those burdens with health care intervention. Such interventions are mindful of ethical dimensions of health and human development.[21] Are DALYs considered to be an ethical measure that is also sensitive—both quantitatively and qualitatively? How do these concepts fit into the ethics of public, global health decision making versus the traditional, doctor-patient-based ethics?[21,22] (See Chapter 2 for other information on this topic).

The 1993 World Bank Report, *Investing in Health*,[23] focused on quantifying and comparing the disease burden borne by diverse populations. The metric created for this purpose was the DALY.[24,25]

Initially introduced by Daniels et al,[26] the *benchmark of fairness* concept queried various equity-related dimensions of health care reform, including provision of universal access to services; comprehensiveness of services; uniformity of benefits; equitable financing as determined by ability to pay value for money (clinical financial efficiency); public accountability; and degree of choice.[26-28] Thailand, Pakistan, Mexico, and Columbia have modified and refined some of these matrices. In Pakistan, for instance, the following benchmarks are used: intersectoral public health; financial- and gender-related barriers to access; comprehensiveness and tiering of benefits; equitable financing; effectiveness, efficiency, and quality of health care; administrative efficiency; democratic accountability; and patient-provider autonomy.[27]

In the setting of low-income and insufficient data, unique thinking and creation of novel benchmarking tools are needed for building greater capacity to monitor and analyze policies from an equity-ethical perspective. In post-apartheid South Africa, another tool—the *equity gauge*—was invented to enable legislators at both the national and subnational levels to monitor the impact of government policy on health systems.[29]

HEALTH-RELATED ETHICS OF GLOBAL POVERTY, DISTRIBUTIVE JUSTICE, AND THE POOR–RICH DIVIDE

One cannot discuss global health ethics without addressing poverty, inequity and injustice. This section will examine some examples of these issues and how they affect the health of people around the world.

Orphans and Other Vulnerable Children of the Urban Slums of Africa

Of the 350 million children under 17 years of age who currently live in sub-Saharan Africa, 43 million (12.3 percent) are orphans.[30] In addition to these children, however, a very large number of nonorphaned children in sub-Saharan Africa are nonetheless highly vulnerable for other reasons; therefore, focusing concern on orphans exclusively would be unfair and unjust. The orphans and other vulnerable children of Africa are the most disadvantaged of any in the world. The dimensions of such disadvantage reach far beyond what usually comes to mind in considering the lives of such children, whether these factors are physical, economic, social, cultural, educational, ethical, or rights-based.

The practical realities of vulnerable children include a broad range of deeply troubling circumstances, including the circumstance of being orphaned, abandoned, or physically handicapped; forced to become a child soldier; being displaced by war or exposed to hazardous work; becoming a victim of human trafficking and other forms of abuse and neglect; living in extremely poor conditions; being homeless, living on the streets; or a combination of these circumstances. To these threats to health and well-being must be added the further burdens imposed by the HIV/AIDS pandemic: Of the 43 million orphans living in sub-Saharan Africa, 28 percent were orphaned as a result of HIV/AIDS.[30]

These vulnerable children can thus be defined as those whose safety, well-being, and development are threatened. Of the many factors contributing to these children's vulnerability, the most important are lack of care and affection, adequate shelter, education, nutrition, or psychological support; and, of course, frequent discrimination.

A useful approach might be to reach beyond the generalizations relating to these children to focus on the extremely vulnerable population of children living in Africa's urban slums. Of people living in the large urban slums of Nairobi—70 percent of that city's population—79 percent live in one-room homes without running water or sanitation and usually without electricity. One can only begin to imagine the extreme difficulties of families trying to build constructive lives under such circumstances; not surprising, therefore, is the exceedingly high mortality rate for children under five years of age: In some areas, this rate reaches 25 percent of children. More than half of these childhood deaths are associated with malnutrition.[31]

To address the needs of those living in the slums, UN Habitat has committed its members to the Millennium Development Goal of improving the well-being of 100 million people dwelling in the urban slums of Africa, simultaneously expressing concern for the orphans and other vulnerable children in those slums.[32]

Given the immense burden on the health and well-being of those children, one can easily understand the existence of multiple approaches to alleviating these children's problems. Indeed, no fixed set of answers exists, and accessible resources fall far short of need for them. Multiple approaches are thus needed and used, and a great challenge is to create coherent interaction among those responses.[33]

One distinct pattern of need is relatively new and under-appreciated. There have been recent advances in the science of early childhood development that are exceedingly important. The National Academy of Science USA[34] and the World Health Organization,[35] report that early caregiver-child interactions, beginning in the early days of life, are strongly foundational determinants of social, psychological, physical, emotional, and cognitive capacities of the young child; a strongly nurturing, loving, protective, stimulating caregiver-child interaction is essential for the child's early development. In contrast, a negligent, unprotective, nonloving interaction can be disruptive, damaging, and produce lifelong negative effects. The nature of these caregiver-child interactions or attachments has been further defined as representing *secure attachment* (which is supportive, nurturing, and loving) or *insecure attachment* (which is negligent and disruptive). Considerable research has been focused on the nature of these attachments and their positive and negative consequences.

Applying these concepts to the circumstances of the lives of vulnerable children in slum settings adds insight not only into the risks to these children's well-being but also into the nature of equity. Let us consider for a moment the place of equity in caring for these children. Equity in child care calls not for equal distribution of care but for delivery of care according to need. Health care programs for vulnerable children in the urban slums are challenged by the extreme scarcity of resources, and active community participation; the aim of these programs is therefore to identify those children most in need and to responding accordingly.

A disturbing equity-related issue is the widespread underappreciation of the importance of early caregiver-child attachments for the foundational development of the child. For example, little local concern is expressed for orphans and other vulnerable children sitting in the trash and mud of an African slum community; the response to this situation is often, *"They are poor, to be sure, and perhaps hungry, but they are not being harmed."* In addition to the potential damage of malnutrition and exposure to infectious disease, the lack of sufficient, positive caregiver-child interactions early in these children's lives does indeed cause them harm. The development of life skills—in particular, the ability to cope with the complex difficulties of their corner of the world—is seriously diminished in these children. Thus, this emerging example illuminates the unseen inequities affecting a large number of children in Africa.

That these children lack opportunity to have a good life is a violation of their human rights, and this deprivation also must not be neglected. Working with UN Habitat in the slums of Nairobi, Bryant and colleagues are addressing this issue in a volume to be published at a later date. Working with local communities, those authors have begun to emphasize these challenges to improving the health and development of these communities. Those in the community have accepted the importance of this issue and are beginning to assess the extent of secure and insecure caregiver-child attachments in specific slum settings. Early observation of the community shows that children who suffer from insecure caregiver-child attachments are more likely to be malnourished than are those with secure attachments. An objective of this community work is to develop a means of spreading across Africa an awareness of the importance of early caregiver-child interactions.

Special attention should be given to the five key strategies (see Table 16-1) discussed in "Framework for the Protection, Care and Support of Orphans and Vulnerable Children Living in a World with HIV and AIDS," which appeared in *Children on the Brink 2004*.[30]

As the World Bank authors state in *Reaching Out to Africa's Orphans*,[33] no established blueprint yet exists for action on behalf of orphans. The modest aim of the authors is to collate and organize the available evidence and contribute to a better understanding of what kinds of interventions and approaches might work in a given country. Such enhanced understanding could provide guidance to agencies involved in responding to the crisis of orphans in sub-Saharan Africa.

Table 16-1. Key strategies for improving the health and development of orphans and other vulnerable children in poor communities worldwide.

- By prolonging the lives of parents and by providing economic, psychosocial, and other support, strengthen the ability of families to protect and care for orphans and other vulnerable children.
- Mobilize and support community-based responses to provide both immediate and long-term assistance to vulnerable households.
- Ensure that orphans and other vulnerable children have access to essential services, such as education, health care, and birth registration.
- Ensure that governments protect the most vulnerable children by improving policies and legislation and by directing resources to communities.
- To create a supportive environment for children affected by HIV/AIDS, raise awareness at all levels through advocacy and social mobilization.

Inequity and Poverty in the Global Health Equation

Inequity is deeply rooted in the soil of poverty, and the oft-expressed question, "Am I poor because I am sick, or am I sick because I am poor?" points to the interpenetrating relation between poverty and global health. Accordingly, global opinion is now focused on the health of the poor along with the ethical notion of inequality in health care. Poverty-oriented economics has thus gained recognition on the world stage.[36] (See Chapter 14 for more information on this topic). Nonetheless, societal discrimination at various levels and predatory unethical practices—prevalent globally, regionally, and locally—still prey on the vulnerable. After long study of AIDS, Mann stated: "The central insight from a decade of hard work against AIDS is that societal discrimination is at the root of individual and community vulnerability to AIDS and other major health problems of the modern world."[37]

In this new millennium, the primary cause of ill health is poverty. Recent climatologic and geologic catastrophes in the first few years of the present millennium—the Indian Ocean tsunami; Hurricane Katrina in the USA; and earthquakes in Turkey, Iran, and Pakistan—garnered global attention to the susceptibility of vulnerable populations—especially the poor—to natural disasters, and massive amounts of aid were offered to help disaster victims. However, such mind-numbing "daily tsunamis" never register on the radar of the same donor communities in the same proportion. For instance, the HIV/AIDS pandemic costs the African subcontinent 1 percent of its gross domestic product each year. Malaria alone kills 2800 Africans a day,[38] and 314 million Africans—nearly twice as many as in 1981—live on less than $1 a day. Moreover, Africa is home to the world's 48 poorest countries, including 24 of the 32 countries ranked lowest in human development.[38] Every week, 10,000 women in the developing world die during childbirth and 200,000 children under the age of five years die from disease. Each day, more than 8000 people die from AIDS-related conditions. In 2005 alone, two million people died from AIDS. Another hallmark of this impoverishment is the observation that an estimated 115 million children in developing countries have no schooling.[38] And even Europe has not been spared: The Roma population, for instance—a people once known as gypsies—is the largest, poorest, and fastest-growing minority worldwide.[38] Table 16-2 outlines a three-step process focused on ethics, which has been proposed for addressing the societal risk factors operating worldwide.[37]

Central to this three-step process is a concept applicable to a wide variety of global health problems: "A careful analysis of the major causes of preventable illness, disability, and premature death—including cancer, heart disease, injuries and violence and infectious disease—shows that they, like AIDS, are linked to societal

Table 16-2. Proposed three-step ethics-based process for addressing societal risk factors operating worldwide.

- Identification of the basic forms of discrimination within one community or nation
- Identification of societal discrimination that leads to risk of HIV exposure and diminished access to health care
- Identification of processes that can reduce this societal discrimination

discrimination and lack of respect for fundamental human rights and dignity."[37]

In 2000, in response to the challenges of poverty and discrimination, 189 countries became signatories to the Millennium Development Goals project, which clearly outlined targets for reducing poverty and other sources of human deprivation as well as promoting eight sustainable development goals.[38–40] (See Table 16-3.)

Private philanthropic foundations have a major ethical and practical role in addressing the problems of global health. The longstanding philanthropic efforts of the Rockefeller Foundation, The Aga Khan Foundation, The Aga Khan Health Services, and other key players[41–43] have now been boosted by more recent contributors, such as Ted Turner, the Bill and Melinda Gates Foundation, and Warren Buffett.

Table 16-3. Sustainable development goals contained within the Millennium Development Goals endorsed by 189 countries in December 2000 at the Millennium Summit in New York.

- Eradicate extreme poverty and hunger. By the year 2015, halve the proportion of people in extreme poverty and the proportion of people who suffer from hunger.
- Achieve universal primary education. By 2015, ensure that all children can complete a full course of primary schooling.
- Promote gender equality and empower women to eliminate gender disparity in primary and secondary education by 2005 and in all levels of education by 2015.
- By the year 2015, reduce child mortality by two thirds.
- By 2015, improve maternal health by reducing the maternal mortality rate by 75 percent.
- By 2015, combat HIV/AIDS, malaria, and other diseases and begin to reverse their spread.
- Ensure environmental sustainability. By 2015, halve the proportion of people without sustainable access to safe drinking water.
- Develop a global partnership for development. Develop further rule-based, predictable, nondiscriminatory trading and financial systems and address the special needs of the least-developed countries.

In 1999, the Bill and Melinda Gates Foundation assumed a major leadership role in the global fight against HIV/AIDS, malaria, tuberculosis, and other underfunded diseases endemic in the developing world. A total of US$6 billion had been pledged by the Foundation until June 2006, when Warren Buffett announced his contribution of some US$38 billion to the Foundation for its global efforts. The Global Fund to Fight AIDS, Tuberculosis, and Malaria promised $4.8 billion to 128 countries, and the [US] President's Emergency Plan for HIV/AIDS Relief (PEPFAR) pledged US$15 billion to help "selected countries." The Global Alliance for Vaccines and Immunization (GAVI) has been involved in 72 countries, using a budget half of which was contributed by the Bill and Melinda Gates Foundation.[44]

Ethical questions abound as to appropriate priorities in distributing health services and funds for these and related services. A recent focus on global health is the complicated, confusing interrelationships between thirty stakeholders—Tanzania, for example, where the HIV/AIDS epidemic highlights ethical dilemmas.[44,45] Aid to intended recipients is often blocked by the "architectural indigestion" that often results from the differing political agendas of multiple donors combined with their often inadequate attention to health ethics.

In response to the mounting evidence and research on social determinants of health inequalities, the WHO Commission on Social Determinants of Health was launched to focus on the world's most vulnerable populations.[46] The Commission seeks to ensure that public policy is based on a vision of the world where people matter most and where social justice is therefore paramount.

The "G8" countries—the United States, Canada, Great Britain, France, Germany, Japan, Italy, and (nominally) Russia—account for roughly half the world's economic activity and dominate the decision making processes of both the World Bank and the International Monetary Fund (IMF).[47] Support from the G8 is therefore critical for improving the key social determinants of health, which include education, housing, sanitation, nutrition, and safe, clean food and water. Intervention by the G8 is pivotal also for reversing the severe debt crises of developing nations (especially those in sub-Saharan Africa), where fragile, destabilized economies are susceptible to internal strife and further crises, health crises foremost among them. The roots of these debt crises are sociopolitical, historical, and economic; for example, postcolonial African nations experimented with Marxism and Socialism, which furthered both the extension of debt and loss of infrastructure. Famine, drought, and wars added more burdens. A recognized effect of deep national debt in the developing countries is the *debt-death link*: The higher the interest payment owing on a nation's debt, the lower is the mean life expectancy of that nation's citizens. This link is now well accepted internationally as a necessary focus of debt relief,[48] especially given that the heavily indebted developing countries spend far more money for arms than for reducing debt: By 1990, for example, sub-Saharan Africa was receiving US$11 billion annually for military weaponry; and developing countries, including those south of the Sahara, sent to the developed countries a staggering US$220 billion more than these developing countries received in aid.[48] Under this scenario, the 1994 World Bank report predicted, the sub-Saharan Black states will require 40 years to reach the level of wealth that existed there 20 years previously.[49] For the world's poorest countries, debt burden is thus the "new slavery."[50] Jubilee 2000, a coalition of more than 90 organizations, including Oxfam, Christian Aid, and the British Medical Association, have spotlighted this relation between the creditor nations and the IMF and World Bank.[8]

These health-related issues become more critical each year as the poor-rich divide increases—so much so that the United Nations Secretary General has called for urgent action to raise the living standards of the world's poor.[51] At the ceremony where he was awarded the Nobel Peace Prize, former US President Jimmy Carter stated that the greatest challenge facing the world is the universal, growing chasm between the richest and the poorest people on earth and that this disparity causes most of the world's unsolved problems, including starvation, illiteracy, environmental degradation, violent conflicts, and unnecessary illnesses from guinea worm to HIV/AIDS.[52]

This enormous, growing disparity is illustrated by many statistics. Of the world's total consumption, the richest fifth of the world's people consume 86 percent of all goods and services, whereas the poorest fifth consumes only 1.3 percent; and the three richest people in the world have assets that exceed the combined gross domestic product of the 48 least-developed countries.[51,53,54] The world's 225 richest individuals (of whom 60 are American) have a combined wealth of more than $1 trillion—equal to the annual income of the poorest 47 percent of the world's population.[51,53,54] The amount of money spent each year by Americans and Europeans on pet food alone—US$17 billion a year—is $4 billion more than the estimated annual amount needed to provide basic health and nutrition for everyone in the world.[51,53,54] The rising economic tide expected to flow from market economics is said to be a force that will "lift all boats"; but "the poor have no boat and are drowning in this tsunami of corporate profit."[55]

Health Care Inequity and Its Worldwide Association with Culture, Race, Ethnicity, and Gender

Global inequities of socioeconomic position and health are disproportionately distributed along racial lines. Disadvantaged groups and countries identifiable by race sustain higher burdens of disease and deprivation than their advantaged cohorts identifiable by race. This inequity exists despite current genomic research, which shows that 99.9 percent of DNA is shared by all human beings, regardless of the anatomic and physiologic aspects of "race"[56] and that genetic variation within socially recognized human populations exceeds the genetic variation between population groups. Race is therefore meaningful only socially, not biologically,[56] and the rational taxonomy traditionally used by anthropologists, epidemiologists, researchers, and nations around the world is clearly outdated.

During the past century, 26 different schemes, most of them motivated by politics of isolation and marginalization, have sought to categorize racial differences in the US population.[57] Over time, several of these schemes have been replaced by others. For instance, Jews were defined as nonwhite along with certain other groups but were "deracialized" later in the century. Similarly, persons of South Asian origin were at first classified as "Hindus"[56] but were later classified as whites regardless of skin tone. In South Africa, the apartheid classified Japanese and Chinese persons—along with other Asians and even Jews—as "colored." Subsequently, with the rising force of the Japanese economy, Japanese persons were classified as "whites" under the apartheid system.

Ethnicity, in comparison, emphasizes the cultural, socioeconomic, religious, and political characteristics of human groups; these characteristics include language, dress, customs, kinship, and historical identification with territory.[58] *Culture* denotes fundamental beliefs, art, language, literature, customs, ideals, and laws in general[5] and provides an inextricable link to morals and ethics of the human species. To violate a person's cultural beliefs and practices is therefore tantamount to assaulting that person's humanity,[5] and imposition of beliefs and practices on an individual or a society is also a violation and is immoral.[5] A cardinal principle of global health ethics is to respect others and uphold their inviolable dignity.

Of course, health disparities based on a person's "race" and skin "color" are prevalent in many countries other than the United States. In Brazil, for instance, the mortality rate among children under 12 months of age is 62.3 for black and brown children as compared with 7.3 for white children.[56] Similarly, in Australia, the life expectancy at birth for nonindigenous males is 75.2 years and is 81.1 years for females, whereas the lifespans of indigenous people are considerably shorter: 56.9 years for males, and 61.7 years for females. In the United States, where most studies on "racial disparities" are conducted, the diabetes-related mortality rate among Native Americans is 27.8 per 100,000—380 percent higher than that of whites (7.3 per 100,000). Black women in the United States have a threefold higher rate of childbirth-related mortality than their white female cohorts, and the rate among Hispanic women is 23 percent higher. Across social lines, similar differences in health outcomes have been shown for asthma, hypertension, heart disease, cancer, diabetes, HIV/AIDS, and end-stage renal disease.

Examples of factors that create barriers to health care—and therefore, inequity—for these disadvantaged populations include lack of economic access to health care, institutional barriers encountered by health care providers, discriminatory health care policies and practices, and lack of language and cultural competency among health care practitioners and policymakers.[56] The Kaiser Permanente National Diversity Council within the Kaiser Permanente Medical Care Program (a large nonprofit-managed care organization headquartered in California) has issued several publications and provider handbooks about techniques for rendering culturally competent care for various populations, including African American, Latino, Southeast Asian, Pacific Islander, gay, bisexual, and transgender patients as well as those with medical disabilities. Nonetheless, except for the United Kingdom, where researchers have substantially documented barriers to health care, data are as yet insufficient to describe these barriers as they exist across Europe and in developing nations, where many "nonwhite" members of society have undergone health care-related discrimination in connection with their ethnicity and culture. Such data are needed to address disparities in health care and in health outcomes; however, they are also susceptible to the hazards inherent in planning delivery of health care on the basis of specified ethnic populations notwithstanding any scientific basis for such "racialization" of disease.

For example, the frequency of the BRCA-1 genetic mutation (present in women with breast cancer) in the general US population is 1 in 1666, whereas the frequency is 1 in 107 among Ashkenazi Jewish Women of Eastern European origin.[56] Identifying female patients with this heritage might therefore facilitate testing that would allow some women to obtain appropriate medical care earlier than would be possible without such testing. However, such targeted testing based on advances in genomic technology can easily lead to both stigmatization and discrimination and raises legitimate ethical questions: Are our genes being singled out as "mutant"? Should the specified female population receive breast screening and "prophylactic" mastectomy?

Specified genetic traits, such as that for sickle cell disease (the first "racialized" disease) might be used inappropriately as a surrogate marker of race. Screening the African American population for sickle cell trait and screening persons of Mediterranean and Southeast Asian ancestry for thalassemia are thus additional examples of issues that raise ethical concerns.

Gender is another factor influencing worldwide disparities in the quality and availability of health care; and a perspective of shared values, equity, and human rights used to transform the health of the global person must challenge historical cultural norms and notions that value males over females. Current measures of aggregate health fail to adequately quantify household assets by gender—a demographic survey marker that has great potential to improve equity in women's and children's health. A seminal paper[59] invoked human rights as well as economic considerations in valuing women's worth.

The burden of disease is carried from one life period to another—from girlhood to motherhood and throughout daughterhood—as multiple male-dominated, paternalistic institutions (political, social, legal, and religious) view women's role as that of procreator over whom males are granted the life-and-death power of decision making. In most nations and societies, the law favors males through male-operated and supported agencies and in the name of religion and morality: Until 1969, for example, Canadian law prohibited distribution of information and materials for contraception, which was regarded as a "crime against morality."[60] In societies where these paternalistic forces operate, women lack power to assert their own priorities and aspirations in making reproductive choices and other health-related decisions. Ownership rights to pregnancy and its termination are vested in the males of these societies; the husband owns proprietary and matrimonial rights, including the legal right of control over the fetus.[60]

Gender-based health disparities are evident also in rates of infant mortality. In Bangladesh, India, Pakistan, and China, more male infants survive to the age of two years than do female infants; more than 1 million girls die each year as a result of being born female.[61] Each year, more than 95 percent of an estimated 20 million unsafe abortions—considered by many as a product of moralistic laws and social injustice—occur in developing countries as a result of repressive colonial laws,[60,62] "religious morality," culture, and misguided ideas about family "nobility."

Disparity—and denial—of reproductive rights around the world and throughout history is evident also in various involuntary sterilization practices. The Nazi practice of "ethnic cleansing" and involuntary sterilization to create an uncontaminated "master race" was one such practice that horrified the civilized world. Similarly appalling is the long history of abusive, nonconsensual sterilization of persons designated as "intellectually subnormal" or classified by other unprofessional, sometimes racist criteria. For many of these vulnerable members of society, reproduction was controlled by the state, which considered their reproduction to be a social menace.[60]

Ethical Case Study: Rights of Mother over the Zygote (Embryo)

The debate over gender-based health care is related to questions of reproductive rights and other issues, such as the sanctity of unborn human life and the relative value of the zygote and mother. In North America, Europe, and certain other countries, viable fetuses are protected *in utero* as "legal persons," entities who are protected by law and who possess legal rights. Some ethical issues in this area are illustrated by the following case:

A court of law orders a pregnant woman with placenta previa to have the fetus delivered by cesarean section. The woman insists on vaginal delivery and refuses elective cesarean section on grounds of religious belief. The obstetrician and the hospital fear that litigation against them will ensue if the fetus dies. A court injunction to perform a cesarean section without the mother's consent is granted. Fortunately, the woman has a successful vaginal delivery.[60]

What are the rights of the fetus, and should they override the mother's rights? In handing down the injunction, did the court violate the rights and autonomy of the mother? Were the caregivers justified in basing their actions on the fear of litigation?

A case such as this was documented along with its negative outcome: A mother and her fetus both died after the mother received a court-ordered, involuntary cesarean section requested by her physicians and the hospital.[60]

This new millennium brings with it great hopes of improving women's rights, health, and educational opportunities. "Just as health care and medical education are critical beacons in the struggle of a community to achieve its highest potential, the status of women and the professions they serve are decisive criteria,"[63] and these criteria are intrinsically related inasmuch as elevated health status is an outcome of elevated societal status.

THE FOUR PRINCIPLES OF ETHICS IN GLOBAL HEALTH AND CULTURE

In the past four decades, both the dialogue of global health ethics and that of clinical bioethics have benefited from articulation of the four principles of ethics, which include autonomy, beneficence, nonmaleficence, and justice. These principles have undergone several challenges, especially within the developing countries milieu,[64–66] but nonetheless provide a common moral language for use as an analytic framework for ethics-related dialogue.

Autonomy (from Greek *autos* self and *nomos* rule) designates a norm of respecting the decision-making capacities of autonomous persons.[66] The proper priority to be given this principle has formed the basis of much debate; in modern dialogue, the original sense of autonomy as self-rule (applied to the independent Greek states) has been extended to diverse meanings including self-governance, liberty rights, privacy, individual choice, freedom of the will, causing one's own behavior, and being one's own person.

Nonmaleficence is a term used to designate a norm of avoiding causation of harm.[66] Throughout the centuries the concepts and practice of nonmaleficence and beneficence have played a central role in medical ethics in all recorded cultures and civilizations. In the setting of global health, the moral objective of providing beneficence (doing good deeds) and avoiding harm assumes production of net benefit to one individual or to society. The maxim "Above all, do no harm" has thus been a foundational part of medical ethics teaching. This concept did not originate within the Hippocratic traditions of medical ethics despite the Hippocratic Oath itself, which states, "I will use treatment to help the sick according to my ability and judgment, but I will never use it to injure or wrong them."[66]

Beneficence—the flip side of nonmaleficence— describes a group of norms for providing benefit and for balancing benefit against risk and cost.[66] Accordingly, acts of mercy, kindness, and charity—colored by altruism, love, humanity, and a sense of obligation— drive global health work and its associated philanthropy.

Justice describes a group of norms for fairly distributing benefit, risk, and cost.[66] Justice is commonly understood as law or lawfulness; in the context of global health, the meaning of "justice" is closer to fairness and is considered a virtue. The concepts of legal justice, criminal justice, distributive justice, social justice, and the fair and equitable allocation of resources and benefits further refine the notion of justice. Philosophical theories and approaches to justice include egalitarianism, communitarianism, libertarianism, and utilitarianism. For constructive reflection on global health policies, various approaches with different emphases should be considered; the diverse problems in global delivery of health care are only partially addressed by any particular theory. Current emphasis on distributive justice focuses on equality, equity, and fairness, especially in allocating benefits and resources.

Aristotle's principle of formal justice or equality— that equals must be treated equally and that unequals must be treated unequally—is found in several theories of justice.[66] Many countries use one or several principles of distributive justice, such as "to each person an equal share," "to each person according to need," "to each person according to effort," "to each person according to contribution," "to each person according to merit," or "to each person according to free market exchanges."[66] In a related line of thinking, also used in constructing benchmarks of fairness, the Rawls-Daniel theories of fair and equal opportunity in health care have gained currency in global health ethics. *Virtue* is a moral quality, which, like character, addresses the ethics of the agent (whether human being, society, or nation). This moral quality is inherent in the human psyche and as such contrasts to the *active* quality of the four ethical principles (autonomy, beneficence, nonmaleficence, and justice), which refer to the ethics of action. Moral virtues and character are expressed in different measures. In contemplating virtue and human character, the ancient Greek philosophers—Socrates, Plato, and Aristotle—identified five character types ranging from the great-souled human being to the moral monster.[67] According to Plato, the cardinal virtues included courage, temperance, wisdom, and justice; and to these cardinal virtues Thomas Aquinas in the 13th century added the Christian values of faith, hope, and charity.[67] However, Aristotle believed that a stupid person could have no true virtue; like other ancient Greek philosophers, Aristotle emphasized perfectionistic ideals and ethics that could not accommodate the equality of democracy.[67]

Many virtues—including compassion, discernment, trustworthiness, integrity, and conscientiousness—are central to health professionals[66] and are equally admirable and desirable at many levels of global health care practice. Within the global binding matrix of values and ethics, these virtues have been made explicit by oaths whose recorded historical roots extend back to the great physician-surgeon Susruta of ancient India.[68] The idealistic, distinct professional ethics and morals incumbent on the practitioners were further refined over centuries. Similarly, the Oath of Hippocrates, the Oath of the Muslim Physicians, and the Oath of Maimonides transcended cultures and boundaries.

The famed physician, alchemist, and Taoist Sun Szu-Miao (AD 581-682) wrote perhaps the oldest ethical text in China, *On the Absolute Sincerity of Great Physicians*. This treatise emphasized compassion, humaneness, self-discipline, education, and rigorous conscientiousness.[69] Value-based ethics clearly dominated and continues to dominate in most nonNorth American cultures.

THE ROLE OF RELIGION IN GLOBAL HEALTH ETHICS: CHRISTIANITY, ISLAM, AND JUDAISM

Ethics are grounded in socio-cultural, philosophical, or religious convictions as well as in conventions deeply ingrained in the social fiber and culture of societies around the world. Health care choices and options are thus immensely influenced by religion. By their very nature, religions possess prescriptive moral ground rules for ethical judgment and fairness. The concept of God is named variously; examples include "the Force" or "the Light." The "Force" notion of God resembles the Heraclitus Logos—a universal "Fire" or energy.

As the cradle of 11 faiths, including the three major monotheistic faiths (Judaism, Christianity, and Islam) as well as Hinduism, Buddhism, Jainism, Confucianism, Shintoism, Baha'i, Taoism, and Zoroastrianism, Asia has a rich recorded tradition of values, ethics, and humanism. Ideals such as love, harmony, tolerance, respect, and reverence were often expressed in theological principles and as a way of life, whereas Western societies emphasized autonomy, justice, and rights—values that may be considered more measurable and practical.

In many societies, religion and culture influence greatly how health care services are perceived, developed, accessed, and built upon. In many cultures around the world, beliefs regarding causation of health and recovery from illness were significantly affected by belief in the power of the "evil eye" as well as other concepts, such as karma, kismet, magic, spells, incantations, possessions by ghosts or spirits (evil and good), jinn, devil, witches, voodoo, departed ancestors, bad humors, and gods. Charismatic and revivalist Christian churches share with others a powerful belief that sin is a cause of disease.

Ecological wisdom and sacredness of the universe (especially earth) is enshrined in many of the major religions along with the unique stature and nobility of the human being. Even now, the quality of life, the environment, consumption, and the ecological crisis are at the center of expanded religious dialogue and response.[70]

On the basis of global population size in 2005—estimated to be 6,446,131,400[71]—the most populous Christian denomination is Roman Catholicism (17.33 percent of the global population), followed by Protestantism (7.03 percent), and Orthodoxy (3.47 percent).[71] On the basis of the same global population estimate, the 1.3-billion-strong Muslim population is estimated to be 20.12 percent; Hindu, 13.34 percent; Buddhist, 5.89 percent; Sikh, 0.39 percent; Jewish, 0.23 percent; other religions, 12.61 percent; nonreligious, 12.03 percent, and atheist, 2.36 percent.[72] All these religions, as well as secularism, have influenced health ethics.

Catholic ethics are rooted in their foundational scripture, the Bible. Health-related Catholic ethics are informed further by more complex doctrines based on exegetical, philosophical deliberation and debate and by papal encyclical documents. Catholic health ethics are rooted also in faith and reason and emphasize the sanctity of life as well as the metaphysical concept of the human being as a composite entity.

The mainstream health ethics of Western culture owes much to Protestantism through behavior and articulation of secular values of body, soul, and spirit.[73] (This precept is shared by Muslims.) The Protestant (i.e., reformed) Christian Church consists of Lutherans, Presbyterians, Baptists, Episcopalians, Anglicans, Pentecostals, Methodists, Mennonites, and others.[73] Offshoots of Protestantism including The Church of Jesus Christ of Latter-Day Saints (Mormons), Seventh Day Adventists, Church of Christ Scientists, and Jehovah's Witnesses have developed distinct theologies and beliefs regarding prevention, illness, and medical care.[73] Some health-related church doctrines are liberal; others are fundamentalist.

Faith, love, fidelity, and the notion of grace temper the four ethical principles of beneficence, nonmaleficence, autonomy, and justice[74] The Christian belief that human life begins prenatally and extends to the afterlife following sojourn in this world is also shared by Muslims who focus on spiritual Islam (i.e., the Sufis and Ismailis). The belief and doctrinal position of the Catholic Church of the "right to life" plays a central, profound role in ongoing ethical debates regarding the beginning and end of life.

The Islamic world community has majority status in several countries of South Asia, Southwest Asia, North Africa, Central Asia, Southeast Asia, and sub-Saharan Africa. In addition, an estimated 5 to 6 million Muslims inhabit Europe, especially France, Chechnya, Kosovo, Albania, Bosnia and Herzegovina, and the Republic of Macedonia. In the United States, Muslims outnumber Jews and Presbyterians. 50 million Muslims live in China, and, if the population of Turkey is included, 84 million live in Europe.[72]

The internal coherence of Islamic theology, cosmology, anthropology, spirituality, faith, and practice has largely been ignored in the West, where the press and other media continue to focus on Islamic fundamentalism and fanaticism. Love, grace, and the yearning for the infinite are woven into the fabric of Muslim thought as much as in Christianity. Science of the soul, ethics, and morality also are tied to Islamic eschatology.

Health ethics in Islam is part of *adab*—proper manners, behavior, comport, etiquette, proper actions, procedure, or ethics as understood generally. Several historical works focus on ethics of rulers, princes, governors, ministers, judges, teachers, and medical students and practitioners.[72] High character, morality, humility, and piety form the core of Islamic ethics. Moderation, balance, and the middle way—the golden mean—are emphasized.[75]

In Islamic thought, a complex but infinite relationship exists between health ethics and spirituality. Like their predecessors in Greece and Persia, the great Muslim physicians of antiquity—al-Razi (Rhazes), Ibn Ridwan (d. 1067), and Ibn Sina (Avicenna, d. 428 A.H./1037 C.E.), whom Sir William Osler called "the prince of physicians"—were interested in the "psyche" (soul). Al-Razi's treatise *Spiritual Medicine*[76] and Avicenna's classic *Cannons* (*Ibn Sina*) traced illness to human behavior and morals.

As the foundational scripture of Islam, the Qur'an is neither a work of systematic theology nor an essay in science of moral discourse, definition, regulations, or laws; instead, it is a sourcebook of faith and external and internal spiritual transformation.[77] The Qur'an confirms the earlier teachings of the Torah and the Bible with regard to ethical and moral injunctions. The Qur'an as a revelation and as God's word was sent as a healing to humanity.[78] The sanctity and value of human life as referenced in the Qur'an is a reflection of Biblical references[79] along with the notion that the human being is created in God's image and is the custodian of nature. Islamic health ethics and bioethics are derived "from a combination of principles, duties and rights, and to a certain extent a call to virtue derived from revelation and tradition."[80] Critical to the understanding of ethics in Islamic thought is its tripartite division into three dimensions, consisting of works, faith, and perfection[81] (or activity, intellectuality, and spirituality).[82] Virtue (ihsan) is part of perfection and is mentioned more than 70 times in the Qur'an in references to both external and ethical good as well as to internal moral and spiritual good.[82]

The Islamic Organization for Medical Sciences (IOMS), located in Kuwait, has long been involved in issues of medical ethics and often interacts on cross-cultural ethical issues with the Council of International Organizations for Medical Sciences (CIOMS), located in Geneva. In 2004, at an IOMS conference in Cairo, the International Islamic Code for Medical and Health Ethics[83] was discussed with reference to the CIOMS International Ethical Guidelines Involving Human Subjects.[84] Specifically, each of the 21 CIOMS guidelines was presented along with a separate section titled "An Islamic Point of View."

These guidelines and their associated Islamic points of view were generally in agreement, but the Islamic statements were strong in their inclusion of religious language, whereas the CIOMS versions were clearly secular. In addition, whereas the major concern examined in the secular context was the nature and quality of the ethical principle in question, Islamic context included determination of whether the actor implementing the guidelines was a virtuous and ethical person. The conference facilitated active dialogue between IOMS and other participating Islamic organizations so as to deepen their mutual understanding and collaboration and develop constructive interaction between Islam and secular organizations. Materials from the conference were published in a book.[85]

The global Jewish population numbers 13 million, of which 5 million reside in the United States and 360,000 in Canada. The majority population of Israel consists of Orthodox, Reformed, and Conservative Jews.[86] The modern source of Jewish bioethics literature originates primarily from Orthodox Jewish sources, in which God's authority is supreme and unchallenged.[87] Moral and ethical deliberations rest on the Jewish law (Halacha), derived from the Torah and the Talmud.[87] The Jewish ethical notions are based on the infinite value of human life and aging. Illness and death are a natural part of life; and improvement of the patient's quality of life, for instance, requires constant commitment.[88] Human beings must act as responsible stewards in preserving their bodies, which actually belong to God. Thus, to save human life, human beings are duty-bound to violate other laws (except those prohibiting murder, incest, and public idolatry).[88] Patient autonomy is thus diminished; however, other rights associated with autonomy are protected. Suicide, euthanasia, withdrawing of treatment, and abortion (when the mother's life or health is not at risk) are prohibited by traditional Judaism.[88]

HUMAN RIGHTS IN RELATION TO GLOBAL HEALTH ETHICS

The visionary WHO constitution, adopted in 1946, emphasizes the central tenet of the "right to health":

The enjoyment of the highest attainable standard of health is one of the fundamental rights of every human being without distinction of race, religion, political belief, economic, or social condition.[89]

The right to health was further strengthened by the Universal Declaration of Human Rights (UDHR), which was signed on December 10, 1948[90] and enshrined the universal principles of freedom, dignity, and rights of individuals embedded in "reason and conscience." Article 25 of the UDHR is visionary in its broad outlook on health of the "global individual" and states that "everyone has the right to a standard of living adequate for the health and well-being of himself [sic], and his [sic] family, including food, clothing, housing, medical care and necessary social services."[90]

Several other declarations and treaties strongly advocated elimination of discrimination against women; bolstered the rights of children; emphasized elimination of all forms of discrimination, torture, and other inhuman or degrading treatment as well as punishment, intolerance, and discrimination based on religion and belief.[91] Ample evidence exists to demonstrate that a violation of any of these rights leads to ill health.

The 1978 WHO Declaration of Alma Ata identified equity, human rights, and social justice as essential elements for achieving health for all.[92] The 1993 World Bank Report titled *Investing in Health*[23] further supported and connected rights-based principles to global health development in alleviating poverty and ill health and granting empowerment through education.

The powerful language and concepts expressed in human rights declarations of global health ethics—including equity, fairness, and justice—have been harnessed by groups of health care providers and lawyers devoted to empowering people globally in issues relating to their health. Groups such as the International Physicians for Prevention of Nuclear War, Physicians for Social Responsibility, Physicians for Human Rights, Médecins Sans Frontières, Médecins du Monde, Global Lawyers and Physicians, the Consortium for Health and Human Rights, Amnesty International, and the [US] National Academy of Sciences Committee on Human Rights have developed effective strategies for promoting health and for preventing and treating diseases and destruction of ecology.[92]

In the new millennium, the language and action of human rights pervades global politics, law, morality, and health and is expanding rapidly—as it should in its role as a premier global health ethics principle. Dialogue on human rights is central for global health governance.

THE ROLE OF SCIENTIFIC RESEARCH IN ADVANCEMENT OF GLOBAL HEALTH ETHICS

Research is a quintessential tool for advancing global health, yet societies and nations worldwide have made uneven progress in the basic sciences, clinical sciences, and epidemiology. And like the research itself, ethical frameworks of research often suffer from lack of political will, poor economics, low levels of education, inadequate human resources, political corruption, and unexercised rights to information and justice.

Moreover, in the current context of global inequity in health research, 87 percent of a total US$12 trillion is spent globally on 16 percent of the world's population,[93] and 10 percent of the global disease burden attracts 90 percent of global expenditures on health research.[94] As an example of governmental priorities skewed away from health research, 66 percent of US government expenditure for research is spent for military research.[95]

Global public health interventions, vaccines, and drug trials (whether randomized, controlled, clustered, or operational) are frequently done without clearly having the good of subjects as an endpoint. Ethical research controls used in developed countries are easily abandoned when studies are done in resource-poor settings. The primary good inheres to the academicians and to the large pharmaceutical companies and global consortia that fund these studies. The intent of intervention is often not to promote sustainability and ongoing involvement in the community but to prove a scientific point and then move on. The process of globalization of research ethics commenced with Article 25 of the Universal Declaration of Human Rights, a pivotal document that emphasizes that the benefits of scientific research, must be accessible and of benefit to all mankind equally so as to address the injustice prevalent in earlier decades.[90] Designed by European physicians as a professional guideline, this physicians' code of ethics was subsequently adopted by the World Medical Assembly at the 1964 Helsinki Meeting. Since then, the "Declaration of Helsinki" has undergone several revisions.[96]

The 1993 World Human Rights conference, held in Vienna, adopted the following template for global cooperation on ethical research:

Everyone has the right to enjoy benefits of scientific progress and its applications . . . and notes that advances, notably in the biomedical and life sciences as well as information technology may have potentially adverse consequences for the integrity, dignity, and human rights, of the individual and calls for international coop-eration to ensure that human rights and dignity are fully respected in this area of universal concern.[97]

The UNESCO (IBC) document titled *Universal Declaration on Human Genome and Human Rights* succinctly affirms this statement and adds the language of nondiscrimination based on genetic characteristics.[98]

The CIOMS/WHO Guidelines reflect a paramount concern for protecting the rights and welfare of research subjects and of vulnerable individuals or groups. These guidelines are equally applicable in developed and developing countries. For instance, guideline 8 states that the research should be responsive to the health of the community and insists on familiarity with community customs, traditions, and priorities.[99] Guideline 15 states that the committees in both the sponsoring and hosting countries are responsible for conducting both scientific and ethical review. Equitable selection of subjects, privacy, and consent also are emphasized.[99–101]

GLOBAL HEALTH ETHICS: PRACTICAL ISSUES AND APPLICATIONS

To understand the practical issues and applications of global health ethics, various historical and ongoing ethical failures should be studied along with the remedial actions taken in response.

The "Doctors' Trial" at Nuremberg (1946–1947) led to indictment of 16 of the 23 Nazi German doctors, seven of whom were later executed by hanging, and nine of whom were imprisoned.[102] In this first-of-its-kind international trial, the physicians were convicted of murder and torture in the conduct of medical experiments on concentration camp inmates.[102] The central facts at issue in the trial related to physiological research experiments, such as high-altitude, hypothermia, and seawater experiments, which were ordered by the State to benefit German fliers and soldiers.[102]

The defense pointed out that ethics were "similarly compromised" during the Statesville Penitentiary experiments on malaria (conducted in Illinois, USA, on more than 800 prisoners) and that no written consent had been given by its subjects (prisoners) although they were supposedly informed and had supposedly consented.[102] With its ten standards, the Nuremberg ethical code was the first to establish the concepts of consent and full disclosure, including risks, benefits, safety, and the right to choose participation, protection of human subjects, avoidance of harm, use of initial animal studies, and a focus on useful research. This code merged Hippocratic ethics—with its maxim *primum non nocere* ("first, do no harm")—and human rights into a single code, thus widening the scope of research ethics. For the first time, consideration focused on the human subject, not the interests of either the researcher or the state.

Ethics violations committed in the United States early in the 20th century have included the use of prisoners as human subjects of research, a subject that has been reviewed extensively.[102] During the Nuremberg trials, the Nazi doctors drew attention to several instances of rights violations by American researchers; from the 1906 cholera experiments upon inmates of the Bilibid Prison in Manila (where fatalities resulted from accidental bubonic plague serum injections) to pellagra studies in Mississippi.[102]

Other ethical violations captured the attention of the American public: testicular implants in San Quentin State Prison, tuberculosis experiments at Denver's National Jewish Hospital, and several post-World War II experiments with plasmapheresis, chemical warfare agents, pain threshold, and hepatitis.[102]

Violations of ethics and human rights have occurred in many countries (including the former Communist countries of Europe) and continue today. Many of these violations have been documented and publicized in published literature.

Strict legislation came into effect in 1976, only after further unethical violations occurred. Examples of such violations included the thalidomide trials, the use of 22 senile patients for live cancer cell studies (at the Jewish Chronic Disease Hospital in New York City), and the Tuskegee syphilis experiments. Despite the Nuremberg pronouncements, researchers—including those working at major pharmaceutical and chemical companies—seemed unable to resist the wealth of test material contained within prisons.[102]

Ethics of Racial Profiling

CASE STUDY 1: RACIAL PROFILING OF BLOOD DONORS

Large inequalities exist globally in the distribution of safe blood: 80 percent of the world's population has access only to 20 percent of the world's blood supply.[103] Moreover, fewer than 30 percent of countries have nationwide blood transfusion services. Family members and paid donors are recognized sources of unsafe blood in approximately 50 percent of blood donations.[104] Each year, an estimated 80,000 to 160,000 people are infected with HIV as a result of receiving a blood transfusion.[105] The worldwide supply of safe transfusion products is thus inadequate, and tainted transfusion products are highly dangerous. Strategies are urgently needed for obtaining safe transfusion products effectively and efficiently. Epidemiologic data showing differences among some donor groups in rates of infection has led to instances of racial profiling in selection of blood donors.

Blood donation is thus an area of medical practice that has raised issues of global health ethics. In the context of national and global health, "racial profiling" and use of "race" and ethnicity for making medical decisions have been the subjects of debate in both national and global health contexts. At present, race is at best an imperfect surrogate associated with many other variables, including language, health beliefs, culture, and socioeconomic status.[57]

In South Africa, a policy of profiling by race, gender, and donor came to light in 2004 after the public learned that South African President Mbeke's blood donation had been discarded as a result of the policy.[106] This revelation raised several ethical questions. One such question was whether profiling by race (or gender) can be a fair and just (ethical) process for ensuring the safety of health care practitioners as well as the safety of persons who receive transfusion products. The urgency of this question was evident in 1999, when antenatal HIV seroprevalence was higher than 20 percent. HIV prevalence in the blood donor pool reached 0.26 percent, and an estimated 26 HIV-infected units had entered the blood supply. Since that time, the procedure for processing blood donations was changed so that it now costs an added $15 per unit. This new procedure avoids racial profiling, but how many nations can afford this added expense? Should it be a national budget priority?

This issue affects all nations regardless of their relative prosperity. In the United States in the early 1980s, for example, Haitian immigrants were identified by the US Centers for Disease Control and Prevention (CDC) as one of four major groups at risk for HIV/AIDS. In 1990, the US Food and Drug Administration refused to accept blood from Haitian donors.[107]

Ethics of Selection for Medical Treatment

The issue of selecting 3 million "lucky" persons globally to receive AIDS treatment by 2005 created an urgent problem for the WHO. The process should ensure transparency, fairness, and equality.[108] In this case, what constitutes distributive fairness? Should patients who have been "accidentally" infected by transfusions, health care workers at high risk, teachers, or tribal leaders have priority in receiving treatment over women and children? How was the transparency and fairness ensured?

Ethics of Research

CASE STUDY 2: A SHORT-TERM AIDS CLINICAL TRIAL IN A DEVELOPING COUNTRY

A pharmaceutical company has a new AIDS drug. The focus of the initial clinical trials is a Latin American country. Participants are selected by "lottery" for a year-long study to be carried out at a local clinic. The protocol requires other components for the multidrug "cocktail."

At the end of the year, the enrolled patients gain weight and can work, earn a living, and look after their household. Their CD4 counts have improved dramatically, and the viral loads are "undetectable." The company stops the trial.[109]

Who benefited from this study? Were the patients appropriately notified that they were participating in a study for one year only and that, after completion of the study, they would be released without drugs and that progress of the AIDS would consequently accelerate?

Was the developing country chosen because of lax ethical guidelines? Would the trial become ethically appropriate if local researchers participated? Were the company and investigators obligated to ensure drug subsidies or free drugs for study participants for a reasonable number of years, considering that drugs are required for lifelong suppression of HIV?

CASE STUDY 3: A PLACEBO-CONTROLLED STUDY IN A DEVELOPING COUNTRY

A study protocol showed that zidovudine (AZT) reduced perinatal transmission of HIV by 65 percent. Use of AZT was therefore considered highly efficacious therapy and rapidly became the standard of care in the United States. NIH and CDC subsequently sponsored randomized, placebo-controlled trials of alternative, less costly protocols of AZT.

Is the use of a placebo-control study protocol ethical in countries or communities where the standard of care is no drug or no other active intervention? Is the use of a placebo-control protocol in this case an example of scientific and imperialistic colonialism? Are the researchers in this case "mosquito scientists," that is, researchers who enter a country to extract blood samples and take them out of the country, releasing the results only at publication of the study?[110,111] Did the researchers consider the culture and health beliefs of the participants outside the United States?

The study rationale was that administering a placebo is justified when effective treatment exists, because placebo-controlled trials are the quickest way to validate drug efficacy. Is this argument valid?

CASE STUDY 4: THE TUSKEGEE SYPHILIS STUDY

The historic Tuskegee study of untreated syphilis was sponsored by the US Public Health Service and lasted for 40 years, beginning in 1932 and ending in 1973.[112–115] A total of 412 impoverished African American men with untreated syphilis were monitored and were compared with 204 disease-free men to determine the natural history of syphilis. The research continued despite availability of penicillin and despite the known fact that penicillin cures syphilis. No informed consent was signed by any of the 412 study participants.

Multiple serious ethical violations were committed in this study and were documented. Did the researchers have a valid argument when they stated that "these poor African American males probably would not have been treated anyway" and that the investigators were therefore "merely observing what would happen"?[112–115]

CASE STUDY 5: RACE AND STUDY DESIGN

In 1997, a total of 16 randomized trials were conducted in several African nations as well as the Dominican

Republic and Thailand to evaluate use effectiveness of a less-costly method of preventing perinatal transmission of HIV. A total of 17,000 pregnant women participated in the trials. In all except one trial, a placebo was used as the control. Subsequently, the study participants gave birth to more than 1,000 babies who were infected with HIV. None of the 16 trials was funded by either the CDC or the NIH.[116]

Did the fact that all participants were nonwhite represent an ethically questionable study design? Was this series of trials an example of exploitation because no benefits accrued to the study population beyond the study period?

CASE STUDY 6: CLINICAL TRIALS IN CHILDREN

A trial of a new antibiotic, trovafloxacin (Trovan, Pfizer, New York, NY), was conducted during a meningitis epidemic in Kano, Nigeria,[117] an impoverished city already devastated by concomitant outbreaks of cholera and measles. In a two-week period, six physicians employed by a large American pharmaceutical company conducted the trial in children by using an oral formulation of Trovan along with a reduced dose of the comparison drug, ceftriaxone. The study perpetrated several ethical breaches, including deviation from protocol, lack of informed consent, inaccurate recordkeeping, inadequate follow-up, and failure to offer subjects a choice of alternative treatment. In addition, no previous research was conducted to study the pharmacokinetics in children. The study thus violated Nigerian law as well as the Helsinki Declaration of Human Rights and the United Nations Convention on the Rights of Children. In its defense, the pharmaceutical company claimed that the study was "a philanthropic act."

Was this trial an example of opportunistic research that unscrupulously exploited the needs of a vulnerable population?

CASE STUDY 7: CLINICAL TRIALS AND THE STANDARD OF CARE

A placebo-controlled arm was included in a Ugandan clinical trial of various regimens of prophylaxis against tuberculosis in HIV-infected adults, most of whom had positive results of tuberculin skin tests.[118] Meanwhile, in the United States, the standard of care for HIV-infected persons with positive tuberculin skin test results called for prophylaxis against tuberculosis.

Should future studies in developing and developed countries include a placebo arm if a standard of care exists for other populations?[119,120]

Defining the Ethical Parameters of Global Health Research

Bhutta's discussion of ethics in global health research from the perspective of the developing world is valuable not only because it points out examples of poorly designed studies, but also because it illustrates studies done properly.[121] Important lessons are also learned from other studies, including the groundbreaking Gambian studies on hepatitis B and *Haemophilus influenzae* type b vaccine[122]; the Gadchiorli neonatal study of suspected sepsis in India[123]; and the randomized controlled trial of the effect of handwashing on child health.[124]

Another admired effort in epidemiology, the International Clinical Epidemiology Network (INCLEN), has successfully developed a sustainable network of clinical epidemiology units in the developing world with technical assistance from European and North American universities.[22,125] Focusing on health research needs in developing countries, where data are meager and often unreliable and where new health research needs and tools are prioritized in the national context, Morrow and Lansang[22] based their equity-oriented approach on the needs of people in developing countries. In the developing world, limited resources, expertise, and capacity for research, as well as poor infrastructure, competing national agendas, and loss of human resources (in the form of internal and external "brain drain") pose tremendous challenges. Implementation of ethical principles and creation of equitable, sustainable, mutually beneficial partnerships focusing on equity and societal needs require innovative solutions. The CIOMS[101] and the Swiss Commission Guidelines[126] clearly enunciated important principles and parameters for culturally sensitive, appropriate research. Central points included in the Swiss guidelines[126] include collective formulation of objectives; building mutual trust; sharing information, responsibility, and responses; developing networks; creating transparency; monitoring and evaluating the collaboration; disseminating and applying results equitably; increasing the research capacity; and building on past achievements.

Ethics of Responsibility

Western technologic, scientific, and informational civilization has created a massive gap in the moral–ethical arena, especially ecological concerns, including eradication of the rainforest; depletion of earth's atmospheric ozone layer; global warming; degradation of air, water, and soil quality; loss of biodiversity; species extinction; misuse of animals; disappearance of wetlands and open lands; and need for wilderness preservation and animal biotechnological interventions.[127]

Geologic deposits of sewage, garbage, and toxic waste provoked the comment, "Surely no creature other than the human being has ever managed to foul its nest in such short order."[128] Powerful industrial and commercial forces have unleashed tremendous hurt onto our biosystems and have shifted the naturally self-rejuvenating balance of the ecosystem—a balance that is closely interwoven with human health. Global health and eco-health are hurt by nations as well as by large corporations operating with unlimited ecological autonomy despite a local and global obligation to act as stewards of the earth and its resources. The WHO report, *Ecosystems and Human Well-being: Health Synthesis*, highlights the complex links between preservation of health and biodiversity, natural ecosystems, and human health and concludes, "Over the past 50 years, humans have changed natural ecosystems more rapidly and extensively than in any comparable period in human history."[129]

CASE STUDY 8: CONFLICT OF INTEREST

In 2000, a group of 30,000 indigenous persons and peasants filed a lawsuit against an oil company operating in Ecuador, accusing the oil company of inflicting irreparable damage to the Amazon rainforest. The lawsuit was dismissed by a US court.[130] Negative consequences of oil exploitation have occurred also in Bolivia, Colombia, Peru, and other Latin American and Asian countries.

In evaluating the merits of this case, consider the following two statements:

- "Oil is a major source of income for Ecuador and since the 1970s has been the 'engine' of the nation's economy, which averages 7 percent growth annually. Per capita income rose from US $290 in 1972 to US $1,200 in 2000, and oil makes up 40 percent of the national budget. Petroecuador, the government-owned company, is responsible for 55 percent of the total oil production."[130]

- Morbidity and mortality rates in oil-producing areas are higher than in communities without this involvement.

What should be the ethical response of the government? What should be the response and responsibility of all oil companies? Does the WHO or the United Nations have a role in this situation? Is this case an example of a human rights violation?

CASE STUDY 9: CONFLICTS OF INTEREST CONCERNING PANDEMICS

In 1918, a total of 20 to 50 million people perished from the "Spanish flu," a strain of influenza, which seems to have been a variant of the avian flu virus.[131] The HIV epidemic has caused more than 13 million children to become orphaned. The late-20th-century limited outbreak of SARS and subsequent threat of pandemic avian influenza refocused global energy on planning and on ethical and legal issues such as equity, access, fair process, vulnerability, civic engagement, and allocation of existing resources globally and locally.[131] Regulation, intellectual property, market incentives, and liability issues have further added more complex ramifications.

In ethical planning regarding higher attack rates in younger, healthy populations and regarding availability of scarce resources, does an altruistic, equity-based process take precedence over a selection process favoring intergenerational group priority, e.g., for the elderly, the frail, the chronically ill, infants, and pregnant females?[131] How should such consideration be applied in sub-Saharan nations? The SARS outbreak in Toronto raised further questions, such as risks to providers and their families. Key ethical issues and underlying values such as individual liberty, protection of the public from harm, proportionality, reciprocity, transparency, privacy, protection of communities from undue stigmatization, duty to provide care, equity, and solidarity have been highlighted.[132]

Therapeutic and Reproductive Cloning and Stem Cell Research: Ethical Challenges

Now that mapping and sequencing of the human genome has enabled human beings to look into the mirror of self cloning, current debate focuses on the science of cloning (especially reproductive cloning), cloning technologies, stem cell research applications, and moral consequences of these activities. This novel encounter with the basic elements of life, prospects of self regeneration, and the ability to choose future progeny has led all religions to ban cloning of an entire human being.

Cloning Californians? The Report of the California Advisory Committee on Human Cloning[133] summarized notes for members of the California State Legislature on the ethics of human cloning and stem cell research and addressed some complex aspects of the debates. Limited stem cell research is currently occurring globally after successful cloning of sheep (despite adverse consequences to the test animals).

At the beginning of this new millennium, a global consensus across nations and faiths states that reproductive cloning should not be allowed. The most robust opposition to all forms of cloning has been declared by the Roman Catholic Church, which is spread across several countries. Differences of opinion between Arab states and other Muslim nations have been expressed. Some of these Muslim countries have conducted highly advanced genomic research, whereas some Arab states are considering a region-wide ban on human cloning. Participants at the November 2003 session of the United Nations General Assembly reached no consensus on the issue of cloning; the General Assembly voted instead to await recommendations from the Organization of the Islamic Conference.[134]

Ethical debate on cloning remains within the matrix of religious beliefs, values, and norms of societies and within the progress of science: increasingly, however, therapeutic cloning is gaining favor as its central concepts and objectives relate to curing disease as well as improving health and quality of life for all humanity. Nonetheless, as of this writing, regenerative cloning has been banned globally by all major religions. Limited research on human cloning for harvesting stem cells is occurring in the United Kingdom, Japan, and the United States. Current thorny, fundamental debate centers on the concept of life itself. Is the embryo a "human being": after the second week of gestation (when differentiation of the sensory system begins), after the third week (when early signs of heartbeat can be detected), when fetal movement occurs as noted by ultrasound (at the tenth week of gestation), or when the fetal movements are first noticed by the mother (at 16 weeks of gestation)?[134]

In Islam, three stages of inception have been defined: the fusion of the "spermed" ovum (zygote stage); implantation; and "ensoulment" at 120 days of inception. Some believe that the latter occurs at the 40th day.[134]

Today, consensus in Islam maintains that any debate on cloning need not rest on scientific merit alone and that advances in science should not be regarded as a threat to religious belief as long as human dignity, values, and cultures are honored.

TOWARD A BRAVE NEW VISION OF GLOBAL HEALTH ETHICS IN THE NEW MILLENNIUM

Kofi Annan's poignant and pragmatic reminder of the "Butterfly Effect" is indeed the new ethical world order:

"Today's real borders are not between nations, but between powerful and powerless, free and fettered, privileged and humiliated. Today, no walls can separate humanitarian or human rights crises in one part of the world from national security crises in another."[135]

The global human being must be the focus of global health ethics as proclaimed by the WHO charter[135] and by the United Nations Charter. If the 19th century was the century of Public health action and the 20th century, that of International Health and the beginning of Global Health, then the 21st century will certainly be defined by a new and more profound awareness of health ethics, rights, equity, fairness, justice, and solidarity, each concept centered on the dignity of the global human being. We entered the new millennium through a "gate of fire"—the tragedy and horror of September 11, 2001, which was masterminded by one global human being. Similarly, genocide and ethnic "cleansing" begins with the killing of one global human being, not for what was done but because of who that individual is.[129] "What begins with failure to uphold the dignity of one life, all too often ends with calamity for entire nations."[135]

Accordingly, the United Nations has outlined three key priorities for the new millennium: *eradicating poverty, preventing conflict,* and *promoting democracy.* These priorities are also key elements in ensuring health advancement. They are of paramount importance if the 21st century is to show improvement over the 20th century, which saw numerous and extensive wars, violence, hatred, poverty, exploitation, ethnic "cleansing," and other human violations that caused millions of people to lose their lives or become permanently injured or displaced.

The ethical values and principles enshrined in the covenants and oaths of the global physician are increasingly being challenged by a new world order that emphasizes consumerism and greed at the expense of health. Historically, like the medical profession's central dictum—that disease and illness transcend boundaries and borders—"cybernations" also transport knowledge and cures across borders and across castes, creeds, religions, and cultures. Certain universal guiding principles and values bind all physicians and health care providers—and even more so the global health physician in unremitting pursuit of health for all. Taylor[68] outlined such ethical principles for the "international physician" in a "free version of the Hippocratic Oath" (see Table 16-4), which still relates well to the global health physician.

Worldwide application of global health ethics requires the competent cooperation of all the world's governments. Currently, however, global public health governance is justifiably perceived as antiquated and structurally weak.[136,137] Ethical reform processes are needed to address national and global governance in this 21st

Table 16-4. Taylor's "Free Version of the Hippocratic Oath."[a]

- I will share the science and art by precept, by demonstration, and by every mode of teaching with other physicians regardless of their national origin.
- I will try to help secure for the physicians in each country the esteem of their own people, and through collaborative work see that they get full credit.
- I will strive to eliminate sources of disease everywhere in the world and not merely set up barriers to the spread of disease to my own people.
- I will work for understanding of the diverse causes of diseases, including social, economic, and environmental.
- I will promote the well-being of mankind in all its aspects, not merely the bodily, with sympathy and consideration for a people's culture and beliefs.
- I will strive to prevent painful and untimely death, and also help parents to achieve a family size conforming to their desires and to their ability to care for their children. In my concern with whole communities I will never forget the needs of its individual members.

[a] Taylor CE. Ethics for an international health profession. *Science* 1966 Aug 12;153(3737):716–20. (Reproduced with permission.)

century amid threatened and spreading global violence, novel health challenges, and loss of many health gains acquired during the past two centuries. Transforming the words of treaties, declarations, and understandings into practical reality cannot take place in a vacuum of autonomy claimed by powerful nations, dictators, or global corporations; indeed, insular self-interests as well as relevant, limited aspects of state sovereignty have recently been relinquished to address transnational health threats such as SARS and avian influenza.

In a collective partnership nurtured by ethics and harmony, civil societies must be reenergized and empowered to protect individual health and rights, because these rights—primarily health security and well-being— are intimately tied to societal obligations. To achieve these goals, ethical concepts operating for the good of all human beings—the global person—have been described by a vocabulary first recorded many centuries ago. Ancient Asian concepts of harmony, tolerance, values, and love can serve as bridges to more concrete practical, secular Western concepts of ethics.[138]

STUDY QUESTIONS

See each case study above for study questions on various global health ethical issues.

ACKNOWLEDGMENTS

Bibliographic assistance was provided by Yvonne Sargent, AA, and Michael W. Bennett, MSLS, AHIP.

Editorial assistance was provided by the staff of the Medical Editing Service of The Permanente Medical Group Physician Education and Development Department: Lila Schwartz, BA, JD; David W. Brown, MLS, MA; Janet H. Startt, MA; and Juan Domingo, BA.

REFERENCES

1. Declaration of Alma-Ata. International Conference on Primary Health Care, Alma-Ata, USSR, September 6–12, 1978 [monograph on the Internet]. [Cited 2006 Apr 6]. http://www.who.int/hpr/NPH/docs/declaration_almaata.pdf.

2. Singer PA, Pellegrino ED, Siegler M. Clinical ethics revisited. *BMC Med Ethics* 2001;2:E1. Epub 2001 Apr 26.

3. Jonsen A. The origins of bioethics in the United States of America. In: Bankowski Z, Bryant JH, eds. *Poverty, vulnerability, the value of human life, and the emergence of bioethics: highlights and papers of the XXVIIIth CIOMS Conference, Ixtapa, Guerrero State, Mexico, 17-20 April 1994.* Geneva: CIOMS; 1994: 38–40.

4. Mainetti JA. Academic and mundane bioethics in Argentina. In: Pellegrino E, Mazzarella P, Corsi P, eds. *Transcultural dimensions in medical ethics.* Frederick, MD: University Publishing Group; 1992:43–55.

5. Pellegrino ED. Prologue: Intersections of Western biomedical ethics and world culture. In: Pellegrino E, Mazzarella P, Corsi P. *Transcultural dimensions in medical ethics.* Frederick, MD: University Publishing Group; 1992:13–9.

6. Velji AM, ed. International health: beyond the year 2000. *Infect Dis Clin North Am* 1995 Jun;9(2):223–461 [entire issue].

7. Global Health Education Consortium [home page on the Internet]. New York: Global Health Education Consortium; c2005 [cited 2006 Jun 26]. www.globalhealth-ec.org

8. Stuck C, Bickley LS, Wallace N, et al. International Health Medical Education Consortium: its history, philosophy, and role in medical education and health development. *Infect Dis Clin North Amer* 1995 Jun;9(2):419–23.

9. Bryant JH. [Opening of the conference]. In: Bankowski Z, Bryant JH, Gallagher J, eds. *Ethics, equity and the renewal of WHO's health-for-all strategy: proceedings of the XXIXth CIOMS Conference, Geneva, Switzerland, 12-14 March 1997.* Geneva: CIOMS, 1997:1–3.

10. Nakajima H. [Opening of the conference]. In: Bankowski Z, Bryant JH, Gallagher J, eds. *Ethics, equity and the renewal of WHO's health-for-all strategy: proceedings of the XXIXth CIOMS Conference, Geneva, Switzerland, 12-14 March 1997.* Geneva: CIOMS, 1997:4–6.

11. Delamothe T. Embargoes that endanger health [editorial]. *BMJ* 1997 Nov 29;315(7120):1393–4.

12. Fort M, Mercer MA, Gish O, eds. *Sickness and wealth: the corporate assault on global health.* Cambridge, MA: South End Press, 2004.

13. Kim JY, Millen JV, eds. *Dying for growth: global inequality and the health of the poor.* Monroe, ME: Common Courage Press, 2000.

14. Bankowski Z, Bryant JH, Gallagher J, eds. *Ethics, equity and the renewal of WHO's health-for-all strategy: proceedings of the XXIXth CIOMS Conference, Geneva, Switzerland, 12–14 March 1997.* Geneva: CIOMS, 1997.

15. Taylor CE. Ethical issues influencing health for all beyond the year 2000. *Infect Dis Clin North Amer* 1995 Jun;9(2): 223–33.

16. Taylor CE. Surveillance for equity in primary health care: policy implications from international experience. *Int J Epidemiol* 1992 Dec;21(6):1043–9.

17. Whitehead M. William Farr's legacy to the study of inequalities in health. *Bull World Health Organ* 2000;78(1):86–7.

18. Gwatkin DR. Health inequalities and the health of the poor: What do we know? What can we do? *Bull World Health Organ* 2000;78(1):3–18.

19. Evans T, Whitehead M, Diderichsen F, et al., eds. *Challenging inequalities in health: from ethics to action.* New York: Oxford University Press, 2001.

20. Brock D. Working Group III. Measurement/surveillance for equity: health status and health systems functions. In: Bankowski Z, Bryant JH, Gallagher J, eds. *Ethics, equity and the renewal of WHO's health-for-all strategy: proceedings of the XXIXth CIOMS Conference, Geneva, Switzerland, 12–14 March 1997.* Geneva: CIOMS, 1997:171–3.

21. Morrow R, Bryant JH. Measuring and valuing human life: cost-effectiveness, equity and other ethics-based issues. In: Bankowski Z, Bryant JH, eds. *Poverty, vulnerability, the value of human life, and the emergence of bioethics: highlights and papers of the XXVIIIth CIOMS Conference, Ixtapa, Guerrero State, Mexico, 17–20 April 1994.* Geneva: CIOMS, 1994:53–6.

22. Morrow RH Jr, Lansang MA. The role of clinical epidemiology in establishing essential national health research capabilities in developing countries. *Infect Dis Clin North Am* 1991 Jun;5(2):235–46.

23. World Bank. World development report 1993: investing in health [monograph on the Internet]. New York: Oxford University Press, 1993 [cited 2006 Jun 29]. http://web.worldbank.

org/WBSITE/EXTERNAL/EXTDEC/EXTRESEARCH/EXTWDRS/0,,contentMDK:20308780~menuPK:604546~pagePK478093~piPK:477627~theSitePK:477624,00.html.

24. Murray CJ. Quantifying the burden of disease: the technical basis for disability-adjusted life years. *Bull World Health Organ* 1994;72(3):429–45.

25. Murray CJ. Understanding DALYs (disability-adjusted life years). *J Health Econ* 1997 Dec;16(6):703–30.

26. Caplan RL, Light DW, Daniels N. Benchmarks of fairness: a moral framework for assessing equity. *Int J Health Serv* 1999; 29(4):853–69.

27. Daniels N, Bryant J, Castano RA, et al. Benchmarks of fairness for healthcare reform: a policy tool for developing countries. *Bull World Health Organ* 2000;78(6):740–8.

28. Daniels N, Flores W, Pannarunothai S, et al. An evidence-based approach to benchmarking the fairness of health-sector reform in developing countries. *Bull World Health Organ* 2005 Jul;83(7):534–40.

29. Ntuli A, Khosa S, McCoy D. The equity gauge [monograph on the Internet]. Salmon Grove (Durban): Health Systems Trust, 1999 [cited 2006 Jun 28]. http://www.hst.org.za/publications/104.

30. Joint United Nations Program on HIV/AIDS, United Nations Children's Fund, and United States Agency for International Development. Children on the brink 2004: a joint report of new orphan estimates and a framework for action [monograph on the Internet]. New York: United Nations Children's Fund, 2004 [cited 2006 May 24]. http:// www.unicef.org/publications/files/cob_layout6-013.pdf.

31. Population and health dynamics in Nairobi's informal settlements: report of the Nairobi Cross-Sectional Slums Survey (NCSS) 2000 [monograph on the Internet]. Nairobi, Kenya: African Population and Health Research Center, 2002 [cited 2006 May 24]. http://www.aphrc.org/publication/aphrc_ncssreport_26april2002_final.pdf.

32. United Nations Human Settlements Programme. *The challenge of the slums: global report on human settlements 2003*. Nairobi, Kenya: United Nations Human Settlements Programme, 2003.

33. Subbarao K, Coury D. Reaching out to Africa's orphans: a framework for public action [monograph on the Internet]. Washington, DC: World Bank, 2004 [cited 2006 May 24]. http://siteresources.worldbank.org/INTHIVAIDS/Resources/375798-1103037153392/ReachingOuttoAfricasOrphans.pdf.

34. Committee on Integrating the Science of Early Childhood Development; Shonkoff JP, Phillips DA, eds. From neurons to neighborhoods: the science of early childhood development [monograph on the Internet]. Washington, DC: National Academy Press, 2000 [cited 2006 May 24]. http://www.nap.edu/books/0309069882/html/.

35. The importance of caregiver-child interactions for the survival and healthy development of young children: a review [monograph on the Internet]. Geneva: Department of Child and Adolescent Health Development, World Health Organization, 2004 [cited 2006 May 24]. http://www.who.int/child-adolescent-health/publications/CHILD_HEALTH/ISBN_92_4_159134_X.htm.

36. Feachem RG. Poverty and equity: a proper focus for the new century. *Bull World Health Organ* 2000;78(1):1–2.

37. Mann J, Tarantola D. The global AIDS pandemic: toward a new vision of health. *Infect Dis Clin North Am* 1995 Jun; 9(2):275–85.

38. World Bank. Annual report 2005 [monograph on the Internet]. Washington, DC: The World Bank; 2005 [cited 2006 Jun 28]. http://web.worldbank.org/WBSITE/EXTERNAL/EXTABOUTUS/EXTANNREP/0,,menuPK:1397243~pagePK:64168427~piPK:64168435~theSitePK:1397226,00.html.

39. World Bank. Development Data Group. Millennium development goals [homepage on the Internet]. Washington, DC: The World Bank, Development Data Group, 2004. [Cited 2006 Jun 28]. http://ddp-ext.worldbank.org/ext/GMIS/home.do? siteId=2.

40. Sachs JD, McArthur JW. The Millennium Project: a plan for meeting the Millennium Development Goals. *Lancet* 2005 Jan 22–28;365(9456):347–53.

41. Velji AM. International health: Beyond the year 2000. *Infect Dis Clin North Am* 1991 Jun;5(2):417–28.

42. Umhau TH, Umhau JC, Morgan RE Jr. National and international health agencies: profile of key players. *Infect Dis Clin North Am* 1991 Jun;5(2):197–220.

43. Howard LM. Public and private donor financing for health in developing countries. *Infect Dis Clin North Am* 1991 Jun;5(2):221–34.

44. Cohen J. The new world of global health. *Science* 2006 Jan 13;311(5758):162–7.

45. Bissell RE. Project selection: many needs, few resources. *Infect Dis Clin North Am* 1995 Jun;9(2):377–89.

46. Marmot M. Social determinants of health inequalities. *Lancet* 2005 Mar 19–25;365(9464):1099–104.

47. Labonte R, Schrecker T, Grupta AS. A global health equity agenda for the G8 summit. *BMJ* 2005 Mar 5;330(7490):533–6.

48. Osuntokun B. A developing-country perspective on the emergence of bioethics. In: Bankowski Z, Bryant JH, eds. *Poverty, vulnerability, the value of human life, and the emergence of bioethics: highlights and papers of the XXVIIIth CIOMS Conference, Ixtapa, Guerrero State, Mexico, 17-20 April 1994*. Geneva: CIOMS, 1994:42–6.

49. World Bank. World development report 1994: infrastructure for development [monograph on the Internet]. New York: Oxford University Press, 1994 [cited 2006 Jun 28]. http://www-wds.worldbank.org/external/default/WDSContentServer/IW3P/IB/1994/06/01/000009265_3970716142907/Rendered/PDF/multi0page.pdf.

50. Abbasi K. Free the slaves [editorial]. *BMJ* 1999 Jun 12; 318(7198):1568–9.

51. Crossette B. Kofi Annan's astonishing facts! *NY Times* [serial on the Internet]. 1998 Sep 27 [cited 2006 Jun 28]:[about 3 screens]. http://www.nytimes.com/learning/general/featured_articles/980928monday.html.

52. Carter J. The Nobel lecture given by the Nobel Peace Prize laureate 2002, Jimmy Carter (Oslo, December 10, 2002) [homepage on the Internet]. [Cited 2006 Jun 28]. [About 6 screens]. http://www.nobel.no/eng_lect_2002b.html.

53. United Nations Development Programme. Human Development Report 2000: human rights and human development [monograph on the Internet]. New York: Oxford University Press, 2000 [cited 2006 Jun 28]. http://hdr.undp.org/reports/global/2000/en/.

54. Handful hog most of the wealth. *Business Times* (Johannesburg, South Africa) [serial on the Internet]. 1998 Sep 13 [cited 2006 Jun 28]. http://www.btimes.co.za/98/0913/world/world04.htm.

55. Mukherjee J. Global injustice. In: Fort M, Mercer MA, Gish O, eds. *Sickness and wealth: the corporate assault on global health*. Cambridge, MA: South End Press, 2004:xv.

56. Lee SS, Mountain J, Koenig BA. The meaning of "race" in the new genomics: implications for health disparities research. *Yale J Health Policy Law Ethics* 2001 Spring;1:33–75.

57. American Anthropological Association [homepage on the Internet]. Arlington, VA: The Association; 1996–2006. [Cited 2006 Jun 28]. American Anthropological Association response to OMB Directive 15: race and ethnic standards for federal statistics and administrative reporting. http://www.aaanet.org/gvt/ombdraft.htm.

58. Barth F. Introduction. In: Barth F, editor. *Ethnic groups and boundaries: the social organization of cultural differences.* Boston: Little Brown, 1969:9–38.

59. Curlin P, Tinker A. Women's health. *Infect Dis Clin North Am* 1995 Jun;9(2):335–51.

60. Cook RJ, Dickens BM, Fathalla MF. *Reproductive health and human rights: integrating medicine, ethics, and law.* Oxford: Clarendon Press, 2003.

61. Grant GP. *The state of the world's children 1992.* New York: Oxford University Press, 1992.

62. World Health Organization. Safe abortion: technical and policy guidance for health systems [monograph on the Internet]. Geneva: The Organization, 2003 [cited 2006 Jun 28]. http://www.who.int/reproductive-health/publication/safe_abortion/safe_abortion.pdf.

63. H.H. The Aga Khan. Inaugural address, November 15, 1990 at Aga Khan University School of Nursing. Quoted in: Velji AM. Preface. *Infect Dis Clin North Am* 1991 Jun;5(2):xii–xv.

64. Gillon R. Medical ethics: four principles plus attention to scope. *BMJ* 1994 Jul 16;309(6948):184–8.

65. Gillon R. Ethics needs principles—four can encompass the rest—and respect for autonomy should be "first among equals." *J Med Ethics* 2003 Oct;29(5):307–12.

66. Beauchamp TL, Childress JF. *Principles of Biomedical Ethics, Fifth Edition.* New York: Oxford University Press, 2001.

67. Pence G. Virtue theory. In: Singer P, ed. *A companion to ethics.* Oxford: Blackwell, 1991:249–58.

68. Taylor CE. Ethics for an international health profession. *Science* 1966 Aug 12;153(737):716–20.

69. Tsai DF. Ancient Chinese medical ethics and the four principles of biomedical ethics. *J Med Ethics* 1999 Aug;25(4):315–21.

70. Center for the Study of World Religions [homepage on the Internet]. Cambridge, MA: The Center, 2005 [last modified 2005 Jun 5; cited 2006 Jun 28]. Tucker ME, Grim J. Series forward: the nature of the environmental crisis; [about 12 screens]. http://www.hds.harvard.edu/cswr/research/ecology/foreword.html.

71. Central Intelligence Agency. The world factbook [monograph on the Internet]. Washington, DC: The Agency, 2006. http://www.cia.gov/cia/publications/factbook/geos/xx.html.

72. Muslim population estimated at 1.1 to 1.2 billion. Wikipedia. Muslim world [homepage on the Internet]. [Cited 2006 Jun 27]. http://en.wikipedia.org/wiki/Muslim_World.

73. Pauls M, Hutchinson RC. Bioethics for clinicians: 28. Protestant bioethics. *CMAJ* 2002 Feb 5;166(3):339–43.

74. Markwell HJ, Brown BF. Bioethics for clinicians: 27. Catholic bioethics. *CMAJ* 2001 July 24;165(2):189–92.

75. "We have made you a community of the middle path." (Qur'an 2:143)

76. Al-Razi. *The spiritual physick of Rhazes.* London: Murray, 1950

77. "But often the Qur'an has been the prisoner of the interpreters rather than their source and guide." Denny FM. Ethics and the Qur'an: community and world view. In: Hovannisian RG, ed. *Ethics in Islam.* Malibu, CA: Undena Publications, 1985:103–21.

78. "We have revealed of the Qur'an that which is a healing and a mercy for those who have faith" (Qur'an 17:82)

79. "Whosoever takes a life except to combat murder and villainy on earth it is as if he killed all humankind; and whosoever saves a life, it is as though all humankind is saved" (Qur'an 5:32)

80. Daar AS, Khitamy BA. Bioethics for clinicians: Islamic bioethics. *CMAJ* 2001 Jan 9;164(1):60–3.

81. True piety is this: "To have faith in God, the Last Day, the Angels, the Book, and the Prophets" (Qur'an 2:177)

82. Chittick WC, trans. *Faith and practice of Islam: three thirteenth century Sufi texts.* Albany, NY: State University of New York Press, 1992.

83. Islam Set. Islamic Organization for Medical Sciences [homepage on the Internet]. [cited 2006 Jul 7]. International Conference on "Islamic Code of Medical Ethics," December, 11–14, 2004; Cairo, Egypt; [about 1 screen]. http://www.islamset.com/ioms/Code2004/index.html.

84. Council for International Organizations of Medical Sciences (CIOMS), World Health Organization, Islamic Organization for Medical Sciences. International ethical guidelines for biomedical research involving human subjects: an Islamic perspective [monograph on the Internet]. Geneva: CIOMS, 2004 [cited 2006 Jul 7]. http://www.islamset.com/ioms/ Code2004/index.html.

85. El-Gendy AR, ed. *International Islamic code for medical and health ethics.* Kuwait: Islamic Organization for Medical Sciences, 2005.

86. Goldsand G, Rosenberg ZR, Gordon M. Bioethics for clinicians: 22. Jewish bioethics. *CMAJ* 2001 Jan 23;164(2):219–22.

87. Felman DM. *Health and medicine in the Jewish tradition: l'hayyim—to life.* New York: Crossroad, 1986.

88. Meier L. Three cardinal principles of Jewish medical ethics. In: Meier L, ed. *Jewish values in health and medicine.* Lanham, MD: University Press of America, 1991.

89. World Health Organization. Constitution of the World Health Organization [monograph on the Internet]. [Cited 2006 Jun 28]. http://www.searo.who.int/LinkFiles/About_Searo_const.pdf.

90. Universal declaration of human rights [monograph on the Internet]. [Cited 2006 Jun 29]. http://www.un.org/Overview/rights.html.

91. Mann JM, Gostin L, Gruskin S, et al. Health and human rights. *Health Hum Rights* 1994 Fall;1(1):6–23.

92. Annas GJ. Human rights and health—the Universal Declaration of Human Rights at 50. *New Engl J Med* 1998 Dec 10;339(24):1778–81.

93. Iglehart JK. The American health care system: expenditures. *New Engl J Med* 1999 Jan 7;340(1):70–6.

94. Commission Health Research for Development. *Health research: essential link to equity development.* New York: Oxford University Press, 1990.

95. Sivard RL. *World Military and Social Expenditures, Sixteenth Edition.* Washington, DC: World Priorities Press, 1996.

96. World Medical Association [homepage on the Internet]. Ferney-Voltaire, France: The Association, 2003 [updated 2004 Oct 9; cited 2006 Jun 29]. World Medical Association declaration of Helsinki; [about 4 screens]. http://www.wma.net/e/policy/b3.htm.

97. United Nations. General Assembly. World Conference on Human Rights. Report of the World Conference on Human

Rights [monograph on the Internet]. Geneva: Office of the United Nations High Commissioner of Human Rights, 1996–2000 [cited 2006 Jun 29]. http://193.194.138.190/huridocda/huridoca.nsf/(Symbol)/A.CONF.157.24+(PART+I).En?OpenDocument.

98. Mayor F. Message from Federico Mayor, Director-General, UNESCO. In: Bankowski Z, Bryant JH, Gallagher J, eds. *Ethics, equity and the renewal of WHO's health-for-all strategy: proceedings of the XXIXth CIOMS Conference, Geneva, Switzerland, 12–14 March 1997.* Geneva: CIOMS, 1997:7.

99. Bankowski Z, Levine RJ. A decade of the CIOMS programme: health policy, ethics and human values: an international dialogue. In: Bankowski Z, Bryant JH, eds. *Poverty, vulnerability, the value of human life, and the emergence of bioethics: highlights and papers of the XXVIIIth CIOMS Conference, Ixtapa, Guerrero State, Mexico, 17–20 April 1994.* Geneva: CIOMS, 1994:13–25.

100. Bankowski Z, Bryant JH, Last JM, eds. *Ethics and epidemiology: international guidelines: proceedings of the XXVth CIOMS Conference, Geneva, Switzerland, 7–9 November 1990: co-sponsored by the World Health Organization.* Geneva: CIOMS, 1991.

101. Council for International Organizations of Medical Sciences. International ethical guidelines for biomedical research involving human subjects: prepared by the Council for International Organizations of Medical Sciences (CIOMS) in collaboration with the World Health Organization (WHO) [monograph on the Internet]. Geneva: CIOMS, 2002 [cited 2006 Jun 29]. http://www.cioms.ch/guidelines_nov_2002_blurb.htm.

102. Hornblum AM. They were cheap and available: prisoners as research subjects in twentieth century America. *BMJ* 1997 Nov 29;315(7120):1437–41.

103. World Health Organization. Regional Office for the Western Pacific [homepage on the Internet]. Manila, Philippines: The Office, 2004 [cited 2006 Jun 29]. WHO: protect the public from contaminated blood: 55th session of The WHO Regional Committee [press release] [about 1 screen]. http://www.wpro.who.int/media_centre/press releases/pr_20040916_3.htm.

104. World Health Organization. Regional Office for the Western Pacific [homepage on the Internet]. Manila, Philippines: The Office, 2004 [cited 2006 Jun 29]. Fact sheets: blood safety and voluntary donations. 2004 Jun 10 [about 2 screens]. http://www.wpro.who.int/media_centre/fact_sheets/fs_20040610.htm.

105. Blood supply and demand [editorial]. *Lancet* 2005 Jun 25–Jul 1; 365(9478):21–51.

106. Henry Kaiser Family Foundation [homepage on the Internet]. Menlo Park, CA: The Foundation, 2004 Dec 7 [cited 2006 Jun 29]. Global challenges: South African blood service to stop calculating donors' risk of HIV infection based on race [about 2 screens]. http://kaisernetwork.org/daily_reports/rep_index.cfm?hint=1&DR_ID=27102.

107. Donor exclusion policy under review. *FDA Consumer* 1990 Jul–Aug;24(6):6.

108. Daniels N. Fair process in patient selection for antiretroviral treatment in WHO's goal of 3 by 5. *Lancet* 2005 Jul 9–15;366 (9480):169–71.

109. Edejer TT. North-South research partnerships: the ethics of carrying out research in developing countries. *BMJ* 1999 Aug 14;319(7207):438–41.

110. Angell M. The ethics of clinical research in the Third World. *New Engl J Med* 1997 Sep 18;337(12):847–9.

111. Lansang MA, Olveda RO. Institutional linkages: strategic bridges for research capacity strengthening. *Acta Trop* 1994 Aug; 57(2–3):139–45.

112. Caplan AL. Twenty years after: The legacy of the Tuskegee Syphilis Study: When evil intrudes. *Hastings Cent Rep* 1993; 22(6):29–32.

113. Edgar H. Twenty years after: The legacy of the Tuskegee Syphilis Study: Outside the community. *Hastings Cent Rep* 1992 Nov–Dec;22(6):32–5.

114. King PA. Twenty years after: The legacy of the Tuskegee Syphilis Study: The dangers of difference. *Hastings Cent Rep* 1992 Nov–Dec;22(6):35–8.

115. Jones JH. The Tuskegee Syphilis legacy AIDS and the black community. *Hastings Cent Rep* 1992 Nov–Dec;22(6): 38–40.

116. Randall V. Race, health care and the law: regulating racial discrimination in health care [monograph on the Internet]. Geneva: United Nations Research Institute for Social Development, 2001 [cited 2006 Jun 29]. http://www.unrisd.org/80256B3C005BCCF9/(httpPublications)/603AC6BDD4C6AF8F80256B6D005788BD?OpenDocument.

117. Stephens J. As drug testing spreads, profits and lives hang in balance. *Washington Post* [serial on the Internet]. 2000 Dec 17; A01 [cited 2006 Jun 29]. [about 6 screens]. http://www.washingtonpost.com/ac2/wp-dyn/A11939-2000Dec15?language=printer.

118. Whalen CC, Johnson JL, Okwera A, et al. A trial of three regimens to prevent tuberculosis in Ugandan adults infected with the human immunodeficiency virus. Uganda-Case Western Reserve University Research Collaboration. *New Engl J Med* 1997 Sep 18;337(12):801–8.

119. Angell M. Ethical imperialism? Ethics in international collaborative clinical research. *New Engl J Med* 1988 Oct 20;319(16): 1081–3.

120. Angell M. The Nazi hypothermia experiments and unethical research today. *New Engl J Med* 1990 May 17;322(20): 1462–4.

121. Bhutta ZA. Ethics in international health research: a perspective from the developing world. *Bull World Health Organ* 2002; 80(2):114–20.

122. Mulholland EK, Hilton S, Adegbola R, et al. Randomized trial of a Haemophilus influenzae type-b tetanus protein conjugate vaccine [corrected] for prevention of pneumonia and meningitis in Gambian infants. *Lancet* 1997 Apr 26;349(9060): 1191–7.

123. Bang AT, Bang RA, Baitule SB, et al. Effect of home-based neonatal care and management of sepsis on neonatal mortality field trial in rural India. *Lancet* 1999 Dec 4;354(9194): 1955–61.

124. Luby SP, Agboatwalla M, Feikin DR, et al. Effect of handwashing on child health: a randomized controlled trial. *Lancet* 2005 Jul 16–22;366(9481):185–7.

125. Neufeld VR, Alger EA. Network is a verb: The experience of the network of community-oriented educational institutions for health sciences. *Infect Dis Clin North Am* 1995 Jun;9(2): 407–18.

126. Commission for Research Partnerships with Developing Countries. Guidelines for research in partnership with developing countries; 11 principles [monograph on the internet]. Berne: Swiss Commission for Research Partnerships with Developing Countries, 1998 [cited 2006 Jun 29]. http://www.kfpe.ch/download/Guidelines_e.pdf

127. Donnelley S. Humans within nature: Hans Jonas and the imperative of responsibility. *Infect Dis Clin North Am* 1995 Jun;9(2): 235–44.

128. White L Jr. The historic roots of our ecologic crisis. *Science* 1967 Mar 10;155(3767):1203–7.

129. World Health Organization. Human health under threat from ecosystem degradation: threats particularly acute in poorer countries [homepage on the Internet]. Geneva: The Organization, 2006 [cited 2006 Jun 29]. [news release]; [about 2 screens]. http://www.who.int/mediacentre/news/releases/2005/pr67/en/print.html.

130. San Sebastian M, Hurtig AK. Oil exploitation in the Amazon basin of Ecuador: a public health emergency. *Rev Panam Salud Publica* 2004 Mar;15(3):205–11.

131. Gostin LO. Medical countermeasures for pandemic influenza: ethics and law. *JAMA* 2006 Feb 1;295(5):554–6.

132. Singer PA, Benatar SR, Bernstein M, et al. Ethics and SARS: lessons from Toronto. *BMJ* 2003 Dec 6;327(7427):1342–4.

133. Markkula Center for Applied Ethics [homepage on the Internet]. Santa Clara, CA: Markkula Center for Applied Ethics, Santa Clara University; 2006 [cited 2006 Jan 23]. Summary notes for members of the California State Legislature on the ethics of human cloning and stem cell research: a report from "California cloning: a dialogue on state regulation" held at Santa Clara University, October 12, 2001; [about 5 screens]. http://www.scu.edu/ethics/publications/cloning.html.

134. World Health Organization. Regional Committee for the Easter Mediterranean. Development of a regional position on human cloning [monograph on the Internet]. [cited 2006 Feb 22]. http://www.ems.org.eg/who_conf/Backgrounddocuments/Cloning.pdf.

135. Annan K. Nobel lecture, Oslo, December 10, 2001 [homepage on the Internet]. [cited 2006 Jan 23]. [About 6 screens]. http://nobelprize.org/peace/laureates/2001/annan-lecture.html.

136. Gostin LO. International infectious disease law: revision of the World Health Organization's International Health Regulations. *JAMA* 2004 Jun 2;291(21):2623–7.

137. Smolinksi MS, Hamburg MA, Lederberg J, ed.; Committee on Emerging Microbial Threats to Health in the 21st Century; Board on Global Health. Microbial threats to health: emergence, detection, and response [monograph on the Internet]. Washington, DC: National Academies Press, 2003. http://darwin.nap.edu/openbook/030908864X/gifmid/R1.gif.

138. Macer D. Bioethics in and from Asia [editorial]. *J Med Ethics* 1999 Aug;25(4):293–5.

Education and Careers in Global Health

17

Thomas E. Novotny

LEARNING OBJECTIVES

- *Understand all the reasons why it is important to study global health.*
- *Develop ideas for ways to teach global health principles.*
- *Understand the many agencies and organizations involved in global health and how to structure a career path.*

GLOBAL HEALTH EDUCATION IN MEDICINE

There is a need today for a greater emphasis on global health in medical education. This section will examine the reasons for this need and then look at some models and content for global health education.

Overview of the Need for Global Health Education

With an increasingly globalized world, medical academia must refocus education to respond to new health challenges and to the growing desire of students who wish to engage these challenges. This educational effort should further support the fundamental altruistic motivations that have attracted the very best minds to the profession of medicine.[1] Attention to global health education is both a response to a shrinking world, replete with global conflicts and opportunities for cooperation, and a driver in the quest for new knowledge—critical knowledge that is needed to address both grand scientific challenges and persistent public health deficiencies. More than any single motivation to expand education

in global health, student interests have encouraged development of more flexible approaches to international learning and experience. Given the globalization of infectious disease and risk factors for noninfectious diseases described in previous chapters, health professionals across disciplines need new curricula, experiential learning, and career development opportunities to support their learning in the 21st century. This chapter will first review the need for global health education; then it will review models and educational pathways for health science students, focusing primarily on medicine, but including public health, basic science, pharmacy, nursing, and other disciplines. The first section will include a description of examples from several medical school programs, with or without public health training components. The second part of the chapter will focus on career tracks and opportunities. These will include government, nongovernment, multilateral organizations, academic, and other possibilities.

GLOBALIZATION OF MEDICAL PRACTICE, RESEARCH, AND EDUCATION

The history of global health was described in detail in Chapter 1, and the idea that medicine and health issues transcend national boundaries is certainly not new. Ill health has negative impacts on global economic and political stability as a result of reduced life expectancy, reduced educational progress, and reduced economic productivity. Poverty and resulting health disparities may result from or be improved by globalization of public health.[2] The global forces for change in medical practice, research, and education are driven by relatively new temporal, spatial, and cognitive dimensions.[3] These dimensions include the transfer of information at high speed around the globe as well as the movement of people across borders, driven by economic forces, conflict, and social change.[4] Research findings may now be more readily available to those with Internet access and library resources, but the challenge of translating these research findings to the needs of resource-poor and highly impacted populations is a vexing dilemma. Specific research and programmatic responses are needed in developing countries to address the dual burden of emerging chronic diseases and the unfinished agendas involving communicable diseases and child health.[5] The 21st century health provider needs an understanding of these dimensions, not just to work abroad, but to also understand the impact of globalization on immigrant and culturally distinct groups who now live in his or her home country.

MOVEMENT OF PEOPLE AND CULTURES

According to United Nations Population Division estimates, there were 175 million migrants in 2000, more than double the total (79 million) in 1960,[6] with more than 40 million migrants estimated in North America alone. In addition, the vast growth in international tourist travel now accounts for one-twelfth of world trade, supporting an economy the size of a middle-income country.[7] Tourism may provide substantial economic benefits to many developing countries, and it may improve cultural understanding among travelers. However, tourism may also bring cultural and environmental disruption as well as infectious diseases across borders. Travelers' health is also now part of global health education, including concerns for safety of international students who work and study abroad.[8]

WORKFORCE NEEDS

Of particular concern to global health is the increasing emigration of health care workers in response to market forces.[9] With the movement of physicians, nurses, and pharmacists out of economically disadvantaged environments to developed countries, there looms a crisis of care in developing countries. For example, Africa bears 25 percent of the world's disease burden but has only 0.6 percent of the world's health care professionals. More than one-third of South African medical school graduates emigrate to the developed world each year; in Zimbabwe, where pharmacists provide substantial primary care, only 40 are trained each year, and in 2001, 60 migrated abroad. Ethical solutions to these manpower flows are needed; these may include educational and institutional incentives that link academia in developed countries to partner institutions in developing countries.

Certainly, models for the contribution of health manpower from better-resourced environments to high-need areas exist. Cuba has been contributing physicians to developing countries for decades as a community service requirement for its new graduates; in fact, it has extended its concern for underserved areas by offering to train US medical students to treat poor urban Americans.[10]

A new and exciting career possibility is based on recommendations from the Institute of Medicine's Board on Global Health.[11] With proposed support from the Presidential Emergency Plan for AIDS Relief, a Global Health Service Corps within the Department of Health and Human Services, modeled on the Peace Corps, could be developed to respond to human resource deficiencies in countries deeply affected by HIV/AIDS. This Corps would consist of full-time, salaried professionals, working side by side with partners on site to provide medical care in clinical, technical, and managerial areas. The intention would be to build local capacity through institutional twinning and education in the 15 hardest hit countries, not simply to provide direct assistance. To attract new US health graduates, a loan-repayment program could be included to help erase higher-education debt, much like the National Health Service Corps debt-repayment program for health commitments in underserved areas. To attract older skilled professionals, a fellowship program could offer competitive awards for those who would seek voluntary service positions abroad. Given the success of the Peace Corps as a diplomatic tool, the Global Health Service Corps could be a critical contribution to solving health manpower problems while providing an outlet for the altruistic spirit of health professionals. At this writing, the Corps is still a legislative proposal in Congress, with hopes attached for submission as a bill in 2007 (see http://newton.nap.edu/catalog/11270.html?onpi_newsdoc04192005 for more information).

RESEARCH OPPORTUNITIES AND RESPONSIBILITIES

Complicating the "brain drain" from developing countries is the enormously changed landscape of philanthropy and investment in global health.[12] Shortages of trained personnel stymie the best intentions of foundations, bilateral donors, the World Bank, and other multinational organizations to bring new resources to the problems of AIDS, tuberculosis, and malaria, as well as to vaccine-preventable diseases. Deteriorating or transitional health systems do not adequately support dissemination of effective pharmaceuticals and vaccines, and traditionally inadequate attention to research on diseases of the poor have ignored development of new drugs, vaccines, diagnostics, and other appropriate technology for poor global populations.

One of the main ethical responsibilities of the health research enterprise is to ensure an equitable response to problems that contribute to the main causes of the global burden of disease and to the vicious cycle of ill health and poverty. The imbalance in research investment has become known as the 10/90 Gap in health research,[13] wherein 90 percent of global health research funding is focused on only 10 percent of the global population. Three main causes for this gap have been identified:

1. Failure of the public sector in high-income countries to allocate funding on the basis of global health priorities
2. Limited capacity for research in many low- and middle-income countries as a result of limited funding, manpower, and progressive policies
3. Limited research by the private sector on neglected diseases and determinants resulting from insufficient commercial incentives

INTERESTS OF STUDENTS

Perhaps the greatest driving force for development of global health educational programs comes from the students themselves.[14] Increased interest in studying abroad coincided in the 1950s with the increase in commercial air travel and the availability of some funding assistance from the pharmaceutical industry. The US Peace Corps energized internationalism and volunteerism in the early 1960s. In 1969, an article in the *Journal of the American Medical Association* reported that 78 percent of incoming students and 85 percent of second-year medical students were interested in international work or study abroad.[15] Although this interest declined in following years, there appears to be increased interest in international education as globalization of health proceeds and as students become aware of health crises and humanitarian needs abroad. For example, the International Federation of Medical Student Associations (IFMSA) has been conducting meetings twice a year involving students from throughout the world, advocating for increased training and attention to experiential learning for the global academic community.[16] IFMSA surveys of students have shown consistent interest in expanded global health education,[17] and IFMSA has developed a guide to developing medical school international health programs.[18]

The American Medical Student Association (AMSA) supports a Global Health Interest Group and International Health Subcommittee, focusing on facilitating medical professional experiences abroad, promoting international health advocacy and education at home, and working to create a more cohesive and engaged international health community.[19] The website features resources to prepare for work and study abroad, links to funding sources, and links to residency programs with a global health perspective.

In surveys done by the Association of American Medical Colleges (AAMC), the percentage of graduating US medical students participating in overseas clinical activities grew dramatically over the last two decades. At least 20 percent of students graduating from US medical schools in 2003 had some form of international learning experiences, compared with only 6 percent of 1984 graduates.[20] More recent AAMC survey data show nearly 50% of graduating medical students participating in international electives in 2005. (See Figure 17-1.)

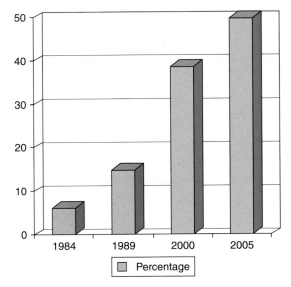

Figure 17-1. Graduating medical students participating in international electives, United States, 1984–2005. (From The Association of American Medical Colleges, 2006.)

An extensive, but sometimes difficult to access, network of resources, organizations, and funding sources supports experiential learning abroad, mostly as electives (see Table 17-1). According to the AAMC, more than 100 of the 125 US allopathic medical schools have some sort of educational opportunity for medical students to participate in global health (Personal Communication, AAMC, July 2006.) The key stimulus cited by some leading educators for the development of global health educational programs is the motivation and desire of health sciences students to address health disparities. This is indeed a passion that can be harnessed through global health education and the development of new knowledge to improve global human welfare.[21]

OUTCOMES OF GLOBAL HEALTH EDUCATION

International travel and experiential learning have traditionally been part of liberal arts education. Outcome assessments of such learning have until recently been quite scarce, but increasingly, the value of study abroad has been linked to needs arising from globalization.[22] These outcomes relate to cognitive flexibility, cultural empathy, personal growth, and problem solving. Results of one outcome study show that students who studied abroad generally showed improvement in intercultural communication skills compared with those who did not study abroad. However, the study abroad experience alone was not the only determinant of cultural competency; prior experiences and training also likely have effects on ultimate outcomes, suggesting that a longer-term,

Table 17-1. Examples of organizations providing resources for health sciences students.

Organization	Resources	Web Link	Comment
American Medical Students Association	Global Health Action Committee: Networking, guides, listserves; Global Pulse International Health Journal	http://www.amsa.org/global/	AIDS, Environment, Human Rights, Leadership, Education
American Medical Women's Association		http://www.amwa-doc.org/	
American Public Health Association	International Health Section; The World Federation of Public Health Associations (WFPHA); DC Global Health Dialogues; Annual meeting job mart	http://www.apha.org/wfpha/global_health.htm	Education and Global Health Resources Unit has internships, student section of organization
American Society of Tropical Medicine and Hygiene	Annual Meeting, Scholarships and Fellowships, Rotations	http://www.astmh.org/	Benjamin H. Kean Traveling Fellowship in Tropical Medicine
Association of American Medical Colleges	Student surveys, guide to medical schools and residencies with global health programs	http://www.aamc.org/students/medstudents/	Supports Fogarty-Ellison Fellowship in International Research
Association of Schools of Public Health	Guide to international programs in schools of public health	http://www.asph.org/document.cfm?page=739	Masters International Program (integrated with Peace Corps)
Global Health Council	Annual meeting job mart, advocacy, small grants, awards, publications	http://globalhealth.org/	University Coalitions for Global Health Resource Group
Global Health Education Consortium	Annual meeting, website, listserve, fact sheets	http://www.globalhealthec.org/	Career guidebooks, curriculum, scholarship, program development guidebook

integrated learning program may be important to optimize outcomes of short and medium-term experiential learning. Longitudinal studies would be very important in evaluating career implications and lasting communication skills resulting from experiential learning.[23]

A 2003 literature review to identify the outcomes of cross-cultural experiences for nursing and medical students reported qualitative and some quantitative data showing positive outcomes for professional development including cultural competence, personal development, clinical learning, and host population benefits.[24] A broadened perspective about the world (and presumably global health) was the most frequently cited outcome of such experiences. However, the review pointed out the dearth of evidence regarding clearly defined outcomes for medical students or for host populations. Another literature review[25] of outcome studies including medical students (n=522) and house staff (n=166) suggested that international health electives may be associated with choosing careers in primary care and focusing careers on underserved populations. Many of the studies reviewed noted positive effects on clinical skills as well as a greater appreciation of the importance of public health, culture, and health care systems. In addition,

the review suggested that participants in experiential learning may be more competent in tropical medicine, potentially supporting better care for both immigrants and travelers. Other reports have confirmed the positive effects of experiential learning on competence with multicultural communities.[26] A randomized control trial of such programs would be essentially impossible, but better long-term follow up studies on participants versus nonparticipants using validated instruments are needed. One long-term follow-up of an integrated didactic/experiential program at Drew University of Medicine and Science reported that of 52 alumni who completed the course as medical students, two-thirds joined national or international relief organizations, and 80 percent returned to the elective site for additional work or cultural experience.[27]

Studies from nonUS institutions show similar results. A Dutch survey of undergraduate medical students reported meaningful learning outcomes for international experiences in medical knowledge, skills, health care organization, society and culture, and personal growth.[28] The International Health and Medical Education Centre at University College London developed Student Selected Modules and International Health electives, combining experience abroad with appropriate didactic training (see the following Section). A preliminary evaluation of this integrated program suggested that the value of experiential learning is enhanced by the integration of such learning with a comprehensive program of teaching about global health.[29]

What Models Exist for Global Health Education?

Until recently, little support for student and resident experiential or didactic learning in medical institutions in the United States has been evident. However, as a result of the growing interest of students in global health, an increasing number of offices to support educational opportunities has developed. Responses to the 2006 survey conducted by the AAMC, the Foundation for Advancement of International Medical Education and Research (FAIMER), and the Global Health Education Consortium (GHEC) indicate that 107 of 125 allopathic US medical schools now support some type of global health educational programs for medical students. Among these, 65 percent offer some form of funding support for students' learning abroad experiences, 87 percent support formal curricular activities, and 31.8 percent have programs to prepare students for international experiences. For example, at the University of California, San Francisco, an Office of International Programs was established in 2004 to develop curriculum, disburse funds for student research and work abroad, arrange experiences and rotations, and develop an Area of Concentration in Global Health (see http://medschool.ucsf.edu/intlprograms/). With a 20 percent time director as well as a program coordinator and support staff, such an office provides mentoring, program development and monitoring, record keeping, and oversight of student international programs, including a careful program of preparation prior to study abroad. Funding is provided from the regular budget as well as from donor sources. The University of Pittsburgh's Global Health Area of Concentration (http://www.zone.medschool.pitt.edu/sites/programs/AOC/globalhealth/default.aspx) features faculty mentorship, a clearinghouse for international learning opportunities, a journal club, an annual symposium, and other services for students. The University of Wisconsin offers an interdisciplinary Certificate in Global Health as collaboration among the schools of medicine and public health, nursing, pharmacy, veterinary medicine, and international studies. Core courses (9 units) and experiential learning characterize this program (http://www.pophealth. wisc.edu/gh/).

Several medical schools are now developing more broad-based global health institutes, incorporating multiple levels of training, research, and service. These institutes respond to a need for coordination of various individual activities, including curriculum, developing service opportunities, linking participants to partner organizations, preparing participants for study and work abroad, administering programs, supporting pursuit of extramural funding, developing a donor base for global health education, and organizing academic enrichment programs. Educational programs may include:

- Undergraduate programs (nonprofessional schools) in international relations, public health, anthropology, etc.
- Certificate programs, applying to both visiting scholars and professional school students who concentrate on global health
- Global Health Professional Tracks for students in medicine, pharmacy, nursing, dentistry, and veterinary medicine
- Masters degrees in global health sciences or clinical research focusing on global health topics
- Areas of Concentration for doctoral students in basic sciences, nursing, or other fields to support research projects in global health
- Clinical scholar programs for residents who wish to expand their clinical training to include research, service, or program work abroad

These institutes depend on high-level commitment from the campus, usually with initial start-up funding to support leadership, administration, and pilot programs. Steering committees consisting of deans, academic leaders, researchers, and development officers oversee development of these institutes, and faculty members are increasingly drawn from across disciplines, not just infectious diseases. Global health is by its nature interdisciplinary, and thus leadership for such institutes must rely on strengths within the health professions but involve disciplines from outside the health sciences. These disciplines include cultural anthropology, foreign policy, ethics, law, international relations, area studies, and so forth. Thus, educational programs based in such institutes will be more effective as interdisciplinary activities. Some examples are provided below.

PRECLINICAL ELECTIVES/COURSES

First-year medical students increasingly are admitted to US medical schools with prior international and multicultural experiences. However, formal didactic education, integrated with experiential learning at some time in the medical curriculum, may now be the best model for assuring global health education for medical students. This may begin in the first year of study with electives or required curricula as part of electives or formal international health topics taught in core courses. Given the changing times, what should be taught in this initial phase of global health education?

In 1993, Heck and Pust reported on a national consensus effort to define the essential international health curriculum for medical schools.[30] They reported frequencies of inclusion for various topics (n=38) among 25 medical schools as well as expert opinion by 22 faculty members on content subjects. Essential topics included malnutrition, family planning and population programs, immunizations, understanding cross-cultural barriers, maternal-child health, sanitation, and community health care. Although all these issues were population-based problems, none of the traditional tropical diseases were in this top-seven list. In addition, the main focal areas of some of the new financial support in global health, AIDS, tuberculosis, and malaria were far down the list. Noncommunicable diseases, including the main contributor (mental health) to the global burden of diseases were not highly ranked. Due to the changing epidemiological landscape, aging, and globalization, new international health curricula must recognize the prevention and control of noncommunicable, chronic health conditions in both high-income and resource-constrained populations. (See Chapter 11.) Critical also to understanding global health is consideration of health systems, macro- and micro-economics, the functions of the multinational and bilateral aid organizations, and increasingly, the priority-setting process of the philanthropic groups now supporting so many global health initiatives. In a follow-up review of the changing curricular environment, Heck described the need for more focused learning about the antecedent factors in global health (see Figure 17-2)[31] and about how one

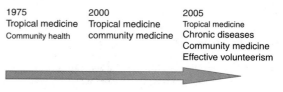

1975	2000	2005
Tropical medicine	Tropical medicine	Tropical medicine
Community health	community medicine	Chronic diseases
		Community medicine
		Effective volunteerism

Curriculum emphasis in international health

Figure 17-3. The changing global health curriculum, 1975–2005. Courtesy of J. Heck, GHEC. From Heck JE. A national consensus on the essential international-health curriculum for medical schools—Author's Postscript. *Update: The GHEC Newsletter 2006.* 1(1). http://www.globalhealth-ec.org/ GHEC/Resources/Newsletter/Vol1Issue1/ClassicsPostscript_ JH.htm. (Reproduced with permission.)

volunteers more effectively. Accordingly, new curricula should focus even less on tropical diseases and more on noncommunicable diseases (see Figure 17-3), with interventions and approaches supported by more rigorous evidence on risks, intervention effectiveness, and technological fixes.[32]

In the United Kingdom, the International Health and Medical Education Centre (IHMEC) at University College London established an "intercalated BSc" in international health for medical students that has required

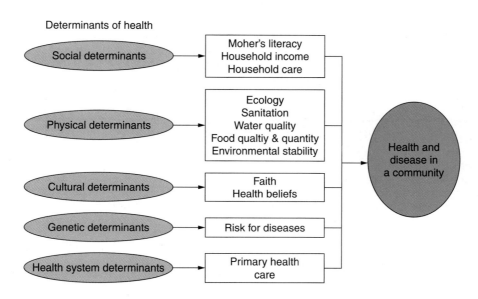

Figure 17-2. Determinants of global health and disease. Courtesy of: Phillip Diller, MD PHD; Jeff Heck, MD; Andrew Bazemore, MD MPH. From Heck JE. A national consensus on the essential international-health curriculum for medical schools—Author's Postscript. *Update: The GHEC Newsletter 2006.* 1(1). http://www.globalhealth-ec.org/GHEC/Resources/ Newsletter/Vol1Issue1/ClassicsPostscript_JH.htm. (Reproduced with permission.)

modules in poverty, inequality, and health; health care in the context of globalization; and human rights and health in the international context. Optional modules included maternal and child health and infectious diseases in developing countries. Other options include courses in anthropology, geography, history, and languages. An elective in the final year is spent in a developing country, health care agency, or educational institution. The goal of this program is to provide medical students with global health education that benefits their practice in the United Kingdom or prepares them for international health careers.[33] An "Elective Pack" published by IHMEC provides essential information for work abroad, including subjects such as development economics, infectious diseases in developing countries, access to essential medicines, nutrition and water, mental health, conflict and health, ethical issues, and practical travel information.[34]

In Sweden, at the Karolinska Institute of Stockholm, there is a five week full-time course offered as the most popular elective course in the curriculum. It covers socioeconomic, cultural, and environmental determinants of health, as well as the global burden of disease and demographic changes. The didactic section is followed by two weeks of experiential learning in developing countries.[35]

In the United States, it would be quite difficult to integrate an extensive list of subjects into a first- or second-year curriculum, given the demands for rigorous basic science education that characterize the first two years of US medical schools. Thus, an elective survey-type course should be offered to all students, and perhaps required of those students who participate in an international health summer elective period between first and second year. For most students, this is the only free time available for language training, cultural immersion, or exposure to medical or research practice abroad prior to the fourth-year elective period. Many students design their own experiential learning for this period, using resources found in Table 17-1, personal contacts established through their faculty and mentors, or through established fee-based programs that might combine language training, clinical "shadowing," or research assistance (see Table 17-2). Medical schools may provide all or partial funding for such programs and may sponsor or give credit for participation in specific programs. Nevertheless, there is ample evidence to support the need for preparatory education prior to engaging in international learning during the summer abroad. Counseling on health and safety should be included in this training to mitigate the potential risks of working and traveling abroad.

The content of preparatory education should include three basic components:

1. Orientation to global health problems, history, actors, systems, successes, and failures

2. Health and physical safety while traveling abroad

3. Cultural sensitivity, professionalism, and diplomacy

In component 1, course material should include basic information on the core health issues influencing the global burden of disease. These might be best presented as expert lectures associated with case studies and one or two readings. Core material should be

Table 17-2. Examples of fee-based, international experiential learning activities for first-year medical students, 2006.

Name of Sponsor	Type of Program	Length of Program	Locations	Address
Child and Family Health International	Language/service	At least 4 weeks		www.cfhi.org
Adventure Education Center	Medical Spanish Program	1–4 weeks	Costa Rica	http://adventurespanish-school.com/
International Health Central American Institute Foundation (IHCAI)	Tropical Medicine, Medical Spanish	4 weeks	Costa Rica	http://www.ihcai.org/
University of Nebraska Medical Center	Medical Spanish/ International Health Course	4 weeks	Guatemala	http://www.unmc.edu/isp
Foundation for Sustainable Development	Language, Service, Research	8–52 weeks		http://www.fsdinternational.org/?q=intlopps/intlopps
Global Service Corps	Service/ learning	2–9 weeks	Tanzania Thailand	http://www.globalser-vicecorps.org/
Interhealth South America	Language/ Service	4 weeks	Ecuador	http://www.interhealth-southamerica.net

presented on the roles and functions of major global health agencies, bilateral donors, and philanthropic organizations. Examples of major successful interventions (smallpox eradication) should be presented as well as less-than-successful historical cases (malaria).

In component 2, extensive pre-trip counseling is needed to reduce risks from infectious diseases, assault, accidents, and sexual harassment.[36,37,38] Protection from HIV infection should be addressed, especially for those students who may work in high-prevalence environments.[39] Immunizations, risk avoidance for personal safety, evacuation and crisis management, insurance coverage, food and water safety, malaria prevention, TB exposure, and logistical issues should all be covered in such orientations. Considerable information can be obtained from web-based sources, including travel warnings and travel safety (www.state.gov), and health issues for travelers (www.CDC.gov).

The University of Arizona offers an 80-hour summer course for medical students and residents who plan to work abroad in the future. Begun in 1982 and revised annually, it is a multidisciplinary, case-based, problem-solving course preparing medical students and primary care residents for health care experiences in developing countries. It focuses on three major issues: infectious diseases, population, and nutrition (http://www. globalhealth.arizona.edu/IHIndex.html). Some universities may emphasize more research in global health; a model 10- to 20-week curriculum emphasizing research skills in global health is shown in Table 17-3.

Table 17-3. Proposed content of multi-disciplinary global health core course (20 weeks; 3 hours per week).

Week	Topic
1	Ethics of Human Research/Vulnerable Populations/IRBs
2	Qualitative Research Methods
3	Epidemiologic Research Methods I: Randomized Trials and Community Interventions
4	Epidemiologic Research Methods II: Observational Study Designs
5	Environmental Health Research Methods
6	Infectious Disease Laboratory Research Methods
7	Health Economics Research Methods
8	Health Policy Research Methods
9	Community Participation, Political Challenges and Constraints to Research
10	Study Implementation and Logistics/Safety Abroad
11–20	Weekly Presentation and In-depth Discussion of Student Research Plans/Protocols

CLINICAL ELECTIVES

Generally speaking, medical students must complete 26 weeks of clinical rotations (sub-internships and required rotations), and most choose a variety of one-month electives to fill out their education and help them choose specialty training. Global health clinical electives in the fourth year are permitted by departments for one month of elective credit, and increasingly, longer electives may be part of areas of concentration or research programs for undergraduate professional students. Most often, these clinical electives do not incorporate any specific integrated preparation. However, at Drew University of Medicine and Science, an elective in international health/tropical medicine combined a six-week classroom and clinical experience with a four-week clinical clerkship assigned in tropical countries. These included Kenya, Zimbabwe, Costa Rica, Colombia, Mexico, Puerto Rico, India, and Peru. As cited above, this program seemed to have a long-term impact on participants.[40] At the University of California, San Francisco (UCSF), students applying for travel funding from the university are required to take either the first-year elective course in global health or a workshop on "'Preparation for Study Abroad."

Other important considerations for such clinical electives are supervision, evaluation, and continuity. Electives in countries where there is a strong research or other academic linkage will foster personal relationships between partner institution faculty members. These can lead to informal or more formal attachments in the form of sabbaticals or perhaps short term teaching and service visits by faculty from US partner schools. These may be facilitated by formal affiliation agreements, which spell out liabilities, supervisory responsibilities, resource needs, and reporting from each side. Often, however, such arrangements are made by handshake or letters of collaboration. Each situation should be considered individually, as formal affiliation agreements may be a daunting barrier to resource-constrained institutions. Still, with sensitivity to mutual needs, written agreements that spell out specific responsibilities for supervision and reporting as part of continual elective programs should be developed. As part of supervision and elective support, some programs provide modest funds to on-site coordinators who can develop housing resources, meet students on arrival, and orient them to the local program and facilities. In particular, orientation to and assurance of student safety must be clearly spelled out. One unfortunate event could ruin years of relationships, create misery for families involved, and terminate institutional support for international electives; liability insurance should be part of the elective activity. For this reason, students who take electives with support from their home university must be oriented in advance as to their limitations, risks, and responsibilities. A signed waiver and a signed commitment to review travel advice on the US Department of State website should be part of the departure package provided to students. (www.state.gov)

AREAS OF CONCENTRATION

An Area of Concentration (AoC) may be considered a "minor" in global health, completed as part of the MD or other health professional degree. The AoC program establishes standards and provides institutional structure for sustained interdisciplinary projects throughout a student's curriculum. Students identify a project and work with faculty advisors to complete a thorough program of preparation and to focus their inquiry. The experiential phase of the program involves completing the project and investigating its links to the practice of medicine. Some students may opt for an additional year of medical school devoted to added study, research, or degree programs. Prior to graduation, students produce and present a tangible legacy, which may be in the form of traditional scholarship such as a scientific paper, but may also be innovative, such as an exhibit, Web-based curriculum module, or new intervention program (http://medschool.ucsf.edu/aoc/). At UCSF, the global health AoC consists of:

- First-year elective survey course in global health
- International experience between first and second year
- Linkage with UCSF mentor during third year
- Global health AoC courses (clinical research and problem-based learning seminar occupying one elective month) in early fourth year
- Two- to five-month project electives OR
- Extra year of research or project work with fellowship support from outside agencies (such as the National Institutes of Health, Centers for Disease Control and Prevention (CDC), and Doris Duke Clinical Research Fellowship)

JOINT DEGREE PROGRAMS

In order to be prepared for careers in global health, health professionals must be able to understand population health and determinants, including demography, economy, and governance. They must be able to develop novel approaches to policy and program implementation in light of globalization, and they must understand the interface between global and local health conditions. Thus, additional education, beyond traditional clinical education, is increasingly required for career preparation in global health. Joint degree programs are one way that health professional students may acquire the necessary perspectives in global health, as appropriate courses, opportunities, and mentorship may not be available in most traditional health science school environments. Joint degree programs supporting education in global health may include:

- Masters in Public Health (MPH), Masters in Health Sciences (MHS), or Masters in Science (MS or MSc). Many health sciences campuses incorporate schools of public health, degree programs in public health, or linkages with off-campus schools of public health. Within these public health programs, there may be program emphases in international health, but often health professional students elect epidemiology as a program focus because of its utility across medical disciplines. The master's degree is often obtained between the third and fourth year of medical school, and ideally would include experiential learning (internships, field work, research) as part of the degree. Distance-based master's degree programs are available, aimed at practicing health professionals, government employees, and others who must maintain employment status while obtaining a degree. The master's degree may be considered a requirement for many career positions in global health. It provides the broad overview of public health practice, skills in health policy and epidemiology, and perspectives on population health that are critical to understanding global health problems. Combined programs may include health policy, public administration, economics, or other specialized career tracks.

- Joint Masters or PhD Programs. Some schools have multiple-year programs leading to MD/MS degrees, joint MD/PhD degrees, MSN/MPH degrees, DDS/MPH degrees, or other combinations. These programs might focus on global health, but they often emphasize methodological training to prepare scientists, researchers, and academics. For example, the Medical Science Training Program (MSTP), funded by the National Institutes of Health, is for students aspiring to careers combining academic medicine and biomedical research.

All such programs have specific required course content areas. For example, the International Program at Johns Hopkins University includes four focus areas: Disease Prevention and Control, Health Systems, Human Nutrition, and Social and Behavioral Interventions. Courses specific to these areas are required in addition to school-wide requirements for course work that include epidemiology, biostatistics, environmental health, public health biology, and management. Additional substantial experiential learning in the form of project work, research, or internship is required for this program (http://www.jhsph.edu/dept/ih).

The MSc at the London School of Hygiene and Tropical Medicine (http://www.lshtm.ac.uk/prospectus/masters/), program in Tropical Medicine and International Health, includes courses on Analysis and Design of Research Studies; diagnosis and management of tropical diseases; and evidence-based medicine and basic epidemiology. The Public Health in Developing

Countries MSc program includes the following requirements:

- **Compulsory:** Epidemiology; Statistics; Health Policy, Process & Power; Health Economics; Principles of Social Research
- **Recommended:** Public Health Lecture Series; Health Promotion; PHDC Student Seminars

Specific masters programs in global health sciences that incorporate some public health disciplines, but extend the boundaries of learning across economics, basic science, political science, anthropology, and behavioral science, are under development at several health sciences campuses. These programs may not be bound by specific requirements of public health schools, and thus may also serve a more focused research training agenda in global health.

The New York University School of Medicine now offers a MPH program in Global Public Health (www.nyu.edu/mph). This program grew from the needs of communities served by international agencies and community-based organizations in New York City. It focuses on:

1. Redefining health in the era of globalization
2. Learning from diverse health systems
3. Reducing barriers and improving health care delivery in diverse settings
4. The process and tools of the trade
5. Local and overseas field work

This program is meant for those with advanced degrees in health, social work, education, public service, law, journalism, and other fields germane to global health. No matter what the timing of extra academic preparation in global health, increasingly the job market demands the special skills and experiential learning provided by these degree programs. In addition, the connections and exposures acquired in these multidisciplinary environments provide the health professional with resources and opportunities later in his or her career. These personal connections cannot be overvalued.

MD WITH THESIS

Many schools of medicine offer programs to provide academic distinction for students who conduct original research of high quality while in medical school. The distinction of MD with Thesis is awarded at graduation to those students who, in addition to fulfilling all of the requirements for the degree of Doctor of Medicine, have completed a research project and have written a thesis approved by a governing committee. Students may conduct thesis research in any of a wide variety of disciplines, including basic sciences, clinical investigation, social sciences, and ethics. The fundamental requirement for such programs is that the work be original and of scholarly quality. To provide ample time for the conduct

of such research, students may officially leave the MD curriculum and complete a separate, nondegree, certificate program during an extra year of work. Typically, certificate programs have some required courses (usually methodological, research ethics, career development) and required products, such as research papers, presentations, and research proposals. These products may focus on global health, and such accomplishments will help set the new physician on a course of academic commitment to global health research.

FELLOWSHIPS

Numerous fellowships are now available to support global health education. These may be as short as one month, but often involve an entire year of commitment. Table 17-4 lists several of the more important fellowship opportunities. The NIH, Doris Duke, and CDC programs are more research oriented, with considerable skills training; the Rotary program is more oriented to language and cultural exchange; and the Kean Fellowship may be for clinical or early experiential learning. Each of these competitive programs provides financial support and requires strong credentials and recommendations from the student's home institution.

RESIDENCY TRACKS

Residency programs are beginning to have tracks in global health research, service, and experiential learning. Perhaps the oldest such activity is the International Health Program (IHP) at Yale University. This program dates to 1981, and was started in response to the relocation of Southeast Asian immigrants to New Haven; volunteer residents caring for them sought additional primary care rotations abroad to help them understand and provide care to these underserved populations. The goals of the IHP were to involve residents within diverse cultural settings, to encourage cost-consciousness using appropriate technology in resource-constrained environments, and to engender a sense of social responsibility. Residents rotated through Haiti, Tanzania, Zimbabwe, Fiji, and several Native America health facilities in the United States. Rotations are four to eight weeks in duration, and available to second-year residents in Internal Medicine. Overall, 20–30 percent of Yale medicine residents participate in the program, supported through departmental funds. This program has developed health professionals who are more likely to care for patients on public assistance and for immigrants; to become primary care rather than specialized physicians; and to look more favorably upon service in developing countries as part of their careers.[41]

At Brigham and Women's Hospital in Boston, Massachusetts, the Howard Hiatt Residency in Global Health Equity and Internal Medicine is a four-year program that leads to certification by the American Board of Internal Medicine (ABIM) and completion of a Masters Degree

Table 17-4. Fellowship opportunities that support global health education for health sciences students.

Name of Fellowship Program	Sponsor	Target Group	Duration	Program Elements
Fogarty-Ellison Program	NIH, AAMC, ASPH	Any upper level health sciences doctoral students	One year	Research abroad in specific NIH-funded sites in developing countries
OC Hubert Student International Fellowship in International Health	CDC Foundation	3rd and 4th year medical and veterinary Students	4–12 weeks	Working with specific CDC staff on priority problem in developing countries
The CDC Experience: Applied Epidemiology Fellowship at CDC	CDC Foundation	4th year medical students	10–12 months	CDC Atlanta-based training in epidemiology; may have some international opportunities
Benjamin H. Kean Traveling Fellowship in Tropical Medicine	American Society of Tropical Medicine and Hygiene	Medical students interested in tropical medicine and international health	Minimum of one month	Financial support for clinical and research electives in the tropics, self designed
Doris Duke Clinical Research Fellowship	Doris Duke Charitable Foundation	3rd or 4th year medical students	One year	Clinical research training; may have international focus
Ambassadorial Scholarship Program	Rotary International Club	Any undergraduate, graduate, or vocational student	One year	To further international understanding and friendly relations among people of different countries

in Public Health through the Harvard School of Public Health, or a comparable degree from another Harvard graduate program.[42] Clinical trainees participate in a novel program that combines rigorous training in internal medicine with the advanced study of social sciences and public heath. The residents are thus able to obtain both the medical and nonmedical skills they need to improve the health of some of the world's most impoverished people, both in the United States and abroad (http://www.brighamandwomens.org/socialmedicine/gheresidency.aspx).

Ozgediz et al.[43] developed a six-week pilot clinical surgical elective for residents in Uganda, following an established General Internal Medicine Rotation for UCSF residents in this country. This rotation may be most easily fit into a research year, after two years of residency training. Now, a Global Health Clinical Scholars Program has been established to support the interests of residents from several different departments at UCSF, including Medicine, Family and Community Medicine, Orthopedic Surgery, General Surgery, Pediatrics, Psychiatry, and others. Included will be didactic training focusing on research skills, cultural anthropology, political economy, and use of appropriate technology. This program will support medical and surgical training, exchanges with host country programs, increased opportunities for research, improved ethical training for residents, and development of programs of sustainable value in research and service. Concurrent with the development of the Global Health Clinical Scholars

Program is a faculty program to both support residents through mentoring and provide opportunities for clinical rotations and research through their personal and professional contacts. Important to this activity is the inclusion of evaluation studies to follow the outcomes of professional activities after such experiences by participating residents.

Content Areas for Global Health Education

Much has been proposed in terms of content for global health education. Pust, Heck, and others cited above have considered the changing epidemiological landscape as well as the changing political economy underlying global health. Risk factors, disease control priorities, the new role of philanthropy, and certainly changing economic perspectives now call for revised and more evidence-based approaches to global health education. Nevertheless, such education should reinforce the altruism and potential for public service that attracts the most dedicated future global health professionals to the field.[44] Basic content in the form of survey courses and basic skills courses may be appropriate for first- or second-year health sciences students, but more focused skill-based, culturally appropriate, experiential, and multidisciplinary training should be part of AoCs, Residency programs, and perhaps faculty re-orientation training programs in global health.

The Disease Control Priorities Project (DCPP), jointly sponsored by the World Bank and the Fogarty

International Center of the US National Institutes of Health and the WHO, outlined intervention strategies and policies to address global health issues for low- and middle-income countries.[45] This review, based on accumulated evidence, cost-effectiveness analyses, and expert consultation, compiled knowledge necessary to assist decision makers in developing countries with interventions to rapidly improve the health and welfare of their populations. The risk factors, intervention-effectiveness and cost-effectiveness, health systems issues, and financing issues addressed in this volume may all be considered as critical information for more advanced trainees in global health.

In addition to specific knowledge about diseases, risk factors, and interventions, language and cultural understanding are core competencies required to become active participants in global health. Other issues to consider include gender, politics, health disparities, global conflict, disaster response, emerging infections, biopreparedness, diplomacy, and the environment.[46] These broad subjects may be touched on in medical school curricula, but most often they require specific coursework, experience, and individual study to fully prepare the health science student for work abroad.

DIDACTIC MATERIAL

Following is a model framework curriculum outline compiled from several sources that can be covered in part in the first-year survey courses described earlier, and in more detail during specific course work within new degree, AoC, or other training activities, including short courses. Specific disease and program targets, including infectious diseases, noncommunicable diseases, injuries, mental health, maternal/child health, and reproductive health can all be addressed through this framework approach.

I. Human Rights, Ethics, Culture, and Diplomacy
A key underlying approach to global health must involve attention to human rights. The UN Universal Declaration of Human Rights, adopted in 1948, calls for rights to health and well-being, including food, clothing, housing, medical care, and necessary social services (http://www.un.org/Overview/rights.html). Understanding this Declaration as the basis for involvement in international health is essential for health professionals.

Further, understanding ethical approaches to research and service in resource-poor environments is essential. Aside from basic bioethical training provided by most medical schools for research and clinical practice in the United States, global health professionals need particular attention to the cultural nuances associated with ethical research and practice.

Culture is "that complex whole which includes knowledge, belief, art, morals, law, custom, and any other capabilities acquired by man as a member of society."[47] It may determine the success or failure of the best laid plans in global health, and should be addressed by all those

planning on work in resource-poor environments. (See Chapter 16.) Basic skills in ethnography may be included in the global health curriculum. Understanding how ethnography is done will assist the learner in valuing cultural perspectives. Understanding culture as a determinant of health is also critical to developing specific approaches to disease prevention and control. These approaches must consider structural factors as well as non-Western belief systems. Experiential learning reinforces the learning of culturally appropriate approaches, but preparing the health worker in advance through case studies and ethics training is important. Language training is essential to both communication and to cultural adaptation. Language may be considered a requirement for global health work.

Health diplomacy may be defined as a political change agent that meets the dual goals of improving global health while maintaining and improving international relations abroad, particularly in conflict areas and resource-poor countries. Health diplomacy begins with a recognition that the most effective health interventions are carried out in an ethical manner sensitive to historical, political, social, economic and cultural differences between nations and peoples. Health professionals as leaders, teachers, and advocates have a responsibility in their work to build relationships, assure attention to human rights, and practice ethically. Global health is in the US national interest as enlightened self-interest. This is based on a concern for biopreparedness (for bioterrorism as well as emerging epidemics), multi-nationalism, and global health diplomacy as essential to maintaining global economic stability as well as peace and the rule of law.[48]

Case studies may be the most effective mode of learning in this module; ethical and cultural problems presented by faculty and researched by students will stimulate discussion and consideration of the context for specific work in global health.

II. Determinants of Health Economics, effectiveness, efficiency, and evidence are critical ingredients in health and development. Understanding basic economics, both at the macro level and at the household level, help orient the health professional towards effective interventions in global health. Income inequality is a major reason for health inequality, but improvements in health can be appreciated without vast expenditures of money if correct approaches and policies can be understood. The DCPP describes cost-effective interventions appropriate for low- and middle-income countries for dozens of risk factors, disease outcomes, and program areas. These may be addressed specifically as case studies, with purposeful multidisciplinary approaches from several perspectives such as financing, health systems, technical requirements, and human resource needs.

Social determinants of health include culture and social structure. Human behavior is wedded to the social environment and must be understood in the context of geopolitics, history, religion, and perhaps most importantly, globalization. Behaviors are dependent on globalizing influences, as pointed out earlier in this chapter, and now, cultural understanding may not be enough to help guide programs and interventions. Understanding market forces and commercial communications may also be necessary for the global health professional.

III. Policy, Governance, and Actors An understanding of policy development processes and global health governance is critical in the changing global health environment. Transnational governance may be seen as a challenge to national sovereignty, discouraging some governments from participation in multinational organizations. However, organizations such as the WHO, the World Trade Organization (WTO), the World Bank Group, the United Nations Development Program (UNDP) are critical to implementing top-down efforts at the national and local levels. In addition, more multinational efforts such as the Global Alliance for Vaccines and Immunization (GAVI) involve multiple actors such as the multinational organizations as well as governments and the philanthropies. These efforts can provide substantial resources but can also affect how national and local agencies work within their own borders. Vertical programs dealing with a single disease eradication priority or age group create demands on human resource-strapped agencies that must be accountable to multiple donors and policy-setting institutions. Sector-wide approaches are an attempt to coordinate donors, and understanding how these approaches work is critical to effective work in global health. A list of the major global health organizations and actors is provided by GHEC on their website (http://www.globalhealthec.org/GHEC/Resources/GHplayers_resources.htm).

Moreover, local, bottom-up approaches must be understood as components of global health programs. Nongovernmental organizations are key to the delivery of health interventions in resource-poor environments, and case studies from such programs should be a component of learning for global health professionals.

Understanding the bilateral approach to foreign assistance is critical as well. The US Agency for International Development (USAID), the UK Department for International Development (DFID), Canadian International Development Agency (CIDA), the Japan International Cooperation Agency (JICA), and the Scandinavian International Development Agency (SIDA) are all important players whose home country agendas, history, and strategic commitments should be understood by global health professionals. These are the "outside-in" agencies which, through donor assistance, can drive policy and priorities with or without the concurrence of host governments.

Philanthropy is now a major component of international health assistance. Key players fund many of the multinational efforts such as GAVI, the Global Fund for AIDS, TB, and Malaria (GFATM), the Stop TB Initiative, Anti-Malaria Initiative in Africa, etc. These contributions are often combined with bilateral donor activities, and thus, global health professionals need extensive orientation as to who is doing what to whom with which partner. A partial list of new global health enterprises is provided in Table 17-5.

Table 17-5. New global health philanthropic activities.

Organization	Focus	Donors
Bill and Melinda Gates Foundation	Global health	Bill and Melinda Gates, Warren Buffet
Global Fund to Fight AIDS, Tuberculosis, and Malaria	Financing treatment and prevention	Governments, foundations, corporations
President's Emergency Plan for AIDS Relief (PEPFAR)	Financing and delivery of HIV/AIDS prevention and treatment	US government
International Finance Facility for Immunization	Financing vaccine delivery/GAVI	UK, France, Italy, Spain, Sweden
Multi-country HIV/AIDS Program	Financing scale-up of existing government and community prevention and treatment efforts	World Bank
Global Alliance for Vaccines and Immunization (GAVI)	Financing and delivery of childhood vaccines	Gates Foundation, governments
Public-Private Partnerships	Drugs, vaccines, microbicides, diagnostics	Philanthropists, governments, industry
Anti-malaria Initiative in Africa	Cut malaria incidence in half by 2010 in 15 countries	US government
United Nations Foundation	Children and women's health	Ted Turner

From Cohen J. The new world of global health. *Science* 2006;311:162–167. (Adapted with permission.)

Thus, a complete understanding of top-down, bottom-up, and outside-in players that address global health problems should be included in curriculum. This will require significant development of case studies, but also direct knowledge of how the multiple actors function at different levels of governance. At this writing, GHEC is compiling case studies and specific curricular tools that will help flesh out such curricula.

IV. Measuring Health, Burden of Disease, and Program Outcomes Quantitative skills are essential in global health science. At the population level, one must understand demographics, population health statistics, and trends. Basic epidemiology, including descriptive statistics, measures of association, and measures of significance should be second nature to global health professionals. In addition, being able to understand the measurement of health burdens is a critical skill. This involves understanding mortality data and the limitations of these data in resource-constrained environments, but also the now-accepted metrics of disability adjusted life years (DALYS), and quality-adjusted life years (QALYS). DALYS combine years lived with disability and years lost to premature death in a single measure. Cost-effectiveness is often measured as US$ per DALY averted. A quality-adjusted life-year (QALY) takes into account both quantity and the quality of life generated by healthcare interventions. QALYs provide a common currency to assess the extent of the benefits gained from a variety of interventions in terms of health-related quality of life and survival. (See Chapter 2.) Basic skills in qualitative research (focus groups, pilot studies, semi-structured interviews) may also be helpful, but perhaps the most important tool in global health is the ability to measure program outcomes. Basic evaluation technology should be part of global health education.

Research projects demand special training in designing and conducting clinical research. Basic skills in research question selection, study design, statistics, sampling and sample size calculation, data management, variable selection, questionnaire development, study populations, and bioethics should be taught in focused courses with careful attention to mentoring and protocol development.[49] These may be separate short courses, or more extensive components of master's training and fellowships. International aspects of clinical research training must specifically address communication, cultural differences, funding, unequal balance of power, and ethics. (See Table 17-3.)

V. Health Systems Health systems are a determinant of health outcomes at several levels. Knowledge about health management, financing, regulation, organizational structure, human resource needs, and allocating resources are critical issues for working in global health. Although most health outcomes depend not so much on health systems as on environment, risk factors, economic factors, and belief systems, functional health systems can assure access to cost-effective interventions, basic primary care, and appropriate technology. Health systems knowledge is essential in knowing how interventions can be implemented and financed. The World Bank and other organizations have invested heavily in health system reforms, and with new interventions in vertical programs as well as sector-wide approaches, the role of the health system must be clearly understood by global health professionals in order to work effectively in the developing world. (See chapter 15.)

Western health care models and their limitations are usually not the best models for developing countries. Nonetheless, pre-paid health care systems (such as Kaiser Permanente), government-funded health insurance, and direct payment models are present in developing countries. Community-based models of participatory governance are also key approaches for understanding health service delivery, and these bottom-up solutions often have the best results in terms of community buy-in.[50]

Most importantly, the public health model for health systems is critical for global health practitioners to understand. This model may not be taught in medical schools, but should be a key component of global health education. In 1920, CEA Winslow defined public health as:

> ...the science and art of preventing disease, prolonging life and promoting health and efficiency through organized community effort for the sanitation of the environment, the control of communicable infections, the education of the individual in personal hygiene, the organization of medical and nursing services for the early diagnosis and preventive treatment of disease, and for the development of the social machinery to insure everyone a standard of living adequate for the maintenance of health, so organizing these benefits as to enable every citizen to realize his birthright of health and longevity.[51]

Public health is an interdisciplinary health system approach with emphasis on preventive strategies, linkage to government and political decision making, and evidence-based adaptation to new challenges. It is a collective effort among people and agencies to identify and address preventable and avoidable adverse health and quality of life outcomes.[52] Financing of public health functions might be considered as global public goods, as this financing is more the responsibility of government than of individuals (as in health insurance systems). However, the collective nature of public health requires the involvement of multiple sectors and financing sources.

VI. Environment and Health The environment and its effects on health may include consideration of natural disasters, climate change, global conflict, migration, and travel medicine as subjects in global health education. Environmental factors may include household,

---

BOX 17-1. PUBLIC HEALTH MISSION

- Prevents epidemics and the spread of disease
- Protects against environmental hazards
- Prevents injuries
- Promotes and encourages healthy behaviors
- Responds to disasters and assists communities in recovery
- Assures the quality and accessibility of health services
    Essential Public Health Services
- Monitor health status to identify community health problems
- Diagnose and investigate health problems and health hazards in the community
- Inform, educate, and empower people about health issues
- Mobilize community partnerships to identify and solve health problems
- Develop policies and plans that support individual and community health efforts

- Enforce laws and regulations that protect health and ensure safety
- Link people with needed personal health services and assure the provision of health care when otherwise unavailable
- Assure a competent public health and personal health care work force
- Evaluate effectiveness, accessibility, and quality of personal and population-based health services
- Research for new insights and innovative solutions to health problems

From Essential Public Health Services Working Group of the Core Public Health Functions Steering Committee, 1994, US Public Health Service. Reproduced with permission.

---

occupational, community, regional, and global influences. Air, water, soil, food, transportation, energy sources, waste, and war are all factors worthy of study. This enormous area of focus is often not included in health sciences education outside of schools of public health, but has significant implications in the success or failure of health interventions. For example, if there is no transportation to rural areas, how can any health technology be available to isolated populations? If there is no water supply or sewage disposal in a refugee camp, how can we prevent diarrheal diseases so that costly drugs and rehydration are not needed? How do we assess the relative risks associated with environmental exposures to pesticides in the face of food shortages in overpopulated areas? Many environmental problems have their origins in poverty, with deficient regulation of occupational exposures, inadequate infrastructure, and mismanagement of water supplies. The health consequences of urbanization and living in mega-cities is particularly evident for the poor, and this subject is worthy of serious attention as environmental science. Again, environmental health is not specifically addressed in most medical school curricula, and thus outside expertise is usually needed to orient future global health professionals to the importance of these issues. (See Chapter 5.)

EXPERIENTIAL LEARNING

Key to the appropriate education of health professionals in global health is experiential learning. As pointed out above, early experiences in professional schools may involve language training, shadowing, or even participation in research abroad. An introductory experience need not be completely academic, but as health sciences students

progress through their clinical training, they may select more intensive approaches such as in the AoC and research fellowships described earlier. For these to be successful, key elements are:

- **Didactic preparation and study:** including cultural anthropology, methodological approaches, language training, and self study
- **Mentoring:** by home institution faculty, and by host country mentors
- **Careful evaluation:** by the scholar of the experiential learning site, and by the mentors of the participating scholar
- **Sustainability:** to assure more than incidental commitment, both to learning and to the service or inquiry engaged
- **Career guidance:** how will the experiential learning fit into career development
- **Return to the community:** the host country/community/institution provides substantial support for the learner—how can there be some return, either through financial support or other material contribution
- **Legacy:** what will be produced and appreciated through the experiential learning activity

Experiential learning in a nonUS site should be required of all students preparing for research or career tracks in global health. This learning should be carefully designed to prevent adverse outcomes, both to the learner and to the host site. Several methods of preparing for experiential learning are possible:

- **Short courses for preparation for study abroad.** These should include orientation to physical safety, prevention of travel-related illnesses, assurance of complete immunization coverage, assurance of evacuation and health insurance, and assurance of cultural orientation to the specific environment. Most schools require students to sign waivers for the risks involved in international travel as part of this orientation.

- **Travel packs.** These include all written material presented in the short course proposed above, with check lists, cultural references, and Web site references to resources.[53]

- **Web-based resources.** These include www.state.gov for travel warnings and safety issues, and http://www.cdc.gov/travel/ for health advice and immunization requirements. GHEC has published a succinct summary of guidelines to prepare for international experiences, available at http://www.globalhealth-ec.org/GHEC/Resources/Newsletter/Vol2Issue1/Fea_IntlExpPrep.htm.[54]

Some key safety issues may be worthy of specific mention.[55]

- A letter of commitment from the host site should be required, spelling out obligations and responsibilities for the local sponsor and the participating student. With larger institutional relationships, formal affiliation agreements may be developed that cover such commitments, but specific experiential opportunities should be spelled out in detail.

- A local contact should be identified, with good phone and e-mail access.

- Evacuation insurance should be provided, with a single phone number access point known to the participant and family contacts at home and host contacts in the field.

- A first aid kit that might include Post-Exposure Prophylaxis for HIV/AIDS (depending on potential exposure) should be provided to the participant. An N-92 mask should be included for use in clinical settings.

- A cell phone or satellite phone might be obtained on entry to the host country. These are now possible in most places, and a Sim card can often be inserted in US-based phones for adaptation abroad. There is no substitute for direct communication.

- Consideration should be given to obtaining Voice-Over-Internet technology, including video transmission if broadband is available for periodic reporting.

- All travelers abroad should register with the US Department of State on the www.state.gov website; this assures the ability to locate participants should there be an emergency situation, natural disaster, or personal crisis. As for participant safety, some institutions prohibit travel to areas where there is a Department of State warning; however, many institutions consider each site

on a case-by-case basis as there are significant variations by regions or even cities within an international setting. A clear policy on this should be established by international education coordinators. (www.state.gov)

A final word about returning resources to the host community or country is in order. In many cases, experiential learning is a burden to host institutions and communities. In actual fact, the resources and generosity of those communities contributes to the learning and academic preparation of the US scholar. Some groups, such as Child and Family Health International [which is a major nongovernmental organization (NGO) providing learning experiences abroad for US health sciences students (www.cfhi.org)], advocate for educational equity through a return of tuition, financial resources, or other benefits to the host communities. These might include small grants, needed goods, or other services. Certainly, both the host country and the hosted scholar can count on long-term benefits through improved cultural understanding and professional development in global health, but a short-term return may be quite important in sustaining the collaborative relationships necessary for equitable experiential learning programs.

CAREER TRACKS IN GLOBAL HEALTH

There is no single formula for engaging in a career in global health. For those in health professions training, it is also important to know that one does not have to be a physician or nurse to productively contribute to global health. Sanitarians, engineers, pharmacists, and certainly basic scientists all have roles that can lead to important global health contributions. This section will briefly describe several approaches to career development in global health.

Personal Aspects of Career Choices: Risks and Benefits

One should begin one's career search with a self examination of motivations and capacity for work and life abroad. International service may imply difficult living and working conditions, strange foods, language challenges, frustrations, future career uncertainties, and risks of disease and physical harm (road accidents are a greater risk than infectious diseases in many settings).[56] Altruism, faith-based motivations, scientific curiosity, commitment to public service, and adventurism may all be driving forces for this career choice, but it is important to prevent the uninformed from inflicting unintentional consequences on themselves, their hosts, their country, or their family. Volunteerism is a great force for human fulfillment and a good way to test the waters abroad, but it must also be conducted in the context of cultural, professional, and political realities that lead to appropriate outcomes and perhaps to sustainable change. Unintended consequences may result from the power imbalance inherent in service by providers from developed countries to developing countries. There are risks for this, and also ethical issues that must be addressed.[57] Given the enormous and growing interest in global health education and experiential learning, one assumes both scientific commitment and dedication to public service as motivation among US health sciences students. In a useful manual entitled, "Finding Work in Global Health," Osborn and Ohmans[58] listed ten myths about global health that might be worthy of consideration. Several of these are presented below with additional discussion:

- *Myth: The demand for global health professionals outweighs the supply.*

  - **Fact:** Although there are health manpower shortages, there are not enough paid positions in organizations to provide solid career tracks for most interested professionals. Instead, one must take a strategic approach to career development that can assure a useful outcome of this interest. This would include appropriate clinical training, extra degrees, and of course, experiential learning.

- *Myth: Working in global health is a good way to find one's self.*

  - **Fact:** This outcome may result from working in global health, but such work is not a cure for career uncertainty or personal crisis. Global health is public service, and not therapy.

- *Myth: You will be able to treat patients.*

  - **Fact:** It is difficult to combine clinical work (licensing abroad is only one issue) with programmatic work. Global health is by its nature *public* health, with nonclinical interventions being the most effective. However, volunteer health professionals still find their place in relief work and occasional clinical service opportunities [for example, Doctors Without Borders (MSF) and faith-based organizations].

- *Myth: You must be a doctor or nurse to work in global health.*

  - **Fact:** This is clearly not the case; technical knowledge, community-based interventions, sanitation, and public health education do not require clinical degrees. However, being an MD is always useful in terms of authority and confidence in most settings.

- *Myth: Volunteering overseas will expand your technical skills.*

  - **Fact:** It can certainly expand one's creativity and perhaps inform one better as to appropriate technology, but it will not improve the sub-specialist's technical acumen in most cases.

- *Myth: More health care is the best solution to health problems in the developing world.*

  - **Fact:** Health care access is usually a good idea, but again, much of the solution to global health problems lies with public health approaches and not individual health care.

Whatever is one's motivation to plan a career in global health, one must also recognize the consequences in terms of family stability and career progression. It may be difficult to find work sites where both spouses have appropriate opportunities; if one is involved in a career commitment in academia or practice, it may be very difficult to progress with interruptions for volunteer or academic work abroad. It may be very discomfiting to raise children in resource-poor settings. On the other hand, such settings provide experiences and challenges that can improve the human spirit. The evidence for this may lie in the reports of returned Peace Corps volunteers, who now number in the tens of thousands (see http://www.geocities.com/ returnedpeacecorpsvolunteers/).

Positioning for Career Choices: Training, Degrees, Organizations, Volunteering

As described above, additional degrees with specific skill development are increasingly desired for work in global health. The timing of this training is variable, but for physicians, additional degrees might be best pursued after the third year of medical school. These degrees could also be completed after residency training or as part of fellowship training for some programs. Specialty training in infectious diseases has been the traditional mode of engagement in global health, but primary care and specialty training in public health are also increasingly appropriate. Subspecialty training may be most useful for those interested in short-term voluntary service activities.

There are many organizations available to those interested in career development in global health. These were listed in Table 17-1, and one should use these for networking and even job fairs. The American Public Health Association, the Global Health Council, the Global Health Education Consortium, the American Society for Tropical Medicine and Hygiene, and nearly all the professional organizations (Pediatrics, Family Practice, Surgery, etc) have international health sections that support student interests as well as professional development in global health. A list of useful Web links is provided in Table 17-6.

The classic way that a practicing or newly certified professional entered a career in global health was through volunteerism. This is less likely to be a successful and rewarding pathway in the 21st century, as even the voluntary organizations now prefer people with appropriate experience. For example, MSF will only accept initial volunteers who can provide six months' service, who have specified clinical training, and who have significant international experience. To gain this experience, experiential learning in professional school may be the best option. With this in hand, voluntary groups will be more

Table 17-6. Web resources for global health.

- World Federation of Public Health Associations (www.wfpha.org)
- World Health Organization (WHO) (www.who.int)
- United Nations Children's Fund (UNICEF) (www.unicef.org)
- African Council for Sustainable Health Development (ACOSHED) (www.acoshed.net)
- Association of Schools of Public Health (www.asph.org)
- Association of Schools of Public Health in the European Region (www.aspher.org)
- Latin American and Caribbean Association of Education in Public Health (www.alaesp.sld.cu/html/informe.htm)
- Asia Pacific Academic Consortium for Public Health (www.apacph.org)
- Global Health Organization (www.globalhealth.org)
- Global Health Reporting (data) (www.globalhealthreporting.org/)
- Bill and Melinda Gates Foundation (www.gatesfoundation.org/GlobalHealth/)
- Office of Global Health Affairs (US Department of Health and Human Services) (www.globalhealth.gov/)

confident in the professional's cultural orientation, flexibility, and dedication. Language training cannot be underemphasized, and this being done in the context of a medical experience would be the best preparation.

Government

Various governmental agencies are actively seeking individuals trained in global health. In this section we will look at a few of these groups in detail.

DEPARTMENT OF HEALTH AND HUMAN SERVICES

Even though the US Department of Health and Human Services (DHHS) is a domestic agency, it has an increasingly important role in global health, with numerous opportunities for career development. Health professionals from across disciplines may serve as Public Health Service (PHS) officers or civilian employees. A partial list of these opportunities includes:

- **The Epidemic Intelligence Service.** This two-year fellowship in applied epidemiology is conducted by the CDC; it is the main workforce for investigation and program application in public health for DHHS, and many US public health leaders are alumni of this program. There is substantial training in basic epidemiology, scientific writing, epidemiologic investigation, analysis, and program evaluation. Substantial international opportunities within the training involve outbreak investigation, HIV/AIDS, malaria, emerging infections, surveillance, immunizations, and other subjects. International applicants may qualify for a fellowship that essentially duplicates this experience, which is directed to US citizens. (http://www. cdc.gov/eis/)

- **Fogarty International Center, NIH.** This is the international component of the NIH; it addresses global health challenges through innovative and collaborative research and training programs and supports and advances the NIH mission through international partnerships. It supports research grants (with collaboration from other NIH institutes), international training programs, regional exchanges of information, and supports specific projects such as DCPP and the Multi-lateral Malaria Initiative, as well as the Fogarty-Ellison International Fellowship. (http://www. fic.nih.gov/)

- **US Public Health Service.** As one of the seven Uniformed Services of the United States, the Corps is a specialized career system designed to attract, develop, and retain health professionals who may be assigned to Federal, State, or local agencies or international organizations. Headed by the Surgeon General, it is a personnel system that integrates within DHHS and other federal agencies (such as the Coast Guard, National Oceanographic and Aeronautic Administration, CDC, NIH, Indian Health Service, Food and Drug Administration, and Health Resources and Services Administration). PHS officers are often deployed in response to emergencies and crises abroad; they may serve as EIS officers in CDC. As in the military, this is a 20-year career for retirement purposes (less service does not count toward retirement), with good training, benefits, and support for career development.

- **Office of Global Health Affairs (Formerly Office of International and Refugee Health).** This staff office to the Secretary of DHHS represents the department to other governments, other federal departments and agencies, international organizations, and the private sector on international and refugee health issues. It develops US policy and strategy positions related to health issues and facilitates collaborative involvement of the US PHS in support of these positions and organizations. Nearly all agencies within DHHS have international offices or key officials focusing on global health—coordinated by this office; thus, within specific agencies, there are global health opportunities serving departmental interests. (www. globalhealth.gov)

- **Global Health Service Corps.** As of this writing, this idea is still only a consideration for funding by the US Congress. However, it is a potentially important career track in global health that could serve many purposes. First, it would provide a highly desirable opportunity for fully trained, early-career US health professionals to contribute to the global public good through government service. Second, it would provide desperately needed expertise to make use of the rapidly increasing global resources for HIV/AIDS from the US government; the Global Fund to Fight AIDS, Tuberculosis, and Malaria; the World Bank; WHO; and others. Third, it would give a positive, human face to the US presence abroad, much as the Peace Corps has done for the last four decades. Finally, it would stimulate training and educational responses to global health challenges within US health sciences schools.[7]

USAID/DEPARTMENT OF STATE/PEACE CORPS

USAID is an independent federal government agency that receives overall foreign policy guidance from the Secretary of State. Its work intends to support long-term and equitable economic growth by advancing US foreign policy objectives for economic growth, agriculture, and trade; global health; and democracy, conflict prevention, and humanitarian assistance. The Bureau of Global Health within USAID provides leadership to improve the quality, availability, and use of essential health services. It focuses on HIV/AIDS, other infectious diseases (such as tuberculosis and malaria), maternal and child health, family planning, environmental health, and nutrition. Much of this work is done through competitively awarded contracts to nongovernmental organizations and some US government agencies such as the CDC and USPHS. For example, PHS officers serve in the Office of Foreign Disaster Assistance at USAID, coordinating across agencies for support to disaster and post-conflict situations. Career opportunities may be direct or through contractors and DHHS agencies. (http://www.usaid.gov/our_work/global_health/)

USAID is gradually becoming more closely integrated with the US Department of State (DOS), the foreign policy arm of the US government. Within this agency, there are rare opportunities for global health careers, but there are clinical opportunities for physicians, nurses, and mid-level practitioners within DOS international facilities, primarily serving DOS employees and programs abroad. (http://www.foreignservicecareers.com/specialist/self_evals/med_jobs.html)

The Peace Corps, a branch of the DOS, has an Office of Medical Services in Washington, DC, serving the public health and clinical needs of volunteers. This is supplemented by mid-level health providers stationed abroad as Peace Corps Medical Officers (PCMOs). In addition, the Peace Corps now has an integrated Masters International (MI) Program with several schools of public health, wherein a prospective student will apply simultaneously to both the Peace Corps and the participating graduate school. After being accepted by both, candidates will complete a year to two years of graduate course work at the respective university while continuing to prepare for work overseas. Each MI Program has its own requirements and will award credit for Peace Corps service accordingly. This is an extraordinary opportunity to acquire a MPH degree (probably not for MD students, but ideal for nursing or mid-level health professionals) while gaining unsurpassed field experience. (http://www.peacecorps.gov/index.cfm?shell=learn.whyvol.eduben.mastersint)

MILITARY

Military service may provide numerous opportunities for global health service, research, and training. For example, the US Army Research Laboratories (ARL) include scientists, engineers, administrators, and support staff, all of whom make valuable contributions both to the ARL's mission and to global health. Often, such laboratories and other military services provide crisis response to natural disasters, first line response to emerging epidemics (for example, avian influenza), and laboratory support for identification and research on potential biopathogens or emerging infections. Post-doctoral research programs are available in military facilities. (http://www.arl.army.mil/main/Main/default.cfm?Action=3)

Nongovernmental Organizations

Nongovernmental organizations perhaps provide the most extensive opportunities for variety in service, research, and practice. These range from direct clinical service providers to specific program contractors and consultants to bilateral and multilateral organizations. Most require substantial training and experience for employment, and most do not have long-term "hard money" career tracks. The Global Health Council (www.globalhealth.org) is an association of health-care professionals and organizations that include NGOs, foundations, corporations, government agencies, and academic institutions that work in global health. The annual meeting of this group is a good opportunity to meet and learn about many NGOs involved in global health. Their website provides a comprehensive list of members.

PRIVATE VOLUNTARY GROUPS/FAITH-BASED ORGANIZATIONS

Volunteerism has been the mainstay for short-term, and sometimes career, involvement in global health. This can take many forms, including faith-based or missionary associated commitments, but also short-term response to emergencies and crises as well as specific clinical specialty needs such as in ophthalmology, maxillo-facial surgery, orthopedic and reconstructive surgery, and cardiac surgery. *Médecins Sans Frontières* (MSF) is perhaps the quintessential private voluntary relief group, having won the Nobel Peace Prize in 1999

Table 17-7. Examples of voluntary organizations with career opportunities in global health.

Organization	Role	Web Link
CARE	Humanitarian organization with roots in post-war emergency assistance and development. Focuses on poverty alleviation through programs in education, health, HIV/AIDS, economic development, nutrition, water and sanitation, and emergency relief.	http://www.care.org/
International Rescue Committee	Global nonprofit charity focusing on emergency relief, rehabilitation, protection of human rights, post-conflict development, resettlement services, and advocacy for those uprooted or affected by conflict and oppression.	http://www.theirc.org/about/
Médecins Sans Frontières (MSF)	International humanitarian aid organization providing emergency medical assistance to populations in danger in more than 70 countries. Opportunities are country specific, and require six-month commitments with previous international experience.	http://www.msf.org/
Operation Giving Back	Provides US surgeons with a database for volunteering abroad. The American College of Surgery created this resource center for surgeons to find information on volunteer opportunities.	http://www.operationgivingback.facs.org/
OXFAM	Oxfam GB is a development, relief, and advocacy organization that works on poverty alleviation and emergency relief globally.	http://www.oxfam.org.uk/index.htm
Project HOPE	Originally the *SS HOPE* hospital ship, now conducts land-based training and education programs on five continents. Implements health education programs, health policy research, and humanitarian assistance in areas of need; responds to disasters, and cooperates with numerous organizations on short-term volunteer opportunities.	http://www.projecthope.org/employment/employment.htm
Rotaplast International	Sponsored by the Rotary Club to address the problem of cleft lip and palate among children worldwide. Facilitates medical missions to provide surgical intervention for children who are not able to receive treatment or who are in need of more complicated medical procedures.	http://www.rotaplast.org/
Unite For Sight	Nonprofit organization that works with communities worldwide to improve eye health and eliminate preventable blindness. Volunteers work with partner eye clinics in developing countries to provide eye care and eye health education programs. Programs implemented worldwide by volunteers working in 90 university and community chapters.	http://www.uniteforsight.org/

as well as many other international awards. The opportunities are too numerous to list completely in this chapter, but Table 17-7 lists examples and the missions of such voluntary organizations.

CONTRACTORS

Private, for profit, or not-for-profit groups may act as contractors for donor organizations, multi-lateral organizations, and governments to carry out specific projects in global health. The headquarters for many of these organizations may be found close to Washington, DC, or near UN agency headquarters in New York and elsewhere. Some, such as Family Health International, are large organizations that focus on a particular area (reproductive health), while others specialize in government-funded projects, often blurring the boundaries between government agencies and the private sector.[59] Many are members of the Global Health Council. Employment is largely task-specific, and consortia of universities, individuals, or other companies may be formed in response

Table 17-8. Examples of contracting organizations serving global health agencies.

Organization	Role	Web Link
Abt Associates	Research and consulting firm focusing on social, economic, and health policy; international development; business research and consulting; and clinical trials and registries.	http://www.abtassociates.com/
Academy for Educational Development	Independent, nonprofit organization focusing on human development, including education (youth), health (HIV), environment, energy, and economic development in the United States and globally.	http://www.aed.org/
Axios	For-profit global consultant group specializing in healthcare systems with a focus on chronic disease management, HIV, and drug delivery; integrating local resources; and private-public partnerships.	http://www.axios-group.com/en/Default.aspx
Chemonics International	For-profit consultant group focusing on management services, technical assistance, research, training, and special expertise in communications, grants management, procurement, and performance monitoring. Agriculture, environment, health, and banking projects.	http://www.chemonics.com/
Family Health International	Nonprofit international public health organization managing research and field activities in more than 70 countries, especially in youth, reproductive health, and HIV programs.	http://www.fhi.org/en/index.htm
JHPIEGO	International health organization affiliated with The Johns Hopkins University focusing on health care services for women and families, including training and support for health care providers in limited-resource settings throughout Africa, Asia, the Middle East, Latin America, and the Caribbean.	http://www.jhpiego.org/
John Snow International	JSI, Inc., and its nonprofit affiliate JSI Research & Training Institute, Inc., are public health research and consulting firms focusing on aging, child health, HIV, health financing and logistics, mental health, quality assurance, and reproductive health.	http://www.jsi.com/
Management Systems International	For-profit consulting organization focusing on private sector development, democracy and governance, environment and natural resources, countries and regions in transition.	http://www.msiworldwide.com/

to task orders to respond to the specific needs of the funding agencies. A partial list of such organizations is shown in Table 17-8. One may obtain a flavor of the range, quantity, and complexity of USAID contractors by accessing the USAID Yellowbook, a compendium of awarded contracts in a given year (see http://www.usaidgov/business/yellowbook/yellowbook01.xls).

Multinational Organizations

Multinational organizations are those comprised of member states (countries), either under the United Nations auspices, or through some other basis of affiliation such as defense or economic cooperation. Career opportunities are difficult to obtain within these organizations, but many have "Young Professional" entry programs, internship opportunities, and opportunities for secundments from government or other agencies through interagency personnel agreements. In many cases, consultants are brought into the agencies as a result of valuable contributions through contractual relationships.

UN Organizations

The United Nations is the world's largest international employer. Its over 60,000 staff members come from all over the world, including about 4,500 from the United States. Among them are health professionals such as sanitarians, physicians, sociologists, nurses, health economists, and health system managers. UN staffing levels are determined by member state contributions

EDUCATION AND CAREERS IN GLOBAL HEALTH / **339**

and nonbudgetary support as well as cultural integration. The United Nations is a complex array of organizations, commissions, and councils, many with a health focus.

The WHO (www.who.int), UNICEF, UNDP, and other health-related multinational agencies are separate autonomous organizations related to the United Nations by special agreements. They have their own membership, legislative and executive bodies, secretariats, and budgets, but they work with the UN and with each other through the Economic and Social Council. Although UN staff are found in nearly every country, the majority work in New York at United Nations headquarters, and in regional or agency headquarters offices in Bangkok, Cairo, Copenhagen, Geneva (WHO), Harare, Manila, Montreal, Nairobi, New Delhi, Paris, Rome, Vienna, and Washington Pan American Health Organization, (PAHO). There are official and unofficial quotas for Americans in these organizations, owing in part to the influence of the world's largest economy on almost all decision making. There is a conscious effort by the Secretariats of these groups to involve Part II countries (developing economies) rather than be influenced predominantly by Part I countries (developed economies).

Most professional positions require an advanced degree, competency in at least two official United Nations languages (Arabic, Chinese, English, French, Russian, and Spanish), and several years of specialized professional experience, much of it gained from service in a particular country or region. Types of employment in United Nations organizations are usually divided into 1) professional positions, and 2) experts and consultants. The experts and consultants are hired for a short term to provide technical advice on specific projects in developing countries. The United Nations and many of its organizations have their own standard application form, though most now accept individual résumés or CVs and many applications can be filled out online (www.jobs.un.org). Some assistance may be provided to US citizens through the Department of State (http://www.state.gov/p/io/empl/).

WORLD BANK

The World Bank, headquartered in Washington, DC, with 7,000 employees, focuses on poverty alleviation, and with it, health and human development (www.worldbank.org).

It works closely with UN agencies and health ministries of member states. Founded as the International Bank for Reconstruction and Development in the wake of World War II and governed by a board of directors with voting power based on gross domestic product (GDP), it has assumed the dominant global role in health development financing since the early 1990s. This grew from the 1993 World Development Report, an annual Bank report that focused for the first time on how health and economic development were inextricably linked.[60] With a loan portfolio of more than $20 billion, and at least $2.5 billion devoted to health related projects, the World Bank influences health policy and works with other partners to support key health interventions. Many of these interventions center around health systems development, but public health projects including infectious diseases, tobacco control, injuries, and mental health have all received investment. The Bank has health professional staff as part of the Human Development Network, with both central office resources and country team professionals who develop health projects.

Research is an extensive Bank activity, especially in health economics, macroeconomics and health, and evidence-based health interventions. The Bank has a Young Professionals program that occasionally admits physicians but requires substantial economics training for these applicants. Consultants have an important role in both project development and implementation. These consultants may be nongovernmental organization employees, university faculty, for-profit companies, or simply individuals with personal contacts within the Bank.

OTHERS

Economic multinational organizations such as the Organization for Economic Cooperation and Development (OECD) with 30 member countries, are committed to the global market economy. Their interests cover economic and social issues from macroeconomics, to trade, education, development, and science and innovation. Health and economics are invariably intertwined, with development dependent on health, and with health expenses and values increasingly of concern to both developed and developing countries. Health economists play a key role in the analyses and publications produced by such organizations, and these publications may drive global health policy and financing.

Another example is the Asia-Pacific Economic Cooperation (APEC), which has a Health Task Force dedicated to sharing information and responding to emerging health issues that directly affect trade, movement of people, tourism, and economic development. Severe Acute Respiratory Syndrome (SARS) and avian flu are of particular interest, and health consultants have been mobilized to help address these regional global health problems.

The World Trade Organization (WTO) is the global international organization dealing with rules of trade between nations. The WTO agreements are negotiated and signed by the bulk of the world's trading nations and ratified in their parliaments. The goal is to help producers of goods and services, exporters, and importers conduct their business. Often, rules on intellectual property rights, especially regarding essential health drugs, may play an important part in health. Although there is no significant representation by health officials in the WTO, there is considerable input by health ministries and health organizations concerned with emergency responses to health crises and health inequity due to lack of availability of essential medicines.

Academia

Research, training, and consultation are all important career tracks for academic health professionals. The range of subjects is limitless, and often academic health professionals may combine occasional work abroad with an active clinical practice. However, international health research in the 21st century may require more specific training in health diplomacy, cultural understanding, health economics, and area studies to prepare researchers and trainers for appropriately collaborative research. Training opportunities in tropical medicine, laboratory diagnostics, vector control, and public health practice are especially important to potential global health research professionals, and these subjects have not been adequately addressed by existing institutions. Thus, some have proposed the establishment of a new academic institution that would provide interdisciplinary training for the next generation of global health scientists.[61]

Given the new philanthropy in global health research and practice, the interests of students, residents, research scientists, and faculty in service and global health equity, and the demands of a globalized economy, academic careers will increasingly focus on global health, and academia must respond with appropriate curriculum, administrative support, and opportunities. The careers on the near and distant horizon in academic global health are exciting, without bounds, and within reach to those who seek them out. We hope this chapter has whetted the appetite of today's students who will be tomorrow's global health leaders.

STUDY QUESTIONS

1. List and describe some of the research opportunities and responsibilities in global health.
2. Describe different ways that the schools of health sciences can be involved in global health education. Choose one method and describe how it could be implemented in your school.
3. List some of the governmental and nongovernmental global health agencies and how they interact in any particular program or area of the world.

REFERENCES

1. Shaywitz DA, Ausiello DA. Global health: a chance for Western physicians to give—and receive. *Am J Med* 2002;113(4): 354–357.
2. Yach D, Bettcher D. The globalization of public health, I: Threats and opportunities. *Am J Public Health* 1998;88: 735–738.
3. Lee, K. Introduction. In: Lee, K. *Globalization and health, an introduction.* London: Palgrave Macmillan, 2003:1–10.
4. Kickbusch I, Buse K. Global influences and global responses: international health at the turn of the twenty-first century. In: Merson M, Black RE, Milles AJ, eds. *International Public Health.* Gaithersburg, MD: Aspen Publications, 2002:701–37.
5. Novotny TE. Why we need to rethink the diseases of affluence. *PLoS Med* 2005;2(5):e104.
6. United Nations Population Division. *The International Migrant Stock: A Global View.* 2002. http://www.iom.int/documents/officialtxt/en/unpd%5Fhandout.pdf.
7. Novotny TE. US Department of Health and Human Services: a need for global health leadership in preparedness and health diplomacy. *Am J Public Health* 2006;96(1):11–3.
8. Sarfaty S, Arnold LK. Preparing for international medical service. *Emerg Med Clin N Am* 2005;23:149–175.
9. Davies A. Health care worker migration: Why should we care? *Migration* March 2006:15–18. http://www.iom.int//DOCUMENTS/PUBLICATION/EN/migration_mar06.pdf.
10. Korcok M. Cuba trains American medical students—to work in US *CMAJ* 2001;164(10):1477.
11. Institute of Medicine, Board on Global Health. *Healers Abroad: Americans Responding to the Human Resource Crisis in HIV/AIDS.* Washington, DC: National Academy Press, 2005.
12. Cohen J. The new world of global health. *Science* 2006; 311: 162–167.
13. Global Forum for Health Research. *Strategic Orientations 2003–2005.* Geneva: World Health Organization, 2003.
14. James D. Going global. *New Physician* 1999;48(6): 290. www.amsa.org/tnp/articlesarticle.cfx?id=290
15. Anonymous. International medical education. *JAMA* 1969; 210(8):1555–57.
16. Bateman C, Baker T, Hoormenborg E, et al. Bringing global issues to medical teaching. *Lancet* 2001;358:1539–1542.
17. Edwards R, Rowson M, Piachaud J. Teaching international health issues to medical students. *Med Educ* 2001;35: 806–810.
18. Evert J, Mautner D, Hoffman I. *Developing Global Health Curricula: A Guidebook for US Medical Schools.* 2006. Global Health Education Consortium. http://www.globalhealth-ec.org/GHEC/Resources/Developing%20GH%20Curricula_Guidebook%20for%20US%20Medical%20Schools.pdf.
19. Global Health Action Committee. www.amsa.org/global
20. Panosian C, Coates TJ. The new medical "missionaries"—grooming the next generation of global health workers. *New Engl J Med* 2006;354(17):1771–1773.
21. Duke University. *Duke Global Health Steering Committee Report. Durham, North Carolina,* June 2005 (revised January 2006).
22. Marcum JA. What direction for study abroad? Eliminate the roadblocks *Chron Higher Educ: Chron Rev* 2001;47(36): B7–B8.
23. Williams TR. Exploring the impact of study abroad on students' intercultural communication skills: adaptability and sensitivity. *J Studies Internat Educ* 2005;9(4):356–371.
24. Mutchnick IS, Moyer CA, Stern DT. Expanding the boundaries of medical education: Evidence for cross-cultural exchanges. *Acad Med* 2003;78(10)/October Suppl:S1–S5.
25. Thompson MJ, Huntington MK, Hunt DD, et al. Educational effects of international health electives on US and Canadian medical students and residents: A literature review. *Acad Med* 2003;78(3):342–347.

26. Godkin MA, Savageau JA. The effect of medical students' international experiences on attitudes toward serving underserved multicultural populations. *Fam Med* 2003;35:273–278.

27. Esfandiari A, Gill G. An international health/tropical medicine elective. *Acad Med* 2001;76(5):516.

28. Niemanstsverdriet S, Majoor GD, van der Vleuten CPM, et al. "I found myself to be a down to earth Dutch girl": a qualitative study into learning outcomes from international traineeships. *Med Educ* 2004;38:749–757.

29. Miranda JJ, Yudkin JS, Willott C. International health electives: Four years of experience. *Trav Med Inf Dis* 2005;3(3): 133–141.

30. Heck JE, Pust R. A national consensus on the essential international health curriculum for medical schools. *Acad Med* 1993; 68(8):596–598.

31. Heck JE. A national consensus on the essential international-health curriculum for medical schools—Author's Postscript. *Update: The GHEC Newsletter*. 2006 1(1). http://www.globalhealth-ec.org/ GHEC/ Resources/Newsletter/Vol1Issue1/ClassicsPostscript_ JH.htm.

32. Beukens P, Keusch G, Belizan J, et al. Evidence-based global health. *JAMA* 2004;291(21):2639–2641.

33. Yudkin JS, Bayley O, Elnour S, et al. Introducing medical students to global health issues: a Bachelor of Science degree in international health. *Lancet* 2003;362:822–824.

34. International Health and Medical Education Centre (IHMEC). *The Elective Pack: The Medical Student's Guide to Essential International Health and Development*. London: International Health and Medical Education Centre, University College London, 2004.

35. Bateman C, Baker T, Hoormenborg E, et al. Bringing global issues to medical teaching. *Lancet* 2001;358:1539–1542.

36. Sarfaty S, Arnold LK. Preparing for international medical service. *Emerg Med Clin N Am* 2005;23:149–175.

37. Edwards R, Rowson M, Piachaud J. Teaching international health issues to medical students. *Med Educ* 2001;35:806–810.

38. Goldsmid JM, Bettiol SS, Sharples N. A preliminary study on travel health issues of medical students undertaking electives. *J Travel Med* 2003;10(3):160–163.

39. Tilzey AJ, Banatvala JE. Protection from HIV on electives: questionnaire survey of UK medical schools. *BMJ* 2002;324: 1010–1011.

40. Esfandiari A, Gill G. An international health/tropical medicine elective. *Acad Med* 2001;76(5):516.

41. Gupta AR, Wells CK, Horwitz RI, et al. The International Health Program: The fifteen-year experience with Yale University's Internal Medicine Residency Program. *Am J Trop Med Hyg* 1999;61(6):1019–1023.

42. Farmer PE, Furin JJ, Katz JT. Global health equity. *Lancet* 2004; 363(9423) 1832–1834.

43. Ozgediz D, Roayaie K, Debas H, et al. Surgery in developing countries—essential training in residency. *Arch Surg* 2005;140; 795–800

44. Taylor CE. International experience and idealism in medical education. *Acad Med* 1994;69(8):631–634.

45. Jamison DT, Breman JG, Measham AR, et al., eds. *Disease Control Priorities in Developing Countries, Second Edition*. Washington, DC: World Bank and Oxford University Press, 2006.

46. Evert J, Mautner D, Hoffman I. *Developing Global Health Curricula: A Guidebook for US Medical Schools*. 2006. Global Health Education Consortium. http://www.globalhealth-ec.org/GHEC/ Resources/Developing%20GH%20Curricula_Guidebook% 20for%20US%20Medical%20Schools.pdf.

47. Scrimshaw SC. Culture, behavior, and health. In: Merson MH, Black RE, Mills AJ, eds. *International Public Health*. Gaithersburg, MD: Aspen Publishers, Inc, 2001.

48. Kickbusch I. Influence and opportunity: Reflections on the US role in global public health. *Health Affairs* 2002;21(6): 131–141.

49. Hulley SB, Cummings SR, Browner WS, et al. (2001) *Designing Clinical Research, Second Edition*. Philadelphia, PA: Lippincott, Williams, and Wilkins, 2001.

50. Hearst N. Community and International Studies. In: Hulley SB, Cummings SR, Browner WS, et al., eds. *Designing Clinical Research, Second Edition*. Philadelphia, PA: Lippincott, Williams, & Wilkins, 2001.

51. Winslow CEA. The untilled fields of public health, *Science* 1920;51(1306): 23–33.

52. Turnock BJ. *Public Health: What It Is and How It Works, Third Edition*. Sudbury, MA: Jones and Bartlett Publishers, 2004.

53. Miranda JJ, Yudkin JS, Willott C. International health electives: Four years of experience. *Trav Med Inf Dis* 2005;3(3): 133–141.

54. Hale WA. Preparing for and international experience. *Update: The GHEC Newsletter* 2006;2(1).

55. Sarfaty S, Arnold LK. Preparing for international medical service. *Emerg Med Clin N Am* 2005;23:149–175.

56. Hall TL. *Global Health: Career Options & Specialization (Revised)*. 2006. http://www.globalhealth-ec.org/GHEC/Resources/ GHCareers.htm.

57. Roberts M. Duffle bag medicine. *JAMA* 2006;295: 1491–1492.

58. Osborn G, Ohmans P. *Finding Work in Global Health, Second Edition*. Saint Paul, MN: Health Advocates Press, 2005.

59. Helton AC, Loescher. NGOs and governments in a new humanitarian landscape (Op-Ed). 2003. Council on Foreign Relations. http://www.cfr.org/publication/6084/ngos_and_governments_ in_a_new_humanitarian_landscape.html.

60. World Bank. *Investing in Health—World Development Indicators*. Washington, DC: Published for the World Bank by Oxford University Press, 1993.

61. Hoetz PJ. Should we establish a North American School of Global Health Science? *Am J Med Sci* 2004;328(2):71–77.

Index